Strategies for the
MCCQE Part II

Strategies for the MCCQE Part II

Mastering the clinical skills exam in Canada

Christopher Naugler, MD, MSc

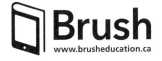

www.brusheducation.ca

Brush Education Inc.
www.brusheducation.ca
contact@brusheducation.ca

Cover design: Dean Pickup; Cover image: Shutterstock/CA-SSIS
Interior design: Carol Dragich, Dragich Design

Library and Archives Canada Cataloguing in Publication
Naugler, Christopher T. (Christopher Terrance), 1967–, author
Strategies for the MCCQE, part II : mastering the clinical skills exam in Canada / Christopher Naugler, MD, MSc.

Includes bibliographical references and index.

Issued in print and electronic formats.

ISBN 978-1-55059-807-0 (softcover).-ISBN 978-1-55059-810-0 (EPUB).-ISBN 978-1-55059-808-7 (PDF).-ISBN 978-1-55059-809-4 (Kindle)

1. Physicians-Licenses-Canada-Examinations-Study guides.
2. Medicine-Canada-Examinations-Study guides. I. Title.

RC58.N38 2019   610.69'5076   C2018-906523-0   C2018-906524-9

We acknowledge the support of the Government of Canada
Nous reconnaissons l'appui du gouvernement du Canada | Canadä

Contributors

Marcia Abbott, BSc, BN, MD
Resident, General Pathology
Department of Pathology and
Laboratory Medicine
University of Calgary

Pavandeep Gill, MD
Resident, General Pathology
Department of Pathology and
Laboratory Medicine
University of Calgary

Alexandra Kirvan, MD, CCFP
Practicing family physician
Clinical lecturer at the Cumming
School of Medicine

**Davinder Sidhu BSc, BPharm,
LLB/JD, MD, FRCPC**
Department of Pathology and
Laboratory Medicine
University of Calgary

Amy Thommasen, MD, FRCPC
Dermatopathology fellow
Department of Pathology and
Laboratory Medicine
University of Calgary

Researchers

Irene Ma, MSc

Leonard Nguyen, PhD

Vijay S. Kandalam, PhD

Developmental reviewers

Melanie Bilbul, MD, CM, BSc
Resident, Psychiatry
McGill University

Rhea B. D'Costa, MD, BHSc (Hon)
Resident, Pediatrics
Queen's University

Tina Felfeli, MD
Resident, Ophthalmology
University of Toronto

Caylea Foster, MD, MSc
Resident, General Pathology
University of Calgary

Natasha Garfield, MD
Program Director, Division of
Endocrinology and Metabolism
McGill University

Emily Lehan, MD
Resident, Pediatrics
Queen's University

Katherine Lines, BSc Pharm, MD
Resident, Psychiatry
Dalhousie University

Alexandra Manning, MD, BEd
Chief Resident, Psychiatry
Dalhousie University

Alicia Nickel, MD
Resident, General Pathology
University of Calgary

Jill Pancer, MD
Division of Endocrinology and
Metabolism
McGill University

Golnaz Roshankar, MD
Resident, General Pathology
University of Calgary

Kirsten Rosler MD, MSc
Resident, General Pathology
University of Calgary

Steven Roy, MD
Chief Resident, Internal Medicine
Northern Ontario School of
Medicine

Calvin Tseng, MD, BSc (Hon)
Resident, General Pathology
University of Calgary

Robby Wang, MD, BHSc
Resident, General Pathology
University of Calgary

Alanna Ward, MD
Resident, Pediatrics
Queen's University

Contents

About this resource

This resource helps you prepare for the Medical Council of Canada's clinical skills exam, the MCCQE Part II, and equivalent exams in other countries, such as the USMLE Step 2 in the United States.

It aims to offer a concise, strategic approach to the exam, based on common entities as the likely targets for the exam and the practical limits of what standardized patients can play.

The clinical presentations in this resource

The clinical presentations in this resource come from the objectives for the exam set by the Medical Council of Canada (MCC). (The MCC publishes its clinical presentations online under its "medical expert" objectives: use the search term *Medical Council of Canada medical expert* in your browser.)

The order of the clinical presentations follows the MCC's online scroll-through order: it starts with the MCC's first clinical presentation and follows the sequence the "next presentation" link establishes.

The resource unpacks each clinical presentation in a series of standard sections.

MCC particular objective(s)

The MCC outlines a particular focus for most of its clinical presentations, which this section summarizes.

MCC differential diagnosis
with added evidence

The MCC lists causal conditions for each clinical presentation, which are presented in this section as an edited and expanded differential diagnosis.

The differential diagnosis is edited (lightly) to exclude uncommon entities.

It is expanded to describe the common presentations of the remaining entities (except where, occasionally, these entities are self-explanatory and need no expansion). So, this section presents the common clinical evidence for the common entities in the MCC's list of causal conditions.

The MCC notes in each clinical presentation that its list of causal entities is not exhaustive. These lists do, however, show the MCC's priorities for the exam—which is why this resource follows them closely.

Strategy for patient encounter

This section describes the elements likely to shape a patient encounter for each clinical presentation, including the likely scenario and the likely tasks. The tasks can include history, physical exam, investigations, or management. Most clinical presentations could engage any of these tasks, so generally this part covers all of them each time.

In clinical presentations where the MCC identifies emergency management as the focus, the resource unpacks steps for emergency management.

This section also sometimes includes "pearls": particular advice gleaned from experience in clinical practice.

How this resource helps you overcome common clinical-exam errors

The Medical Council of Canada reports several common clinical-exam errors, including:

- not recognizing urgent presentations
- peppering patients with closed-ended, yes-no questions
- not listening for, or looking for, evidence to rule out differential diagnoses
- counselling patients with rote, directive, generic information

This resource helps you overcome these common errors by:

- summarizing the MCC's objectives for each clinical presentation, which highlight when urgent presentations are at issue, and unpacking steps in emergency management where relevant
- modelling open-ended questions
- clarifying diagnostic goals for history taking, physical exams, and investigations
- modelling approaches to counselling that target the particular situation of patients and enable them to make their own, informed decisions

---

Exam basics

Exam format

You can read about the format of the MCCQE Part II on the MCC's website.

The exam takes place over 2 days and involves a series of encounters with standardized patients. An examiner is present during each encounter (you should ignore the examiner, except when the examiner speaks to you).

The first day has 8 encounters, each 14 minutes long.

The second day has 4 encounters, each 6 minutes long and each combined with a 6-minute reading or written-answer task (the encounters may come before or after the reading or written-answer tasks).

Any clinical presentation can form the focus of either kind of encounter.

The use of standardized patients places some strategic constraints on the exam. For example:

- Only people age 16 and older can play standardized patients. So, in pediatric cases, the patient will likely be an adolescent, a child absent on some pretext (leaving the parents to discuss the concern), or a simulated neonate.
- Psychiatric disorders are easier to simulate than disorders with physical symptoms, which increases the likelihood of a psychiatric disorder on the exam.

Overall goal: find evidence, use evidence

Your overall goal is to gather evidence, and use this evidence to focus on what is relevant and useful to the individual case at hand.

Read the case instructions carefully

Each patient encounter begins with a set of written instructions that describe a scenario and specify the tasks you need to perform.

You have 2 minutes to go over these.

- Glean context from the instructions. For example, they may contain laboratory test results, or information about the patient's age or occupation, which may be relevant to the differential diagnosis. The instructions may also specify a setting for the encounter, such as an office, emergency room, or hospital ward, which can be important to patient management (e.g., an unstable patient in an outpatient setting needs immediate transfer to an emergency department).
- Do only the tasks specified by the instructions.
- If an instruction says to "assess" a patient, start by taking a history. Do a physical exam only if warranted by the evidence.

Always take these first steps

Always:

- Introduce yourself to the patient.
- Ask the patient for consent to interview and examine them. Be aware that consent may depend on culturally sensitive care, which the patient may not clarify until you ask.
- Offer the patient a chaperone for the encounter.
- Wash your hands.

Use history taking to help the patient talk

Standardized patients have information to tell you that is designed to narrow your differential diagnosis. Use open-ended questions, as opposed to yes-no questions, to let the patient talk.

And then listen.

Make notes sparingly

You will be supplied with a pen and paper at the exam (you're not allowed to bring your own). You can use these for notes during history taking, but keep your focus on your patient. Make eye contact with the patient as they talk. If you take notes, be strategic—for example, sum up distinguishing symptoms or red flags with single words.

Focus on diagnostic evidence in physical exams

Approach physical exams with as much focus as possible. Consider what evidence you have in hand—for example, from the instructions for the patient encounter, or from history taking. Let this information guide the physical exam, so that you pursue diagnostic manoeuvres relevant to the specific patient.

Talk your way through physical exams

Describe your procedures and findings as you perform a physical exam, including normal findings. This allows the examiner to understand your process.

Always:

- Obtain the patient's permission to conduct a physical exam.
- Drape the patient appropriately.

Focus on relevant investigations

Order investigations that narrow the differential diagnosis, based on evidence from the scenario instructions, the history, and/or the physical exam. Don't order every possible investigation.

Tailor management to the patient

Provide next steps and information that target the situation of the particular patient. This means you need to ask the patient for relevant details about their situation, such as work, recreation, and dietary routines. Think of these details as a way to begin a conversation with the patient about changes to their routines that could help them.

Listen for redirection when you're stuck

There may be times that you blank on a scenario, or nerves get in your way. If you are seriously off track, the examiner may try to redirect you. Be aware of attempts at redirection and adjust your approach accordingly.

If you draw a blank on history taking, remember that you can always ask about medications, allergies, family and personal medical history, and the psychosocial impact of the presenting problem.

Prepare for particular challenges

Patients who require culturally sensitive care

Any patient encounter may engage the need for culturally sensitive care. When you ask permission to interview and examine a patient, a refusal from the patient may stem from this. When a patient withholds consent, engage in a straightforward, respectful conversation about the patient's expectations for care. For example:

- Express confidence in your ability to help the patient.
- Describe specific procedures and investigations you may need to perform in the context of the patient's case.
- Ask the patient how to proceed with their permission (e.g., by providing a same-sex doctor).
- Do your best to meet the patient's expectations while protecting the patient's health and safety.

Patients who are reluctant to talk

Some standardized patients may show reluctance to talk, to test your ability to elicit information on sensitive topics. In these situations:

- Acknowledge the patient's reluctance to talk (e.g., "It seems like you are having some difficulty talking about your health concern.")
- Offer empathy and reassurance (e.g., "Some problems are hard to talk about. It's okay to feel unsettled. I want to help you, not judge you.").
- Express confidence in your ability to help the patient.
- Show your ability to listen respectfully: allow the patient to talk at their own pace.

Abusive patients

Some standardized patients may be angry. In these situations:

- Remain calm.
- Acknowledge the patient's anger.
- Express confidence in your ability to help the patient.

- Ensure your safety and the safety of others. It may be appropriate to assess for homicidal ideation (e.g., "When someone is as upset and angry as you are, they sometimes think about harming others. What thoughts have you had about harming others?"). Seek an emergent admission to a psychiatry ward in the case of homicidal ideation.
- Offer clear next steps. For example, state that you need the patient to answer some questions, so you can better understand their situation.

Noncompliant patients

The health concerns of some standardized patients may stem from noncompliance with prescribed medications.

For example, uncontrolled diabetes can contribute to a variety of presenting problems, such as incontinence, hypertension, and diplopia. Patients may have uncontrolled diabetes because they are not taking their medication, due to forgetfulness or financial constraints.

In any noncompliant patient, seek the reasons for noncompliance.

- In forgetful patients, discuss possible strategies to help with compliance. For example, how could they set up reminders for themselves? How well do they cope with day-to-day tasks in general? What family or friends could they call on for assistance? In patients who are not coping and who do not have social supports, consider community supports such as home care services.
- In patients who cannot afford their medications, express empathy and seek details about the patient's situation. Consider referring the patient to social service agencies, which can help with financial assistance and skills such as budgeting.

Patients with needs beyond the stated scenario

Some standardized patients may have issues in addition to those described in the instructions for the patient encounter. These issues will likely be obvious. They will test your ability to observe, and respond to, a patient's most pressing needs. In these situations, first pursue the presenting issue identified in the instructions, and then ask whether the patient has other concerns. Allow what the patient tells you to refocus the encounter.

Dissenting health-care professionals

The exam may test your ability to manage conflict with other health-care professionals who disagree with your decisions about a patient's care. Use evidence to negotiate these situations:

- Take a position based on evidence, and defend it calmly and rationally.

- Offer to monitor the patient's situation and revisit your decisions as the evidence warrants.

Abdominal distension

MCC particular objective

Differentiate ascites from bowel obstruction.

MCC differential diagnosis
with added evidence

ASCITES

ASCITES IN GENERAL

Signs and symptoms: normal bowel sounds; "shifting dullness" on percussion of the abdomen

Investigations: abdominal ultrasound to detect ascitic fluid

Exudative: low serum-to-ascites albumin gradient (e.g., peritoneal carcinomatosis)

MALIGNANCY

Signs and symptoms: history of abdominal or pelvic malignancy; palpable abdominal mass; enlarged lymph nodes

Investigations: ascites specimen for cytology and culture (the culture rules out bacterial infection)

Transudative: high serum-to-ascites albumin gradient (e.g., portal hypertension)

PORTAL HYPERTENSION

Causes of portal hypertension include congestive heart failure, liver disease, and pancreatitis.

CONGESTIVE HEART FAILURE

Signs and symptoms: severe shortness of breath; elevated jugular venous pressure; edema in the abdomen and legs; pink phlegm; heart murmurs and extra cardiac sounds

> History of heart disease or risk factors for heart disease (diabetes, hypertension, hyperlipidemia, and smoking) or hepatic vein thrombosis (Budd-Chiari syndrome)

Investigations: chest X-ray to detect pulmonary edema; NT-proBNP level; echocardiogram imaging to distinguish forms of heart failure; cardiac stress testing, either with exercise or pharmacological agent

LIVER DISEASE

Signs and symptoms: jaundice; abdominal pain, swelling; palpable, tender liver; swelling in the legs and ankles; systemic symptoms (anorexia, weight loss, weakness, fatigue); itching; easy bruising

> History of chronic alcohol abuse; chronic infection with hepatitis B virus (HBV) or hepatitis C virus (HCV), or risk factors for these infections (unprotected sex, intravenous drug abuse, blood transfusions, tattoos, body piercings, imprisonment, workplace exposure to body fluids); hemochromatosis; autoimmune conditions; α_1-antitrypsin deficiency; primary biliary cirrhosis; congestive heart failure

Investigations: tests for liver enzymes (elevated AST, ALT) and liver function (elevated bilirubin; possible abnormal PT/INR); viral serologic tests to detect HBV, HCV; Doppler ultrasound; CT scan; MRI; transient elastography; liver biopsy

PANCREATITIS

Signs and symptoms: constant upper abdominal pain that radiates to the back (sitting up and leaning forward may reduce the pain; pain occurs with coughing, vigorous movement, deep breathing); shortness of breath; nausea, vomiting; hypotension; fever; jaundice; abdominal tenderness

> History of gallstones or chronic alcoholism (usual); hyperlipidemia; hypercalcemia; change of medication

Investigations: serum amylase and lipase (levels are ≥ 3 times the upper limit of normal levels; elevated lipase indicates pancreatic damage); possible elevated calcium; possible elevated cholesterol; possible elevated ALT (this indicates associated liver inflammation); chest X-ray (this may show left-sided or bilateral pleural effusion; atelectasis); abdominal X-ray (this may show calcifications within pancreatic ducts, calcified gallstones, or localized ileus of a segment of small intestine); ultrasound

BOWEL DILATATION

Mechanical obstruction (e.g., adhesions, volvulus)

Signs and symptoms (in general): abnormal bowel sounds (increased in early bowel obstruction, decreased in late bowel obstruction); palpable hernia or bowel obstruction

> History of abdominal or pelvic surgery; inflammatory bowel disease (ulcerative colitis or Crohn disease); hernia (abdominal, femoral, or inguinal)

Paralytic conditions (e.g., toxic megacolon, neuropathy)

TOXIC MEGACOLON

Signs and symptoms: fever, shock, decreased bowel sounds; history of inflammatory bowel disease, colonic infection (*C. difficile*)

Investigations: elevated WBCs

NEUROPATHY

Examples of diseases with neuropathic effects that can lead to bowel dilation include scleroderma and diabetes.

OTHER

Abdominal mass

Signs and symptoms: abdominal pain, change in bowel habits, constitutional symptoms (fever, weight loss, night sweats), palpable abdominal mass

Investigations: ultrasound, CT scan

Irritable bowel syndrome[1]

Irritable bowel syndrome is commonly diagnosed by applying the Rome criteria.

Signs and symptoms (Rome criteria): at least 2 symptoms, present for ≥ 1 day/week for ≥ 3 months

> Symptoms: pain associated with defecation, pain associated with a change of stool frequency, pain associated with a change in stool consistency

Organomegaly (e.g., hepatomegaly)

Signs and symptoms (in general): palpable liver or spleen

Investigations: ultrasound

Pelvic mass (e.g., ovarian cancer)

OVARIAN CANCER

Signs and symptoms: postmenopausal female (more common); asymptomatic in early stage (usual); abdominal bloating, discomfort, distention (ascites); ovarian or pelvic mass; urinary urgency, frequency; abnormal vaginal bleeding; fatigue; gastrointestinal symptoms (nausea, heartburn, diarrhea, constipation, early satiety); shortness of breath

Investigations: transvaginal and abdominal ultrasound; CA 125 blood test; pelvic/abdominal CT scan; analysis of ascitic fluid; biopsy

Strategy for patient encounter

The likely scenario is a patient with ascites or bowel obstruction. The specified tasks could engage history, physical exam, investigations, or management.

History

Start with open-ended questions about the abdominal distension and associated symptoms: When did the abdominal distension start? How constant is it? What other symptoms do you have? Listen for evidence consistent with particular entities (e.g., pain with defecation, or changes in stool frequency or consistency in irritable bowel syndrome; jaundice, systemic symptoms, and swollen legs in liver disease; palpable mass with changes in bowel habits in abdominal or pelvic mass).

Take a medical history. Listen for heart disease, liver disease, or pancreatitis (these suggest ascites); and cancer or bowel surgery (these suggest bowel obstruction); and scleroderma and diabetes (these suggest bowel dilation). Ask about a history of irritable bowel syndrome (relevant to functional bloating, which is diagnosed in patients who do not meet the criteria for irritable bowel syndrome, but have had a recurrent feeling of bloating or visible distention for at least 3 days per month for at least 3 months). Ask about a history of psychosocial distress, depression, and anxiety.

Physical exam

Examine the abdomen, looking for masses and ascites. Auscultate the heart for murmurs and extra sounds. Perform a rectal exam to look for masses. In women, perform a pelvic exam to look for masses.

(State that you will perform a pelvic and/or rectal exam. Since these exams are not performed on standardized patients, the examiner will likely interrupt, ask what you are looking for, and provide findings.)

Investigations

Order a complete blood count (CBC), celiac serology, liver function tests, 3 views of the abdomen, and an abdominal ultrasound. Order other tests if a specific diagnosis is suggested from the history and physical exam. H_2 breath testing following a carbohydrate load is commonly used to diagnose small intestinal bacterial overgrowth (SIBO). Patients with ascites require paracentesis for diagnosis (cytology for tumour cells; cell count and culture to rule out spontaneous bacterial peritonitis) and for symptom relief. In suspected SIBO or celiac disease, refer the patient for endoscopy and biopsy.

Management
Patients with bowel obstruction require emergency referral to a general surgeon. Patients with functional bloating are managed with exercise, diet, simethicone, and possibly other medications for irritable bowel syndrome. Tricyclic antidepressants are frequently used to treat functional abdominal pain.

REFERENCE

1 Lacey B, Mearin F, Chang L, et al. Rome IV functional gastrointestinal disorders: disorders of gut-brain interaction. 4th ed. Vol. 2. Raleigh, NC: Rome Foundation; 2017. Chapter 11, Functional bowel disorders; 1393–1407.

2

Abdominal or pelvic mass

MCC particular objective
Recognize features of a mass that indicate the need for immediate intervention.

MCC differential diagnosis
with added evidence

ORGANOMEGALY

Hepatomegaly
Signs and symptoms: palpable, enlarged liver; signs of congestive heart failure (severe shortness of breath; elevated jugular venous pressure; edema in the abdomen and legs; pink phlegm; heart murmurs and extra cardiac sounds); signs of infection or malignancy (fever, enlarged lymph nodes)

> History of congestive heart failure; hepatic vein thrombosis (Budd-Chiari syndrome); myeloproliferative disorders;

hepatitis, or risk factors for hepatitis B virus (HBV) or hepatitis C virus (HCV) infection (unprotected sex, intravenous drug abuse, blood transfusions, tattoos, body piercings, workplace exposure to body fluids); lipid storage disease (e.g., Gaucher disease)

Investigations: abnormal serum liver function tests (this indicates liver disease)

Splenomegaly

Signs and symptoms: palpable, enlarged spleen

History of viral infection (especially mononucleosis), myeloproliferative disorders, lymphoma, liver disease, hemolytic anemia

Investigations: abnormal serum liver function tests (this indicates liver disease); blood tests to detect hemoglobinopathy, hemolytic anemia; heterophile antibody test to detect mononucleosis; abnormal differential and blood smear in the case of hematologic malignancy

Enlarged kidneys (e.g., cysts, hydronephrosis)

Signs and symptoms: palpable, enlarged kidneys

History of oliguria, hypertension; personal or family history of polycystic kidney disease, renal stones

Investigations: elevated creatinine (this indicates renal impairment)

NEOPLASM (BENIGN OR MALIGNANT)

Lymphoma or sarcoma

Signs and symptoms (in general): constitutional symptoms (weight loss, fever, night sweats), enlarged lymph nodes, palpable abdominal mass

Investigations: peripheral blood smear to detect blasts or cancer cells; bone marrow examination to detect excess blasts or cancer cells

Gastrointestinal tumour (e.g., gastric, colon, pancreas, hepatoma, gastrointestinal stromal tumour)

Signs and symptoms (in general): weight loss, abdominal pain, blood in the stool, change in bowel habits, family history of gastrointestinal cancer, palpable abdominal mass

Investigations: elevated CEA, elevated CA 19-9

Gynecologic tumour (e.g., ovarian, uterine)— see below

Renal or adrenal neoplasm

Signs and symptoms (in general): flank pain, constitutional symptoms (weight loss, night sweats), blood in the urine, hypertension (this suggests renal tumour), palpable abdominal mass

Neuroblastoma

Neuroblastoma usually affects children younger than 5 years.

Signs and symptoms: abdominal pain; swelling of the legs; palpable, painless mass

GYNECOLOGIC

Ovary (e.g., benign or malignant mass)

Signs and symptoms (in general): pelvic pain; pain on intercourse; menstrual irregularities; change in bowel or bladder habits; family or personal history of gynecological or breast cancer

> Malignant ovarian masses: constitutional symptoms (fever, weight loss, night sweats)

Investigations (for malignancy): elevated CA 125

Fallopian tube (e.g., ectopic pregnancy)

ECTOPIC PREGNANCY

Signs and symptoms: symptoms of pregnancy and/or positive pregnancy test; pelvic pain; vaginal bleeding; painful intercourse; shoulder pain; palpable tubal mass; pelvic tenderness and pain associated with 1 or both adnexa

> Severe symptom: syncope

Risk factors: previous ectopic pregnancy, pelvic inflammatory disease, pregnancy during intrauterine device (IUD) use

Investigations (pathognomonic): β-hCG above discriminatory zone (> 1500–2000 mIU/mL) **with** transvaginal ultrasound findings of a lack of intrauterine gestational sac, complex (mixed solid and cystic) masses in the adnexa, and free fluid in the cul-de-sac

Uterus (e.g., leiomyoma, pregnancy)

LEIOMYOMA

This is the most common pelvic tumour in women.

Signs and symptoms: commonly asymptomatic; premenopausal (usual); heavy or prolonged menstrual bleeding; pelvic, abdominal pressure; pain on intercourse; urinary symptoms (incontinence; frequent urination; difficulty emptying the bladder); constipation; pelvic mass or enlarged, irregular uterus on bimanual palpation

Risk factors: family history of leiomyoma; African descent

Investigations: ultrasound to detect mass ≥ 1 cm in diameter

PREGNANCY

Signs and symptoms: amenorrhea, especially during childbearing years (some experience spotting); sexual activity, especially without contraception or with inconsistent use of contraception; nausea, vomiting (common early sign); breast enlargement and tenderness; increased frequency of urination without other urinary symptoms; fatigue

Investigations: blood or urine β-hCG

BLADDER OR PROSTATE CONDITIONS (E.G., URINARY RETENTION, CANCER)

Signs and symptoms (in general): change in urinary habits (reduced urination in prostate conditions; blood in the urine; reduced and/or frequent urination in bladder conditions; new-onset nocturia in adults); palpable bladder mass, or enlarged or irregular prostate on palpation

Investigations: urine cytology; CT scan or cytoscopy to detect bladder mass

OTHER

Pancreatic pseudocyst

Signs and symptoms: history of pancreatitis (usual), fever, abdominal tenderness, palpable abdominal mass

Abdominal aortic aneurysm

Signs and symptoms: back pain; abdominal pain; syncope; palpable pulsatile midabdominal mass

Risk factors: history of smoking; family history of abdominal aortic aneurysm; previous aneurysms; hypertension

Abdominal wall masses

Signs and symptoms: abdominal pain; change in bowel or bladder habits; renal obstruction; constitutional symptoms (weight loss, fever, fatigue, night sweats)

Strategy for patient encounter

The likely scenario is a patient with urinary retention associated with an abdominal or pelvic mass. The specified tasks could engage history, physical exam, investigations, or management.

History

Start with open-ended questions about the mass: When did you discover it? How did you discover it? Where is it? How has it changed since you discovered it? Listen for evidence that helps localize and characterize the mass, and in particular for evidence of growth in the mass.

Ask about associated symptoms. Listen for pain; constitutional symptoms (these suggest malignancy: fever, weight loss, night sweats, fatigue); and urinary symptoms (these suggest gynecological, bladder, or prostate conditions). Ask about nausea, vomiting, constipation, and diarrhea, and about changes in menstruation. Take a medication history, looking especially for narcotics, opiates, and anticholinergic medications (these may cause urinary retention or constipation). Ask whether the patient could be pregnant. Take a medical and surgical history.

Physical exam

Obtain the patient's vital signs, looking for hypotension and fever. Perform an abdominal exam (remember to check for an abdominal aortic aneurysm). Perform a rectal exam, looking for masses and blood. In women, perform a pelvic exam, looking for ovarian or uterine masses.

(State that you will perform a rectal and/or pelvic exam. Since these exams are not performed on standardized patients, the examiner will likely interrupt, ask what you are looking for, and provide findings.)

Investigations

In women of childbearing age, order a pregnancy test. Order an abdominal ultrasound, CT scan, and tests for tumour markers. Initial laboratory studies may include a complete blood count (CBC) and urinalysis, and tests for electrolytes, creatinine, liver function, and pregnancy. Order a plain kidneys-ureters-bladder (KUB) X-ray to look for constipation, obstruction, and free intraperitoneal air. Order an abdominal CT scan with contrast to evaluate for bowel or pelvic pathology, and organomegaly. In suspected bowel mass, refer the patient to a surgeon or gastroenterologist for colonoscopy.

Management

Stabilize any patient with a life-threatening cause (e.g., ruptured abdominal aortic aneurysm). Treat the specific entity identified. Most patients with a mass require referral to a general surgeon, urologist, or gynecologist as appropriate. Discontinue any contributing medications.

3

Hernia (abdominal wall and groin)

MCC particular objectives

Pay particular attention to the physical examination.
Identify the type of hernia.
Determine if the hernia is incarcerated, because incarcerated hernias require emergent (not elective) repair.

MCC differential diagnosis
with added evidence

INCARCERATED HERNIA IN GENERAL

Any hernia can become incarcerated.

Signs and symptoms: nausea, vomiting, pain, constipation

CONGENITAL HERNIA

Inguinal hernia (infants)

Signs and symptoms: bulge in the internal or external inguinal ring or within the scrotum; bulge that may disappear at rest, and that recurs with crying or straining with a bowel movement

Umbilical hernia (infants and children)

Signs and symptoms: mass that protrudes through the umbilicus, which may be more pronounced with straining; mass that is easily reducible (generally)

ACQUIRED HERNIA

Inguinal hernia

DIRECT

Signs and symptoms: inguinal swelling; swelling that aches and enlarges with straining (usually); palpable bulge above the inguinal canal and **medial** to the internal inguinal ring

INDIRECT

Signs and symptoms: male patient (common); inguinal swelling; swelling that aches and enlarges with straining (usually); palpable bulge above the inguinal canal and **lateral** to the internal inguinal ring

Femoral hernia

Signs and symptoms: female patient (more common); bulge in the upper thigh; palpable bulge below the inguinal ligament

Umbilical hernia

Signs and symptoms: mass that protrudes through the umbilicus, which may be more pronounced with straining

Ventral (incisional) hernia

Signs and symptoms: abdominal bulge that becomes more pronounced on straining; obesity (common)

> History of abdominal surgery (common), postoperative wound infection (very common)

Strategy for patient encounter

The likely scenario is a patient with a groin mass. The specified tasks could engage history, physical exam, investigations, or management.

History

Use open-ended questions to establish the patient's symptoms: When did you notice the mass? How does the mass change with lying down or straining? (A mass that disappears when the patient is supine, and enlarges with straining, is typical for hernia.) What other symptoms do you have? Listen for sudden severe pain, nausea, vomiting, and constipation (these suggest incarcerated hernia). Ask about constitutional symptoms (fever, weight loss, fatigue, night sweats), which are consistent with infection and malignancy. Ask about recent injuries to the abdomen or groin. Take a history of abdominal surgeries.

Physical exam

Perform an abdominal exam. Look for redness and tenderness around an umbilical hernia. Examine for an inguinal hernia by inspecting the femoral and inguinal areas for bulges while the patient is standing. Ask the patient to perform a Valsalva maneuver and observe for the accentuation of any hernia masses. Insert a finger into the external inguinal ring and ask the patient to cough, feeling for a bulge. Repeat this on the other side. Examine the scrotal sack for a mass separate from the testes.

(State that you will examine the scrotal sack. Since this exam is not performed on standardized patients, the examiner will likely interrupt, ask what you are looking for, and provide findings.)

Investigations
Investigations are usually not needed. However, ultrasound can help diagnose a scrotal mass in a male patient or an inguinal hernia in a female patient.

Management
Strangulated hernias are a medical emergency. The patient requires immediate admission, stabilization, and surgical intervention. For other hernias, refer the patient to a general surgeon.

Some infants have umbilical hernias. These generally close as the children grow. Refer children with umbilical hernias to surgery if the hernia is painful, larger than 1.5 cm in diameter, still present at age 4 years, or incarcerated.

Pearls
Inguinal hernias occur primarily in men (9:1 male:female ratio), and are most common in patients aged 40 to 59.

4

Acute abdominal pain

MCC particular objective
Identify patients who need emergency medical or surgical treatment.

MCC differential diagnosis
with added evidence

LOCALIZED PAIN

Upper abdominal region

BILIARY TRACT DISEASE
Signs and symptoms: middle-aged woman (more common) (mnemonic: **4Fs**—female, fat, fertile, forties); epigastric pain, often

after eating (the pain is generally constant and often radiates to the right shoulder); right-sided subcostal pain that is worse on deep inhalation; obesity; history of pregnancy

Cancer or primary biliary cholangitis: fatigue, weight loss

Obstructive biliary disease: jaundice

Investigations: elevated ALP, bilirubin (this indicates biliary obstruction); elevated aminotransferases (AST, ALT) (this indicates liver injury); ultrasound or CT scan to detect gallstones; MRCP to detect bile duct obstruction

PANCREATITIS

Signs and symptoms: constant upper abdominal pain that radiates to the back (sitting up and leaning forward may reduce the pain; pain occurs with coughing, vigorous movement, deep breathing); shortness of breath; nausea, vomiting; hypotension; fever; jaundice; abdominal tenderness

History of gallstones or chronic alcoholism (usual); hyperlipidemia; hypercalcemia; change in medication

Investigations: serum amylase and lipase (levels are ≥ 3 times the upper limit of normal levels; elevated lipase indicates pancreatic damage); possible elevated calcium; possible elevated cholesterol; possible elevated ALT (this indicates associated liver inflammation); chest X-ray (this may show left-sided or bilateral pleural effusion; atelectasis); abdominal X-ray (this may show calcifications within pancreatic ducts, calcified gallstones, or localized ileus of a segment of small intestine); ultrasound

PEPTIC ULCER DISEASE, GASTRITIS

PEPTIC ULCER DISEASE

Signs and symptoms: constant midepigastric pain, often relieved with eating or with antacids; weight loss

Investigations: test for *H. pylori*; endoscopy to detect ulcer or inflammation of the gastric lining

GASTRITIS

Signs and symptoms: upper abdominal pain; burning, aching pain; pain that is better or worse with eating; feeling of fullness in the upper abdomen with eating; nausea, vomiting

Risk factors: *Helicobacter pylori* infection; regular use of acetylsalicylic acid (ASA), ibuprofen, naproxen; alcohol use; stress; autoimmune disorders (Hashimoto disease, type 1 diabetes)

GASTROESOPHAGEAL REFLUX DISEASE

Signs and symptoms: burning chest pain radiating into the throat (often with a bitter taste in the mouth or regurgitation of food into the mouth; often worse with lying down; often better with standing up or taking antacids; worse with spicy food, coffee, alcohol, fatty foods, peppermint); acid damage to teeth

Risk factors: obesity, pregnancy

ACUTE HEPATITIS

Signs and symptoms: viral-like illness; abdominal pain; jaundice; palpable, tender liver

History of infection with hepatitis A virus (HAV), hepatitis B virus (HBV), hepatitis C virus (HCV) or risk factors for these infections (autoimmune conditions, unprotected sex, intravenous drug abuse, blood transfusions, tattoos, body piercings, workplace exposure to body fluids); toxic ingestion (e.g., acetaminophen); adverse drug reaction (e.g., change of medication)

HCV: often asymptomatic

Investigations: elevated AST, ALT, bilirubin; abnormal PT/INR; positive viral serologic tests (e.g., HAV, HBV, HCV)

CARDIOTHORACIC CONDITION (REFERRED PAIN)

Signs and symptoms: cough, shortness of breath

Heart exam: extra heart sounds or pericardial rub

Lung exam: abnormal breath sounds, absent breath sounds, or lung rales on auscultation; solid sounds on percussion

Risk factors for heart and lung disease: personal or family history of heart and lung disease; hyperlipidemia; diabetes; smoking; occupational exposure to smoke or other lung irritants

Investigations: elevated cardiac enzymes (e.g., troponin), chest X-ray, ECG

MUSCULOSKELETAL CONDITION

Signs and symptoms: palpable abnormalities and point tenderness in abdominal muscles and spine

History of recent trauma, overuse of abdominal muscles, chronic musculoskeletal problems

Lower abdominal pain

APPENDICITIS

Signs and symptoms: child (often); periumbilical pain that migrates over several days to localize in the right lower quadrant; anorexia; fever; localized pain over the McBurney point on abdominal palpation

Investigations: elevated WBCs; ultrasound or CT scan to detect distended appendix

MESENTERIC LYMPHADENITIS

Mesenteric lymphadenitis is a common differential diagnosis with appendicitis.

Signs and symptoms: lower abdominal pain; abdominal tenderness (particularly in the right lower quadrant); fever; diarrhea; nausea, vomiting

Investigations: normal appendix on CT scan (this may be useful in distinguishing mesenteric lymphadenitis from appendicitis)

DIVERTICULITIS

Signs and symptoms: constant left lower quadrant abdominal pain; abdominal tenderness; fever; nausea, vomiting; change in bowel habits (constipation and/or diarrhea)

Risk factors: advanced age, obesity, smoking, poor diet, lack of exercise

Investigations: CT scan

INCARCERATED HERNIA

Signs and symptoms: mass or swelling in the abdomen, groin, or upper thigh; rapid-onset acute pain at the site of the mass or swelling; nausea, vomiting; constipation; history of abdominal surgery (this is common in ventral hernias); obesity (this is a risk factor for ventral hernias)

Investigations: ultrasound, CT scan

PELVIC INFLAMMATORY DISEASE

Signs and symptoms: lower abdominal and pelvic pain; pain during intercourse; fever; urinary symptoms; vaginal discharge; irregular menstruation; pelvic tenderness and pain associated with 1 or both adnexa

History of gonorrhea, chlamydia, or risk factors for them (multiple partners, unprotected sex); intrauterine device (IUD); childbirth; gynecologic procedure

Investigations: cultures for gonorrhea and chlamydia; ultrasound (this has normal findings)

ECTOPIC PREGNANCY

Signs and symptoms: symptoms of pregnancy and/or positive pregnancy test; pelvic pain; vaginal bleeding; painful intercourse; shoulder pain; palpable tubal mass; pelvic tenderness and pain associated with 1 or both adnexa

Severe symptom: syncope

Risk factors: previous ectopic pregnancy, pelvic inflammatory disease, pregnancy during intrauterine device (IUD) use

Investigations (pathognomonic): β-hCG above discriminatory zone (> 1500–2000 mIU/mL) **with** transvaginal ultrasound findings of a lack of intrauterine gestational sac, complex (mixed solid and cystic) masses in the adnexa, and free fluid in the cul-de-sac

OVARIAN CONDITION (E.G., TORSION OR RUPTURED CYST)

Signs and symptoms: pelvic pain; pain during intercourse; change in bowel habits; nausea, vomiting; fever; worsening or sudden onset of pain (this may indicate ovarian torsion); pelvic tenderness and pain associated with 1 or both adnexa

Investigations: enlarged ovary or ovaries on pelvic ultrasound or laparoscopy

URINARY TRACT INFECTION

Signs and symptoms: frequent urination; painful urination; pelvic pain and/or flank pain; fever; tenderness over the bladder

Investigations: urinalysis, urine culture

RENAL COLIC

Signs and symptoms: colicky flank pain; nausea, vomiting; fever; history of kidney stones (common); extreme tenderness at the costovertebral angle on abdominal examination; hematuria

Investigations: KUB X-ray; ureter ultrasound, abdominal CT scan

INFLAMMATORY BOWEL DISEASE

Signs and symptoms: younger than 30 (usually); family history of inflammatory bowel disease; fluctuating symptoms with periods of exacerbation and remission; diarrhea (possibly with nocturnal waking); blood in the stool; abdominal pain; weight loss; fever; fatigue; right lower quadrant and periumbilical pain; extraintestinal manifestations (e.g., uveitis, arthritis)

> Crohn disease: right lower quadrant mass, inflammation of the eyes, arthritis

Investigations: elevated CRP (this suggests active inflammation); fecal calprotectin; colonoscopy with biopsy (this is a standard diagnostic procedure); CT scan or MRI (findings: diagnostic structural changes associated with inflammatory bowel disease)

BOWEL OBSTRUCTION

Signs and symptoms: crampy abdominal pain; nausea, vomiting; change in bowel habits (diarrhea or constipation); abdominal distention; palpable mass; increased bowel sounds (this suggests early obstruction; bowel sounds may be decreased in later obstruction); history of colonic diseases (diverticulitis, colon cancer, inflammatory bowel disease)

Risk factors for adhesions: abdominal surgery

Risk factors for paralytic ileus: narcotic medications, chronic neuromuscular disease, diabetes

Investigations: abdominal X-ray to detect distended bowel with air-fluid levels; CT scan to identify etiology of obstruction

DIFFUSE ABDOMINAL PAIN

Generalized peritonitis

BACTERIAL PERITONITIS

Signs and symptoms: fever, abdominal pain, generalized abdominal tenderness, guarding on physical examination, rebound tenderness, ascites

> History of abdominal surgery, diverticulitis, appendicitis, recent colonoscopy, inflammatory bowel disease, peptic ulcer disease, pancreatitis, liver disease, pelvic inflammatory disease, peritoneal dialysis, ovarian cyst or mass

Investigations: elevated WBCs; blood and peritoneal cultures

Ruptured abdominal aortic aneurysm

Signs and symptoms: older than 60 (usual); abdominal, back pain; syncope; pulsatile mass; tachycardia; hypotension

Risk factors: history of smoking; family history of abdominal aortic aneurysm; previous aneurysms; hypertension

Investigations: decreased hemoglobin (this may not arise in the context of acute bleeding); ultrasound, CT scan, MRI

Ischemic bowel disease

Signs and symptoms: abrupt-onset abdominal pain; abdominal tenderness; nausea, vomiting; fever; blood in the stool; hypotension (this is possible in acute ischemia); localized tenderness (in early presentations) or peritoneal signs (in late presentations) on abdominal exam

> History of pancreatitis, bowel cancer, inflammatory bowel disease, inherited clotting disorders, diseases of blood vessels (peripheral vascular disease, cardiovascular disease, atherosclerosis), diabetes, use of oral contraceptives

Investigations: PT/INR; PTT; elevated lactate (this is possible with ischemic injury); angiography by CT scan or MRI to detect clots; colonoscopy, laparotomy

Gastroenteritis

Signs and symptoms: abrupt-onset diarrhea; crampy abdominal pain; nausea, vomiting; fever; headache; muscle aches; epigastric tenderness on abdominal examination

Risk factors: exposure to persons with similar symptoms or to large groups of people (common: most cases are viral); eating undercooked or contaminated foods, or raw fluids (these are risk factors for bacterial infection)

Irritable bowel syndrome[1]

Irritable bowel syndrome is commonly diagnosed by applying the Rome criteria.

Signs and symptoms (Rome criteria): at least 2 symptoms, present for
≥ 1 day/week for ≥ 3 months
  Symptoms: pain associated with defecation, pain associated
  with a change of stool frequency, pain associated with a
  change in stool consistency

Strategy for patient encounter

The likely scenario is a patient with sudden-onset abdominal
pain. The specified tasks could engage history, physical exam, investigations, or management.

History

Start with open-ended questions to obtain a pain history: Where
is the pain? When did the pain start? How constant is it? How
long does it last? Where does the pain radiate? What kind of
pain is it (e.g., sharp, dull, or throbbing)? How severe is the pain?
What makes the pain better or worse? Listen for evidence consistent with particular entities (e.g., constant upper abdominal pain,
worse with coughing, that radiates to the back in pancreatitis;
pelvic pain made worse with intercourse in pelvic inflammatory
disease, ectopic pregnancy, and ovarian conditions; diffuse abdominal and back pain in ruptured abdominal aortic aneurysm).

Use open-ended questions to establish associated symptoms:
What other symptoms do you have? Listen for evidence associated with particular entities (e.g., viral-like symptoms with
jaundice in acute hepatitis; lower abdominal mass or swelling
in hernia; urinary symptoms, vaginal discharge, and irregular
menstruation in pelvic inflammatory disease). Ask about constitutional symptoms (fever, weight loss, night sweats, fatigue).
Ask about syncope or presyncope (these suggest a surgical emergency). Ask whether the patient is vomiting blood or bleeding
from the rectum (bright red blood or black, tarry stools).

Take a medical and medication history: What conditions have
you been diagnosed with? What medications do you take? Listen for conditions associated with particular entities (see the information this resource lists in the MCC differential diagnosis),
and for erythromycin and nonsteroidal antiinflammatory drugs
(NSAIDs). Ask about the patient's sexual history, listening for
risk factors for pelvic inflammatory disease. Ask about symptoms
of irritable bowel syndrome.

Physical exam

Obtain the patient's vital signs, looking for fever, hypotension, and tachycardia. Examine the heart (relevant to cardiac ischemia) and lungs (pneumonia). Examine the abdomen, looking for masses and tenderness (including rebound tenderness), and listen for bowel sounds. Look specifically for Murphy sign (this suggests cholecystitis), Carnett sign (relevant to abdominal wall pain), and the psoas sign (appendicitis). Perform a rectal exam, looking for fecal impaction, palpable masses, and occult blood. In women, perform a pelvic examination (relevant to ectopic pregnancy, vaginitis, and pelvic inflammatory disease).

(State that you will perform a rectal and/or pelvic exam. Since these exams are not performed on standardized patients, the examiner may interrupt, ask what you are looking for, and provide findings.)

Investigations

Order a complete blood count (CBC), to look for infection and anemia. Order a urinalysis, and tests for electrolytes, creatinine, liver function, and lipase. In patients with right upper quadrant pain, order an ultrasound. In patients with right and left lower quadrant pain, order a CT scan. Order a urine pregnancy test in women of childbearing age. In suspected ectopic pregnancy, order a transvaginal ultrasound. In patients at risk of sexually transmitted infection, test for chlamydia and gonorrhea.

Management

Stabilize any patient with unstable vital signs. Additional management depends on the entity diagnosed: keep in mind the most

CHECKLIST

Sources of acute abdominal pain by location

LEFT UPPER QUADRANT	RIGHT UPPER QUADRANT	RIGHT LOWER QUADRANT	LEFT LOWER QUADRANT
Esophagus	Pulmonary system	Appendix	Diverticula
Stomach	Urinary system	Urinary system	Urinary system
Pancreas	Hepatobiliary system	Colon	
Spleen		Pelvis	
Kidneys			
Intestines			

common and serious sources of pain for each anatomic location (see the checklist). Refer the patient to surgery as appropriate.

REFERENCE

1 Lacey B, Mearin F, Chang L, et al. Rome IV functional gastrointestinal disorders: disorders of gut-brain interaction. 4th ed. Vol. 2. Raleigh, NC: Rome Foundation; 2017. Chapter 11, Functional bowel disorders; 1393–1407.

5

Abdominal pain (children)

MCC particular objectives

Identify patients who need emergency medical or surgical treatment.

Recognize that nonorganic causes are the most common causes.

MCC differential diagnosis
with added evidence

LOWER ABDOMINAL PAIN

Appendicitis

Signs and symptoms: periumbilical pain that migrates over several days to localize in the right lower quadrant; anorexia; fever; localized pain over the McBurney point on palpation

Investigations: elevated WBCs; ultrasound or CT scan to detect distended appendix

Constipation

Signs and symptoms: recurrent abdominal pain; straining at hard stools; poor fluid intake; frequent, painful urination (this suggests urinary tract infection, which is a possible complication); palpable stool on abdominal exam; impacted stool on rectal exam; anal fissures

Gastroenteritis

Signs and symptoms: abrupt-onset diarrhea; crampy abdominal pain; nausea, vomiting; fever; headache; muscle aches; epigastric tenderness on abdominal examination

Risk factors: exposure to persons with similar symptoms or to large groups of people (most cases are viral); eating undercooked or contaminated foods, or raw fluids (these are risk factors for bacterial infection)

Mesenteric lymphadenitis

Mesenteric lymphadenitis is a common differential diagnosis with appendicitis.

Signs and symptoms: lower abdominal pain; abdominal tenderness (particularly in the right lower quadrant); fever; diarrhea; nausea, vomiting

Investigations: normal appendix on CT scan (this may be useful in distinguishing mesenteric lymphadenitis from appendicitis)

Inflammatory bowel disease

Signs and symptoms: younger than 30 (usually); family history of inflammatory bowel disease; fluctuating symptoms with periods of exacerbation and remission; diarrhea (possibly with nocturnal waking); blood in the stool; abdominal pain; weight loss; fever; fatigue; right lower quadrant and periumbilical pain; extraintestinal manifestations (e.g., uveitis, arthritis)

> Crohn disease: right lower quadrant mass, inflammation of the eyes, arthritis

Investigations: elevated CRP (this suggests active inflammation); fecal calprotectin; colonoscopy with biopsy (this is a standard diagnostic procedure); CT scan or MRI (findings: diagnostic structural changes associated with inflammatory bowel disease)

Inguinal hernia (incarcerated)

Signs and symptoms: mass or swelling in the groin; rapid-onset acute pain at the site of the mass or swelling; nausea, vomiting; constipation

Investigations: ultrasound, CT scan

Urinary tract infection

Signs and symptoms: frequent urination; painful urination; pelvic pain and/or flank pain; fever; tenderness over the bladder

Investigations: urinalysis, urine culture

Gynecological cause in pubertal children

Common causes include dysmenorrhea, pelvic inflammatory disease, ectopic pregnancy, and ovarian torsion.

GENERALIZED PAIN

Peritoneal inflammation

Signs and symptoms: fever, abdominal pain, generalized abdominal tenderness, guarding on physical examination, rebound tenderness, ascites

> History of abdominal surgery, appendicitis, inflammatory

bowel disease, peptic ulcer disease, pancreatitis, liver disease, recent colonoscopy

Investigations: elevated WBCs; blood and peritoneal cultures

Bowel

INFANTILE COLIC

Signs and symptoms: age 2 weeks to 4 months (common); crying in the late afternoon or evening; crying > 3 hours per day, > 3 days per week, for ≥ 3 weeks (mnemonic: **rule of 3**)

History of low birth weight, maternal smoking during pregnancy

No evidence of viral or bacterial illness; child abuse; malabsorption; failure to gain weight; frequent or bloody diarrhea; fever

OBSTRUCTION

Signs and symptoms: crampy abdominal pain; nausea, vomiting; change in bowel habits (diarrhea or constipation); abdominal distention; palpable mass; increased bowel sounds (this suggests early obstruction; bowel sounds may be decreased in later obstruction); history of colonic diseases (diverticulitis, colon cancer, inflammatory bowel disease)

Volvulus (surgical emergency): bilious vomiting

Risk factors for adhesions: abdominal surgery

Risk factors for paralytic ileus: narcotic medications, chronic neuromuscular disease, diabetes, cystic fibrosis

Investigations: abdominal X-ray to detect distended bowel with air-fluid levels; CT scan to identify etiology of obstruction

Malabsorption

Signs and symptoms: frequent or bloody diarrhea; failure to gain weight; family history of similar problems; low weight and height for age; reduced muscle and fat (these suggest malnutrition); enlarged liver or spleen (these suggest chronic malabsorption); skin breakdown around the anus (this suggests chronic diarrhea)

Irritable bowel syndrome[1]

Irritable bowel syndrome is commonly diagnosed by applying the Rome criteria.

Signs and symptoms (Rome criteria): at least 2 symptoms, present for ≥ 1 day/week for ≥ 3 months

Symptoms: pain associated with defecation, pain associated with a change of stool frequency, pain associated with a change in stool consistency

FLANK PAIN

Pyelonephritis

Signs and symptoms: frequent urination, painful urination, fever, tenderness over the costovertebral angle

Investigations: elevated WBCs; urinalysis, urine culture, blood culture to identify causative organism

Kidney stones

Signs and symptoms: colicky flank pain; nausea, vomiting; fever; history of kidney stones (common); extreme tenderness at the costovertebral angle on abdominal examination; hematuria

Investigations: KUB X-ray; ureter ultrasound, abdominal CT scan

PERIUMBILICAL RECURRENT ABDOMINAL PAIN

Signs and symptoms: age 4 to 16 years (common); recurrent pain centred around the umbilicus

EPIGASTRIC PAIN

Gastroesophageal reflux disease

Signs and symptoms: burning chest pain radiating into the throat (often with a bitter taste in the mouth or regurgitation of food into the mouth; often worse with lying down; often better with standing up or taking antacids; worse with spicy food, coffee, alcohol, fatty foods, peppermint); acid damage to teeth

Risk factors: obesity, pregnancy

Peptic ulcer disease

Signs and symptoms: constant midepigastric pain, often relieved with eating or with antacids; weight loss

Investigations: test for *H. pylori*; endoscopy to detect ulcer or inflammation of the gastric lining

Biliary tract disease

Signs and symptoms: epigastric pain, often after eating (the pain is generally constant and often radiates to the right shoulder); right-sided subcostal pain that is worse on deep inhalation; obesity; history of pregnancy

    Cancer or primary biliary cholangitis: fatigue, weight loss

    Obstructive biliary disease: jaundice

Investigations: elevated ALP, bilirubin (this indicates biliary obstruction); elevated aminotransferases (AST, ALT) (this indicates liver injury); ultrasound or CT scan to detect gallstones; MRCP to detect bile duct obstruction

Strategy for patient encounter

This patient encounter will likely involve a parent discussing a child who is absent on some pretext (e.g., a nurse is weighing the child in another room) or an older adolescent (the minimum age to play standardized patients is 16). The following notes assume the scenario is a parent discussing a child.

The specified tasks could engage history, physical exam, investigations, or management.

History

Start with open-ended questions to obtain a pain history: Where is your child's pain? When did the pain start? How constant is it? How long does it last? Where does the pain radiate? What kind of pain is it (e.g., sharp, dull, throbbing)? How severe is the pain? What makes the pain better or worse? Listen for evidence consistent with particular entities (e.g., pain with periumbilical onset over several days that has localized in the right lower quadrant in appendicitis; recurrent pain associated with defecation, or changes in stool frequency or consistency, in irritable bowel syndrome; constant midepigastric pain relieved with eating or antacids in peptic ulcer disease).

Use open-ended questions to establish associated symptoms: What other symptoms does your child have? Listen for evidence consistent with particular entities (e.g., abrupt-onset diarrhea with fever, vomiting, and muscle aches in gastroenteritis; diarrhea and failure to gain weight in malabsorption; frequent, painful urination in urinary tract infection).

Take a medication history (listen especially for erythromycin). Ask about diseases that run in the family (listen for sickle cell disease, cystic fibrosis, inflammatory bowel disease, celiac disease).

In postmenarcheal girls, ask about menstrual history and sexual activity.

Physical exam

Obtain the patient's vital signs (looking for fever and hypovolemia). Observe the patient for pain behaviour (e.g., colic, reluctance to move, guarding). Examine the heart, lungs, and abdomen. Examine the external genitalia looking for penile and scrotal abnormalities in boys, and vaginal discharge in girls. In sexually active girls, perform a bimanual exam looking for tenderness and adnexal masses. Examine the skin for jaundice.

(State that you will examine the child and perform these procedures. Because an actual pediatric patient is unlikely, and because genital and pelvic exams are not performed on standardized patients in any case, the examiner may interrupt, ask what you are looking for, and provide findings.)

Investigations

For all patients, order a complete blood count (CBC), urinalysis, and abdominal plain films. Ultrasound examination is useful for diagnosing gynecologic causes. Order a pregnancy test in postmenarcheal girls.

Management

Treat any specific causes identified. These are often age dependent (see the checklist). In children with abdominal guarding, rebound tenderness, or trauma, and in patients whose pain has no obvious etiology, consult a pediatric surgeon.

CHECKLIST

Common causes of abdominal pain in children

YOUNGER THAN 1 YEAR	1 TO 5 YEARS	6 TO 11 YEARS	12 TO 18 YEARS
Gastroenteritis	Gastroenteritis	Gastroenteritis	Appendicitis
Constipation	Appendicitis	Appendicitis	Gastroenteritis
Urinary tract infection	Constipation	Constipation	Constipation
Intussusception	Urinary tract infection	Functional pain	Dysmenorrhea
Volvulus	Intussusception	Urinary tract infection	Mittelschmerz
Incarcerated hernia	Volvulus	Trauma	Pelvic inflammatory disease
Hirschsprung disease	Trauma	Pneumonia	Ectopic pregnancy
	Mesenteric lymphadenitis	Mesenteric lymphadenitis	Ovarian/testicular torsion

REFERENCE

1 Lacey B, Mearin F, Chang L, et al. Rome IV functional gastrointestinal disorders: disorders of gut-brain interaction. 4th ed. Vol. 2. Raleigh, NC: Rome Foundation; 2017. Chapter 11, Functional bowel disorders; 1393–1407.

6

Chronic abdominal pain

MCC particular objectives
None stated.

MCC differential diagnosis
with added evidence
CHRONIC ABDOMINAL PAIN IN GENERAL
Definition: abdominal pain lasting > 3 months

UPPER ABDOMINAL PAIN

Gastric cancer
Signs and symptoms: constitutional symptoms (fever, weight loss, night sweats); constant abdominal pain; enlarged lymph nodes; smoking; personal or family history of cancer; epigastric mass on abdominal exam

Investigations: CT scan of abdomen, endoscopy with biopsy

Ulcer and nonulcer dyspepsia
Signs and symptoms: constant midepigastric pain, often relieved with eating or with antacids; weight loss

Investigations: test for *H. pylori*; endoscopy to detect ulcer or inflammation of the gastric lining

Biliary disease
BILIARY TRACT DISEASE
Signs and symptoms: middle-aged woman (more common) (mnemonic: **4Fs**—female, fat, fertile, forties); epigastric pain, often after eating (the pain is generally constant and often radiates to the right shoulder); right-sided subcostal pain that is worse on deep inhalation; obesity; history of pregnancy

    Cancer or primary biliary cholangitis: fatigue, weight loss

    Obstructive biliary disease: jaundice

Investigations: elevated ALP, bilirubin (this indicates biliary obstruction); elevated aminotransferases (AST, ALT) (this indicates liver injury); ultrasound or CT scan to detect gallstones; MRCP to detect bile duct obstruction

Pancreatic disease

PANCREATITIS

Signs and symptoms: constant upper abdominal pain that radiates to the back (sitting up and leaning forward may reduce the pain; pain occurs with coughing, vigorous movement, deep breathing); shortness of breath; nausea, vomiting; hypotension; fever; jaundice; abdominal tenderness

>History of gallstones or chronic alcoholism (usual); hyperlipidemia; hypercalcemia; change of medication

Investigations: serum amylase and lipase (levels are ≥ 3 times the upper limit of normal levels; elevated lipase indicates pancreatic damage); possible elevated calcium; possible elevated cholesterol; possible elevated ALT (this indicates associated liver inflammation); chest X-ray (this may show left-sided or bilateral pleural effusion; atelectasis); abdominal X-ray (this may show calcifications within pancreatic ducts, calcified gallstones, or localized ileus of a segment of small intestine); ultrasound

Hepatic disease

Patients with compensated cirrhosis may be asymptomatic.

Hepatitis C virus (HCV) is often asymptomatic.

Signs and symptoms: jaundice; abdominal pain, swelling; palpable, tender liver; swelling in the legs and ankles; systemic symptoms (anorexia, weight loss, weakness, fatigue); itching; easy bruising

>History of chronic alcohol abuse; chronic infection with hepatitis B virus (HBV) or HCV, or risk factors for these infections (unprotected sex, intravenous drug abuse, blood transfusions, tattoos, body piercings, imprisonment, workplace exposure to body fluids); hemochromatosis; autoimmune conditions; a_1-antitrypsin deficiency; primary biliary cirrhosis; congestive heart failure

Investigations: tests for liver enzymes (elevated AST, ALT) and liver function (elevated bilirubin; possible abnormal PT/INR); viral serologic tests to detect HBV, HCV; Doppler ultrasound; CT scan; MRI; transient elastography; liver biopsy

Cardiothoracic conditions (referred pain)

Signs and symptoms: cough, shortness of breath

>Heart exam: extra heart sounds or pericardial rub

>Lung exam: abnormal breath sounds, absent breath sounds, or lung rales on auscultation; solid sounds on percussion

Risk factors for heart and lung disease: personal or family history of heart and lung disease; hyperlipidemia; diabetes; smoking; occupational exposure to smoke or other lung irritants

Investigations: elevated cardiac enzymes (e.g., troponin), chest X-ray, ECG

LOWER ABDOMINAL PAIN

Bowel disease

INFLAMMATORY BOWEL DISEASE

Signs and symptoms: younger than 30 (usually); family history of inflammatory bowel disease; fluctuating symptoms with periods of exacerbation and remission; diarrhea (possibly with nocturnal waking); blood in the stool; abdominal pain; weight loss; fever; fatigue; right lower quadrant and periumbilical pain; extraintestinal manifestations (e.g., uveitis, arthritis)

> Crohn disease: right lower quadrant mass, inflammation of the eyes, arthritis

Investigations: elevated CRP (this suggests active inflammation); fecal calprotectin; colonoscopy with biopsy (this is a standard diagnostic procedure); CT scan or MRI (findings: diagnostic structural changes associated with inflammatory bowel disease)

DIVERTICULAR DISEASE

DIVERTICULITIS

Signs and symptoms: constant left lower quadrant abdominal pain; abdominal tenderness; fever; nausea, vomiting; change in bowel habits (constipation and/or diarrhea)

Risk factors: advanced age, obesity, smoking, poor diet, lack of exercise

Investigations: CT scan

IRRITABLE BOWEL SYNDROME[1]

Irritable bowel syndrome is commonly diagnosed by applying the Rome criteria.

Signs and symptoms (Rome criteria): ≥ 2 symptoms, present for ≥ 1 day/week for ≥ 3 months

> Symptoms: pain associated with defecation, pain associated with a change of stool frequency, pain associated with a change in stool consistency

Genitourinary disease

ENDOMETRIOSIS

Signs and symptoms: pelvic pain associated with menstruation (very common); excessive bleeding during menstruation; pain during intercourse; pain during urination or bowel movements; tenderness on pelvic exam; normal findings on abdominal exam (common)

Risk factors: family history of endometriosis; nulliparity; personal history of pelvic inflammatory disease

Investigations: ultrasound to detect ovarian cysts (common finding); laparoscopy with biopsy

TUMOUR (BENIGN OR MALIGNANT)
Signs and symptoms: weight loss; abdominal pain; blood in the stool; palpable abdominal or pelvic mass
Investigations: elevated CEA, elevated CA 19-9

URINARY TRACT INFECTION
Signs and symptoms: frequent urination; painful urination; pelvic pain and/or flank pain; fever; tenderness over the bladder
Investigations: urinalysis, urine culture

PELVIC INFLAMMATORY DISEASE
Signs and symptoms: lower abdominal and pelvic pain; pain during intercourse; fever; urinary symptoms; vaginal discharge; irregular menstruation; pelvic tenderness and pain associated with 1 or both adnexa

History of gonorrhea, chlamydia, or risk factors for them (multiple partners, unprotected sex); intrauterine device (IUD); childbirth; gynecologic procedure

Investigations: cultures for gonorrhea and chlamydia; ultrasound (this has normal findings)

Strategy for patient encounter

The likely scenario is a patient with chronic abdominal pain. The specified tasks could engage history, physical exam, investigations, or management.

History

Use open-ended questions to take a history of the patient's pain, associated symptoms, psychosocial stressors, and medical conditions.

- **Pain:** Where is the pain? What is the pain like? How constant is it? What makes it better and worse? Make particular note of the location of the pain: this is key evidence in narrowing a diagnosis. Listen for radiating pain (e.g., to the right shoulder in biliary disease; to the back in pancreatic disease); constant versus intermittent pain (episodic pain suggests inflammatory bowel disease, irritable bowel syndrome, or endometriosis); pain made better by eating (ulcer and nonulcer dyspepsia), sitting up and leaning forward (pancreatic disease); and pain made worse with eating (biliary disease), deep breathing (pancreatic disease), and menstruation (endometriosis).

- **Associated symptoms:** What other symptoms do you have? Listen for evidence consistent with particular entities (e.g., constitutional symptoms and enlarged lymph nodes in gastric cancer; constipation and/or diarrhea in bowel disease; vaginal discharge and irregular menstruation in pelvic inflammatory disease). Ask about symptom relationship to dietary factors, especially milk and milk products (lactose intolerance), gluten (celiac disease), and soft drinks and fruit juice (fructose and sorbitol intolerance). Ask about gastroesophageal reflux. Ask about the presence of red flags (see the checklist).
- **Psychosocial stressors:** What stresses have you recently experienced? Listen for major stressors, such as divorce, job loss, and death of a family member. Ask about a history of physical or sexual abuse.
- **Medical history:** What conditions have you been diagnosed with? Listen for cancer, hepatitis B or C virus infection (HBV, HCV), lung disease, heart disease, hyperlipidemia, and diabetes. Ask about previous abdominal surgeries. Ask about prescription and illicit drug use, and alcohol intake.

CHECKLIST
Red flags for chronic abdominal pain
Fever
Anorexia
Weight loss
Pain that wakes the patient
Blood in the stool or urine
Jaundice
Edema
Abdominal mass
Organomegaly

Physical exam

Obtain the patient's vital signs, looking for fever and tachycardia. Examine the patient for the presence of jaundice, rashes, and peripheral edema. Listen to the heart and lungs, looking for abnormal sounds (relevant to referred cardiothoracic pain). Perform an abdominal exam, looking for masses, tenderness, and organomegaly. Perform a rectal exam looking for tenderness, masses, and blood. In women, perform a pelvic exam, looking for tenderness and masses.

(State that you will perform a rectal and/or pelvic exam. Since these exams are not performed on standardized patients, the examiner may interrupt, ask what you are looking for, and provide findings.)

Investigations

Order a urinalysis and complete blood count (CBC), and tests for liver function, C-reactive protein (CRP), and lipase. Order a test for *Helicobacter pylori* (stool antigen or urea breath test). Consider ordering imaging (abdominal ultrasound or CT scan with contrast).

Management

Refer patients with red flags, or patients older than 50 with new abdominal pain, for upper gastrointestinal endoscopy and colonoscopy. Manage any specific disorders identified.

For patients with functional abdominal pain, consider non-opioid analgesics, H_2 receptor blockers, proton pump inhibitors, or tricyclic antidepressants. Consider referral for relaxation training, biofeedback, and cognitive behavioural therapy. Encourage a balanced diet, regular exercise, and stress reduction.

Pearls

Patients with Barrett esophagitis need long-term follow-up because of the risk of progression to esophageal cancer.

> **TIP**
>
> **Tailoring information to individual patients**
>
> The MCC identifies providing generic information as a common exam error.
>
> To avoid this error, ask patients about aspects of their lives that might affect their condition. Provide information that targets their situation and engage the patient in figuring out next steps.
>
> For example, better management of stress might be relevant for this case. Ask the patient for an example of a stressful situation they encountered last week. What steps could help relieve that situation?

REFERENCE

1 Lacey B, Mearin F, Chang L, et al. Rome IV functional gastrointestinal disorders: disorders of gut-brain interaction. 4th ed. Vol. 2. Raleigh, NC: Rome Foundation; 2017. Chapter 11, Functional bowel disorders; 1393–1407.

7

Anorectal pain

MCC particular objectives
Inquire about risk factors and symptoms suggestive of underlying disease.

MCC differential diagnosis
with added evidence

ANORECTAL DISEASE

Inflammatory bowel disease
Signs and symptoms: younger than 30 (usually); family history of inflammatory bowel disease; fluctuating symptoms with periods of exacerbation and remission; diarrhea (possibly with nocturnal waking); blood in the stool; abdominal pain; weight loss; fever; fatigue; right lower quadrant and periumbilical pain; extraintestinal manifestations (e.g., uveitis, arthritis)

>Crohn disease: right lower quadrant mass, inflammation of the eyes, arthritis

Investigations: elevated CRP (this suggests active inflammation); fecal calprotectin; colonoscopy with biopsy (this is a standard diagnostic procedure); CT scan or MRI (findings: diagnostic structural changes associated with inflammatory bowel disease)

Fissures, fistulas
Signs and symptoms: pain with bowel movements; small amounts of bright red blood following bowel movements; anal fissures or fistulas on physical exam

Hemorrhoids
Signs and symptoms: anal pain (if hemorrhoids are thrombosed); anal bleeding (bright red blood), often following a bowel movement; hemorrhoids on physical exam

DERMATOLOGIC DISEASE

Psoriasis
Signs and symptoms (general): nail pitting; current or prior erythematous scaly rashes; family history of psoriasis or similar skin conditions; history of other autoimmune diseases

>Anal psoriasis: pain during bowel movements; anal bleeding; excessive anal dryness and itching

Contact dermatitis or atopic dermatitis

Signs and symptoms: redness, itchiness, dry cracked skin, blisters, swelling, burning

MALIGNANCY

Signs and symptoms: weight loss, abdominal pain, blood in the stool, constipation, change in stool calibre, personal or family history of colorectal cancer, palpable mass (anal or rectal)

Investigations: colonoscopy; CEA

INFECTION

Sexually transmitted infections

Signs and symptoms: lower abdominal and pelvic pain; pain during intercourse; fever; urinary symptoms (often); vaginal or urethral discharge (anal discharge in anal sex); irregular menstruation

Risk factors: unprotected sex, multiple sexual partners

Investigations: positive cultures for gonorrhea and/or chlamydia

Bacterial, fungal, or parasitic infections

BACTERIAL INFECTIONS IN GENERAL

Food-borne bacterial infections are a more common source of anorectal pain than fungal or parasitic infections.

Signs and symptoms: nausea, vomiting, abdominal pain, diarrhea, fever

Risk factors: ingesting raw meat, poultry, seafood, or eggs, or unpasteurized milk, or contaminated water; travel (e.g., travel to developing countries, camping); close exposure to birds or reptiles; antibiotic use (which can lead to *Clostridium difficile* infection)

FUNGAL AND PARASITIC INFECTIONS IN GENERAL

These are less likely to cause anorectal pain, except in severe infection.

Risk factors for severe infection: AIDS; other factors causing immunosuppression (e.g., chemotherapy)

TRAUMA

Examples of causes include occupational trauma, intimate partner violence, and sexual assault. If the trauma comes from a high-force injury, associated pelvic fracture is possible.

Investigations: proctoscopy, sigmoidoscopy

COCCYGEAL PAIN

Signs and symptoms: female patient (more common); pain that is worse with standing from a sitting position; history of prolonged sitting on hard surfaces; history of trauma (falling on the coccyx); obesity

Strategy for patient encounter

The likely scenario is a patient with anorectal pain. The specified tasks could engage history, physical exam, investigations, or management.

History

Start with open-ended questions about the onset of the pain: When did the pain start? What is the quality of the pain? How constant is it? Listen for recent-onset versus chronic pain (chronic pain suggests a chronic disorder such as anorectal disease); pain isolated to the anus versus pain involving other areas (e.g., abdominal pain in inflammatory bowel disease; crampy pain in bacterial infection; pain from pelvic fracture in trauma); and constant versus episodic pain (episodic pain, triggered by bowel movements, suggests anal fissures, fistulas, or hemorrhoids; episodic pain triggered by standing after sitting suggests coccygeal pain; constant pain suggests an unremitting condition such as trauma).

Ask open-ended questions to establish associated symptoms: What other symptoms do you have? Listen for evidence consistent with particular entities (e.g., small amounts of bright red blood following bowel movements in anal fissures, fistulas, and hemorrhoids; blood in the stool with constitutional symptoms in malignancy; nausea and diarrhea in bacterial infection; vaginal and/or anal discharge in sexually transmitted infection). Ask about constipation.

Ask about risk factors for underlying disease (see the checklist). Ask about trauma, including sexual trauma.

Obtain a medication history, focusing on medications known to cause constipation: antidepressants, antipsychotics, levodopa, antihistamines, antacids, and iron supplements. Ask about recent antibiotic use (relevant to *Clostridium difficile* infection).

> **CHECKLIST**
> **Risk factors for underlying disease in anorectal pain**
> Family history of inflammatory bowel disease
> Family history of psoriasis
> Family history of colorectal cancer
> Unprotected sex, multiple sexual partners (sexually transmitted infection)
> AIDS or other immunosuppressive factors (infection)

Physical exam

Obtain the patient's vital signs, looking for fever and hypotension. Examine the abdomen for masses. Examine the anus for masses, bleeding, hemorrhoids, and anal fissures. Perform a rectal exam looking for masses.

(State that you will examine the anus and perform a rectal exam. Since these exams are not performed on standardized patients, the examiner may interrupt, ask what you are looking for, and provide findings.)

Investigations

Order a complete blood count (CBC) to look for anemia and infection. Order other specific tests as indicated (see the information this resource lists in the MCC differential diagnosis).

Management

If the patient has a benign cause of anorectal pain (e.g., hemorrhoids or anal fissures), advise conservative treatment: increased fibre, increased exercise, stool softeners, analgesics, and sitz baths. In the absence of an obvious benign cause, refer the patient for proctoscopy or colonoscopy to rule out malignancy and inflammatory bowel disease.

8

Allergic reactions and atopy

MCC particular objective

Pay particular attention to findings suggestive of anaphylaxis.

MCC differential diagnosis
with added evidence

ANAPHYLAXIS

Signs and symptoms: personal or family history of anaphylaxis; hives; itchiness; peripheral edema; tongue or throat swelling; wheezing; stridor; shortness of breath; tachycardia; cardiovascular collapse; hypotension

URTICARIA OR ANGIOEDEMA

From drugs
Signs and symptoms: drug allergies, change in medication

From food
Signs and symptoms: food allergies, exposure to a known food allergen
Investigations: skin prick testing or serum specific IgE testing

From parasites
Signs and symptoms: history of travel, camping
Investigations: stool analysis to detect ova and parasites

From physical stressors (e.g., cold, exercise)
CRYOGLOBULINEMIA
Signs and symptoms: history of urticaria on exposure to cold; joint pain; positive ice test (applying ice to the skin provokes urticaria); constitutional symptoms (fatigue, weight loss)

> History of autoimmune disease (e.g., arthritis, vasculitis); infection with hepatitis B virus (HBV) or hepatitis C virus (HCV), or risk factors for these infections (autoimmune conditions, unprotected sex, intravenous drug abuse, blood transfusions, workplace exposure to body fluids, tattoos, body piercings)

Investigations: specific laboratory testing for cryoglobulinemia

HYPOTHYROIDISM
Signs and symptoms: history of hypothyroidism or symptoms of hypothyroidism (decreased reflexes, dry skin, weight gain, impaired cognition)
Investigations: elevated thyrotropin (TSH)

EXERCISE-INDUCED URTICARIA
Signs and symptoms: hives during or following exercise

Congenital
URTICARIA PIGMENTOSA
Signs and symptoms: lesions that blister when rubbed; lesions exacerbated by nonsteroidal antiinflammatory drugs (NSAIDs), narcotics, alcohol
Investigations: elevated serum tryptase, elevated urine histamine, lesion biopsy

ATOPIC DERMATITIS
Signs and symptoms: rash that is aggravated by soap, water, dry environments, exposure to allergens; highly pruritic rash; personal or

family history of atopic dermatitis, asthma, allergies; wheezing (this suggests coexisting asthma, nasal polyps)

    Children (rash location): face, scalp, hands, feet

    Adults (rash location): the popliteal fossa, antecubital fossa

RESPIRATORY ALLERGY (E.G., DUST MITES, POLLEN)

Signs and symptoms: wheezing; rhinitis; cough; seasonal symptoms; personal or family history of allergies; allergic "shiners"; eczema; red, watery sclera; nasal polyps; rash

Strategy for patient encounter

The likely scenario is a patient with atopic dermatitis. The specified tasks could engage history, physical exam, investigations, or management.

Anaphylaxis is possible in this clinical presentation. No matter what tasks the instructions for the encounter specify, start by checking the patient's airway and hemodynamic status.

Airway and hemodynamic status

Check the patient's airway, breathing, and circulation (mnemonic: **ABCs**), looking for hypotension and tachycardia.

Check for key symptoms (e.g., itchiness, swelling, shortness of breath).

Note that a patient presenting with allergic symptoms can develop anaphylaxis minutes or hours after the triggering event. Stay alert to changes in the condition of any patient who presents with urticaria or angioedema.

Provide emergency care to any patient with unstable vital signs, including administration of epinephrine and transfer to an emergency department.

History

Ask about the nature of the allergy: Have you been diagnosed with allergies? Have you been exposed to a known trigger? Is this the first time? What was the suspected exposure? When did it occur? Symptoms within 2 hours of exposure suggest an IgE-mediated process.

Ask about the patient's symptoms, and listen especially for vomiting, diarrhea, gastrointestinal pain, itching, wheezing, and coughing (these may indicate anaphylaxis). Note symptoms consistent with particular entities (e.g., hives following exercise in exercise-induced urticaria; itchy rash with wheezing in atopic dermatitis; seasonal cough and rhinitis in respiratory allergy).

Ask about new medications, especially penicillin and ACE inhibitors.

Physical exam

Examine the skin for urticaria, angioedema, and rash.

Investigations

In the case of anaphylaxis, no immediate testing is indicated. Pursue investigations for nonemergent allergies as indicated (see the checklist).

Management

In suspected atopic dermatitis, counsel the patient to avoid too-frequent bathing and exposure to known allergens. Patients should use mild soaps and moisturize their skin frequently (e.g., twice a day).

CHECKLIST

Recommended allergy evaluations

FOOD ALLERGY
Allergy testing is not indicated for mild atopic dermatitis or isolated respiratory symptoms. Serum IgE testing and skin-prick testing can confirm suspected allergens, but are not indicated for food intolerances that are not IgE mediated.

INHALANT ALLERGY
Serum IgE tests or skin-prick testing are the preferred methods of testing for inhalant allergens (e.g., pollen, fungus, dust mites).

LATEX
This is tested by serum IgE.

DRUGS
Use skin-prick testing for penicillin reaction. Use serum antigen-specific IgE testing for other drugs.

VENOM
Use skin-prick testing or serum antigen-specific IgE testing.

9

Attention, learning, and school problems

MCC particular objective

Pay particular attention to interdisciplinary management and ongoing supportive care.

MCC differential diagnosis
with added evidence

DEVELOPMENTAL DISORDERS (E.G., ATTENTION DEFICIT HYPERACTIVITY DISORDER, SPECIFIC LEARNING DISORDER, AUTISM SPECTRUM DISORDER)

DEVELOPMENTAL DISORDERS IN GENERAL

Signs and symptoms: family history of developmental delay, disorders, or impairments; history of complications during gestation (e.g., toxin exposure such as alcohol or smoking) and/or delivery, including premature birth; growth abnormalities; neurological abnormalities; dysmorphic features; hypothyroidism; lead poisoning

ATTENTION DEFICIT HYPERACTIVITY DISORDER[1(pp59-60)]

Signs and symptoms (children younger than 17 years): hyperactive-impulsive symptoms and/or inattention symptoms; symptoms that are present before age 12; symptoms with significant impact on the child's day-to-day life in a variety of contexts (e.g., home, school)

> Hyperactive-impulsive symptoms (examples): excessive fidgeting, talking, restlessness; inability to play quietly or wait turns
>
> Inattention symptoms (examples): marked frequency of careless mistakes, not listening, forgetfulness, distractibility; marked difficulty with activities that require organization, sustained attention

SPECIFIC LEARNING DISORDER[1(pp66-67)]

Specific learning disorder is often identified during school years, but may only become a problem in later academic life, with heavier workloads and timed tests.

Signs and symptoms: significantly impaired key academic skills (e.g., reading, spelling, grammar, punctuation, numbers, and math); persistent impairments (e.g., impairments endure for months and despite steps to remediate)

AUTISM SPECTRUM DISORDER[1(pp50-51)]

Signs and symptoms: deficits in social interaction and communication; repetitive, stereotyped behaviours (motor and/or vocal); restricted interests; sensory problems; presence of symptoms in all contexts (e.g., home, school); presence of symptoms from early childhood

SENSORY IMPAIRMENT (E.G., HEARING OR VISION IMPAIRMENT)

SENSORY IMPAIRMENT IN GENERAL

Signs and symptoms: differences in development compared to other children; problems with social interactions with other children

HEARING IMPAIRMENT

Signs and symptoms: problems identifying the source of a sound; language or speech delays; blocked (from impacted wax or mass) or nonmobile (from chronic effusion) tympanic membranes

VISION IMPAIRMENT

Signs and symptoms: frequent injuries; problems with self-feeding; abnormal pupil reflexes or optic fundi (possible)

NEUROLOGICAL DISORDERS (E.G., SEIZURE DISORDER, FETAL ALCOHOL SPECTRUM DISORDER)

NEUROLOGICAL DISORDERS IN GENERAL

Signs and symptoms: family history of neurological disorders; history of complications during gestation (e.g., toxin exposure such as alcohol or smoking) and/or delivery; growth abnormalities; dysmorphic features; hypothyroidism; lead poisoning

SEIZURE DISORDER

Signs and symptoms: personal or family history of seizures; behavioural and other abnormalities

FETAL ALCOHOL SPECTRUM DISORDER

Signs and symptoms: history of exposure to alcohol in utero

Pathognomonic dysmorphic features: small eye openings; thin upper lip; smooth philtrum; maxillary hypoplasia; small lower jaw; short upturned nose; flat nasal bridge; abnormal ear position or formation

Other features: growth deficits before and after birth (at birth: low weight; short length; head circumference ≤ tenth percentile); defects in the heart, kidneys, bones; deformities in joints, limbs, extremities; neurobehavioural impairments

MENTAL HEALTH DISORDERS

Signs and symptoms: personal or family history of psychiatric conditions (e.g., anxiety, major depressive disorder); excessive worry;

loss of interest in friends and usual activities; changes in sleep habits; hallucinations or delusions; suicidal thoughts; history of adverse experience (emotional, physical, or sexual abuse; recent stress such as death of a friend or family member), or substance abuse

PSYCHOSOCIAL STRESSORS (E.G., HUNGER, ADVERSE CHILDHOOD EXPERIENCE)

Hunger can be a sign of neglect. Other signs and symptoms of neglect include not attending school regularly; poor hygiene, dental care; and reports by the child suggesting lack of physical and/or emotional care at home.

Examples of adverse experiences include abuse, and death of a friend or family member.

CHRONIC MEDICAL DISEASE (E.G., OBSTRUCTIVE SLEEP APNEA)

OBSTRUCTIVE SLEEP APNEA

Signs and symptoms: excessive or loud snoring; disturbed sleep (e.g., not feeling rested in the morning); obesity (common); allergic rhinitis (sneezing, runny nose, eye irritation); morning headache; palpable masses in the oral cavity or neck

Investigations: sleep study (polysomnography); hypertrophic adenoid tissue on lateral neck X-ray

DISORDERS RELATED TO SUBSTANCE ABUSE AND ADDICTION

Signs and symptoms: personal or family history of substance abuse; excessive worry; loss of interest in friends and usual activities; adverse experience (e.g., abuse, death of a friend or family member); physical evidence (track marks on the arms, nasal septum perforation); tachycardia; tremor and/or sweating

Strategy for patient encounter

This patient encounter could involve a parent discussing behaviour problems in their child, where the child is absent on some pretext (e.g., another caregiver has taken the child for a walk, because the child was upset), or an adult discussing their own problems at university or work. The following notes assume the scenario is a parent discussing a child.

The specified tasks could engage history, physical exam, investigations, or management.

History

Use open-ended questions to establish evidence about the child's symptoms, medical history (including gestation, birth, and development), family history, and the presence of psychosocial stressors.

- **Symptoms:** Please tell me about the problems your child is experiencing. How old was your child when these problems began? In what contexts do the problems occur? What impact do they have on your child's school performance and relationships with family and friends? Listen for evidence consistent with particular entities (e.g., symptoms of hyperactivity or inattention at school and at home that began before age 12, and that significantly impair the child's academic performance, in attention deficit hyperactivity disorder; delayed speech development compared to other children and problems interacting with other children in hearing impairment; excessive worry, sleep disturbance, and loss of interest in friends and activities in mental health disorder).

- **Gestation, birth, and developmental history:** What complications were there during the pregnancy for this child? What complications were there during the delivery? What was the gestational age of your child at birth? How does your child's development compare with children of the same age? Listen for prenatal exposures (e.g., tobacco, drugs, alcohol); perinatal complications or infections; and evidence of developmental delays.

- **Medical history:** What conditions has your child been diagnosed with? Listen for key entities (see the MCC differential diagnosis), including hypothyroidism. Ask about medications the child takes and about potential substance abuse by the child.

- **Family history:** What conditions run in your family? Listen for developmental, neurological, and mental health disorders. Ask about a family history of drug abuse.

- **Psychosocial stressors:** Ask about a history of child abuse and recent psychosocial stressors such as a death in the family.

Physical exam

Obtain the child's height, weight, and head circumference. Plot these on a growth chart. Obtain the child's vital signs. Examine the child for dysmorphic features. Perform a complete neurological exam, including assessment of vision and hearing.

Stay alert to signs of neglect and abuse.

(State that you will examine the child. Because an actual pediatric patient is unlikely, the examiner may interrupt, ask what you are looking for, and provide findings.)

Investigations

Order tests for serum lead level and thyrotropin (TSH) levels. Consider referring the child for audiology and optometric testing. If the child has dysmorphic features, consider genetic testing and/or a genetics consultation (e.g., for fragile X syndrome). In

---

QUICK REFERENCE

Behaviour-rating scales

The Canadian Paediatric Society lists screening tools for a variety of behaviour disorders potentially relevant to this clinical presentation, including anxiety, attention deficit hyperactivity disorder (including assessment of coexisting conduct problems and oppositional defiant disorder), autism spectrum disorder, and depression. It's good general preparation for the exam to familiarize yourself with this list and plan for what tools you would recommend for different situations.

The table that follows shows select examples of these screening tools, some of which are free and some for purchase.

SCREENING TOOL	AGE RANGE	DISORDERS ASSESSED	WHO COMPLETES, HOW LONG
Conners Rating Scales	3–17 years	Conduct and learning problems, physical symptoms, ADHD symptoms, anxiety	Parent, patient, teacher 5–20 minutes
SNAP-IV Parent and Teacher Rating Scale	5–18 years	ADHD, oppositional defiant disorder, aggression	Parent, patient, teacher 5–10 minutes
Autism Spectrum Screening Questionnaire (ASSQ)	7–16 years	Autism spectrum disorders	Parent and teacher 10 minutes
Patient Health Questionnaire 9 (PHQ-9)	12–18 years	Depression	Parent, patient, teacher 5–15 minutes

suspected obstructive sleep apnea or restless legs syndrome, order overnight polysomnography.

Assess the child for developmental disorders and coexisting conditions with behaviour-rating scales (see the quick reference), filled out by parents, family members, teachers, or caregivers, as appropriate. Ask to examine school report cards and examples of schoolwork.

Management
Identify any modifiable conditions (toxic exposure, neglect), and treat any coexisting medical conditions (e.g., hypothyroidism, obstructive sleep apnea).

All cases of attention and learning problems require a multidisciplinary approach involving family, educators, and ongoing supportive care.

In patients with attention deficit hyperactivity disorder (ADHD), prescribe psychostimulant medication (monitor appetite, weight, and blood pressure), refer for behavioural therapy, and consider referral to a multidisciplinary clinic for ADHD.

There is no specific treatment for autism. Management includes behavioural therapy and treating any associated conditions (e.g., depression, ADHD).

Management of fetal alcohol spectrum disorder includes supports for learning and behaviour, and addressing any ongoing maternal addiction issues.

REFERENCE

1 American Psychiatric Association. Diagnostic and statistical manual of mental disorders. 5th ed. Arlington, VA: American Psychiatric Association; 2013. 991 p.

10

Upper gastrointestinal bleeding

MCC particular objective

Determine and manage the hemodynamic status of the patient.
Resuscitate if necessary.

MCC differential diagnosis
with added evidence

ULCERATIVE OR EROSIVE PROCESSES

Peptic ulcer disease

Signs and symptoms: constant midepigastric pain, often relieved with
eating or with antacids; weight loss

Investigations: test for *H. pylori*; endoscopy to detect ulcer or
inflammation of the gastric lining

Esophagitis

Signs and symptoms: difficulty swallowing or pain with swallowing;
food becoming impacted in the esophagus, especially foods that are
solid or difficult to chew; acid reflux; oral *Candida* infection; oral ulcers;
epigastric tenderness (this could arise from associated peptic ulcer
disease or reflux)

> History of food allergies or environmental allergies
> (e.g., pollen); factors causing immunosuppression, such as
> HIV, cancer, immunosuppressant medications, autoimmune
> disease, malnutrition (immunosuppression creates a
> higher risk for bacterial, viral, and fungal infections of the
> esophagus); use of antiinflammatories and bisphosphonates
> (these present a particular risk if they are not swallowed
> properly and remain in the esophagus)

Investigations: upper GI series (barium swallow) or endoscopy

Gastritis

Signs and symptoms: constant epigastric pain that may be relieved
by antacids; constitutional symptoms (fever, night sweats, weight
loss, fatigue); epigastric tenderness; history of using gastric irritants
(antiinflammatories, smoking, alcohol)

Investigations: test for *H. pylori*

PORTAL HYPERTENSION

Signs and symptoms: enlarged or tender liver; enlarged spleen;
abdominal masses; ascites

History of cirrhosis (common) (risk factors: alcohol abuse, hepatitis); portal vein thrombosis (less common) (risk factors: chronic liver disease, prothrombin *G20210A* mutation)

Investigations: endoscopy to detect esophageal varices

TRAUMA (E.G., MALLORY-WEISS TEAR)

Signs and symptoms: coughing; severe or prolonged hiccups; recurrent vomiting or retching; abdominal pain; history of trauma to the chest or abdomen

Investigations: endoscopy

TUMOURS

Signs and symptoms: epigastric pain; difficulty swallowing or pain with swallowing; food becoming impacted in the esophagus, especially foods that are solid or difficult to chew; acid reflux; constitutional symptoms (fever, night sweats, weight loss, and fatigue); smoking; alcohol use; personal or family history of malignancy; palpable abdominal mass

Investigations: CT scan, MRI; endoscopy with biopsy

Strategy for patient encounter

The likely scenario is an alcoholic patient vomiting blood. The likely task is emergency management.

Emergency management

AIRWAY AND HEMODYNAMIC STATUS

Check the patient's airway, breathing, and circulation (mnemonic: **ABCs**). Look in particular for hypotension and tachycardia. Begin resuscitation as required: administer red cell transfusions and bolus(es) of isotonic crystalloid solution to maintain systolic blood pressure at > 100 mmHg.

TIP

Working with nurses to provide emergency care

The MCC identifies unclear directions to nurses as a common exam error.

To avoid this error, work out some standard directions for nurses in emergency scenarios. Emergency scenarios are likely to involve nurses, and likely to involve similar procedures to stabilize the patient. For example, if 1 nurse is present:

- Ask the nurse to take the patient's vital signs and obtain intravenous access.
- You start ventilation.

If 2 nurses are present:

- Ask for the first name of each nurse present.
- Ask a specific nurse by name to start ventilation.
- Ask a specific nurse by name to take the patient's vital signs and obtain intravenous access.

HISTORY

Use open-ended questions to establish the history of the bleeding and associated symptoms: When did the bleeding start? How much blood is there? What is the nature of the blood? What other symptoms do you have? Listen for evidence consistent with particular entities (e.g., blood with a "coffee grounds" appearance and constant midepigastric pain in peptic ulcer disease; recent-onset bleeding with bright red blood, and abdominal pain or chest pain, following trauma, coughing, vomiting, or hiccups in Mallory-Weiss tear; epigastric pain and difficulty swallowing with constitutional symptoms in tumour). Ask about bleeding from the rectum (tarry stools or bright red blood).

Obtain a medical history, looking for peptic ulcer disease, liver disease (relevant to portal hypertension), HIV and allergies (esophagitis), and cancer (tumour). Ask about abdominal surgery.

Obtain a medication history, looking in particular for clopidogrel, warfarin, nonsteroidal antiinflammatory drugs (NSAIDs), aspirin, selective serotonin reuptake inhibitors (SSRIs), and corticosteroids. Ask about smoking, alcohol abuse, and use of illicit drugs.

PHYSICAL EXAM

Obtain the patient's blood pressure in supine and standing positions to look for orthostatic changes. Examine the abdomen for signs of liver disease, abdominal tenderness, masses, and surgical scars. Perform a rectal exam looking for melena or bright red blood (the presence of melena is consistent with upper gastrointestinal bleeding; bright red blood indicates lower gastrointestinal bleeding).

(State that you will perform a rectal exam. Since this exam is not performed on standardized patients, the examiner will likely interrupt, ask what you are looking for, and provide findings.)

INVESTIGATIONS

Order a complete blood count (CBC), and tests for prothrombin time/international normalized ratio (PT/INR), partial thromboplastin time (PTT), creatinine, blood urea nitrogen (BUN), and liver function. Order a test for *Helicobacter pylori* (stool antigen or urea breath test). Order blood typing and cross-matching. Order an emergency endoscopy: this may identify a source of bleeding, and also allow treatment of any discovered lesions with epinephrine injection, thermocoagulation, application of clips, or banding.

MANAGEMENT

For patients with coagulopathy, give transfusions with fresh frozen plasma. For patients with low platelet counts, give platelet transfusions.

If bleeding remains uncontrolled after medical or endoscopic treatment, refer the patient to surgery. Discontinue any NSAIDs. Treat *H. pylori* infection, if present. Assess the patient's risk of rebleeding (this risk increases with older age, the presence of shock, and with increasing comorbidities).

PEARLS

Patients with cirrhosis should have regular upper-endoscopy screening to identify the presence or development of esophageal varices. The recommended frequency of screening depends on findings of the initial screening.

11

Lower gastrointestinal bleeding

MCC particular objectives

Determine the hemodynamic status of the patient and the need for immediate specialized care.

Identify patients at high risk of colorectal cancer for colonoscopy.

MCC differential diagnosis
with added evidence

COLORECTAL CANCER OR POLYPS

Signs and symptoms: weight loss, abdominal pain, blood in the stool, constipation, change in stool calibre, personal or family history of colorectal cancer, palpable mass (anal or rectal)

Investigations: CEA, colonoscopy

DIVERTICULOSIS

Signs and symptoms: often asymptomatic, history of diverticular disease, painless rectal bleeding

ANGIODYSPLASIA

Signs and symptoms: older age (usual), rectal bleeding

ANORECTAL DISEASE

FISSURES, HEMORRHOIDS

Signs and symptoms: small amounts of bright red blood following bowel movements; pain, irritation; constipation

FISTULAS, ABSCESSES

These are often related to inflammatory bowel disease.

Signs and symptoms: history of inflammatory bowel disease (e.g., Crohn disease, ulcerative colitis), diarrhea, blood in the stool, abdominal pain, weight loss, fever, fatigue

ENTEROCOLITIS

Signs and symptoms: abdominal pain, cramping, tenderness; diarrhea; nausea, vomiting; rectal bleeding

Investigations: colonoscopy

BRISK BLEEDING FROM THE UPPER GASTROINTESTINAL TRACT

Signs and symptoms: blood in the stool; epigastric pain; difficulty or pain with swallowing; acid reflux; food becoming impacted in the esophagus, especially foods that are solid or difficult to chew

History of trauma to the chest or abdomen; liver disease (esophageal varices and/or impaired production of clotting factors)

Investigations: endoscopy or barium swallow

RECTAL TRAUMA

If the trauma comes from a high-force injury, associated pelvic fracture is possible.

Risk factors: substance abuse, intimate partner violence, homelessness, occupational hazards

Investigations: proctoscopy, sigmoidoscopy

Strategy for patient encounter

The likely scenario is a hemo-dynamically unstable patient in the emergency room. The likely task is emergency management.

Emergency management

AIRWAY AND HEMODYNAMIC STATUS

Check the patient's airway, breathing, and circulation (mnemonic: **ABCs**). Look in particular for hypotension and tachycardia. Begin resuscitation, as required: administer bolus(es) of isotonic crystalloid solution to maintain systolic blood pressure at > 100 mmHg.

HISTORY

Use open-ended questions to establish the history of the rectal bleeding and associated symptoms: What is the nature of the blood? What other symptoms do you have? Listen for bright red blood, versus clots, versus dark tarry stools (melena); and for vomiting of blood (this suggests an upper gastrointestinal source—vomiting without blood may indicate an intestinal blockage), abdominal pain (colorectal cancer, inflammatory bowel disease, enterocolitis), and constitutional symptoms (malignancy).

Ask about a recent colonoscopy with polypectomy (relevant to a postpolypectomy bleed), prior abdominal or pelvic radiation (radiation colitis), and a history of alcoholism or chronic liver disease (portal hypertension with varices).

Obtain a medical history, looking for colorectal cancer, diverticular disease, hemorrhoids, inflammatory bowel disease, and liver disease. Obtain a medication history, looking specifically for acetylsalicylic acid (ASA) and nonsteroidal antiinflammatory drugs (NSAIDs).

PHYSICAL EXAM

Obtain the patient's blood pressure in supine and standing positions to look for orthostatic changes. Look for abdominal tenderness and masses. Look for stigmata of liver disease. In patients without hematemesis, perform a nasogastric lavage to rule out an upper gastrointestinal tract source of blood. Perform a rectal exam to look for masses and the presence of frank blood. (State that you will perform a rectal exam. Since this exam is not performed on standardized patients, the examiner will likely interrupt, ask what you are looking for, and provide findings.)

INVESTIGATIONS

Order a complete blood count (CBC) to assess for anemia. Order liver function tests (liver disease), and tests for prothrombin time/international normalized ratio (PT/INR), creatinine, and electrolytes. Urgent colonoscopy is the main method of establishing a diagnosis, and treatment (e.g., banding) may be administered at the same time. If urgent colonoscopy is not possible or does not yield a diagnosis, consider a tagged red blood cell scan (technetium-99m-labelled red blood cells) or mesenteric angiography to localize a source of bleeding.

MANAGEMENT

For anemic patients, order blood transfusion. The transfusion threshold may vary depending on comorbidities and can be as low as 7 g/dL in patients without cardiac disease. Consider platelet transfusions to keep the platelet count above 50, and vitamin K or fresh frozen plasma to keep the PT/INR at or below 1.5. Consult general surgery or gastroenterology for colonoscopy, and general surgery for consideration of surgical correction of a bleeding source.

PEARLS

The most common cause of lower gastrointestinal bleeding is diverticulosis, followed by hemorrhoids, ischemic colitis, postpolypectomy bleed, inflammatory bowel disease, cancer or polyps, and vascular ectasia.

12

Blood in sputum (hemoptysis)

MCC particular objective

Determine if the patient requires urgent intervention and stabilization, or if the patient requires further investigation to rule out serious underlying disease.

MCC differential diagnosis
with added evidence

AIRWAY DISEASE

Inflammatory (e.g., bronchiectasis, bronchitis)

BRONCHIECTASIS

Signs and symptoms: long-standing symptoms, productive cough, shortness of breath, chest pain, fever, general physical wasting

Investigations: CT scan to detect abnormal bronchial tree dilatation

BRONCHITIS

Signs and symptoms: productive cough, shortness of breath, fever, minimal hemoptysis, abnormal lung sounds (wheezing, crackles, rhonchi)

> Chronic bronchitis: symptoms of acute bronchitis lasting > 3 months, with exacerbations (this identifies chronic bronchitis); history of asthma, chronic obstructive pulmonary disease; general physical wasting

Neoplasm (e.g., bronchogenic carcinoma)

BRONCHOGENIC CARCINOMA

Signs and symptoms: constitutional symptoms (fever, weight loss, night sweats, fatigue); abnormal lung sounds on auscultation; areas of dullness on percussion of the chest; enlarged lymph nodes

Risk factors: smoking, asbestos exposure

Investigations: chest X-ray and CT scan; biopsy

Other (e.g., foreign body, trauma)

FOREIGN BODY

Signs and symptoms: history of inhaling a foreign body; wheezing (possible: this suggests a partially obstructed bronchus)

Investigations: chest X-ray or CT scan

TRAUMA

Signs and symptoms: absence of lung sounds (this suggests pneumothorax); tender spine, ribs, spleen; history of a medical procedure (e.g., bronchoscopy)

PULMONARY PARENCHYMAL DISEASE

Infectious disease (e.g., tuberculosis, necrotizing pneumonia)

TUBERCULOSIS

Signs and symptoms: constitutional symptoms (fever, weight loss, night sweats, fatigue), chest pain

Risk factors: contact with tuberculosis-infected individuals; use of intravenous street drugs; factors causing immunosuppression (HIV infection, cancer, immunosuppressant medications, autoimmune disease, and malnutrition); hypoxia

Investigations: positive tuberculin skin test (purified protein derivative) in suspected latent TB; sputum mycobacterial culture, PCR of sputum in suspected active TB; chest X-ray

NECROTIZING PNEUMONIA

Signs and symptoms: rapid onset and progression of symptoms; rapidly worsening shortness of breath; fever; hypoxia; recent history of pneumonia

Investigations: CBC to detect leukopenia (leukopenia may rapidly worsen); chest X-ray to detect lung consolidation

Inflammatory or immune disease (e.g., vasculitis)

VASCULITIS

Signs and symptoms: personal or family history of vasculitis; cutaneous vasculitis (polyarteritis nodosa: palpable purpura, petechiae, ulcers); abnormal lung sounds; neuropathy (numbness, weakness); hematuria in pulmonary-renal syndrome (e.g., Goodpasture syndrome)

Investigations: elevated serum ANCA; CT scan to detect diffuse alveolar infiltrates; anti-GBM; biopsy

Other (e.g., coagulopathy)

COAGULOPATHY

Signs and symptoms: use of anticoagulants; history of liver disease (this can lead to deficits in clotting factor production); bruising and petechiae on the skin and in the mouth

Investigations: elevated PT/INR; serum liver enzyme tests to detect liver disease

CARDIAC OR VASCULAR DISEASE

Pulmonary embolus with infarction

Signs and symptoms: sharp chest pain; shortness of breath; cough (possibly with blood); hypoxia; possible unilateral swelling of the lower limbs (this indicates deep vein thrombosis); elevated pulse and respiratory rate; arrhythmias; lung rales on auscultation; lower-lung dullness on percussion; motor or sensory deficits

Risk factors: heart failure; cancer; surgery; prolonged immobility (e.g., long plane trips); smoking; estrogen replacement therapy; oral contraceptives; current pregnancy; previous deep vein thrombosis, embolism, or stroke; family history of embolism

Investigations: elevated D-dimer level; area of reduced pulmonary perfusion on V/Q scan; CT angiography to detect blocked vessel

Elevated pulmonary capillary pressure (e.g., mitral stenosis, left ventricular failure)

ELEVATED PULMONARY CAPILLARY PRESSURE IN GENERAL

Signs and symptoms: chest pain; shortness of breath; history of heart disease (especially acute myocardial infarction or ischemia); hypoxia; lung rales; heart murmur (this suggests mitral valve stenosis)

Investigations: chest X-ray to detect pulmonary edema; ECG; echocardiogram

Pulmonary arteriovenous malformation

Signs and symptoms: often asymptomatic until bleeding begins; shortness of breath on exertion; localized abnormal lung sounds (this suggests the location of the pulmonary arteriovenous malformation); orthodeoxia (characteristic: this is oxygen desaturation with upright position)

Long-standing hypoxia: digital clubbing, cyanosis

Investigations: elevated hemoglobin (this indicates long-standing hypoxia); imaging to detect pulmonary arteriovenous malformations

Strategy for patient encounter

The likely scenario is a patient with hemoptysis. The specified tasks could engage history, physical exam, investigations, or management.

An actively bleeding patient is possible in this clinical presentation. No matter what tasks the instructions for the encounter specify, start by checking the patient's airway and hemodynamic status.

Airway and hemodynamic status

Check the patient's airway, breathing, and circulation (mnemonic: **ABCs**). Look in particular for hypotension and tachycardia. Begin resuscitation, as required: administer bolus(es) of isotonic crystalloid solution to maintain systolic blood pressure at > 100 mmHg.

In cases of massive hemoptysis, mortality is secondary to asphyxiation (and not exsanguination). It is thus essential to protect the airway with intubation (if necessary). If the source of hemoptysis is known (e.g., right-sided bronchiectasis), have the patient lie on the side of the source (e.g., right lateral decubitus position).

TIP

Working with nurses to provide emergency care

The MCC identifies unclear directions to nurses as a common exam error.

To avoid this error, work out some standard directions for nurses in emergency scenarios. Emergency scenarios are likely to involve nurses, and likely to involve similar procedures to stabilize the patient. For example, if 1 nurse is present:

- Ask the nurse to take the patient's vital signs and obtain intravenous access.
- You start ventilation.

If 2 nurses are present:

- Ask for the first name of each nurse present.
- Ask a specific nurse by name to start ventilation.
- Ask a specific nurse by name to take the patient's vital signs and obtain intravenous access.

History

Use open-ended questions to establish the key features of the case.

- **History and timing of the hemoptysis:** How much blood are you coughing up? How often? Listen for evidence of massive hemoptysis (> 200 mL per day), which is a medical emergency. (Note that bleeding can start and stop unpredictably: patients may not be bleeding when you see them.) Ask about the nature of the blood (e.g., bright red, blood-tinged sputum, "coffee grounds").
- **Associated symptoms:** What other symptoms do you have? Listen for evidence consistent with particular entities (e.g., productive cough, shortness of breath, and fever in bronchitis; constitutional symptoms and enlarged

lymph nodes in bronchogenic carcinoma; constitutional symptoms and chest pain in tuberculosis).

- **Medical and medication history:** What conditions have you been diagnosed with? What medications do you take? Listen for tuberculosis, vasculitis, liver disease, heart disease, cancer, pulmonary embolism, and HIV and other conditions that cause immune-system suppression; for anticoagulants, acetylsalicylic acid (ASA), and nonsteroidal antiinflammatory drugs (NSAIDs); and for estrogen replacement therapy and oral contraceptives (relevant to pulmonary embolism). Ask about recent medical procedures, such as bronchoscopy (relevant to trauma).
- **Exposures:** What is your history with asbestos exposure? What is your smoking history? Listen for possible occupational exposures to asbestos (e.g., from work in asbestos mining, construction, firefighting, industrial work, shipyard work), and for a history of smoking or exposure to secondhand smoke.

Physical exam
Perform a physical exam, focusing on the respiratory system, and the head and neck.

Investigations
In all patients, order a chest X-ray or CT scan of the chest; a complete blood count (CBC) to assess for anemia; and tests for serum electrolytes, creatinine, and prothrombin time/international normalized ratio (PT/INR). In possible pulmonary embolus, order a V/Q scan.

Management
Admit patients reporting massive hemoptysis to hospital. For anemic patients, order blood transfusion. The transfusion threshold may vary depending on comorbidities and can be as low as 7 g/dL in patients without cardiac disease. Consider platelet transfusions to keep the platelet count above 50, and vitamin K or fresh frozen plasma to keep the PT/INR at or below 1.5. Consult general surgery, gastroenterology, or respirology, as appropriate, for bronchoscopy or endoscopy. Bronchoscopy or endoscopy will

facilitate diagnosis, biopsy, and possible treatment (e.g., banding of varices). Refer patients who may need surgery to a thoracic or general surgeon.

13

Blood in urine (hematuria)

MCC particular objectives
Interpret a urinalysis, paying attention to differentiating glomerular from nonglomerular causes.

Describe initial management.

MCC differential diagnosis
with added evidence

RENAL CONDITION

Glomerular disease (e.g., systemic lupus erythematosus, hemolytic uremic syndrome, vasculitis)

GLOMERULAR DISEASE IN GENERAL
Investigations: abnormal findings on urine microscopy (dysmorphic red blood cells, proteinuria, and red cell casts); elevated creatinine; decreased serum complement level

SYSTEMIC LUPUS ERYTHEMATOSUS
Signs and symptoms: personal or family history of systemic lupus erythematosus; malar rash; arthritis; cytopenias
Investigations: elevated ANA titre; elevated dsDNA level

HEMOLYTIC UREMIC SYNDROME
This commonly follows infection from Shiga toxin-producing *Escherichia coli*.

Signs and symptoms: gastrointestinal symptoms (abdominal pain, bloody diarrhea); anemia (fatigue, weakness, pallor); neurologic symptoms (irritability, confusion, seizures); peripheral edema (this is a sign of renal failure); thrombocytopenia
Investigations: low platelet count; elevated PT/INR; schistocytes on blood smear; microangiopathic hemolytic anemia

VASCULITIS

Signs and symptoms: personal or family history of vasculitis; cutaneous vasculitis (polyarteritis nodosa: palpable purpura, petechiae, ulcers); abnormal lung sounds; neuropathy (numbness, weakness); hematuria in pulmonary-renal syndrome (e.g., Goodpasture syndrome)

Investigations: elevated serum ANCA; CT scan to detect diffuse alveolar infiltrates; anti-GBM; biopsy

Nonglomerular disease (e.g., acute interstitial nephritis, renal tumour, exercise)

NONGLOMERULAR DISEASE IN GENERAL

Signs and symptoms: possible history of autoimmune disorders

Investigations: normal findings on urine microscopy, normal creatinine, normal serum complement level

ACUTE INTERSTITIAL NEPHRITIS

This is the usual cause of nonglomerular disease.

Signs and symptoms: fever; rash; joint pain; use of diuretics, antibiotics, analgesics (usual); history of autoimmune disorders

Investigations: urine eosinophils (their presence is suggestive); urinalysis (normal findings for RBCs, proteinuria, and red cell casts); blood tests (normal creatinine, normal complement level); renal biopsy (definitive)

RENAL TUMOUR

Signs and symptoms: flank pain, constitutional symptoms (weight loss, night sweats), hypertension (this can indicate certain renal tumours), palpable renal mass

Investigations: CT scan, ultrasound

EXERCISE

This is hematuria that occurs after strenuous exercise and resolves with rest.

POSTRENAL CONDITION (E.G., STONES, BLADDER TUMOUR, BENIGN PROSTATIC HYPERPLASIA, CYSTITIS)

KIDNEY STONES

Signs and symptoms: flank pain, history of kidney stones

Investigations: intravenous urography, ultrasound, CT scan

BLADDER TUMOUR OR BENIGN PROSTATIC HYPERPLASIA

Signs and symptoms: change in urinary habits (reduced urination in prostate conditions; blood in the urine; reduced and/or frequent urination in bladder conditions); bladder mass or enlarged prostate on palpation

Investigations: urine cytology; CT scan or cytoscopy to detect bladder mass

CYSTITIS

Signs and symptoms: increased frequency of urination; painful urination; pelvic and/or flank pain; fever; tenderness over the bladder

Investigations: urinalysis, urine culture

HEMATOLOGIC CONDITION (E.G., COAGULOPATHY, SICKLE CELL HEMOGLOBINOPATHY)

COAGULOPATHY

Signs and symptoms: use of anticoagulant medication; history of liver disease (this can lead to deficits in clotting factor production); bruising and petechiae on the skin and in the mouth

Investigations: elevated PT/INR; serum liver enzyme tests to detect liver disease

SICKLE CELL DISEASE

Signs and symptoms: family history of sickle cell disease; painful swelling of the hands and feet

Investigations: CBC to detect anemia, sickle cells; positive sickle cell screen; abnormalities on peripheral blood smear; abnormalities on hemoglobin electrophoresis

Strategy for patient encounter

The likely scenario is a patient with hematuria. The specified tasks could engage history, physical exam, investigations, or management.

History

Use open-ended questions to establish symptoms associated with the hematuria: What symptoms do you have in addition to the blood in your urine? Listen for evidence consistent with particular entities (e.g., gastrointestinal and neurologic symptoms in hemolytic uremic syndrome; constitutional symptoms in urologic malignancy or infection; frequent and painful urination in cystitis or urinary tract infection).

If pain is present, ask how constant it is (intermittent colicky pain suggests stones).

Use open-ended questions to take a medical and medication history: What conditions have you been diagnosed with? What medications do

---

CHECKLIST

Risk factors for urologic malignancy

Male

Older than 35

History of smoking

Exposure to benzenes or aromatic amines (through, for example, work in chemical manufacturing)

you take? Listen for kidney or bladder disease, and kidney stones; and for use of nonsteroidal antiinflammatory drugs (NSAIDs) and anticoagulants. Ask about a history of pelvic irradiation. Ask about risk factors for malignancy (see the checklist).

Physical exam

Obtain the patient's vital signs, looking for hypertension. Examine the abdomen and pelvis. On men, perform a prostate exam, looking for prostate abnormalities (relevant to benign prostatic hyperplasia, prostatitis, and prostate cancer). On women, perform a pelvic exam, looking for atrophic vaginitis, masses, and uterine bleeding.

(State that you will perform a prostate or pelvic exam. Since these exams are not performed on standardized patients, the examiner will likely interrupt, ask what you are looking for, and provide findings.)

Investigations

Order a urine sample for microscopic examination and urine culture to assess the presence of:

- pyuria and/or bacteriuria
- casts and/or dysmorphic red cells (these suggest a glomerular cause)
- intact red cells and the absence of casts (this suggests a nonglomerular cause)

Significant hematuria is defined as 3 or more red blood cells per high power field. In microscopic hematuria, order a CT urography. In patients with poor renal function, or in pregnant patients, order renal and pelvic ultrasounds instead of CT scans.

Management

Many patients will not have an identifiable cause. These patients should have annual urinalysis with a repeat workup performed within 3 to 5 years.

Refer patients with risk factors for malignancy to a urologist for cystoscopy (see the checklist). Urine cytology has lower sensitivity, but may also be useful in patients with risk factors for malignancy.

Refer patients with hypertension, elevated serum creatinine, dysmorphic red blood cells, cellular casts, or proteinuria to a nephrologist.

Refer patients who have masses for biopsy.

Pearls
Malignancy is present in up to 5% of patients with microscopic hematuria and up to 40% of patients with gross hematuria.

14

Hypertension

MCC particular objectives
Identify patients with urgent or emergent hypertension.

Assess cardiac risk factors and existing target organ damage.

MCC differential diagnosis
with added evidence
HYPERTENSION IN GENERAL
Definition: ≥ 135/85 mmHg for nondiabetic individuals; ≥ 130/80 mmHg for diabetic individuals

PRIMARY
Signs and symptoms: often asymptomatic, headache
Risk factors: family history of hypertension; lack of exercise; high-sodium diet; obesity

SECONDARY
Renal parenchymal disease (e.g., kidney injury, polycystic kidney disease)
KIDNEY INJURY
Signs and symptoms: history of kidney disease, chronic renal failure, and/or current renal dialysis; bilateral lower limb swelling; shortness of breath; paroxysmal nocturnal dyspnea; orthopnea
Risk factors: diabetes, diabetic complications, and/or inadequate monitoring; hypertension; smoking .
Investigations: renal function tests (elevated creatinine, reduced calcium, elevated phosphate), reduced vitamin D

POLYCYSTIC KIDNEY DISEASE

This is the most common inherited cause of kidney disease.
It may not be detected in patients younger than 30.

Signs and symptoms: family history of polycystic kidney disease; hypertension with pain (abdomen, flank, lower back); hematuria; urinary tract infections (UTIs)

Investigations: renal ultrasound; genetic testing; serum creatinine and GFR to assess disease; urine tests (hematuria, micro or gross; culture to detect UTI or cyst infection)

Metabolic or endocrine conditions (e.g., adrenal adenoma or hyperplasia, thyroid conditions)

FUNCTIONAL ADRENAL ADENOMA OR HYPERPLASIA

Adrenal adenoma is usually asymptomatic. Secretion of cortisol (Cushing syndrome), aldosterone (hyperaldosteronism), or catecholamines (pheochromocytoma) might result in hypertension.

Signs and symptoms: round face, pronounced abdominal weight, hump on the upper back, thin arms and legs, stretch marks, acne (these are signs of Cushing syndrome); hypokalemia (sign of hyperaldosteronism); episodes of palpitations, diaphoresis, anxiety (signs of pheochromocytoma)

Investigations: 24-hour urine free cortisol or 1 mg dexamethasone suppression test (Cushing syndrome); plasma aldosterone:renin ratio (hyperaldosteronism); 24-hour urine collection for catecholamines and metanephrines (pheochromocytoma); CT scan to detect adrenal mass

HYPERTHYROIDISM

In the context of hypertension, hyperthyroidism typically exhibits high diastolic blood pressure.

Signs and symptoms: history of hyperthyroidism or symptoms of hyperthyroidism (changes in menstrual patterns, enlarged thyroid, tachycardia, palpitations, diarrhea, muscle weakness, tremor, hyperactive reflexes, weight loss, sweating, thinning hair)

Investigations: elevated thyrotropin (TSH)

HYPOTHYROIDISM

Signs and symptoms: history of hypothyroidism or symptoms of hypothyroidism (decreased reflexes, dry skin, weight gain, impaired cognition)

Investigations: elevated thyrotropin (TSH)

Vascular conditions (e.g., unilateral renal artery stenosis, coarctation of the aorta)

UNILATERAL RENAL ARTERY STENOSIS

Signs and symptoms: personal or family history of renal disorders; renal artery bruits; signs and symptoms of diabetes (personal or family history of diabetes; history of diabetic complications and/or inadequate monitoring; polydipsia, polyuria, weight loss)

Investigations: elevated creatinine; urinalysis (to detect proteinuria, eosinophils, and WBCs or white cell casts); fasting glucose or HbA_{1c} test to detect diabetes

COARCTATION OF THE AORTA

Signs and symptoms: weaker pulse in the legs than in the arms; heart murmur

Investigations: CT scan of the chest and/or abdomen

Catecholamine excess (e.g., pheochromocytoma, drug-induced conditions)

CATECHOLAMINE EXCESS IN GENERAL

Signs and symptoms: cardiac rate and rhythm abnormalities (possible)

Investigations: elevated catecholamine level on 24-hour urine collection; CT scan to detect adrenal mass

PHEOCHROMOCYTOMA

Signs and symptoms: tachycardia; pallor; headaches; shortness of breath; symptoms that occur in brief spells (up to 20 minutes) with no symptoms between (these spells may be mistaken for panic attacks)

DRUG-INDUCED CATECHOLAMINE EXCESS

Associated drugs include nonsteroidal antiinflammatory drugs (NSAIDs); anabolic steroids; erythropoietin; cocaine and other stimulants; and thyroxine replacements.

Obstructive sleep apnea

Signs and symptoms: excessive or loud snoring; disturbed sleep (e.g., not feeling rested in the morning); obesity (common); allergic rhinitis (sneezing, runny nose, eye irritation); morning headache; palpable masses in the oral cavity or neck

Investigations: sleep study (polysomnography); hypertrophic adenoid tissue on lateral neck X-ray

Strategy for patient encounter

The likely scenario is a patient in the emergency room with headache and high blood pressure. The specified tasks could engage history, physical exam, investigations, or management.

In this patient encounter, stay alert to risk factors for hypertension (see the checklist).

CHECKLIST

Risk factors for hypertension

Older age

African descent

Obesity

Male

Lack of physical activity

Tobacco use

High-sodium diet

Alcohol abuse

Emotional stress

History

Although most hypertensive adults have primary (essential) hypertension, it is important to rule out secondary causes. Ask about snoring (obstructive sleep apnea), a personal or family history of kidney disease, a history of adrenal tumour, and a history of thyroid disease. Ask about symptoms of high blood pressure (headaches, shortness of breath, nosebleeds, chest pain, numbness or weakness, vision changes, back pain). Take a drug and medication history, looking particularly for oral contraceptives, decongestants, caffeine, cocaine, and amphetamines. Assess the patient for cardiac risk factors: ask about a family history of heart disease, a personal history of dyslipidemia, and whether the patient smokes. Check for other risk factors for hypertension: ask about the patient's exercise routines, alcohol use, and recent emotional stressors. Ask about a family history of hypertension, focusing on age of onset.

Physical exam

Obtain the patient's vital signs, including blood pressure in both arms (see the checklist for interpreting blood pressure readings). Obtain the patient's weight and height, and calculate their body mass index (BMI). Examine the patient's cardiac and respiratory systems. Perform a fundoscopic exam.

CHECKLIST
Interpreting blood pressure readings

- **Normal blood pressure:** < 120/80 mmHg
- **Elevated blood pressure:** systolic 120–129 mmHg, diastolic < 80 mmHg
- **Stage 1 hypertension:** systolic 130–139 mmHg or diastolic 80–89 mmHg
- **Stage 2 hypertension:** systolic ≥ 140 mmHg or diastolic ≥ 90 mmHg

Investigations

Assess for potential secondary causes: order a urinalysis, and a test for urinary catecholamines, and tests for serum creatinine, electrolytes, and thyrotropin (TSH). Assess for additional cardiovascular risks: order a lipid panel, and a fasting glucose or glycated hemoglobin (HbA_{1c}) test to screen for diabetes. Assess for end organ damage: order a test for microalbuminuria and an electrocardiogram (ECG). In suspected underlying left ventricular dysfunction, consider an echocardiogram to assess cardiac structure and function.

Management

Identify any existing hypertensive emergency. This is defined as systolic blood pressure > 180 mmHg and/or diastolic blood pressure > 120 mmHg, with end organ dysfunction (aortic dissection, acute coronary syndrome, stroke, encephalopathy, acute renal failure, pulmonary edema, eclampsia). Treat hypertensive emergencies with intravenous medications; the choice of medication depends on the context (e.g., nitroglycerin in pulmonary edema or acute coronary syndrome; labetalol in aortic dissection).

Counsel all patients on lifestyle modifications, including reduced sodium intake, regular exercise, maintaining a healthy weight, and limiting alcohol intake. Counsel the patient to follow a diet rich in fruits, vegetables, whole grains, poultry, fish, and low-fat dairy. Treat any secondary causes and manage additional cardiovascular risk factors (e.g., smoking cessation).

Most patients will also require antihypertensive medication. First-line therapy is often a thiazide diuretic (e.g., hydrochlorothiazide). Thiazide diuretics or calcium channel blockers are often more effective in patients of African descent and older individuals than other antihypertensives. ACE inhibitors or angiotensin II receptor blockers are other first-line medications, and may be a better choice in patients with diabetes or chronic liver disease.

TIP

Tailoring information to individual patients

The MCC identifies providing generic information as a common exam error.

To avoid this error, ask patients about aspects of their lives that might affect their condition. Provide information that targets their situation and engage the patient in figuring out next steps.

For example, diet and exercise changes, and smoking cessation, might be relevant for this case:

- Ask what the patient ate yesterday for breakfast, lunch, and supper. Use this to personalize guidelines on dietary changes they need to make.

- Ask what the patient did for exercise last week. Discuss short-term goals with the patient: What could the patient do next week to exercise every day? (For example, when could the patient fit in a 30-minute walk?)

- In a patient who smokes, express your concern with their continued smoking. Ask what experience they have had with methods to quit. Provide information about other methods, as appropriate. Ask if there is a method they would like to pursue now, and describe the support you can offer them.

15

Hypertension in childhood

MCC particular objective
Distinguish primary from secondary hypertension.

MCC differential diagnosis
with added evidence

HYPERTENSION IN CHILDHOOD IN GENERAL
In children, hypertension from a secondary cause is usual.
In adolescents, essential hypertension is more likely, but secondary causes must be ruled out.

NEONATES AND YOUNG INFANTS

Renal artery thrombosis after umbilical artery (UA) catheter
Signs and symptoms: history of umbilical artery catheterization (rare); renal artery bruits

Investigations: elevated creatinine; urinalysis (to detect proteinuria; eosinophils; WBCs or white cell casts)

Coarctation of the aorta
Signs and symptoms: pale skin; failure to thrive; presence of symptoms since birth (often); family history of coarctation of the aorta; weaker pulse in the legs than in the arms; heart murmur

   Turner syndrome (common associated condition): female; small stature; skeletal abnormalities

Investigations: CT scan of the chest and/or abdomen

Congenital renal disease
Signs and symptoms: failure to thrive, family history of hereditary renal disease

Investigations: elevated creatinine; urinalysis (to detect proteinuria; eosinophils; WBCs or white cell casts); ultrasound or CT scan to detect abnormalities in renal size or shape

Renal artery stenosis
Signs and symptoms: failure to thrive, renal artery bruits, family history of hereditary renal disease

Investigations: elevated creatinine; urinalysis (to detect proteinuria; eosinophils; WBCs or white cell casts); ultrasound or CT scan to detect abnormalities in renal size or shape

CHILDREN AGED 1 TO 10 YEARS

Renal disease

Signs and symptoms: failure to thrive, family history of hereditary renal disease

Investigations: elevated creatinine; urinalysis (to detect proteinuria; eosinophils; WBCs or white cell casts); ultrasound or CT scan to detect abnormalities in renal size or shape

Coarctation of the aorta—see above

CHILDREN OLDER THAN 10 YEARS

Essential hypertension

Signs and symptoms: often asymptomatic, headache

Risk factors: family history of hypertension; lack of exercise; high-sodium diet; obesity

Renal disease

Signs and symptoms: failure to thrive; family history of hereditary renal disease; symptoms and signs of diabetes (personal or family history of diabetes; history of diabetic complications and/or inadequate monitoring; polydipsia, polyuria, and/or weight loss)

> Poststreptococcal glomerulonephritis: history of group A β-hemolytic streptococcus infection

Investigations: elevated creatinine; urinalysis (to detect proteinuria; eosinophils; WBCs or white cell casts); ultrasound or CT scan to detect abnormalities in renal size or shape; fasting glucose or hemoglobin A_{1c} test to detect diabetes

Coarctation of the aorta—see above

Strategy for patient encounter

The likely scenario is hypertension discovered on routine exam. It may involve an adolescent (the minimum age to play standardized patients is 16), or parents discussing a child who is absent on some pretext (e.g., a nurse is weighing the child in another room). The following notes assume the patient is an adolescent.

The specified tasks could engage history, physical exam, investigations, or management.

History

Start by checking for symptoms of hypertensive emergency: headache, vomiting, and altered level of consciousness.

Use open-ended questions to establish the patient's medical history, including birth, growth, and developmental history: What conditions have you been diagnosed with? What complications occurred during your birth? What complications did you have as you grew and developed? Listen for a history of kidney, heart, or endocrine disease; and for evidence of failure to thrive.

Use open-ended inquiry to establish the patient's diet: Please tell me what you ate yesterday and today. How typical is this diet for you? Listen for evidence of a diet high in fat and sodium (e.g., full of fast food).

Ask about maternal smoking during pregnancy (this increases risk of hypertension in the child); a family history of hypertension and cardiovascular disease; snoring (a symptom of sleep apnea); and symptoms of hyperthyroidism (heat intolerance, tachycardia, and weight loss).

Take a drug and medication history, looking especially for amphetamines, anabolic steroids, cocaine, phencyclidine, caffeine, and oral contraceptives.

Physical exam

Obtain the patient's vital signs, weight, and height. Calculate the patient's body mass index (BMI). Confirm that hypertension is present: compare the patient's blood pressure measurement with a table of normal pressures for the age, height, weight, and sex of the patient (see the quick reference on blood pressure tables). Measure blood pressure in both arms (it should be equal) and in 1 leg in prone position (it should be slightly higher in the leg). Unequal arm pressures, or a lower blood pressure in the leg, may indicate coarctation of the aorta. Palpate the femoral pulses (decreased pulses may also indicate coarctation of the aorta). Listen for abdominal bruits (relevant to renovascular disease). Look for acne, hirsutism, striae, moon facies, and truncal obesity (relevant to Cushing syndrome).

QUICK REFERENCE

Blood pressure tables for children and adolescents

As general preparation for the exam, review tables on child and adolescent blood pressure. In the context of the exam, if hypertension is present, it will likely be obvious, not borderline.

The US National Institutes of Health published a standard reference in 2005, "The Fourth Report on the Diagnosis, Evaluation, and Treatment of High Blood Pressure in Children and Adolescents," which is available online.

Investigations

In children with hypertension, order a complete blood count (CBC), tests for serum creatinine and electrolytes, a renal ultrasound, and urinalysis. Consider ordering a urine drug screen if illicit drug use is a possibility. Order a fasting glucose or glycated hemoglobin (HbA_{1c}) test to screen for diabetes. Order a lipid panel to look for dyslipidemia. Order an echocardiogram to examine heart structure and function. Refer the patient for, or perform, a retinal examination to look for retinal damage. In suspected sleep apnea, order polysomnography.

Management

Counsel the patient on lifestyle modifications: weight reduction if the patient is overweight or obese; regular physical activity; a diet rich in fresh fruit and vegetables, and fibre; avoidance of alcohol and tobacco; and sodium reduction (1.2 g/day in children 4 to 8 years old, 1.5 g/day in children older than 8 years). Most children will require antihypertensive medication.

To diagnose hypertension in a pediatric patient, the patient must present with a high blood pressure reading for at least 3 visits in a row. Arrange follow-up appointments, and consider ambulatory and home monitoring of blood pressure. Consider referring the patient to a pediatrician.

TIP

Tailoring information to individual patients

The MCC identifies providing generic information as a common exam error.

To avoid this error, ask patients about aspects of their lives that might affect their condition. Provide information that targets their situation and engage the patient in figuring out next steps.

For example, diet and exercise changes might be relevant for this case:

- Ask what the patient ate for breakfast today. Use this to personalize guidelines on dietary changes they need to make.
- Ask what the patient did for exercise last week. Discuss short-term goals with the patient: What could the patient do next week to exercise every day? (For example, when could the patient fit in a 30-minute walk?)

Pearls

Children 3 years of age and older should have their blood pressure measured at every office visit.

16

Hypertension disorders of pregnancy

MCC particular objective
Identify patients with eclampsia and preeclampsia, and take urgent action.

MCC differential diagnosis with added evidence

HYPERTENSION DISORDERS OF PREGNANCY IN GENERAL
Signs and symptoms:
Preeclampsia: blood pressure > 140/90 mmHg, and proteinuria or other symptoms
Eclampsia: preeclampsia and neurological symptoms

CHRONIC HYPERTENSION WITH OR WITHOUT PREECLAMPSIA OR ECLAMPSIA
Signs and symptoms: preexisting hypertension; headaches; changes in vision; decreased urine output; seizures (this is a sign of eclampsia)
Investigations: CBC (to detect thrombocytopenia, hemolytic anemia); renal function tests; chest X-ray to detect pulmonary edema; urinalysis

GESTATIONAL HYPERTENSION WITH OR WITHOUT PREECLAMPSIA OR ECLAMPSIA
Signs and symptoms: headaches, changes in vision, seizures, **no** history of preexisting hypertension
Investigations: CBC (to detect thrombocytopenia, hemolytic anemia); renal function tests; chest X-ray to detect pulmonary edema; urinalysis

Strategy for patient encounter
The likely scenario is a pregnant patient with hypertension discovered on prenatal exam. The specified tasks could engage history, physical exam, investigations, or management.

History
Ask if the patient has a history of hypertension. Ask if previous pregnancies were complicated by hypertension or preeclampsia. Ask about cerebral and visual disturbances.

Physical exam

Obtain the patient's vital signs. Nonsevere hypertension in pregnancy is defined as systolic blood pressure of 140–159 mmHg and/or diastolic blood pressure of 80–109 mmHg. Severe hypertension is defined as systolic blood pressure ≥ 160 mmHg and/or diastolic blood pressure ≥ 110 mmHg. Examine the lungs for edema, and the abdomen for right upper quadrant pain (relevant to preeclampsia).

Investigations

Order investigations to look for eclampsia and preeclampsia. Order a 24-hour urine collection looking for urine protein (≥ 0.3 g in preeclampsia, and ≥ 5 g in eclampsia). Order liver function tests and a complete blood count (CBC) to look for thrombocytopenia. Order an ultrasound of the fetus to look for intrauterine growth restriction.

Management

Refer the patient to an obstetrician for management and follow-up. Antihypertensive therapy is recommended for patients with systolic blood pressure ≥ 140 mmHg or diastolic blood pressure ≥ 90 mmHg. Start antihypertensive therapy with oral labetalol, methyldopa, long-acting nifedipine, or other beta-blockers (acebutolol, metoprolol, pindolol, and propranolol). ACE inhibitors and angiotensin receptor blockers should not be used in pregnant women.

Pearls

Hypertension affects 7% of pregnancies in Canada.

17

Hypotension, shock

MCC particular objectives

Pay particular attention to the presence or absence of shock. General life-saving measures are usually indicated, regardless of the underlying cause.

MCC differential diagnosis
with added evidence

HYPOTENSION IN GENERAL

Definition: systolic blood pressure < 90 mmHg or systolic blood pressure < 60 mmHg

CARDIAC OUTPUT DIMINISHED

Hypovolemia

HEMORRHAGE

Causes include recent massive blood loss from trauma or the disruption of a large internal blood vessel.

THIRD SPACE LOSS

Signs and symptoms: history of congestive heart failure, chronic liver disease, recent extensive burns, renal disease, overzealous fluid replacement

Investigations: blood tests (albumin, sodium, creatinine, CBC)

Cardiac dysfunction

INTRINSIC

MYOPATHY (E.G., ISCHEMIC CONDITION)

Signs and symptoms: chest pain (usual; this is a symptom of myocardial infarction, which is generally the cause of cardiogenic shock), sweating, pallor, shortness of breath, abnormal heart sounds

Investigations: elevated troponin; ECG; chest X-ray to detect cardiac enlargement and pulmonary edema

RHYTHM ABNORMALITIES

Signs and symptoms: tachycardia or bradycardia; light-headedness; fainting; shortness of breath

Investigations: ECG

MECHANICAL ABNORMALITIES

Signs and symptoms: heart murmurs (these suggest valvular abnormalities or cardiac shunt)

EXTRINSIC OR OBSTRUCTIVE

PULMONARY EMBOLUS

Signs and symptoms: sharp chest pain; shortness of breath; cough (possibly with blood); hypoxia; possible unilateral swelling of the lower limbs (this indicates deep vein thrombosis); elevated pulse and respiratory rate; arrhythmias; lung rales on auscultation; lower-lung dullness on percussion; motor or sensory deficits

Risk factors: heart failure; cancer; surgery; prolonged immobility (e.g., long plane trips); smoking; estrogen replacement therapy; oral contraceptives; current pregnancy; previous deep vein thrombosis, embolism, or stroke; family history of embolism

Investigations: elevated D-dimer level; area of reduced pulmonary perfusion on V/Q scan; CT angiography to detect blocked vessel

TENSION PNEUMOTHORAX

Signs and symptoms: history of trauma or recurrent spontaneous pneumothorax; absence of breath sounds on auscultation; deviated trachea

PERICARDIAL DISEASE

Signs and symptoms: increased jugular venous pressure, multiple heart sounds, pulsus paradoxus (decrease of ≥ 10 mmHg in systolic pressure with inspiration); history of conditions that can lead to fluid accumulation in the pericardial space, which compresses the heart and causes hypotension (cardiac surgery, trauma to the chest, myocardial infarction, pericarditis)

Investigations: echocardiogram to detect pericardial effusion

AORTIC DISSECTION

Signs and symptoms: intense "ripping" chest pain; tachycardia; different pulses in the arms versus the legs; heart murmur

Risk factors: long-standing hypertension; hereditary connective tissue disorders (especially Marfan syndrome); deceleration trauma; abdominal aortic aneurysm; arteritis; pregnancy

Investigations: elevated troponin; CT scan, echocardiogram, or MRI

VENA CAVAL OBSTRUCTION

Signs and symptoms: tachycardia; edema of the lower extremities (this indicates inferior vena cava syndrome)

History of malignancy (especially renal cell carcinoma); liver transplantation or other invasive procedures involving the inferior vena cava; hepatic vein thrombosis (Budd-Chiari syndrome); coagulopathy; use of oral contraceptives; pregnancy

Investigations: elevated hemoglobin (this indicates polycythemia, which is a related condition); abnormal serum liver enzyme tests (this indicates Budd-Chiari syndrome); CT scan with contrast to detect obstruction of the vena cava

DISTRIBUTIVE CONDITIONS

Sepsis

Definition: infection with systemic inflammatory response, dysfunction of ≥ 1 organ system

Signs and symptoms: fever or hypothermia; tachycardia; tachypnea; infection (most common: pneumonia, abdominal infection, kidney infection, bacteremia)

> Severe: oliguria; mental status changes; shortness of breath; extreme hypotension, unresponsive to fluid replacement (this indicates septic shock)

Risk factors: very young or very old; compromised immune system; wounds, burns; catheterization, intubation

Investigations: CBC with differential; cultures (blood, CSF, urine) to detect causative organism; ABG to detect acidosis; elevated creatinine; chest X-ray to detect pulmonary edema

Anaphylaxis

Signs and symptoms: personal or family history of anaphylaxis; hives; peripheral edema; swelling; tongue or throat swelling; wheezing; stridor; shortness of breath; tachycardia; cardiovascular collapse; hypotension

Inadequate tissue oxygenation

Signs and symptoms: bradycardia

> History of autonomic dysfunction (e.g., multiple system atrophy, Parkinson disease, tabes dorsalis, stroke); use of beta-blockers; spinal cord injury (common: the injury is usually acute); Addison disease or symptoms of Addison disease (muscle weakness, weight loss, skin hyperpigmentation)

Investigations (Addison disease): decreased serum cortisol; elevated serum ACTH

Postprandial hypotension

This occurs in up to one-third of older adults and is caused by blood redistribution to the gastrointestinal tract after eating.

Signs and symptoms: dizziness, faintness, or falls following meals

Strategy for patient encounter

The likely scenario is a patient in the emergency room with hypotension. The likely task is emergency management.

Emergency management

AIRWAY AND HEMODYNAMIC STATUS

Check the patient's airway, breathing, and circulation (mnemonic: **ABCs**). Begin resuscitation, as required: give oxygen, insert 2 large bore intravenous lines, give a 1 litre bolus of crystalloid, and then reassess the patient's vital signs.

HISTORY

Perform a history and physical exam at the same time.

Use open-ended questions to establish the patient's symptoms, and their duration and possible triggers: What symptoms do you have? How long have you had the symptoms? How constant are they? What triggers have you noticed for the symptoms? Listen for evidence consistent with particular entities (e.g., long-standing symptoms, such as light-headedness and fatigue, in chronic conditions such as congestive heart failure; chest pain, shortness of breath, and sweating triggered by exertion in cardiac myopathy; chest pain alleviated by leaning forward in pericarditis; hives and itching triggered by known allergens in anaphylaxis; presyncope after eating in postprandial hypotension).

Ask about a history of anaphylaxis and known triggers; recent infections and symptoms of infection (fever, cough, pain); recent blood loss (relevant to anemia); and recent severe vomiting or diarrhea (relevant to dehydration). Ask about a history of Addison disease and thyroid disease. Ask about a history of cardiac problems. Ask female patients if they are pregnant. Ask about medications, especially antihypertensives and anticoagulants.

TIP

Working with nurses to provide emergency care

The MCC identifies unclear directions to nurses as a common exam error.

To avoid this error, work out some standard directions for nurses in emergency scenarios. Emergency scenarios are likely to involve nurses, and likely to involve similar procedures to stabilize the patient. For example, if 1 nurse is present:

- Ask the nurse to take the patient's vital signs and obtain intravenous access.
- You start ventilation.

If 2 nurses are present:

- Ask for the first name of each nurse present.
- Ask a specific nurse by name to start ventilation.
- Ask a specific nurse by name to take the patient's vital signs and obtain intravenous access.

PHYSICAL EXAM

If the patient can stand, measure their blood pressure both supine and standing. Assess the patient's peripheral perfusion (symptoms of poor perfusion include cold, clammy skin and delayed capillary refill). Assess the patient's mental status for confusion. Assess heart rate and rhythm. Listen to the lungs for rales and wheezing. Assess the skin (including lips) for hives and swelling. Look for sources of infection.

INVESTIGATIONS

Order a complete blood count (CBC) (relevant to anemia and infection). Order tests for blood glucose (relevant to hypoglycemia and hyperglycemia), creatinine, and electrolytes. Order a urinalysis, and blood and urine cultures. Order an electrocardiogram (ECG) for all patients. For possible cardiac patients, consider an echocardiogram to assess cardiac function, an exercise test to assess for ischemic heart disease, and a 24-hour Holter monitor. Order a chest X-ray and urinalysis (infection). Consider other specific tests (see the information this resource lists in the MCC differential diagnosis).

MANAGEMENT

Treat any specific disorders identified. Consult a critical-care physician and admit the patient to an intensive care unit (ICU) for monitoring and treatment.

18

Breast masses and enlargement

MCC particular objectives
None stated.

MCC differential diagnosis
with added evidence

MALIGNANT BREAST MASSES

DUCTAL CARCINOMA IN SITU
Signs and symptoms: palpable breast mass (this occurs in 10% of patients); nipple discharge (occasionally); microcalcifications on mammogram (this is usually how it is detected)

LOBULAR CARCINOMA IN SITU
This has a higher risk of subsequent invasive breast carcinoma.

Signs and symptoms: **no** specific clinical presentation; **no** palpable lump; incidental breast biopsy finding (this is usually how it is detected); rarely visible on mammogram

INVASIVE BREAST CANCER
Signs and symptoms: women (most common), older age (the risk increases with age); palpable mass; nipple inversion; skin redness or dimpling; nipple discharge

> History of estrogen replacement therapy in postmenopausal women; excessive alcohol consumption; lack of physical activity; obesity

Risk factors: increasing age; family history of breast cancer and/or *BRCA1* and *BRCA2* mutations

Investigations: mammogram, biopsy

NONMALIGNANT BREAST MASSES

Fibrocystic change
Signs and symptoms: tender, bilateral lumps that fluctuate in size and tenderness with menstrual cycle; possible green or dark brown nipple discharge

Infection
Signs and symptoms: pain; redness; breast tenderness; fever and flu-like symptoms; unilateral symptoms, sometimes confined to a small segment of the breast; redness; tenderness; skin warmth; tender lymph nodes in the ipsilateral axilla

Risk factors: current lactation, nipple piercings, breast implants, tuberculosis

Investigations: ultrasound

GYNECOMASTIA

Physiological (newborns, adolescents, elderly)

PHYSIOLOGICAL GYNECOMASTIA IN GENERAL

Most male infants have some degree of gynecomastia at birth due to the effect of maternal estrogen. The gynecomastia generally goes away by 2 to 3 weeks of age.

Gynecomastia is common during puberty and in the elderly.

Pathological (e.g., testosterone deficiency or increased estrogen production, medications)

TESTOSTERONE DEFICIENCY

Signs and symptoms: use of antiandrogen medications (e.g., flutamide, finasteride) (these treat prostate enlargement and prostate cancer); use of spironolactone (this treats hypertension and edema); possible hypogonadism; history of liver disease, Klinefelter syndrome, hypothyroidism

Investigations: testosterone, thyrotropin (TSH)

INCREASED ESTROGEN PRODUCTION

Signs and symptoms: use of medications that increase estrogen levels (e.g., estrogen, spironolactone, verapamil, cimetidine); history or symptoms of hypothyroidism (decreased reflexes, dry skin, weight gain, impaired cognition); symptoms of pituitary tumour (headaches, vision changes); testicular abnormalities (hypogonadism, asymmetry, masses)

Investigations: abnormal LH levels; elevated estradiol levels; abnormal thyrotropin (TSH); MRI scan of the brain to detect pituitary tumour

MEDICATIONS

Medications known to cause gynecomastia include antiandrogen drugs, anabolic steroids, diazepam, tricyclic antidepressants, some antibiotics, spironolactone, cimetidine, digoxin, calcium channel blockers, and methadone.

Strategy for patient encounter

The likely scenario is an older woman with a breast mass. The specified tasks could engage history, physical exam, investigations, or management.

History

Use open-ended questions to obtain a history of the mass the patient has detected: When did you discover the mass? How has it changed? What other symptoms do you have? Listen for evidence consistent with particular entities (e.g., nipple inversion, nipple discharge with skin redness, or dimpling in invasive breast cancer; fluctuating bilateral lumps with breast tenderness in fibrocystic change; fever with breast pain and redness in infection). Ask if the symptoms are related to the menstrual cycle. Ask about risk factors for breast cancer (see the checklist). Take a medication history, looking for estrogen, oral contraceptives, selective serotonin reuptake inhibitors (SSRIs), haloperidol, spironolactone, and digoxin.

CHECKLIST

Risk factors for breast cancer

GENERAL RISK FACTORS	SPECIFIC RISK FACTORS FOR HEREDITARY BREAST CANCER
First-degree relative with breast or ovarian cancer	Breast cancer diagnosed at age 35 or younger
Personal history of atypical ductal hyperplasia or lobular carcinoma in situ	"Triple negative" (ER, PR, HER2 receptors) breast cancer diagnosed at age 60 or younger
Personal history of breast or ovarian cancer	Male breast cancer
More than 1 alcoholic drink per day	2 primary breast cancers with at least 1 diagnosed at age 50 or younger
Current or prior use of hormone therapy or oral contraceptives	Ovarian cancer at any age
Menarche before age 12	Breast or ovarian cancer and Ashkenazi Jewish heritage
Menopause after age 55	Family member with confirmed BRCA1 or BRCA2 mutation
Nulliparity	
Older than age 35 at first delivery	1 breast cancer and 1 ovarian cancer in first-degree relatives
High breast density on mammography	2 first-degree relatives with breast cancer diagnosed at age 50 or younger
Thoracic radiation exposure	2 first-degree relatives with ovarian cancer
	3 breast cancers in first-degree relatives, with 1 diagnosed at age 50 or younger

---

Physical exam

Obtain the patient's vital signs, looking for fever. Perform a breast exam. In addition to palpation of the breast tissue, remember to inspect for asymmetry, note the presence or absence of nipple discharge, and note skin changes. Inspect the axillae, supraclavicular area, and chest wall.

Investigations

Breast masses should be evaluated by mammography in women aged 30 and older. Ultrasound is more sensitive in women younger than 30. For all masses, order an ultrasound-guided core needle biopsy.

Management

Refer patients with malignant breast masses to surgery for excisional biopsy or mastectomy. Refer patients with risk factors for hereditary breast cancer (see the checklist) for *BCRA1* and *BCRA2* gene testing.

19

Breast discharge

MCC particular objective

Differentiate galactorrhea from other causes of breast discharge.

MCC differential diagnosis
with added evidence

GALACTORRHEA

Idiopathic

Signs and symptoms: bilateral discharge (usual)
Investigations: elevated prolactin (possible)

Hyperprolactinemia

PHYSIOLOGIC

Signs and symptoms: current pregnancy; recent stress; recent nipple stimulation; history of hypothyroidism or symptoms of hypothyroidism (decreased reflexes, dry skin, weight gain, impaired cognition)

DRUG-INDUCED

Examples of drugs include atypical antipsychotics, selective serotonin reuptake inhibitors (SSRIs), or monoamine oxidase inhibitors (MAOIs); and herbal supplements (fennel, anise, or fenugreek seed).

PITUITARY TUMOUR

Signs and symptoms: menstrual abnormalities; infertility; vision changes and/or headaches

Investigations: LH, FSH, ACTH; MRI of the brain

BREAST NEOPLASM

Signs and symptoms: breast pain or swelling; unilateral discharge (often); palpable mass in the breast and/or axilla

Risk factors: personal or family history of breast cancer; smoking; hormone replacement therapy

Investigations: cytology of breast discharge; mammogram

Strategy for patient encounter

The likely scenario is a postmenopausal woman with nipple discharge. The specified tasks could engage history, physical exam, investigations, or management.

History

Start with open-ended questions about the onset and colour of the discharge: When did the discharge start? How did it start? What colour is it? Listen, in particular, for evidence of red flags (see the checklist). Ask about a history of pregnancy and lactation:

> CHECKLIST
> **Red flags for nipple discharge**
> Spontaneous
> Unilateral
> Bloody
> Involves a single duct
> Associated with a mass

Are you pregnant now? Have you been pregnant recently? Have you been lactating? In patients who do not think they are pregnant, ask about symptoms of possible current pregnancy (sexually active, amenorrhea, nausea, breast tenderness). Ask about possible symptoms of a pituitary tumour (headaches, vision changes, menstrual changes) and hypothyroidism (dry skin, weight gain). Obtain a medication history, looking especially for verapamil, cimetidine, metoclopramide, estrogen, oral contraceptives, opiates, antipsychotics, monoamine oxidase inhibitors (MAOIs), neuroleptics, selective serotonin reuptake inhibitors (SSRIs), and tricyclic antidepressants. Ask about herbal supplements.

Physical exam

Perform a physical exam, including breast, thyroid, and vision exam. Note the colour of any discharge, the presence of breast masses, and duct involvement.

(State that you will perform a breast exam. Since breast exams are not routinely done on standardized patients, the examiner may interrupt, ask what you are looking for, and provide findings.)

Investigations

In patients with bilateral milky discharge, order a pregnancy test to rule out pregnancy. If this is negative, order tests for prolactin (relevant to pituitary tumour) and thyrotropin (TSH) (hypothyroidism). If red flags are present, send a sample of the discharge for cytology, and order a mammogram and breast ultrasound. Abnormal prolactin should be followed up with an MRI of the pituitary.

Management

Patients with pathologic discharge should be referred to a surgeon for duct excision.

20

Burns

MCC particular objective

Manage major thermal trauma.

MCC differential diagnosis

The MCC notes that burns can be thermal, electrical, chemical, or radiation injuries.

Strategy for patient encounter

This encounter will likely test your skills in emergency management of a patient with acute extensive burns.

Emergency management

ASSESS AIRWAY AND HEMODYNAMIC STATUS

Stabilize the patient's airway, breathing, and circulation (mnemonic: **ABCs**) as necessary.

TAKE A HISTORY

Take a history at the same time as you perform other tasks.

Ask the patient or accompanying caregivers how the burn happened. Obtain a brief medical history (including allergies). Determine the patient's tetanus immunization status.

REMOVE THE PATIENT'S CLOTHING

This ensures the burning process has stopped. Cool the burnt area with cool, running water for 20 minutes.

> **TIP**
>
> **Working with nurses to provide emergency care**
>
> The MCC identifies unclear directions to nurses as a common exam error.
>
> To avoid this error, work out some standard directions for nurses in emergency scenarios. Emergency scenarios are likely to involve nurses, and likely to involve similar procedures to stabilize the patient. For example, if 1 nurse is present:
> - Ask the nurse to take the patient's vital signs and obtain intravenous access.
> - You start ventilation.
>
> If 2 nurses are present:
> - Ask for the first name of each nurse present.
> - Ask a specific nurse by name to start ventilation.
> - Ask a specific nurse by name to take the patient's vital signs and obtain intravenous access.

ESTABLISH LARGE-BORE INTRAVENOUS ACCESS

Be prepared to administer fluid resuscitation. Go through burned skin if necessary.

TEST ARTERIAL BLOOD GASES (ABG)

Administer oxygen or hyperbaric oxygen to patients with elevated carboxyhemoglobin.

CALCULATE THE BURN AREA

Estimate the total body surface area (TBSA) burned as follows (mnemonic: **rule of 9s**):
- each arm: 9%
- face and/or scalp: 9%
- back: 18%
- front: 18%

- each leg: 18%
- perineum: 1%
- any area as big as the patient's own hand: 1%

CHECK FOR INHALATION INJURY

Ask the patient or accompanying caregivers about risk factors for inhalation injury: Were you inside a burning building? Were you involved in an explosion? Did you lose consciousness? Does your voice sound different?

Examine the patient for traces of carbon around the nose and mouth, and in the throat or sputum; burned or singed facial hair and facial swelling; and stridor, hoarseness, black sputum, or respiratory distress.

ADMIT OR TRANSFER THE PATIENT TO A BURN UNIT, AS WARRANTED

Patients require treatment in a burn centre if they have:

- burns to 20% or more TBSA (any age)
- burns to 10% or more TBSA (younger than 10 years or older than 50 years)
- Full-thickness burns to more than 5% TBSA (any age) (see the checklist on assessing burn depth)
- Superficial partial-thickness burns or full-thickness burns to the hands, feet, face, perineum, genitalia, or major joints (any age)
- inhalation injury (any age)

CHECKLIST
Assessing burn depth

- **Superficial burns:** dry, painful, minor blisters; red skin; brisk capillary return
- **Superficial partial-thickness burns:** moist, painful, red, broken blisters; brisk capillary return
- **Deep partial-thickness burns:** moist, painless, white-or-red mottled, sloughed skin; sluggish capillary return
- **Full-thickness burns:** dry, painless, charred skin or white skin; absent capillary return

---

PROVIDE ONGOING FLUID SUPPORT, AS WARRANTED

Patients who require treatment in a burn unit also require fluid support for the first 24 hours after injury (use Hartmann's solution).

Use the Parkland formula to calculate the patient's 24-hour fluid requirement:

$$4 \text{ cc} \times \% \text{ TBSA burned} \times \text{weight in kg}$$

Give half the calculated amount in the first 8 hours from time of injury, and half in the subsequent 16 hours.

TREAT PAIN
Provide immediate pain relief (e.g., intravenous morphine 0.1 mg/kg in titrated boluses).

PREVENT SECONDARY INFECTION
Administer systemic antibiotics and tetanus prophylaxis.

Dress the patient's wounds (apply topical antibiotic ointment on facial burns and topical silver sulfadiazine on other burns).

21

Hypocalcemia

MCC particular objectives
None stated.

MCC differential diagnosis
with added evidence

HYPOCALCEMIA IN GENERAL
Definition: total calcium < 2.1 mmol/L or ionized calcium < 1.1 mmol/L

Signs and symptoms: unusual sensations or loss of feeling in the fingers, toes, and around the mouth; itchy areas on the body; tetany; fatigue; depression; papilledema

LOSS OF CALCIUM FROM THE CIRCULATION

Hyperphosphatemia (e.g., renal insufficiency)
RENAL INSUFFICIENCY
Signs and symptoms: history of kidney disease, chronic renal failure, and/or current renal dialysis; bilateral lower limb swelling; shortness of breath; paroxysmal nocturnal shortness of breath; orthopnea

Risk factors: diabetes, diabetic complications, and/or inadequate monitoring; hypertension; smoking

Investigations: renal function tests (reduced calcium, elevated phosphate, elevated creatinine), reduced vitamin D

Pancreatitis

Signs and symptoms: constant upper abdominal pain that radiates to the back (sitting up and leaning forward may reduce the pain; pain occurs with coughing, vigorous movement, deep breathing); shortness of breath; nausea, vomiting; hypotension; fever; jaundice; abdominal tenderness

> History of gallstones or chronic alcoholism (usual); hyperlipidemia; change of medication

Investigations: serum amylase and lipase (levels are $\geq$ 3 times the upper limit of normal levels; elevated lipase indicates pancreatic damage); possible elevated cholesterol; possible elevated ALT (this indicates associated liver inflammation); chest X-ray (this may show left-sided or bilateral pleural effusion and/or atelectasis); abdominal X-ray (this may show calcifications within pancreatic ducts, calcified gallstones, or localized ileus of a segment of small intestine); ultrasound

Osteoblastic metastases

Signs and symptoms: history of cancer, especially breast or prostate; point tenderness over bones on physical exam

Investigations: elevated phosphate; X-ray or bone scan to detect metastases

Rhabdomyolysis

Signs and symptoms: use of street drugs (especially cocaine, heroin, and amphetamines), statin medications, or anesthetics (i.e., during recent surgery); muscle weakness; recent severe trauma; fever and/or hypotension (possible: these are signs of malignant hyperthermia following anesthesia)

Investigations: elevated creatine kinase; elevated serum or urine myoglobin; elevated phosphate

DECREASED VITAMIN D PRODUCTION OR ACTION

Kidney injury—see renal insufficiency, above

Rickets

Signs and symptoms: children younger than 3 years (most common); skeletal abnormalities (bowed legs; thick wrists and ankles); pain in the back, pelvis, legs

> History of premature birth; delayed growth; malnutrition; exclusive breast feeding without vitamin D supplementation

Investigations: reduced serum vitamin D

Malabsorption

Signs and symptoms: muscle wasting (possible)

> History of celiac disease, surgical removal of part of the small bowel, chronic diarrhea, weight loss

Investigations: CBC (to detect anemia); tTG antibodies (this is a sign of celiac disease); decreased serum vitamin D

DECREASED PARATHYROID HORMONE PRODUCTION OR ACTION

Signs and symptoms: history of thyroidectomy, parathyroidectomy, autoimmune hypoparathyroidism, or polyglandular autoimmune syndrome

Investigations: decreased PTH; > 1 type of endocrine deficiency (testosterone, FSH, LH, ACTH, thyrotropin) (this is a sign of polyglandular autoimmune syndrome)

LOW MAGNESIUM

Signs and symptoms: history of hypomagnesemia; use of diuretics, especially thiazide diuretics; diet low in green leafy vegetables

Investigations: decreased magnesium

Strategy for patient encounter

The likely scenario is a patient in the emergency room with low calcium found on blood work. The specified tasks could engage history, physical exam, investigations, or management.

History

In this patient encounter, you will likely know from the outset that the patient has hypocalcemia, based on already-done blood work. (Many patients with hypocalcemia are asymptomatic and the problem is discovered with blood testing.)

If the scenario does not specify hypocalcemia (e.g., it might only specify a calcium disorder), begin the history by establishing the patient's symptoms. Ask about numbness and tingling, especially in the fingers and toes or around the mouth; muscle cramping, twitching, or stiffness; seizures; spasms in the throat or difficulty breathing (this indicates laryngospasm, bronchospasm); and fatigue or depression.

Ask about risk factors for hypocalcemia: history of neck surgery (hypoparathyroidism), chronic renal disease, and diabetes (this is a risk factor for renal failure).

Use open-ended questions to take a medical history, and medication and drug history: What conditions have you been diagnosed with? What medications and recreational drugs do you take? Listen for kidney disease, hypertension, gallstones, hyperlipidemia, cancer, celiac disease, and conditions that affect parathyroid hormone (see the information this resource lists in the MCC's differential diagnosis); and for statins, diuretics, and street drugs.

Physical exam

Assess the patient's mental function during your history (confusion or delirium may be manifestations of hypocalcemia). Perform a neurological exam, looking for increased reflexes, Trousseau sign, and Chvostek sign (see the checklist).

Examine the eyes for papilledema. Examine the heart and lungs for congestive heart failure.

CHECKLIST
Trousseau sign and Chvostek sign
- **Trousseau sign:** Inflate a blood pressure cuff above the systolic blood pressure for 3 minutes. This induces carpal spasm.
- **Chvostek sign:** Tap the facial nerve anterior to the earlobe and just below the zygomatic arch. This induces spasm of the facial muscles.

Investigations

Order the following tests for all patients: serum total calcium or ionized calcium, creatinine, phosphorus, magnesium, parathyroid hormone (PTH), and vitamin D.

Remember that the result for total calcium must be corrected for serum albumin level, because calcium is tightly bound to albumin in the circulation. The equation to use is:

$$\text{Corrected } Ca^{2+} = \text{Total } Ca^{2+} + [0.02 \times (40 - \text{albumin})]$$

Note that if Ca^{2+} is in mmol/L, albumin must be in g/L.

Look for 1 of the following patterns of test results:
- High PTH, high phosphorus, high creatinine: renal failure
- High PTH, low or normal phosphorus, normal creatinine: vitamin D deficiency or pancreatitis
- Low PTH, high phosphorus, normal creatinine: hypoparathyroidism or hypomagnesemia

Order an electrocardiogram to look for prolonged QT interval.

Management

The initial emergency treatment is intravenous (IV) calcium: 10 ampules of 10% calcium gluconate in 900 mL of dextrose 5% in water (D5W), resulting in a 1 mg/mL solution. Infuse this at a rate of 1 to 3 mg/kg/hr. After the patient's symptoms have resolved and their calcium level is within the normal range, taper IV therapy over 24 to 48 hours, and, concurrently, start oral calcium (1 to 2 grams elemental calcium in total, administered over 2 doses or 3 doses per day) and vitamin D.

22

Hypercalcemia

MCC particular objectives
None stated.

MCC differential diagnosis
with added evidence

HYPERCALCEMIA IN GENERAL

Definition: total calcium ≥ 2.63 mmol/L or ionized calcium ≥ 1.4 mmol/L

Signs and symptoms: fatigue, depression, constipation, vomiting, bone pain, confusion, history of kidney stones

INCREASED INTESTINAL ABSORPTION

Increased intake (e.g., milk-alkali syndrome)

Causes include use of calcium supplements (milk-alkali syndrome has been associated with ≥ 2 g of elemental calcium per day) and a diet high in calcium (e.g., high in milk and cream).

Investigations: decreased PTH

Vitamin D–mediated condition (e.g., sarcoidosis)
SARCOIDOSIS

Sarcoidosis can cause hypercalciuria and hypercalcemia through calcitriol (the active form of vitamin D).

Signs and symptoms: lymphadenopathy (a mass in the middle of the mediastinum is the most common lesion), fever, fatigue, weight loss, lung symptoms (dry cough, shortness of breath, wheezing, chest pain)

> Other (for this context): aggravated hypercalcemia on exposure to the sun; increased intestinal calcium absorption; serum calcitriol concentrations that are not reduced on intake of calcium

Risk factors: age 20 to 40, African descent, family history of sarcoidosis

Investigations: decreased PTH; elevated 1,25-dihydroxyvitamin D_3 (calcitriol)

INCREASED BONE RESORPTION

Malignancy

Signs and symptoms: history of cancer, especially cancer of the breast or prostate, or multiple myeloma

Investigations: decreased PTH

Hyperparathyroidism

Signs and symptoms: often asymptomatic; bone pain; nephrolithiasis; fractures; proximal muscle weakness (often in the lower extremities); depression; lethargy; confusion, dementia

> Contributing drugs: thiazide-type diuretics, lithium, corticosteroids, bisphosphates

Risk factors: postmenopausal woman; chronic kidney disease; vitamin D deficiency; kidney transplant recipient; elderly with depression; family history of hyperparathyroidism

Investigations: ALP; BUN; creatinine; vitamin D; 24-hour urine collection for calcium; dual-energy X-ray absorptiometry (bone mineral density); ultrasound or parathyroid sestamibi scan (for localization)

> Primary hyperparathyroidism: elevated serum calcium; normal or elevated PTH
>
> Secondary hyperparathyroidism (this may occur in the context of vitamin D deficiency): normal/low serum calcium; extremely elevated PTH
>
> Tertiary hyperparathyroidism (this may occur in the context of chronic kidney disease): normal/elevated calcium; elevated PTH after treatment of secondary hyperparathyroidism

Hyperthyroidism

Signs and symptoms: history of hyperthyroidism or symptoms of hyperthyroidism (changes in menstrual patterns, enlarged thyroid, tachycardia, palpitations, diarrhea, muscle weakness, tremor, hyperactive reflexes, weight loss, sweating, thinning hair)

Investigations: decreased thyrotropin (TSH)

Immobilization

Examples of causes include spinal cord injury; stroke; and long-bone fracture, especially in children.

Investigations: decreased PTH

DIMINISHED EXCRETION (E.G., DIURETICS)

DIURETICS

The cause is thiazide-type diuretics.

Investigations: decreased urinary calcium, decreased serum PTH, increased serum vitamin D

Strategy for patient encounter

The likely scenario is a patient with hypercalcemia found on an insurance-company check. The specified tasks could engage history, physical exam, investigations, or management.

Pay particular attention to the setting for this patient encounter, which may be described in the instructions. In outpatient settings, the most common cause of hypercalcemia is hyperparathyroidism. In hospital (inpatient) settings, the most common cause is malignancy.

History

In this patient encounter, you will likely know from the outset that the patient has hypercalcemia, based on already-done blood work.

If the scenario does not specify hypercalcemia (e.g., it might only specify a calcium disorder), begin the history by establishing the patient's symptoms. The symptoms of hypercalcemia are classically described by the somewhat pejorative mnemonic "stones, bones, abdominal moans, and psychic groans." Ask about a history of kidney stones. Ask about bone pain, and the presence of arthritis and osteoporosis. Ask about nausea, vomiting, anorexia, weight loss, constipation, abdominal pain, and a history of pancreatitis. Ask about impaired concentration and memory, confusion, lethargy, and muscle weakness.

Use open-ended questions to obtain a medical and medication history: What conditions have you been diagnosed with? What medications do you take? Listen for malignancy, hyperthyroidism, Paget disease, sarcoidosis, tuberculosis, hepatitis, and AIDS; and for possible contributory medications (thiazide diuretics, lithium, and theophylline). Ask about excessive intake of calcium supplements (relevant to milk-alkali syndrome).

Physical exam

Obtain the patient's vital signs, looking for hypertension. Determine the patient's volume status. Perform a neurological exam.

Investigations

Order a test for serum total calcium or ionized calcium. Remember that the result for total calcium must be corrected for serum albumin level, because calcium is tightly bound to albumin in the circulation. The equation to use is:

$$\text{Corrected } Ca^{2+} = \text{Total } Ca^{2+} + [0.02 \times (40 - \text{albumin})]$$

Note that if Ca^{2+} is in mmol/L, albumin must be in g/L.

Order an electrocardiogram (ECG) to check for shortened QT interval. Order tests to assess serum lipase (relevant to pancreatitis), serum thyrotropin (TSH) (hyperthyroidism), serum parathyroid hormone (PTH) (hyperparathyroidism), and serum creatinine and electrolytes (renal function).

Management

Most cases of hypercalcemia are due to hyperparathyroidism or malignancy. Patients with hyperparathyroidism have elevated PTH levels. Refer these patients to an ear, nose, and throat (ENT) surgeon for an urgent parathyroidectomy. In patients with reduced parathyroid hormone (PTH), malignancy is the most common diagnosis (especially lung, breast, and multiple myeloma). In malignancy-related hypercalcemia, begin treatment with intravenous (IV) zoledronate or pamidronate, and monitor the patient's hemodynamic and electrolyte status.

Patients with elevated calcium are often significantly dehydrated. Emergency treatment includes aggressive hydration with IV normal saline. Consider treatment with a loop diuretic once the patient is replete and there is evidence of volume overload.

23

Cardiac arrest

MCC particular objective
Initiate immediate cardiac life support.

MCC differential diagnosis
with added evidence

CORONARY ARTERY DISEASE
Signs: ST elevation on the cardiac monitor or defibrillator

CARDIAC CONDUCTION ABNORMALITIES
Signs: VT or VF on the cardiac monitor or defibrillator

MYOCARDIAL ABNORMALITIES
This is typically identified on autopsy.

NONCARDIAC CAUSES (E.G., PULMONARY EMBOLUS)

PULMONARY EMBOLISM
Signs and symptoms: sharp chest pain; shortness of breath; cough (possibly with blood); hypoxia; possible unilateral swelling of the lower limbs (this indicates deep vein thrombosis); elevated pulse and respiratory rate; arrhythmias; lung rales on auscultation; lower-lung dullness on percussion; motor or sensory deficits

Risk factors: heart failure; cancer; surgery; prolonged immobility (e.g., long plane trips); smoking; estrogen replacement therapy; oral contraceptives; current pregnancy; previous deep vein thrombosis, embolism, or stroke; family history of embolism

Investigations: elevated D-dimer level; area of reduced pulmonary perfusion on V/Q scan; CT angiography to detect blocked vessel

HYPOXIA
Signs: cyanosis of ≥ 1 extremities; low oxygen saturation on pulse oximetry (but be aware that low oxygen saturation will be present as a consequence of the cardiac arrest itself)

TENSION PNEUMOTHORAX
Signs: absence of breath sounds over 1 or both lungs on auscultation, deviated trachea

ACIDOSIS
Investigations: low pH on ABG test

HYPO- OR HYPERKALEMIA
Investigations: abnormal electrolyte concentrations on ABG test, normal ECG findings

TOXINS
Common overdose drugs include tricyclic antidepressants, beta-blockers, calcium channel blockers, and cocaine.

HYPOVOLEMIA
Common causes are severe dehydration or bleeding.

CARDIAC TAMPONADE
Common causes are chest trauma and recent myocardial infarction.

Strategy for patient encounter

The likely scenario is a patient in the emergency room with cardiac arrest. The likely task is emergency management (initiating cardiac life support).

Emergency management

AIRWAY AND HEMODYNAMIC STATUS
Perform a primary survey for airway, breathing, and circulation. Be aware of possible cervical spine injury and maintaining cervical stabilization. If the patient has no pulse, begin chest compressions at a rate of 100 to 120 per minute. If breathing is absent, begin ventilation at a rate of 10 per minute using a bag-valve mask. If bag-mask ventilation is not adequate, insert an advanced airway device: laryngeal mask airway (LMA), Combitube, or endotracheal intubation. Confirm placement of the airway device by observation and confirming the presence of lung sounds in 4 lung fields. Attach electrocardiogram (ECG) leads and identify the patient's rhythm. Establish intravenous (IV) or intraosseous (IO) access. Follow the appropriate advanced cardiac life support (ACLS) protocol for the rhythm identified. Look for reversible causes.

HISTORY
Obtain a brief history from accompanying caregivers, witnesses, and first responders. Ask about clinical features relevant to the arrest: What did you notice about the patient before the arrest? What was the patient doing when the arrest happened? Does the

patient have a history of coronary artery disease? (Check for a sternotomy scar.) What treatment did the patient receive before arriving at the hospital?

Consider stopping cardiopulmonary resuscitation (CPR) if ACLS produces no response after 20 minutes of efficient resuscitation (no return of spontaneous circulation, no shockable rhythm, no reversible causes).

MANAGEMENT IN CASES OF DEATH

If the patient is deceased, talk to the family.

First, offer condolences and determine the extent of the family's understanding of the medical condition of their relative.

Determine if the patient is an organ donor. The family may know the answer to this. If not, they may have the patient's wallet, which might contain the patient's driver's license (which often lists organ donor status) or an organ donor card.

If the patient is not a donor, counsel the family about the possibility of organ donation. If the family consents to donation, determine which organ(s) they are consenting to.

TIP

Working with nurses to provide emergency care

The MCC identifies unclear directions to nurses as a common exam error.

To avoid this error, work out some standard directions for nurses in emergency scenarios. Emergency scenarios are likely to involve nurses, and likely to involve similar procedures to stabilize the patient. For example, if 1 nurse is present:

- Ask the nurse to take the patient's vital signs and obtain intravenous access.
- You start ventilation.

If 2 nurses are present:

- Ask for the first name of each nurse present.
- Ask a specific nurse by name to start ventilation.
- Ask a specific nurse by name to take the patient's vital signs and obtain intravenous access.

TIP

Truth telling

This case engages the need for truth telling. Truth telling involves communicating difficult information clearly.

- Ask about friends, family, or spiritual mentors who could provide support. Help the family make a plan to contact these people, or to use community support services or hospital spiritual care services.
- Use direct, clear language. Make eye contact. Avoid technical terms and jargon.
- Check for understanding. Answer any questions.
- Revisit the family's plan for seeking support.

If the patient is an organ donor or the family consents to donation, contact the organ transplant team.

24

Chest pain

MCC particular objective
Exclude life-threatening entities.

MCC differential diagnosis
with added evidence

CARDIOVASCULAR CONDITIONS

Ischemic

ACUTE CORONARY SYNDROME

Some patients present with atypical pain (this is more common in women).

Signs and symptoms: squeezing pain that radiates to the left arm or jaw (often); pain that started with exertion or exercise and has not subsided; decreased oxygen saturation

> Left heart failure: extra cardiac sounds and lung rales on auscultation
>
> Right heart failure: edema in the feet and legs

Risk factors: personal or family history of cardiac disease; high cholesterol; hypertension; diabetes; smoking; renal failure; anemia; electrolyte abnormalities

Investigations: 12-lead ECG (possible findings: ST-segment elevation, T-wave inversion); CBC to detect anemia; creatinine; electrolytes; elevated troponin (this may take 4 to 6 hours to appear); chest X-ray

STABLE ANGINA PECTORIS

Some patients present with atypical pain.

Signs and symptoms: pain on exertion or exercise that subsides with rest or nitroglycerin medication; squeezing pain that radiates to the left arm or jaw (often); decreased oxygen saturation

> Left heart failure: extra cardiac sounds and lung rales on auscultation
>
> Right heart failure: edema in the feet and legs

Risk factors: high cholesterol; smoking; hypertension; diabetes; family history of cardiac disease; anemia; electrolyte abnormalities

Investigations: 12-lead ECG; CBC to detect anemia; electrolytes; chest X-ray (this is normal)

Nonischemic

AORTIC ANEURYSM

Signs and symptoms: pain in the chest or midback, often described as tearing pain; shortness of breath; cough; hoarse voice; difficulty swallowing

Risk factors: hypertension, Marfan syndrome

Investigations: ultrasound, MRI, or CT scan

PERICARDITIS

Signs and symptoms: sudden-onset stabbing chest pain; pain made worse with inhalation or lying down, made better with sitting up or leaning forward (usual); radiation of pain to the neck, arms, left shoulder, and especially to the trapezius muscle; pericardial rub on auscultation (usual)

> History of recent viral illness; infection (e.g., tuberculosis), autoimmune disease (e.g., systemic lupus erythematosus, rheumatoid arthritis, scleroderma), uremia, myocardial infarction, aortic dissection, chest wall trauma, thoracic surgery

Diagnosis: ECG; chest X-ray for pericardial effusion

PULMONARY OR MEDIASTINAL CONDITIONS

Pulmonary embolism or pulmonary infarct

PULMONARY EMBOLISM

Signs and symptoms: sharp chest pain; shortness of breath; cough (possibly with blood); hypoxia; possible unilateral swelling of the lower limbs (this indicates deep vein thrombosis); elevated pulse and respiratory rate; arrhythmias; lung rales on auscultation; lower-lung dullness on percussion; motor or sensory deficits

Risk factors: heart failure; cancer; surgery; prolonged immobility (e.g., long plane trips); smoking; estrogen replacement therapy; oral contraceptives; current pregnancy; previous deep vein thrombosis, embolism, or stroke; family history of embolism

Investigations: elevated D-dimer level; area of reduced pulmonary perfusion on V/Q scan; CT angiography to detect blocked vessel

Pleuritis

Signs and symptoms: chest pain aggravated by breathing; shortness of breath; fever; decreased oxygen saturation; areas of lung consolidation on auscultation (this suggests pneumonia)

Risk factors: viral or bacterial infection; autoimmune disease, especially rheumatoid arthritis; tuberculosis; heart surgery

Investigations: CBC to detect elevated WBCs, chest X-ray

Pneumothorax

Signs and symptoms: sudden-onset shortness of breath with pain; absence of breath sounds over 1 lung on auscultation; deviated trachea (this suggests a tension pneumothorax)

Risk factors: prior pneumothorax; chronic obstructive pulmonary disease; smoking; emphysema

Investigations: chest X-ray

Malignancy

Signs and symptoms: shortness of breath (often; this symptom is consistent with a space-occupying lesion); constitutional symptoms (fever, weight loss, night sweats, fatigue)

Risk factors: smoking, exposure to asbestos, history of cancer

Investigations: CT scan of the lungs

GASTROINTESTINAL CONDITIONS

Esophageal spasm or esophagitis

ESOPHAGEAL SPASM

Signs and symptoms: squeezing chest pain, difficulty swallowing, regurgitation of food

ESOPHAGITIS

Signs and symptoms: difficulty swallowing or pain with swallowing; food becoming impacted in the esophagus, especially foods that are solid or difficult to chew; acid reflux; oral *Candida* infection; oral ulcers; epigastric tenderness (this could arise from associated peptic ulcer disease or reflux)

> History of food allergies or environmental allergies (e.g., pollen); factors causing immunosuppression, such as HIV, cancer, immunosuppressant medications, autoimmune disease, malnutrition (immunosuppression creates a higher risk for bacterial, viral, and fungal infections of the esophagus); use of antiinflammatories and bisphosphonates (these present a particular risk if they are not swallowed properly and remain in the esophagus)

Investigations: upper GI series (barium swallow) or endoscopy

Peptic ulcer disease

Signs and symptoms: constant midepigastric pain, often relieved with eating or with antacids; weight loss

Investigations: test for *H. pylori*; endoscopy to detect ulcer or inflammation of the gastric lining

Mallory-Weiss syndrome

Common causes include vomiting, coughing, hiccups, and abdominal trauma (e.g., a fall, car accident).

Signs and symptoms: abdominal pain, vomit with blood

Investigations: endoscopy

Biliary disease or pancreatitis

BILIARY DISEASE

Signs and symptoms: middle-aged woman (more common) (mnemonic: **4Fs**—**f**emale, **f**at, **f**ertile, **f**orties); epigastric pain, often after eating (the pain is generally constant and often radiates to the right shoulder); right-sided subcostal pain that is worse on deep inhalation; obesity; history of pregnancy

> Cancer or primary biliary cholangitis: fatigue, weight loss
> Obstructive biliary disease: jaundice

Investigations: elevated ALP, bilirubin (this indicates biliary obstruction); elevated aminotransferases (AST, ALT) (this indicates liver injury); ultrasound or CT scan to detect gallstones; MRCP to detect bile duct obstruction

PANCREATITIS

Signs and symptoms: constant upper abdominal pain that radiates to the back (sitting up and leaning forward may reduce the pain; pain occurs with coughing, vigorous movement, deep breathing); shortness of breath; nausea; vomiting; hypotension; fever; jaundice; abdominal tenderness

> History of gallstones or chronic alcoholism (usual); hyperlipidemia; hypercalcemia; change of medication

Investigations: serum amylase and lipase (levels are $\geq$ 3 times the upper limit of normal levels; elevated lipase indicates pancreatic damage); possible elevated calcium; possible elevated cholesterol; possible elevated ALT (this indicates associated liver inflammation); chest X-ray (this may show left-sided or bilateral pleural effusion; atelectasis); abdominal X-ray (this may show calcifications within pancreatic ducts, calcified gallstones, or localized ileus of a segment of small intestine); ultrasound

ANXIETY DISORDERS[1(pp189-234)]

Examples of anxiety disorders listed in the *Diagnostic and Statistical Manual of Mental Disorders* (*DSM-5*) include generalized anxiety disorder, panic disorder, separation anxiety disorder, social anxiety disorder, and specific phobia. Anxiety disorders can provoke panic attacks (e.g., exposure to a phobic object). In the case of panic disorder, panic attacks occur spontaneously.

Signs and symptoms: history of anxiety disorder and/or symptoms consistent with a panic attack; history of social or emotional triggers for symptoms (possible); lack of evidence for other causes, including hyperthyroidism (anxiety can mimic other conditions and is therefore a diagnosis of exclusion)

> Panic attack: symptoms that peak within minutes; symptoms that can include palpitations, accelerated heart rate,

shortness of breath, chest pain, dizziness, numbness or tingling, fear of losing control, fear of dying

CHEST WALL PAIN (E.G., COSTOCHONDRITIS)

COSTOCHONDRITIS

Signs and symptoms: chest wall trauma; consistent pain with specific movements; pain on palpation of the ribs, sternum, and/or sternoclavicular joints

Strategy for patient encounter

The likely scenario is a patient in the emergency room with chest pain. The specified tasks could engage history, physical exam, investigations, or management, and will likely involve interpreting an electrocardiogram.

No matter what tasks the instructions for the encounter specify, the first step in any patient with chest pain is to check the patient's airway and hemodynamic status.

Stay alert to red flags for serious causes of chest pain (see the checklist). The likely cause in this encounter is acute ST-elevation myocardial infarction (STEMI).

> **CHECKLIST**
> ### Red flags for serious causes of chest pain
> Abnormal vital signs
> Signs of hypoperfusion
> Shortness of breath
> Hypoxemia
> Asymmetric breath sounds or pulses
> New heart murmur
> Pulsus paradoxus > 10 mmHg

Airway and hemodynamic status

Check the patient's airway, breathing, and hemodynamic status. Provide emergency management to stabilize the patient as required. Ensure any unstable patient is in a monitored setting with good peripheral intravenous (IV) access.

History

Use open-ended questions to take a pain history, establish associated symptoms, and take a medication history. Check risk factors for coronary artery disease and venous thromboembolism.

- **Pain history:** When did the current episode of chest pain start? What is the character of the pain? Where is it located? What makes the pain better? What makes it worse? What triggered the pain? Listen for evidence consistent with particular entities (e.g., unremitting, squeezing chest pain that radiates to the left arm or jaw, and that started with exertion, in acute coronary syndrome; sudden-onset stabbing chest pain that radiates to the trapezius muscle, made better by leaning forward in pericarditis). Unless the patient volunteers the information, specifically ask if the pain is present with respiration (this suggests pericarditis, pleuritis), with swallowing (esophageal condition), with exercise (cardiovascular condition), or with changes in position (pericarditis, pancreatitis).

- **Associated symptoms:** What other symptoms do you have? Listen for evidence consistent with particular entities (e.g., shortness of breath, cough, and difficulty swallowing in aortic aneurysm; shortness of breath and unilateral calf swelling in pulmonary embolism; shortness of breath and fever in pleuritis; shortness of breath, nausea, vomiting, and fever in pancreatitis).
- **Medication and drug history:** What medications do you take? What recreational drugs do you take? Listen especially for cocaine, triptans, and phosphodiesterase inhibitors.
- **Risk factors for coronary artery disease:** Ask about hypertension, hyperlipidemia, diabetes, smoking, and a family history of premature cardiovascular disease (onset before age 55 in men and age 60 in women).
- **Risk factors for venous thromboembolism:** Ask about immobilization, recent surgery, malignancy, pregnancy, and family history of venous thromboembolism.

Physical exam

Note the general appearance of the patient (pallor, sweating, cyanosis, anxiety). Palpate pulses in both arms and both legs, measure blood pressure in both arms, and measure pulsus paradoxus. Examine the neck for venous distention and increased hepatojugular reflux. Note the carotid pulses, and examine the neck for an enlarged thyroid and lymphadenopathy. Auscultate the lungs for breath and adventitious sounds. Auscultate the heart for heart sounds, splitting, pericardial friction rubs, murmurs, and gallops. Examine the abdomen for tenderness, organomegaly, and masses.

Examine the legs for signs of deep vein thrombosis (swollen calf that is erythematous, tender, and > 3 cm larger than the other calf when measured 10 cm distal to the tibial tuberosity), edema, and peripheral pulses.

Investigations

Order an electrocardiogram (ECG) and interpret the result, looking especially for ST elevation. Order pulse oximetry and a chest X-ray. In possible acute coronary syndrome (this will include most patients), order a test for serum troponin. In possible pulmonary embolism, order a D-dimer test.

Because a single normal set of cardiac markers does not rule out a cardiac cause, patients whose symptoms suggest an acute coronary syndrome should have serial measurement of the cardiac marker troponin and ECGs at least 6 hours apart. Some clinicians follow these tests (acutely or within several days) with a stress ECG or a stress imaging test. Drug treatment (acetylsalicylic acid and clopidogrel) is begun while awaiting results of the second troponin level, unless there is a clear contraindication (see the checklist on contraindications). A diagnostic trial of sublingual nitroglycerin or an oral liquid antacid does not adequately differentiate myocardial ischemia from gastroesophageal reflux disease or gastritis. Either drug may relieve symptoms of either disorder.

Troponin will be elevated in all acute coronary syndromes causing cardiac injury, and often in other disorders that damage the myocardium (e.g., myocarditis, pericarditis, aortic dissection involving coronary artery flow, pulmonary embolism, heart failure, severe sepsis). Creatine kinase (CK) may be elevated due to damage to any muscle tissue, but CK-MB elevation is

---

CHECKLIST

Contraindications to fibrinolysis in acute myocardial infarction

Systolic blood pressure > 180 mmHg, diastolic blood pressure > 110 mmHg

Aortic dissection

History of structural central nervous system disease

Significant closed head injury or facial trauma in the past 3 months

Recent stroke

Intraocular bleeding

Major trauma, surgery, or gastrointestinal or genitourinary bleed in the past 6 weeks

Bleeding or clotting problems, or taking an oral anticoagulant

Cardiopulmonary resuscitation longer than 10 minutes

Pregnancy

Advanced or terminal cancer, or severe liver or kidney disease

---

specific to damage to the myocardium. However, troponin is now the standard marker of cardiac muscle injury. ST-segment abnormality on ECG may be nonspecific or due to antecedent disorders, so comparison with previous ECGs is important.

Management

Treat any identified disorders. As preparation for the exam, review current treatment guidelines for acute myocardial infarction. Remember the mnemonic "MONA treats MIs." MONA stands for morphine, oxygen, nitrates, and aspirin. Begin fibrinolytic therapy within 30 minutes of hospital arrival, and, if available, initiate primary percutaneous coronary intervention (PCI) within 90 minutes of hospital arrival. On hospital discharge ensure the patient is prescribed aspirin, a $P2Y_{12}$ inhibitor, a beta-blocker, an ACE inhibitor or angiotensin receptor blocker (ARB), and a statin. Counsel on tobacco cessation. Refer the patient to a cardiac rehabilitation service.

REFERENCE

1 American Psychiatric Association. Diagnostic and statistical manual of mental disorders. 5th ed. Arlington, VA: American Psychiatric Association; 2013. 59–60. 991 p.

25

Bleeding, bruising

MCC particular objective

Recognize that some presentations are self-limiting.

MCC differential diagnosis
with added evidence

LOCALIZED BLEEDING (E.G., EPISTAXIS, LACERATION)

HEMOSTASIS DISORDERS

Platelet or blood vessel disorders (e.g., von Willebrand disease, collagen disorder, medication-induced disorder)

VON WILLEBRAND DISEASE

Signs and symptoms: family history of von Willebrand disease

Investigations: decreased von Willebrand factor on vWF antigen test; decreased ristocetin cofactor activity assay (this indicates a functional problem with von Willebrand factor)

COLLAGEN DISORDER

Signs and symptoms: history of collagen vascular disease (e.g., Ehlers-Danlos syndrome); hypermobile joints; hyperelastic skin; skin that tears easily

Investigations: genetic test for collagen vascular disease

MEDICATION-INDUCED DISORDER

Signs and symptoms: recent use of anticancer drugs, antibiotics (especially sulfonamide, penicillin, cephalosporin, rifampin, and vancomycin), heparin, digoxin, thiazide diuretics, H_2 antagonists, phenytoin, valproic acid, carbamazepine, oral anticoagulants, antiplatelet agents

Coagulation disorders (e.g., factor VIII deficiency, vitamin K deficiency, fibrinolysis)

FACTOR VIII DEFICIENCY

Signs and symptoms: family history of hemophilia, hemarthrosis

Investigations: decreased factor VIII or factor IX

VITAMIN K DEFICIENCY

Signs and symptoms: use of warfarin; diet restricting vitamin K intake (rare); conditions that cause fat malabsorption (celiac disease, Crohn disease, chronic pancreatitis, cystic fibrosis, small bowel surgery)

Investigations: elevated INR

FIBRINOLYSIS

Signs and symptoms (disseminated intravascular coagulopathy): history of recent, severe infection, especially sepsis; recent heat stroke; current pregnancy or recent delivery; organ transplant or recent blood transfusion; pancreatitis; malignancy; hepatic failure

Investigations: peripheral blood smear to detect red blood cell fragments (diagnostic); decreased platelets on CBC; elevated D-dimer level; elevated INR; elevated PTT; decreased plasma fibrinogen

Strategy for patient encounter

The likely scenario is a patient with prolonged bleeding on injury. The specified tasks could engage history, physical exam, investigations, or management.

An actively bleeding patient is possible in this clinical presentation. No matter what tasks the instructions for the encounter specify, start by checking for active bleeding and follow up with an assessment of the patient's vital signs as indicated.

Active bleeding and vital signs

If the patient is actively bleeding, check the patient's airway, breathing, and hemodynamic status (mnemonic: **ABCs**). Provide emergency management, if indicated (e.g., apply pressure and gauze to the site of bleeding; apply a tourniquet to a limb to control life-threatening bleeding; apply nasal packing for epistaxis).

History

Use open-ended inquiry to take a history of the bleeding: How easily do you bleed? Listen for bleeding after minor injuries or dental work that is difficult to stop. Ask about bleeding that has required surgical intervention, blood transfusion, or replacement therapy. Ask about a family history of bleeding problems. In women, ask about a history of menorrhagia, or hysterectomy for postpartum bleeding.

Use open-ended questions to obtain a medical and medication history: What conditions have you been diagnosed with? What medications do you take? Listen for hemostasis disorders; for conditions associated with vitamin K deficiency (celiac disease, Crohn disease, chronic pancreatitis, cystic fibrosis, and small bowel surgery); and for medications associated with bleeding and bruising (see the information this resource lists in the MCC's differential diagnosis).

Physical exam

Examine the skin and mucous membranes for petechiae and bruising. Examine the joints for hemarthroses. Examine the abdomen for hepatosplenomegaly.

Investigations

Order a complete blood count (CBC) and peripheral blood smear to look for anemia and thrombocytopenia. Order tests for prothrombin time/international normalized ratio (PT/INR) and partial thromboplastin time (PTT) to look for clotting factor deficiencies.

Order a coagulopathy screen (or hemostasis screen), which would generally include:

- circulating anticoagulant (inhibitory screen)
- factor assays (factors II, V, VII, VIII, IX, X, XI, XII, XIII)
- inhibitor screen or assay
- 50:50 mixing study
- von Willebrand factor workup (von Willebrand factor antigen, von Willebrand factor activity)

Consider platelet function studies to look for platelet disorders.

Management

Consider referring the patient to a hematologist for assistance with management, especially in ongoing suspicion of a bleeding disorder despite a nondiagnostic workup.

26

Prevention of venous thrombosis

MCC particular objectives
Recognize patients who may be at risk of venous thrombosis.
Assess the risk and intervene as warranted.

MCC differential diagnosis
with added evidence

STASIS (E.G., HOSPITALIZATION, TRAVEL)

ENDOTHELIAL INJURY (E.G., PREVIOUS THROMBOSIS)

HYPERCOAGULABILITY (E.G., DRUGS, CANCER, INHERITED OR ACQUIRED CONDITIONS)
DRUGS
Examples include chemotherapy and heparin.

CANCER
Metastatic cancer is particularly associated with hypercoagulability.

INHERITED CONDITIONS
SICKLE CELL DISEASE
Signs and symptoms: family history of sickle cell disease; painful swelling of the hands and feet
Investigations: CBC to detect anemia, sickle cells; positive sickle cell screen; abnormalities on peripheral blood smear; abnormalities on hemoglobin electrophoresis

CONGENITAL CLOTTING FACTOR ABNORMALITIES
These include protein C deficiency, protein S deficiency, antithrombin III deficiency, and factor V Leiden deficiency.
Signs and symptoms: family history of thrombosis; thrombosis starting at a young age; recurrent thrombosis

ACQUIRED CONDITIONS
Examples include hypercoagulability due to pregnancy, smoking, old age, use of oral contraceptives, and use of estrogen replacement therapy.
Investigations: positive lupus anticoagulant test, positive anticardiolipin antibody test

Strategy for patient encounter

The likely scenario is a patient with a personal history of blood clots who is seeking advice. The specified tasks could engage history, physical exam, investigations, or management.

History

Ask about risk factors for venous thrombosis: a personal or family history of venous thrombosis; prolonged immobilization; recent surgery; current pregnancy; use of oral contraceptives or hormone replacement therapy; smoking; personal history of cancer, heart failure, inflammatory bowel disease; and age older than 60. Check for current signs and symptoms of deep vein thrombosis (e.g., recent stroke or uncontrolled severe hypertension; red, painful, warm, and/or swollen calf), and pulmonary embolism (shortness of breath, pleuritic chest pain, tachycardia, hemoptysis). In women, ask about recurrent pregnancy loss (this is a possible sign of an inherited coagulation defect).

Physical exam

Obtain the patient's height and weight, and calculate their body mass index (BMI).

Perform a physical exam, focusing on the legs (relevant to deep vein thrombosis) and lungs (pulmonary embolism).

In the leg exam, check in particular for a swollen calf that is erythematous, tender, and > 3 cm larger than the

---

TIP

Tailoring information to individual patients

The MCC identifies providing generic information as a common exam error.

To avoid this error, ask patients about aspects of their lives that might affect their condition. Provide information that targets their situation and engage the patient in figuring out next steps.

For example, diet and exercise changes, and smoking cessation, might be relevant for this case:

- Ask what the patient ate yesterday for breakfast, lunch, and supper. Use this to personalize guidelines on dietary changes they need to make.

- Ask what the patient did for exercise last week. Discuss short-term goals with the patient: What could the patient do next week to exercise every day? (For example, when could the patient fit in a 30-minute walk?)

- In a patient who smokes, express your concern with their continued smoking. Ask what experience they have had with methods to quit. Provide information about other methods, as appropriate. Ask if there is a method they would like to pursue now, and describe the support you can offer them.

other calf when measured 10 cm distal to the tibial tuberosity. In the lung exam, check in particular for lung rales on auscultation, and lower-lung dullness on percussion.

Investigations

Consider investigations for underlying conditions as appropriate (e.g., age-appropriate cancer screening for unprovoked venous thromboembolism).

Management

In asymptomatic patients at risk of venous thrombosis, suggest lifestyle changes such as weight loss, exercise, and smoking cessation. Consider compression stockings.

Treat deep vein thrombosis or pulmonary embolism with anticoagulant therapy (in hemodynamically unstable patients with pulmonary embolism, treat with intravenous thrombolysis). Prescribe low molecular weight heparin and overlap this therapy with warfarin or direct oral anticoagulants (dabigatran, rivaroxaban; there is no need to overlap in the case of apixaban or edoxaban). Treatment is continued for 3 to 6 months. Consider indefinite treatment or a change to acetylsalicylic acid (ASA) in patients with an underlying coagulopathy or nonmodifiable risk factors.

27

Adult constipation

MCC particular objectives

None stated.

MCC differential diagnosis
with added evidence

DIET, LIFESTYLE

Causes include recent changes in diet; recent decrease in activity level; low-fibre diet; and inadequate hydration.

IRRITABLE BOWEL SYNDROME[1]

Irritable bowel syndrome is commonly diagnosed by applying the Rome criteria.

Signs and symptoms (Rome criteria): ≥ 2 symptoms, present for ≥ 1 day/week for ≥ 3 months

> Symptoms: pain associated with defecation, pain associated with a change of stool frequency, pain associated with a change in stool consistency

DRUG-INDUCED CONDITION

Drugs known to cause constipation include opioids, iron supplements, antidepressants, antipsychotics, levodopa, antihistamines, and antacids.

NEUROGENIC CONDITION (CENTRAL OR PERIPHERAL)

SPINAL CORD INJURY

Signs and symptoms: history of trauma, infection, or malignancy; leg weakness; fatigue; lack of coordination

AMYOTROPHIC LATERAL SCLEROSIS (ALS)

Signs and symptoms: onset in a limb or extremity; weakness, cramps, twitching, muscle wasting (lower motor neuron involvement); walking difficulty due to spasticity (upper motor neuron involvement); general fatigue; reduced exercise tolerance; possible language dysfunction

> Bulbar onset, which may precede limb weakness: swallowing difficulty, slurred speech, jaw jerking, increased gag reflex; tongue twitching (very specific for ALS)

Investigations: EMG, nerve conduction study, MRI

SPINA BIFIDA

This is congenital and diagnosed at birth.

MULTIPLE SCLEROSIS

Signs and symptoms: variable depending on lesion location

> Spinal cord: sensory or motor dysfunction; Lhermitte sign (paresthesias radiating down the extremities or trunk with neck flexion); bowel, bladder or erectile dysfunction

> Brainstem: double vision; swallowing, speech difficulties; vertigo; pseudobulbar palsy

> Cerebrum: cognitive impairment; depression; upper motor neuron signs; unilateral motor or sensory deficits

> Cerebellum: problems with balance and coordination; vertigo

> Other symptoms: tonic spasms; fatigue; pain; exercise intolerance; temperature sensitivity; painful unilateral loss of visual acuity

Risk factors: younger than 50, female

Investigations: brain and spinal cord MRI, including advanced MRI techniques, with established occurrence of multiple episodes; CSF fluid analysis

PARKINSON DISEASE

Signs and symptoms (mnemonic **TRAP**): **t**remor at rest; **r**igidity of the lower limbs; **a**kinesia, bradykinesia; **p**ostural instability

> Other symptoms: cognitive impairment; dementia; shuffling gait with stooped posture and loss of arm swing; micrographia; hypophonia; masklike facies, "pill rolling"; lack of blinking; orthostatic hypotension

> History of use of antipsychotics, antiemetics; toxin ingestion (e.g., carbon monoxide, cyanide); head trauma; vascular disease; other neurodegenerative disease (e.g., Lewy body dementia, Huntington disease); brain tumour, hydrocephalus; metabolic conditions (e.g., hypoparathyroidism, Wilson disease, chronic liver failure); infections that spread to the brain (HIV/AIDS, syphilis, prion disease, toxoplasmosis, encephalitis lethargica, progressive multifocal leukoencephalopathy)

STROKE

Signs and symptoms: history of stroke, or signs and symptoms consistent with stroke (e.g., unilateral neurologic defects)

Risk factors: hypertension, dyslipidemia, diabetes, coagulopathy

MYOPATHIC CONDITION

Signs and symptoms: child (usual, but still rare); history of long-standing constipation; increased anal tone on physical examination

Investigations: positive for myopathy on rectal biopsy

METABOLIC CONDITION

HYPOTHYROIDISM

Signs and symptoms: history of hypothyroidism or symptoms of hypothyroidism (cold intolerance, decreased reflexes, dry skin, weight gain, impaired cognition)

Investigations: elevated thyrotropin (TSH)

DIABETES

Signs and symptoms: personal or family history of diabetes; history of diabetic complications and/or inadequate monitoring; polydipsia, polyuria, and/or weight loss

Investigations: fasting glucose or HbA_{1c} test

PREGNANCY

Signs and symptoms: amenorrhea, especially during childbearing years (some experience spotting); sexual activity, especially without contraception or with inconsistent use of contraception; nausea or vomiting (common early sign); breast enlargement and tenderness; increased frequency of urination without other urinary symptoms; fatigue

Investigations: blood or urine β-hCG

OBSTRUCTIVE LESIONS

Signs and symptoms: constitutional symptoms (fever, weight loss, night sweats, fatigue); rectal bleeding or blood in the stool; increased bowel sounds (this can indicate early obstruction; bowel sounds may be decreased in later obstruction); possible enlarged lymph nodes in the groin; possible palpable abdominal mass

> History of colorectal carcinoma (this is a source of intrinsic lesions); carcinoma, sarcoma, lymphoma (these are sources of extrinsic lesions)

Investigations: colonoscopy, X-ray

ANORECTAL DISEASE

ANAL FISSURES OR HEMORRHOIDS

Signs and symptoms: history of anal fissures or hemorrhoids; small amounts of bright red blood following bowel movements; anal pain or irritation; anal fissures and/or hemorrhoids on physical exam

ANAL FISTULAS OR ABSCESSES

Signs and symptoms: history of inflammatory bowel disease (e.g., Crohn disease, ulcerative colitis); blood in the stool; abdominal pain; weight loss; fever; fatigue; fistulas and/or abscesses on physical exam

INFLAMMATORY BOWEL DISEASE

Signs and symptoms: younger than 30 (usually); family history of inflammatory bowel disease; fluctuating symptoms with periods of exacerbation and remission; diarrhea (possibly with nocturnal waking); blood in the stool; abdominal pain; weight loss; fever; fatigue; right lower quadrant and periumbilical pain; extraintestinal manifestations (e.g., uveitis, arthritis)

> Crohn disease: right lower quadrant mass, inflammation of the eyes, arthritis

Investigations: elevated CRP (this suggests active inflammation); fecal calprotectin; colonoscopy with biopsy (this is a standard diagnostic procedure); CT scan or MRI (findings: diagnostic structural changes associated with inflammatory bowel disease)

Strategy for patient encounter

The likely scenario is an adult patient with constipation. The specified tasks could engage history, physical exam, investigations, or management.

Be aware of risk factors for constipation (female, older age, inactivity, low caloric intake or low-fibre diet, polypharmacy, low income, low education level).

History

Start with open-ended questions about the onset, frequency, and quality of stools: When did the constipation start? How often do you have a bowel movement? What is the size and consistency of the stools? If the patient is female, ask if digital splinting of the vagina is necessary to have a bowel movement (this indicates pelvic floor dysfunction). Ask about other symptoms the patient has. Listen in particular for red flags (see the checklist) and constitutional symptoms (these suggest malignancy).

Use open-ended questions to take a medical and medication history: What conditions have you been diagnosed with? What medications do you take? Listen for neurogenic conditions, hypothyroidism, diabetes, cancer (colorectal carcinoma, other carcinoma, sarcoma, lymphoma), hemorrhoids, and irritable bowel syndrome; and for medications that cause constipation (see the information this resource lists in the MCC differential diagnosis). Ask about a family history of bowel cancer and inflammatory bowel disease. Ask whether the patient uses laxatives.

> **CHECKLIST**
>
> **Red flags in constipation**
>
> New-onset constipation in an elderly patient
>
> Anemia (symptoms: fatigue, pallor, dizziness, shortness of breath, tachycardia)
>
> Rectal bleeding or positive fecal occult blood test
>
> Family history of bowel cancer or inflammatory bowel disease
>
> Tenesmus
>
> Weight loss

Physical exam

Focus the physical exam on the abdomen and rectum. Look for abdominal masses, liver enlargement, and a palpable colon. Inspect the perineum for fissures, rectal prolapse, and hemorrhoids. Perform a digital rectal examination, looking for masses and fecal impaction.

(State that you will perform these exams. Since examinations of the rectum and perineum are not performed on standardized patients, the examiner will likely interrupt, ask what you are looking for, and provide findings.)

Investigations

Routine investigations in patients without red flags (see the checklist) are usually not indicated. If the diagnosis is uncertain, order a chest X-ray and abdominal films (flat and upright) to confirm the diagnosis of obstipation. In suspected anemia, consider ordering a complete blood count (CBC). In older patients, test the stool for occult blood. In suspected hypothyroidism, order a test for thyrotropin (TSH). Consider tests for electrolytes and calcium to rule out a metabolic cause. In patients older than 50, consider colonoscopy to rule out colorectal cancer.

> **TIP**
>
> ### Tailoring information to individual patients
>
> The MCC identifies providing generic information as a common exam error.
>
> To avoid this error, ask patients about aspects of their lives that might affect their condition. Provide information that targets their situation and engage the patient in figuring out next steps.
>
> For example, diet and exercise changes might be relevant for this case:
>
> - Ask what the patient ate yesterday for breakfast, lunch, and supper. Use this to personalize guidelines on dietary changes they need to make.
> - Ask what the patient did for exercise last week. Discuss short-term goals with the patient: What could the patient do next week to exercise every day? (For example, when could the patient fit in a 30-minute walk?)

Management

In patients without red flags, provide counselling on increasing dietary fibre and fluid intake, increasing exercise, and using laxatives as needed (magnesium hydroxide, lactulose, polyethylene glycol). If red flags are present, refer the patient to a gastroenterologist or surgeon for colonoscopy.

REFERENCE

1 Lacey B, Mearin F, Chang L, et al. Rome IV functional gastrointestinal disorders: disorders of gut-brain interaction. 4th ed. Vol. 2. Raleigh, NC: Rome Foundation; 2017. Chapter 11, Functional bowel disorders; 1393–1407.

28

Pediatric constipation

MCC particular objectives
None stated.

MCC differential diagnosis
with added evidence

PEDIATRIC CONSTIPATION IN GENERAL
The MCC notes that most pediatric constipation has a nonorganic cause.

NEONATES AND INFANTS

Diet-induced constipation
Signs and symptoms: formula feeding; introduction of solid foods; iron supplementation; possible impacted stool in rectum

Anatomic condition
Signs and symptoms: family history of Hirschsprung disease; passage of meconium > 48 hours after delivery; tight anal sphincter; empty rectum; palpable abdominal fecal mass
> Older children: abdominal distention; failure to thrive

Investigations: positive rectal biopsy

OLDER CHILDREN

Diet-induced constipation
The common cause is a diet low in fibre and fluid, and/or high in calcium.

Psychologically induced constipation
Signs and symptoms: excessive worry; loss of interest in friends and usual activities; changes in sleep habits; hallucinations or delusions; suicidal thoughts
> History of emotional, physical, or sexual abuse; substance abuse; recent stresses (e.g., death of a friend or family member)

Risk factors: family history of mental health disorders

Anatomic condition (e.g., bowel obstruction)

BOWEL OBSTRUCTION

Signs and symptoms: crampy abdominal pain; nausea, vomiting; change in bowel habits (diarrhea or constipation); abdominal distention; palpable abdominal mass; increased bowel sounds (this can indicate early obstruction: bowel sounds may be decreased in later obstruction); history of colonic diseases (diverticulitis, colon cancer, inflammatory bowel disease)

Risk factors: paralytic ileus (narcotic medications, chronic neuromuscular disease, diabetes), adhesions (abdominal surgery)

Investigations: abdominal X-ray

Neurologic condition

Signs and symptoms: symptoms of spinal cord injury (e.g., history of trauma; leg weakness; fatigue; lack of coordination); decreased anal tone and lack of stool in the rectum (usual); absent cremasteric reflex (in males) (usual); absent anal wink (in both sexes) (usual); decreased muscle tone and reflexes in the lower extremities (usual)

Endocrine or metabolic condition

DIABETES

Signs and symptoms: personal or family history of diabetes; history of diabetic complications and/or inadequate monitoring; polydipsia, polyuria, and/or weight loss

Investigations: fasting glucose or HbA_{1c} test

HYPOTHYROIDISM

Signs and symptoms: history of hypothyroidism or symptoms of hypothyroidism (cold intolerance, decreased reflexes, dry skin, weight gain, impaired cognition)

Investigations: elevated thyrotropin (TSH)

Other condition (e.g., celiac disease, cystic fibrosis)

CELIAC DISEASE

Signs and symptoms: family history of celiac disease, or signs and symptoms of celiac disease (chronic abdominal pain, rashes)

Investigations: positive serum anti-tTG (with IgA level); duodenal biopsy to detect villous blunting

CYSTIC FIBROSIS

Signs and symptoms: family history of cystic fibrosis; recurrent pneumonia; shortness of breath; productive cough; failure to thrive; fever; wheezing on lung auscultation

Investigations: positive sweat chloride test

Strategy for patient encounter

The likely scenario is a parent discussing a young child with constipation. The child will be absent on some pretext (e.g., a nurse is taking the child's vital signs and weight in another room). The specified tasks could engage history, physical exam, investigations, or management.

History

Start with open-ended questions about the frequency and quality of stools: How often does your child have a bowel movement? What is the size and consistency of the stools? Ask about other symptoms the child has and listen for evidence consistent with particular entities (e.g., mental health issues in psychologically induced constipation; nausea and vomiting in bowel obstruction; increased thirst and urine production in diabetes; chronic abdominal pain and rash in celiac disease; recurrent pneumonia, productive cough, and failure to thrive in cystic fibrosis).

Use open-ended questions to take a medical and medication history: What conditions has your child been diagnosed with? What surgeries has your child had? What medications does your child take? Listen for Hirschsprung disease, mental health issues, abdominal surgery, neuromuscular disease, spinal cord injury, colonic disease, diabetes, hypothyroidism, celiac disease, and cystic fibrosis; and for medications associated with constipation (e.g., opioids). Ask what conditions run in the family.

Ask about toileting behaviour (e.g., timing of bowel movements, toilet avoidance). Ask about diet, especially intake of dietary fibre.

Physical exam

Obtain the child's vital signs, looking for any abnormal signs. Measure the child's height, weight, and head circumference, and plot these on a growth chart. Examine the abdomen for tenderness and palpable stool in the large bowel. Perform a neurological exam, looking for decreased anal tone, absent anal wink, and lower limb weakness. Perform a rectal exam to look for impacted stool in the rectum.

(State that you will perform these exams. Because an actual pediatric patient is unlikely, and rectal exams are not performed on standardized patients in any case, the examiner may interrupt, ask what you are looking for, and provide findings.)

Investigations

If a rectal examination is not possible, consider abdominal X-ray to confirm constipation. If constipation is confirmed by exam or radiography, then no further investigations are needed.

Management

Rule out secondary causes (e.g., cystic fibrosis: pneumonia, failure to thrive; celiac disease: chronic abdominal pain, rash; Hirschsprung disease: bloating, failure to thrive). Stay alert to red flags (see the checklist). Treatment of functional constipation starts with disimpaction by enemas, rectal suppositories, or oral agents (polyethylene glycol, lactulose, mineral oil, senna). This is followed by maintenance medications (polyethylene glycol, lactulose) and increased dietary fibre.

> **CHECKLIST**
> ## Red flags in pediatric constipation
> Abnormal anatomy
> Signs or symptoms of hypothyroidism
> Signs or symptoms of cystic fibrosis
> Signs or symptoms of diabetes
> Findings on neurological exam
> Poor growth
> Bilious vomiting
> Ileus

Pearls

Most patients (95%) have functional constipation characterized by infrequent, large-calibre stools.

29

Contraception

MCC particular objective

Discuss options for contraception.

MCC list of contraceptive methods

NONPERMANENT CONTRACEPTION

Hormonal contraception

ORAL CONTRACEPTIVES

Failure rate: 1% per year if taken as prescribed (3% compliance failure)

Potential complications:

> Estrogen effects: worse migraines, increased body weight, higher blood pressure, aggravation of uterine fibromas, nausea

> Progesterone effects: depression, acne, more body hair, breast tenderness

> Risk factors for complications: smoking, preexisting coagulopathy

No protection from sexually transmitted infections (STIs)

Drug interactions (the following may decrease the effectiveness of oral contraceptives): antacids; H_2 blockers; proton pump inhibitors; antiepileptic drugs; Rifabutin and Rifampicin (antibiotics); antiretroviral drugs; St. John's wort (herbal medication)

PROGESTERONE IMPLANT, PATCH, OR INJECTION (E.G., DEPO-PROVERA)

Failure rate: 0.1% per year

Potential complications:

> Progesterone effects: depression, acne, increased body hair, breast tenderness

> Risk factors for complications: none

No STI protection

Drug interactions: antiepileptic drugs may decrease effectiveness

Barrier methods

CONDOM

Failure rate: 3% per year if consistently used (some inconvenience is involved)

Potential complications: latex allergy or reaction

STI protection

No drug interactions

DIAPHRAGM

Failure rate: 6% per year

Potential complications: increased urinary tract infections; allergy to latex or nonoxyl-9 (the active ingredient in spermicidal jelly)

Possibly some STI protection

No drug interactions

VAGINAL SPONGE

Failure rate: 12% per year if consistently used (some inconvenience is involved)

Potential complications: allergy to nonoxyl-9; vaginal irritation or dryness; increased urinary tract infections

No STI protection

No drug interactions

Intrauterine device (IUD)

Failure rate: 1% per year

Potential complications:

> Copper IUD: cramping, midcycle bleeding, heavy periods
>
> Copper or progesterone IUD: ectopic pregnancy, pelvic inflammatory disease, perforation, expulsion
>
> Risk factors for complications: chlamydia or gonorrhea; previous ectopic pregnancy

No STI protection

No drug interactions

Other (e.g., abstinence)

ABSTINENCE

Abstinence, if maintained, has no risk of failure or complications.

If not maintained, however—especially if the person involved is not prepared for sex—the chance of pregnancy averages around 5% per act of sexual intercourse, and increases to 25% in the 2 days before ovulation. Lack of preparation also provides no protection from STIs.

PHYSIOLOGIC METHODS (RHYTHM, COITUS INTERRUPTUS)

Failure rate: 25% per year (note that rhythm requires regular menstrual cycles)

Potential complications: none

Risk factors for complications: none

No STI protection

No drug interactions

PERMANENT CONTRACEPTION

Male sterilization (vasectomy)

Failure rate: < 1%

Potential complications: postvasectomy pain; **no** reliable evidence for increased risk of prostate cancer, dementia, or heart disease, despite earlier reports of an association

Risk factors for complications: none

No STI protection

No drug interactions

Female sterilization (tubal ligation)

Failure rate: < 1%

Potential complications: surgical complications (e.g., reactions to anesthetic, wound infection, blood loss)

> Risk factors for complications: previous pelvic or abdominal surgery; obesity; diabetes

No STI protection

No drug interactions

Strategy for patient encounter

The likely scenario is a couple seeking contraception information. The specified tasks could engage history, physical exam, investigations, or management.

History

Start with open-ended questions to obtain a general medical history and medication history: What conditions have you been diagnosed with? What medications do you take? In women, listen for venous thromboembolism, myocardial infarction, and stroke (these suggest coagulopathy, which oral contraceptives can make worse); and medications that interact with oral contraceptives (e.g., antacids, antiretroviral drugs, antiepileptics). In both patients, listen for allergies (relevant to some barrier methods). Check risk factors for combination oral contraceptives (see the checklist).

CHECKLIST

Contraindications for combination oral contraceptives

Venous thromboembolism

Thrombogenic mutations

Ischemic heart disease

Current breast cancer

Migraine with aura

Older than 35 and smoking more than 15 cigarettes per day

Uncontrolled hypertension (≥ 160/100 mmHg

Take a menstrual history. Ask about previous methods of contraception and previous pregnancies. Ask about smoking.

Check risk factors for sexually transmitted infections (STIs): unprotected sex with multiple partners or new partners; working in the sex trade; sexual contact with sex workers; age 15 to 24; prior STIs; alcohol or drug abuse; and forced sexual intercourse.

Physical exam
Obtain the woman's vital signs, looking for hypertension. Ask when she last had a Pap test, and perform a Pap smear, if indicated by provincial guidelines.

(If indicated, state that you will perform a Pap smear, in keeping with provincial guidelines. Since this exam is not performed on standardized patients, the examiner will likely interrupt and acknowledge this step.)

Investigations
Order a pregnancy test.

If either patient has risk factors for STIs, swab for gonorrhea and chlamydia.

Management
Counsel both partners (the likely scenario is a couple seeking information). Discuss contraception options and emergency backup. Counsel all women who smoke to stop before starting oral contraceptives. Women older than 35 who smoke should not be prescribed combined oral contraceptives. The choice of contraceptive technique should take into account the patients' preferences and the presence of contraindications.

30

Cough

MCC particular objective

Distinguish benign from serious causes that require full investigation and further management.

MCC differential diagnosis
with added evidence

ACUTE COUGH

Infectious cough

PNEUMONIA

This is the key concern with infectious cough.

Signs and symptoms: shortness of breath; cough; purulent sputum; chest pain on coughing or deep breaths; fatigue; tachypnea; tachycardia; decreased oxygen saturation; lung crackles on auscultation; lung dullness on percussion

> Children: fever

> Elderly: confusion, low body temperature

Risk factors: very old, very young, smoking, immune compromise (e.g., due to chronic illness), hospitalization

Investigations: chest X-ray to detect consolidation

Irritant-induced cough

Common irritants include tobacco smoke, pollen, dust, and animal dander.

Signs and symptoms: history of environmental allergies or asthma; runny nose or postnasal drip; exposure to known allergens

Other condition (e.g., cardiac condition)

CARDIAC CONDITION

Signs and symptoms: chest pain (often); shortness of breath; personal or family history of cardiac disease (e.g., myocardial infarction, pericarditis, congestive heart failure); abnormal heart sounds; lung rales

> Congestive heart failure: increased jugular venous pressure, dependent edema

> Pericarditis: autoimmune disease, uremia

Investigations: elevated cardiac enzymes (e.g., troponin) (this suggests myocardial infarction); ECG; chest X-ray to detect possible pulmonary edema

CHRONIC COUGH (LASTING 3 WEEKS OR LONGER)

Upper respiratory condition

Signs and symptoms: postnasal drip; frequent throat clearing; sinus pain on palpation (this suggests sinusitis); mucous in the oropharynx and/or cobblestone appearance to the mucosa; normal lung sounds

Pulmonary condition

CHRONIC BRONCHITIS

Signs and symptoms: frequent exposure to irritants (e.g., workplace exposure; firsthand or secondhand smoke), wheezing

Investigations: reduced capacity on pulmonary function testing

COUGH-VARIANT ASTHMA

Signs and symptoms: worse symptoms after exercise and/or on exposure to irritants (e.g., workplace exposure; firsthand or secondhand smoke), wheezing

Investigations: lung hyperinflation on chest X-ray

BRONCHOGENIC CARCINOMA

Signs and symptoms: history of smoking (usual); constitutional symptoms (fever, weight loss, night sweats, fatigue); enlarged lymph nodes in the neck and axilla

Investigations: chest X-ray to detect mass

INTERSTITIAL LUNG DISEASE

Investigations: prominent interstitium on CT scan of the lungs; reduced capacity on pulmonary function testing

Gastrointestinal condition (e.g., gastroesophageal reflux)

GASTROESOPHAGEAL REFLUX DISEASE

Signs and symptoms: burning chest pain radiating into the throat (often with a bitter taste in the mouth or regurgitation of food into the mouth; often worse with lying down; often better with standing up or taking antacids; worse with spicy food, coffee, alcohol, fatty foods, peppermint), acid damage to teeth

Risk factors: obesity, pregnancy

Cardiac condition—see above

Other condition (e.g., drug-induced condition, work-related exposure)

DRUG-INDUCED CONDITION

Examples of drugs include ACE inhibitors and oxymetazoline (Afrin).

WORK-RELATED EXPOSURE

Examples of exposures are dust (e.g., farming, demolition),

particulates (e.g., metal work), smoke (e.g., firefighting), and chemicals (e.g., laboratory work, construction).

Signs and symptoms: cough that occurs or worsens at work

Strategy for patient encounter

The likely scenario is an adult patient with a history of cough. The specified tasks could engage history, physical exam, investigations, or management.

History

Start with open-ended inquiry about the cough: How long have you had it? What triggers have you noticed? What other symptoms do you have? The duration defines the cough as acute (less than 3 weeks), subacute (3 to 8 weeks), or chronic (more than 8 weeks). Listen for aggravating factors such as smoke (including smoking), occupational or recreational exposures, exertion, and cold air; and symptoms consistent with particular entities (e.g., heart burn in gastroesophageal reflux; shortness of breath in pneumonia; chest pain in cardiac conditions). Ask about the presence and quality of sputum. Ask about constitutional symptoms (fever, fatigue, night sweats, weight loss).

Use open-ended questions to take a medical and medication history: What conditions have you been diagnosed with? What medications do you take? Listen for asthma, gastroesophageal reflux, environmental allergies, cancer, tuberculosis, and AIDS; and for possible contributing medications (ACE inhibitors, beta-blockers). Ask about recent colds. Ask about a family history of environmental allergies or asthma.

Ask about exposure to tuberculosis and endemic fungal diseases. Take a travel history.

Physical exam

Examine the nose for obstruction and discharge. Examine the throat, oropharynx, the external acoustic meatus, and the tympanic membranes. Auscultate the heart and lungs.

Investigations

For cough lasting more than 2 weeks, order a chest X-ray. Consider pulmonary function testing to diagnose asthma. If the cough is productive, consider submitting a sputum culture for microscopic analysis.

Management

Management will depend on the specific cause identified. Remember that the 3 most common causes are rhinosinusitis (e.g., allergies), asthma, and gastroesophageal reflux (GERD). Treatment for asthma includes inhaled glucocorticoids and bronchodilators. Treatment for GERD includes proton pump inhibitors or H_2 blockers. Treatments for postnasal drip include antihistamines, glucocorticoids, and decongestants. For cough without a specific cause, consider the use of cough suppressants.

TIP

Management of workplace risks and exposures

This clinical presentation may involve a workplace exposure. The MCC objectives for the exam identify work-related health issues as an important area of clinical practice.

In a suspected work-related health issue:

- Clarify the aspects of the patient's workplace that pose risks.
- Consider ways to reduce the patient's risks, including, if necessary, recommending the patient change jobs.
- Identify risks with potential impacts on the health and safety of the patient's coworkers, and report these to public health authorities.

31

Cyanosis, hypoxia

MCC particular objective

Determine if hypoxia or hypoxemia is present.

MCC differential diagnosis
with added evidence

CENTRAL CYANOSIS OR HYPOXIA

CENTRAL CYANOSIS OR HYPOXIA IN GENERAL

Signs and symptoms: mental status changes; bluing of the lips and mucous membranes; tachycardia (except for opioid overdose); tachypnea (except for opioid overdose)

High alveolar-arterial (A-a) gradient

SHUNTING (E.G., TETRALOGY OF FALLOT, ACUTE RESPIRATORY DISTRESS SYNDROME)

TETRALOGY OF FALLOT

Signs and symptoms: newborn or infant; heart murmur

Investigations: decreased oxygen on ABG; characteristic heart defects on chest X-ray, echocardiogram; right ventricular hypertrophy on ECG

ACUTE RESPIRATORY DISTRESS SYNDROME (ARDS)

Signs and symptoms: recent critical illness (e.g., sepsis; severe pneumonia; major trauma; serious smoke or chemical inhalation); severe shortness of breath

Investigations: decreased oxygen on ABG; bilateral infiltrates on chest X-ray

VQ (VENTILATION-PERFUSION) MISMATCH (E.G., CYSTIC FIBROSIS, PULMONARY EMBOLUS)

CYSTIC FIBROSIS

Signs and symptoms: family history of cystic fibrosis; recurrent pneumonia; shortness of breath; productive cough; failure to thrive; fever; wheezing on lung auscultation

Investigations: positive sweat chloride test

PULMONARY EMBOLISM

Signs and symptoms: sharp chest pain; shortness of breath; cough (possibly with blood); hypoxia; possible unilateral swelling of the lower limbs (this indicates deep vein thrombosis); elevated pulse and respiratory rate; arrhythmias; lung rales on auscultation; lower-lung dullness on percussion; motor or sensory deficits

Risk factors: heart failure; cancer; surgery; prolonged immobility (e.g., long plane trips); smoking; estrogen replacement therapy; oral contraceptives; current pregnancy; previous deep vein thrombosis, embolism, or stroke; family history of embolism

Investigations: elevated D-dimer level; area of reduced pulmonary perfusion on V/Q scan; CT angiography to detect blocked vessel

DIFFUSION IMPAIRMENT (E.G., RESTRICTIVE LUNG DISEASE)

RESTRICTIVE LUNG DISEASE

Signs and symptoms: dry cough (usual), progressive exertional shortness of breath (usual)

Risk factors: family history of restrictive lung disease; occupational exposure to asbestos or heavy metals (e.g., construction, farming, mining)

Normal A-a gradient

HYPOVENTILATION (E.G., OPIOID OVERDOSE)

OPIOID OVERDOSE

Signs and symptoms: bradycardia; constricted pupils; confusion, stupor, or coma; nystagmus; gait disturbance; history of opioid abuse, or signs of abuse (track marks on the arms)

HIGH ALTITUDE

Signs and symptoms: current or recent exposure to high altitudes; shortness of breath; elevated pulse

PERIPHERAL CYANOSIS OR HYPOXIA (E.G., LOW CARDIAC OUTPUT, COLD EXPOSURE)

PERIPHERAL CYANOSIS OR HYPOXIA IN GENERAL

Definition: cyanosis of ≥ 1 extremities

LOW CARDIAC OUTPUT

Signs and symptoms: history of congestive heart failure; shortness of breath; increased jugular venous pressure; dependent edema; livedo reticularis; lung rales on auscultation; heart murmurs or extra sounds on auscultation

Investigations: ECG; pulmonary edema on chest X-ray

COLD EXPOSURE

Patients suffering from cold exposure have hypothermia.

Strategy for patient encounter

The likely scenario is an adult patient with central cyanosis (V/Q mismatch or diffusion impairment). The specified tasks could engage history, physical exam, investigations, or management.

History

Use open-ended questions to obtain a history of the cyanosis. When was it first noted and by whom? How constant is it? What parts of the body does it affect? Listen for acute versus gradual onset (acute onset suggests a recent trigger such as an embolus or overdose); intermittent versus constant symptoms (intermittent symptoms suggest reversible causes such as pulmonary embolus); symptoms in the extremities only (this suggests peripheral cyanosis) versus the central body (central cyanosis). Obtain a smoking history. Obtain a medical and medication history, looking for recent critical illness, cardiovascular disease, and lung disease, and drugs associated with hypoventilation (opioids), methemoglobinemia (nitrites, topical anesthetics, dapsone, phenytoin, sulfonamides, metoclopramide), and sulfhemoglobinemia (e.g., sulfonamides, sulfasalazine).

Physical exam
Examine the patient for the pattern of cyanosis (central versus peripheral). Perform a full physical examination paying special attention to the cardiorespiratory system.

Investigations
Order a test for arterial blood gases (ABG).

You will probably be asked to calculate the alveolar-arterial gradient. This is estimated as:

$$[150 \text{ mmHg} - (5/4 \times \text{PaCO}_2)] - \text{PaO}_2$$

A normal A-a gradient is:

$$(\text{age} \div 4) + 4$$

See the checklist for the differential diagnosis of increased and normal A-a gradients. Consider methemoglobinemia or sulfhemoglobinemia in patients with cyanosis and normal oxygenation. Methemoglobinemia and sulfhemoglobinemia are both diagnosed by cooximetry.

Management
Treat the underlying cause identified. Methemoglobinemia is reversible with methylene blue, with or without ascorbic acid. In cases of sulfhemoglobinemia, or when methylene blue is contraindicated in methemoglobinemia, treatment with hyperbaric oxygen prevents tissue hypoxia.

CHECKLIST
Interpretation of A-a gradient
Increased in:
- right-to-left intrapulmonary shunt
- congestive heart failure
- pneumonia
- pulmonary embolism
- atelectasis
- obstructive lung disease (e.g., asthma, chronic obstructive pulmonary disease)
- pneumothorax
- interstitial lung disease

Normal in:
- hypoventilation
- neuromuscular disorders
- central nervous system disorders
- high altitudes

32

Limp in children

MCC particular objective

Rule out the most serious diagnoses, which are usually unilateral.

MCC differential diagnosis
with added evidence

CONGENITAL CONDITIONS

Lower limbs, spine

HIP DYSPLASIA

Signs and symptoms: long-standing limp with no pain (usual); walking on the toes of the foot (this is especially true in older children); limited range of motion in the hips; 1 leg shorter than the other (often)

Investigations: bilateral hip X-ray to detect subluxation of 1 or both hips

COXA VARA

Signs and symptoms: waddling gait with no pain (usual); mild discrepancy in limb length

Investigations: bilateral hip X-ray to detect unilaterally prominent greater trochanter

ACQUIRED CONDITIONS

Infection

SEPTIC ARTHRITIS

Signs and symptoms: fever (often); severe pain, usually in 1 joint
> History of recent joint injury and/or surgery; structural joint abnormality; recent or current infections (e.g., genitourinary, pulmonary, skin); systemic disease (e.g., diabetes mellitus, liver disease, malignancy, chronic kidney disease); use of immunosuppressants; **no** vaccine for *Haemophilus influenzae type b* (Hib)

Investigations: elevated WBCs; very high CRP; synovial fluid analysis (WBCs, Gram stain, culture)

VIRAL SYNOVITIS

Signs and symptoms: low-grade fever (usual); pain (this is not as severe as in septic arthritis), usually in 1 joint; history of recent viral illness (usual)

Investigations: X-ray, ultrasound of affected joint to detect effusion

Inflammation

JUVENILE IDIOPATHIC ARTHRITIS

Signs and symptoms: swollen, tender joints; skin rash; iritis

Investigations: normal WBCs; moderately high CRP; X-ray of affected joints to detect bony overgrowth, decreased joint space, decreased bone density

Tumour

Signs and symptoms: weakness in the lower limbs; possible palpable mass in the abdomen, pelvis, back

> Malignant: constitutional symptoms (fever, weight loss, night sweats, fatigue)
>
> Benign: often asymptomatic

Investigations: WBCs; CRP; X-ray, CT scan, MRI, and/or nuclear scan

OTHER

Growing pains

Signs and symptoms: bilateral leg pain; pain that occurs only at night; no pain or limp during the day

Pain amplification syndromes

Signs and symptoms: pain in several parts of the body (e.g., headache, abdominal pain); pain from light touching of the skin

> History of sedentary lifestyle, inadequate sleep

Strategy for patient encounter

This patient encounter will likely involve an adolescent (the minimum age to play standardized patients is 16) who has growing pains. The specified tasks could engage history, physical exam, investigations, or management.

History

Use open-ended questions to obtain a history of the limp: When did it start? What other symptoms do you have? Listen for evidence consistent with particular entities (e.g., long-standing limp with no pain in hip dysplasia; sudden-onset fever and unilateral severe pain in infection; lower-limb weakness and constitutional symptoms in malignant tumour).

Note that the MCC includes slipped capital femoral epiphysis in clinical presentation 72 (oligoarthralgia), where the presenting symptom is pain. It would be wise to also consider this disorder in the differential diagnosis for this clinical presentation (pediatric limp), because it can cause altered gait (limping, 1 leg turned outward, and/or waddling gait) and is the most common hip disorder in adolescents.

If the patient has pain, ask how constant it is. Listen for suggestive patterns of pain (e.g., pain only at night suggests growing pains; hip pain that becomes worse with physical activity suggests slipped epiphysis). Pay particular attention to the presence of red flags for septic arthritis (see the checklist). Ask about possible trauma associated with the symptoms. Screen for possible child abuse.

Physical exam

Obtain the patient's vital signs, looking for fever. Observe the patient's gait while walking and running. Palpate the legs, hips, and pelvis for tenderness. Examine the patient for bruising, swelling, redness, and deformities. Assess the active and passive range of motion in each joint.

Perform the following specific tests:

- **Trendelenburg sign:** Ask the patient to stand on the affected limb and lift the unaffected limb from the floor. A positive sign is when the pelvis drops down toward the unaffected side.
- **Galeazzi sign:** In the supine position, the patient flexes their hips and knees, with knees together. Assess for leg length discrepancy by noting if 1 knee is lower than the other.
- **Test for flexion, abduction, and external rotation (FABER test):** With the patient supine, flex, abduct, and externally rotate the hip joint. A positive test is when pain occurs in the sacroiliac joint.
- **Pelvic compression test:** With the patient supine, compress the iliac wings toward each other looking for pain in the sacroiliac joint.
- **Psoas sign:** With the patient lying on their side, passively extend the hip. Pain indicates a positive test.

Investigations

Order anteroposterior and lateral X-rays of both lower extremities.

In suspected hip effusion, order a hip ultrasound. A bone scan should be ordered if other imaging is negative. In suspected septic arthritis (see the checklist), aspirate the joint and submit the specimen for Gram stain, culture, and cell count. In suspected osteomyelitis, obtain blood and bone cultures. Order a complete blood count (CBC) and C-reactive protein (CRP) level to assess for infection, inflammatory arthritis, and malignancy.

CHECKLIST
Red flags for septic arthritis
Severe, unilateral joint pain
Temperature > 38.5°C
Refusal to bear weight on the affected leg
ESR > 40 mm/hour or CRP level > 2.0 mg/dL
WBCs > 12.0×10^9/L

Management

Management will depend on the specific entity identified. Consider referring the patient to a pediatrician or orthopedic surgeon.

33

Developmental delay

MCC particular objective

Use a validated developmental screening tool to identify domains of developmental delay (children may have delay in 1 or more domains).

MCC differential diagnosis
with added evidence

GLOBAL DEVELOPMENTAL DELAY

Neurological disorders (e.g., fetal alcohol spectrum disorder, cerebral dysgenesis)

Signs and symptoms (in general): neurological abnormalities, growth abnormalities, dysmorphic features

History of seizures; complications during gestation (e.g., toxin exposure such as alcohol) and/or delivery

Genetic and metabolic disorders (e.g., trisomy 21, congenital hypothyroidism)

TRISOMY 21 (DOWN SYNDROME)

Signs and symptoms: characteristic dysmorphic features (small head, flattened facial features, protruding tongue, upward slanting eyes, small hands and feet, short fingers, single crease on the palms of the hands)

> Other: ligamentous laxity

Risk factors: older maternal age, siblings with Down syndrome

Investigations: karyotyping, X-rays of target areas to assess development

CONGENITAL HYPOTHYROIDISM

This is generally diagnosed at birth: newborn thyroid screening is a requirement in most of North America.

Signs and symptoms: often asymptomatic at birth, jaundice, frequent choking, large tongue, puffy appearance to the face

Investigations: thyrotropin (TSH), thyroxine

Toxic exposures (e.g., lead)

LEAD

A common source of lead exposure is deteriorating lead paint in pre-1979 houses.

Signs and symptoms: neurological abnormalities, growth abnormalities

Investigations: elevated serum lead level

Severe psychosocial deprivation

Examples include childhood institutionalization, severe abuse, and/or severe neglect.

SPEECH AND LANGUAGE DELAY

Hearing impairment

Signs and symptoms: problems identifying the sources of sounds; complications during gestation (e.g., toxin exposure such as alcohol) and/or delivery; blocked tympanic membranes (e.g., from impacted wax or mass) or nonmobile tympanic membranes (from chronic effusion) (possible)

Investigations: hearing test

Autism spectrum disorder (when associated with atypical social and behavioural features)[1(pp50–51)]

Signs and symptoms: deficits in social interaction and communication; repetitive, stereotyped behaviours (motor and/or vocal); restricted interests; sensory problems; presence of symptoms in all contexts (e.g., home, school); presence of symptoms from early childhood

Developmental language disorder

Signs and symptoms: impaired language skills for a child's age (e.g., impairments with mastery of vocabulary, sentence structure, conversation); impairments with significant impact on the child's day-to-day life; presence of impairments from early childhood

MOTOR DELAY

Cerebral palsy

Signs and symptoms: history of complications during gestation (e.g., toxin exposure such as alcohol) and/or delivery; abnormal posture and/or physical movement; growth abnormalities

Muscular dystrophies

MUSCULAR DYSTROPHY

Common types of muscular dystrophy include Duchenne (more common in males), Becker, facioscapulohumeral, and myotonic.

Signs and symptoms: frequent falls; difficulty getting up from sitting or lying; difficulty running, jumping; waddling gait; walking on the toes; muscle pain, stiffness; large calf muscles

Risk factors: family history of muscular dystrophy

Investigations: muscle biopsy, increased creatine kinase, EMG, genetic testing

Developmental coordination disorder

Signs and symptoms: impaired motor skills for a child's age; impairments with significant impact on the child's day-to-day life; presence of impairments from early childhood

Strategy for patient encounter

This encounter will likely involve parents discussing a child who has less language than the child's same-age peers. The child will be absent on some pretext (e.g., a nurse is taking the child's vital signs and weight in another room).

A complete general physical exam is warranted in this patient encounter, including a full neurological exam. But an actual pediatric patient is unlikely, and the MCC's particular objective focuses on developmental screening tools. So, the scenario for this patient encounter will likely specify screening for development delay and not physical exam. It could also specify investigations or management.

History

A detailed history is key to identifying potential developmental problems. Use open-ended questions to establish the child's symptoms, prenatal history, birth history, family history, social context, and toxic exposures.

- **Symptoms:** What concerns do you have about your child's development? Inquire about specific symptoms in the child including aggression, self-injury, hyperactivity, inattention, anxiety, depression, sleep problems, unusual or repetitive behaviours, lack of friends, and poor school performance.
- **Prenatal history:** What complications did you (the mother) have during the pregnancy for this child? Listen for prenatal infections, prenatal toxic exposures (e.g., alcohol), and abnormal results from prenatal screening.
- **Birth history:** What complications did you have during the delivery of this child? What was the gestational age of your child at birth? What was your group B streptococcus status? What was the child's Apgar score?
- **Family history:** What conditions run in your family? Listen for a family history of developmental delay and/or genetic abnormalities.
- **Social history:** What is your financial situation? What is your living situation? Listen for evidence of poverty and unstable living conditions. Ask whether the family has a history of neglect or abuse (e.g., emotional, physical, sexual), or a history of substance abuse. Ask if there is consanguinity between the parents.
- **Toxic exposures:** What concerns do you have about toxic exposures for your child? Listen for concerns about lead and other toxins.

Developmental screening

Use a validated screening tool to assess the child for developmental delay (see the quick reference).

QUICK REFERENCE

Developmental screening tools

The MCC specifies a validated multidomain developmental screening tool for this clinical presentation. A variety of tools are possible. Know which tool you would recommend, depending on the case scenario.

The Denver II screening tool is widely used, and available for free download from Denver Developmental Materials, Inc.

The Canadian Paediatric Society lists several multidomain screening tools. Here, for example, are screening tools for younger children, which fit the likely scenario for this patient encounter. Note that factors such as age range and completion time will affect their fit with different situations.

SCREENING TOOL	AGE RANGE	TIME TO COMPLETE
Ages and Stages Questionnaires (ASQ)	4 months–5 years	10–20 minutes
Child Development Inventory	15 months–16 years	30–50 minutes
Nipissing District Developmental Screen	Infant–6 years	Less than 5 minutes
Parents' Evaluation of Developmental Status (PEDS)	Birth–11 years	Less than 10 minutes

You can read descriptions of these tools online. Note that none are available for free, except for the Nipissing District Developmental Screen, which is free to clinicians in Ontario.

Investigations

Order hearing and vision tests. Consider karyotyping to detect chromosomal abnormalities and fluorescence in situ hybridization (FISH) for microdeletions. Order a test for thyrotropin (TSH) to look for hypothyroidism. Order a screening panel for metabolic disorders, including serum glucose, electrolytes, lactate, ammonia, liver function tests, pyruvate, albumin, triglycerides, uric acid, quantitative amino acids, and creatine kinase, as well as urine organic acids. Consider a head CT scan and electroencephalogram (EEG).

Management

Refer children with any identified delays for diagnostic assessment and intervention. Identify any modifiable conditions (toxic exposure, neglect). Consider referring patients to medical genetics for further investigations.

Pearls

Note that developmental assessment is an ongoing process involving screening, surveillance, and definitive diagnostic assessment. Screening should occur at each regular pediatric visit using a validated screening tool. Surveillance involves parental interview and direct observation in the office.

REFERENCE

1 American Psychiatric Association. Diagnostic and statistical manual of mental disorders. 5th ed. Arlington, VA: American Psychiatric Association; 2013. 59–60. 991 p.

34

Adults with developmental disabilities

MCC particular objectives

Identify common physical, mental, and behavioural issues.

Pay particular attention to:

- known disparities in health status and health care for adults with developmental disabilities
- adapting communication to the patient's level
- interdisciplinary coordination of care

MCC differential diagnosis
with added evidence

The focus of this clinical presentation is to identify and manage common health issues in adults with developmental disabilities.

GENERAL HEALTH ISSUES AND RISKS

Abuse and neglect

Risk factors: older age; female; noncompliance with medication; mental illness; lack of follow-up with medical appointments; repeated emergency room visits or hospital admissions; lack of a social network; dependence on a caregiver; living alone; inadequate housing; poverty; unexplained weight loss or failure to thrive; poor grooming and/or hygiene

Atypical presentations of serious illness and/or pain (e.g., infection, trauma)

Signs and symptoms: change in mood or personality; irritability; change in appetite; change in sleep habits

COMMON HEALTH ISSUES AND RISKS BY ETIOLOGY

DEVELOPMENTAL DISABILITIES IN GENERAL

The MCC objectives for the exam focus on the disorders in the following breakdown.

The MCC notes that developmental disability may be idiopathic.

Genetic syndromes (e.g., Down syndrome)

DOWN SYNDROME

Susceptibilities and risks: hearing loss; obstructive sleep apnea; ear infections; cataracts; severe refractive errors; ongoing problems stemming from congenital heart defects; gastrointestinal atresia; hip dislocation; thyroid disease; risks related to reproductive health

Autism spectrum disorder

Susceptibilities and risks: depression, anxiety, bipolar disorder, psychosis, diabetes, gastrointestinal disorders, epilepsy, sleep disorders, high cholesterol, high blood pressure, obesity

Fetal alcohol spectrum disorder

Susceptibilities and risks: health issues linked to poverty and/or homelessness (people with fetal alcohol spectrum disorder often have cognitive and behavioural issues that lead to unemployment and inadequate housing); cognitive issues such as attention and memory deficits; behavioural issues such as poor impulse control

Brain injury (e.g., cerebral palsy)

CEREBRAL PALSY

Susceptibilities and risks: seizures, respiratory infections, gastroesophageal reflux, obesity, dental diseases, urinary tract infections, osteoporosis

Central nervous system infection

Susceptibilities and risks: seizures, memory problems, cognitive changes

Strategy for patient encounter

The likely scenario is a mentally challenged adult with a recent decline in function, whose caregiver is present. Screening and case findings will likely figure prominently in this encounter, because atypical presentations of serious illnesses are common among individuals with developmental disabilities. It is also important to remember that these individuals often have complex health issues, and are often underdiagnosed.

A complete general physical exam is warranted in this patient encounter, as a way to screen for possible multiple health issues, including trauma. But the exam's time limitations will likely eliminate it as a task. The scenario will more likely specify history, investigations, or management.

History

The MCC's objectives for the exam identify the following as key elements for this history: assessing the patient's level of intellectual and adaptive functioning; and communicating appropriately.

Validated scales to assess intellectual and adaptive functioning are best administered by psychologists. The case scenario may therefore provide the results of psychologist-administered tests for you to interpret (see the quick reference on intellectual and adaptive functioning scales).

Clear and simple language is useful for every patient, but it is especially important for adults with developmental disabilities. Prepare a strategy in advance of the exam for communicating with people at different levels of functioning. For example, for patients with severe developmental disabilities, ask whether you can speak to family or caregivers (with the patient's permission, ask family or caregivers directly for information, or consult family

---

QUICK REFERENCE

Scales for assessing intellectual functioning and adaptive functioning

INTELLECTUAL FUNCTIONING SCALES	ADAPTIVE FUNCTIONING SCALES
Stanford-Binet Intelligence Scales, Fifth Edition (SB5)	Adaptive Behavior Assessment System, Second Edition (ABAS-II)
Universal Nonverbal Intelligence Test (UNIT)	Comprehensive Test of Adaptive Behavior (CTAB)
Wechsler Adult Intelligence Scale, Fourth Edition (WAIS-IV)	Scales of Independent Behavior Revised (SIB-R)
	Vineland Adaptive Behavior Scales, Second Edition (Vineland-II)

Know how to interpret results from these tests.

and caregivers on strategies they have found helpful for communicating with the patient). Consider how to phrase questions and ideas clearly and simply (see the tip on communication).

Use open-ended questions to establish the patient's disability and current symptoms: What disability do you have? How have you been feeling? Why have you come to see me? Listen for evidence consistent with particular entities, especially common entities such as arthritis, urinary tract infection, dysmenorrhea, constipation, and dental disease (these are all possible causes of decline in function); and for difficulties communicating and/or changes in behaviour (these may indicate the presence of pain). Remain aware that complex issues and atypical presentations are likely.

> **TIP**
>
> ## Communicating with clear and simple language
>
> Avoid jargon. For example, say *urinary tract infections* instead of *UTIs*.
>
> Check for understanding. For example, does the patient know what a urinary tract infection is? If not, give some basic information.
>
> Rephrase. For example, try *pee* instead of *urine*.
>
> Break questions down into concise, single-idea components. For example, don't ask: *What prescription medications do you take?* Instead ask: *Have you seen a doctor before? Has a doctor told you to take medicine? What medicine?*

Screen for risk factors for abuse and neglect: How often do you need to see a doctor? Where do you live? Who lives with you? Who helps you when you need help? How do you get the money you need? Listen for evidence of frequent trips to emergency, living alone, social isolation, and financial and housing insecurity.

Investigations

In all patients, order a complete blood count (CBC) to assess for anemia and infection, and urinalysis to look for urinary tract infection.

In patients with Down syndrome, order a test for thyrotropin (TSH), to screen for thyroid disease.

Note that men with developmental disabilities have an increased risk of hypogonadism. In young adult men, consider ordering a serum testosterone level to screen for this.

Remember that cancer screening is often missed in patients with developmental disabilities, including screening for prostate cancer, breast cancer, and colon cancer. Order screening, as appropriate.

Management

Treat any identified underlying disorder.

Psychiatric disorders are common in patients with developmental disorders, but can be difficult to diagnose. Consider referring the patient to a psychiatrist.

Encourage regular physical activity and supplementation with oral vitamin D.

Patients with developmental disabilities need interdisciplinary care. Aim to create systematic follow-up with these patients to coordinate their care, including:

- up-to-date immunizations for influenza, *Streptococcus pneumoniae*, human papillomavirus (HPV), hepatitis A virus (HAV), and hepatitis B virus (HBV)
- regular medication reviews to reduce or eliminate medications that are no longer necessary
- assessment for abuse and neglect (report abuse and neglect to the police, and refer patients to community support agencies as necessary)
- capacity for consent, which needs regular reassessment
- care plans, including advance directives
- regular dental care
- regular vision and hearing assessments

35

Acute diarrhea

MCC particular objectives

Identify risk factors associated with specific causes.

Assess for complications (volume loss, electrolyte abnormalities).

MCC differential diagnosis
with added evidence

ACUTE DIARRHEA IN GENERAL

Definition: abrupt-onset disturbance of stool frequency or stool consistency

INFECTION

GASTROENTERITIS IN GENERAL

Signs and symptoms: abrupt-onset diarrhea; crampy abdominal pain; nausea, vomiting; fever (this suggests viral infection); blood in the stool (this suggests bacterial infection)

VIRUSES

Common viruses include norovirus and rotavirus.

Risk factors: contact with infectious people

BACTERIA

Common bacteria include *Campylobacter*, *Salmonella*, *Shigella*, *Escherichia coli*, and *Clostridium difficile*.

Risk factors: ingesting undercooked or contaminated foods, or raw fluids; hospitalization, recent antibiotic use (*Clostridium difficile*)

PARASITES

Common parasites include *Giardia* and *Cryptosporidium*.

Risk factors: contact with infants in day care; AIDS; men having sex with men; coming from a community with a waterborne parasite outbreak; travel to mountainous regions and/or tropical countries

Investigations: stool examination for ova and parasites

DRUGS OR TOXINS

DRUGS

Examples include laxatives; antacids containing magnesium; antibiotics; and nonsteroidal antiinflammatory drugs (NSAIDs).

SHIGA TOXIN

Signs and symptoms of *E. coli* infection: abdominal pain, blood in the stool, **no** fever

PREFORMED TOXINS

Signs and symptoms: symptoms that develop within 6 hours of ingesting contaminated food (e.g., undercooked meat, poorly refrigerated food)

Investigations: stool culture to detect enteric pathogens

ISCHEMIC CONDITION

This typically occurs in patients with risk factors for mesenteric ischemia.

Signs and symptoms: abdominal pain, bloody diarrhea, **no** risk factors for infection

Risk factors (mesenteric ischemia): congestive heart failure, arrhythmia, atherosclerosis, heart failure, chronic kidney failure

Investigations: CT scan; sigmoidoscopy, colonoscopy, arteriography (these are the best methods to definitively identify ischemia-related intestinal injury)

INFLAMMATORY BOWEL DISEASE

Signs and symptoms: younger than 30 (usually); family history of inflammatory bowel disease; fluctuating symptoms with periods of exacerbation and remission; diarrhea (possibly with nocturnal waking); blood in the stool; abdominal pain; weight loss; fever; fatigue; right lower quadrant and periumbilical pain; extraintestinal manifestations (e.g., uveitis, arthritis)

> Crohn disease: right lower quadrant mass, inflammation of the eyes, arthritis

Investigations: elevated CRP (this suggests active inflammation); fecal calprotectin; colonoscopy with biopsy (this is a standard diagnostic procedure); CT scan or MRI (findings: diagnostic structural changes associated with inflammatory bowel disease)

METABOLIC DISEASE (E.G., HYPERTHYROIDISM)

HYPERTHYROIDISM

This results in hyperdefecation (not diarrhea per se).

Signs and symptoms: history of hyperthyroidism or symptoms of hyperthyroidism (changes in menstrual patterns, enlarged thyroid, tachycardia, palpitations, diarrhea, muscle weakness, tremor, hyperactive reflexes, weight loss, sweating, thinning hair)

Investigations: decreased thyrotropin (TSH)

Strategy for patient encounter

The likely scenario is acute diarrhea in a recent traveller. The specified tasks could engage history, physical exam, investigations, or management.

History

Ask about the duration of the diarrhea: When did it start? How many bowel movements per day? How does this differ from usual? What is the consistency of the bowel movements? Is there blood or pus? Ask about medical and surgical history, medications, and allergies. Ask about systemic symptoms (fever, weight loss, fatigue, night sweats) that may indicate malignancy or chronic infection. Ask about a history of travel and exposure to others with diarrhea. Take a medical and medication history, listening in particular for bowel disease and immunodeficiency (e.g., HIV, steroid use).

Physical exam

Obtain the patient's vital signs, looking for fever (this suggests infection) and to assess the patient's volume status (hypotension suggests dehydration). Examine the abdomen, looking for tenderness and increased bowel sounds.

Investigations

Testing is not necessary for most cases of acute diarrhea in developed countries. Consider stool cultures and stool examination for ova and parasites in patients with diarrhea lasting more than 7 days, especially in cases of bloody diarrhea, severe dehydration, immunosuppressed patients, patients who have been camping, or during outbreaks. Consider testing for *Clostridium difficile* toxins in patients with recent hospitalization and/or recent antibiotic use. In severely dehydrated patients, order tests for serum creatinine and electrolytes.

Management

Treat dehydration with oral (or if needed parenteral) rehydration. Consider loperamide or simethicone for symptomatic treatment of nonspecific diarrhea. Consider antibiotic treatment for traveller's diarrhea (quinolone or azithromycin, depending on local susceptibility patterns and travel history). Treat other infections based on culture results.

Pearls

Remember that some causes of infectious diarrhea are reportable to public health authorities, including *Campylobacter, Salmonella, Shigella*, enterohemorrhagic *Escherichia coli* (EHEC), *Vibrio cholerae, Cryptosporidium*, and *Giardia*.

36

Chronic diarrhea

MCC particular objective

Focus the history on contrasting large and small bowel diarrhea.

MCC differential diagnosis
with added evidence

CHRONIC DIARRHEA IN GENERAL

Definition: disturbance of stool frequency or consistency for > 4 weeks

STEATORRHEA

Luminal

PANCREATIC INSUFFICIENCY

Signs and symptoms: chronic weight loss, nausea, diarrhea; pale or clay-coloured stools; fatty or oily stools

Investigations: serum enzyme levels; fecal fat test; abdominal CT scan, MRI, or ultrasound to detect damage or injury to the pancreas

CHOLESTASIS

Signs and symptoms: abdominal pain; nausea, vomiting; jaundice; itchiness; palpable, tender liver and/or gallbladder; history of liver disease, gallstones, cancer; current pregnancy

Investigations: abnormal liver enzyme tests; elevated bilirubin; abdominal ultrasound

ILEAL DISEASE OR RESECTION

Common reasons for extensive resection are diseases, infarction, and congenital anomalies.

Severe diarrhea and bile acid malabsorption result when > 100 cm of the ileum is resected.

BACTERIAL OVERGROWTH

This is excess bacteria in the small intestine, which damages the intestinal mucosa.

Signs and symptoms: abdominal fullness; pain, cramps; bloating; weight loss; watery diarrhea; fatty stools

Investigations: breath test for hydrogen; CBC; blood chemistry; vitamin levels; fecal fat test; biopsy or culture of the small bowel; X-ray of the small bowel

Mucosal

LACTASE DEFICIENCY

Signs and symptoms: abdominal distension; abdominal pain; diarrhea; symptom correlation with eating dairy products

Investigations: hydrogen breath test; lactose tolerance blood test

CELIAC DISEASE

Signs and symptoms: family history of celiac disease, or signs and symptoms of celiac disease (chronic abdominal pain, rashes)

Investigations: positive serum anti-tTG (with IgA level); duodenal biopsy to detect villous blunting

LARGE BOWEL CONDITIONS

Secretory diarrhea (e.g., villous adenoma)

VILLOUS ADENOMA

This is a neoplastic colon polyp.

Signs and symptoms: often asymptomatic; hematochezia with anemia; diarrhea; constipation; flatulence; pencil-thin stools; intense cramping (this indicates torsion or large adenomas); palpable mass on digital rectal exam

> Common locations: rectum, rectosigmoid

Risk factors: family history of colon polyps and cancer

Investigations: endoscopy (villous adenomas are cauliflower-like projections); biopsy (larger adenomas are associated with severe dysplasia)

Inflammatory diarrhea

INFLAMMATORY BOWEL DISEASE

Signs and symptoms: younger than 30 (usually); family history of inflammatory bowel disease; fluctuating symptoms with periods of exacerbation and remission; diarrhea (possibly with nocturnal waking); blood in the stool; abdominal pain; weight loss; fever; fatigue; right lower quadrant and periumbilical pain; extraintestinal manifestations (e.g., uveitis, arthritis)

> Crohn disease: right lower quadrant mass, inflammation of the eyes, arthritis

Investigations: elevated CRP (this suggests active inflammation); fecal calprotectin; colonoscopy with biopsy (this is a standard diagnostic procedure); CT scan or MRI (findings: diagnostic structural changes associated with inflammatory bowel disease)

INFECTION

Causes include viruses (e.g., norovirus, rotavirus), bacteria, and parasites.

Signs and symptoms: fever (this suggests viral infection); blood in the stool (this suggests bacterial infection)

Risk factors:

> Viral: contact with infectious people
>
> Bacterial: ingesting undercooked or contaminated foods, or raw fluids
>
> Parasitic: contact with infants in day care; AIDS; men having sex with men; coming from a community with a waterborne parasite outbreak; travel to mountainous regions and/or tropical countries

OTHER (E.G., RADIATION, ISCHEMIC COLITIS)

INTESTINAL LINING INJURY, INFLAMMATION IN GENERAL

Signs and symptoms: excretion of large volumes of water; abdominal pain, cramping

Investigations: X-ray with barium; colonoscopy or sigmoidoscopy to assess the extent of intestinal lining damage

RADIATION

An example is treatment for ovarian cancer.

ISCHEMIC COLITIS

Causes include atherosclerosis; hypotension (e.g., from heart failure, major surgery, trauma, shock); venous thrombosis; bowel obstruction (hernia, scar tissue, tumour); surgery (cardiac, vascular, gastrointestinal, gynecological); vasculitis; systemic lupus erythematosus; sickle cell disease; use of cocaine, methamphetamine.

Risk factors: older than 60; clotting disorders (factor V Leiden); high cholesterol; previous abdominal surgery; surgery involving the aorta; heavy exercise (e.g., marathon running)

Motility disorder (e.g., irritable bowel syndrome)

IRRITABLE BOWEL SYNDROME[1]

Irritable bowel syndrome is commonly diagnosed by applying the Rome criteria.

Signs and symptoms (Rome criteria): ≥ 2 symptoms, present for ≥ 1 day/week for ≥ 3 months

> Symptoms: pain associated with defecation, and/or change in stool frequency, and/or a change in stool consistency

SMALL BOWEL CONDITIONS

Osmotic diarrhea

Osmotic diarrhea is primarily a result of unabsorbable, water-soluble solutes remaining in the bowel and retaining water.

It is associated with sugar intolerance and large consumption of sugar substitutes.

Secretory diarrhea

NEUROENDOCRINE TUMOUR (E.G., CARCINOID)

INERT NEUROENDOCRINE TUMOURS

Signs and symptoms: pain, luminal bleeding, gastrointestinal obstruction

ACTIVE, MALIGNANT CARCINOIDS

These may exert carcinoid syndrome (excessive release of serotonin hormone and other chemicals, which dilates blood vessels, accelerates intestinal transit, and has other effects).

Signs and symptoms (carcinoid syndrome): telangiectasias; cutaneous flushing of the head and neck; difficulty breathing; cardiac problems; abdominal cramps; diarrhea

Investigations: blood and urine tests to detect serotonin and other chemicals; imaging of the abdomen, chest, heart

NEOPLASIA (E.G., LYMPHOMA)

LYMPHOMA

Signs and symptoms (non-Hodgkin): constitutional symptoms (fatigue, fever, night sweats, weight loss), enlarged lymph nodes, chest pain, coughing, shortness of breath

> Hodgkin lymphoma (less common): constitutional symptoms (fatigue, fever, night sweats, weight loss); enlarged lymph nodes; itching; pain on drinking alcohol, or increased sensitivity to alcohol

Investigations: blasts or cancer cells on peripheral blood smear; excess blasts or cancer cells on bone marrow examination

MUCOSAL

Examples of causes of damage to the mucosal lining include ulcerative colitis, Crohn disease, infections, bacteria overgrowth, and ischemia.

Signs and symptoms: abdominal pain, cramping; fever; diarrhea; fatigue

Investigations: CBC to detect inflammatory markers; barium X-ray of the small bowel; fecal fat analysis

Motility disorders (e.g., diabetic neuropathy)

DIABETIC NEUROPATHY

Signs and symptoms: personal or family history of diabetes; history of diabetic complications and/or inadequate monitoring; polydipsia, polyuria, and/or weight loss

> Autonomic neuropathy: indigestion, nausea, diarrhea, constipation, dizziness, urinating difficulty, erectile dysfunction, vaginal dryness
>
> Motor neuropathy: weakness, fatigue, wasting, cramps, twitching, decreased reflexes, myokymia
>
> Sensory neuropathy: numbness, burning, or stabbing pain; tingling; gait and balance difficulty; temperature intolerance; hyperalgesia

Strategy for patient encounter

The likely scenario is a young adult with chronic diarrhea. The specified tasks could engage history, physical exam, investigations, or management.

History

This clinical presentation has a wide differential diagnosis. A useful first step is differentiating between large and small bowel diarrhea to narrow the possible entities.

Use open-ended questions to establish the duration and severity of the diarrhea, and accompanying symptoms: When did the diarrhea start? How many bowel movements do you have per day? How does this differ from usual? What is the consistency of the bowel movements? Is there blood or pus in the stools? What other symptoms have you noticed? Listen for features of small bowel disease versus large bowel disease (small bowel: voluminous, watery stools possibly with fat; large bowel: frequent smaller-volume stools, which may be accompanied by blood, mucus, pus, and lower abdominal pain); and for systemic symptoms (fever, weight loss, fatigue, night sweats), which may indicate malignancy or chronic infection. Pay particular attention to symptoms commonly associated with irritable bowel syndrome (pain with defecation, pain with changes in stool form or frequency).

Take a general medical and surgical history. Ask about medications and allergies. Ask about a history of travel.

Physical exam

Perform a full physical exam looking for extraabdominal signs of disease (episcleritis in inflammatory bowel disease; exophthalmia in hyperthyroidism; dermatitis herpetiformis in celiac disease;

lymphadenopathy in malignancy). Examine the abdomen for bowel sounds, tenderness, and masses. Perform a rectal exam looking for anal fistulae (relevant to Crohn disease), masses, and impacted stool. Perform occult blood testing on the stool sample you extract with your glove.

(State that you will perform a rectal exam. Since rectal exams are not done on standardized patients, the examiner will likely interrupt, ask what you are looking for, and provide findings, including occult blood findings.)

Investigations

Order a complete blood count (CBC), and tests for albumin level, C-reactive protein (CRP), liver function, electrolytes, and thyrotropin (TSH). Consider an anti–tissue transglutaminase (anti-tTG) antibody test (with IgA level) for celiac disease. Consider tests for fecal pH (< 5.5 suggests lactose intolerance), fecal electrolyte levels (to distinguish secretory from osmotic diarrhea), fecal calprotectin (this is relevant to inflammatory bowel disease), *Clostridium difficile* stool toxin (in patients with recent antibiotic use), and stool examination for ova and parasites (in patients with travel to endemic areas).

Management

Treat any specific entities identified. Refer the patient for colonoscopy and biopsies if no specific diagnosis is identified. Empiric antidiarrheal therapy can be considered in patients when a specific treatment is not available. Irritable bowel syndrome is treated first with diet and lifestyle changes (managing stress, increasing dietary fibre, drinking plenty of fluids, exercising regularly, getting adequate sleep). More severe cases may require laxatives; antidiarrheal medications; anticholinergics; tricyclic antidepressants or selective serotonin reuptake inhibitors (SSRIs) (in patients with coexisting depression); or pain medications such as pregabalin or gabapentin.

REFERENCE

1 Lacey B, Mearin F, Chang L, et al. Rome IV functional gastrointestinal disorders: disorders of gut-brain interaction. 4th ed. Vol. 2. Raleigh, NC: Rome Foundation; 2017. Chapter 11, Functional bowel disorders; 1393–1407.

37

Pediatric diarrhea

MCC particular objective

Pay particular attention to signs of hypovolemia, dehydration, and electrolyte abnormalities.

MCC differential diagnosis
with added evidence

INFECTION

VIRAL GASTROENTERITIS

This is a common concern, typically in children 2 months to 2 years.
It resolves within 1 week.

Signs and symptoms: abrupt-onset watery, nonbloody diarrhea; crampy abdominal pain; nausea, vomiting; fever (> 38°C); headache; muscle aches; epigastric tenderness on abdominal examination

BACTERIAL ENTERITIS

This typically occurs in children older than 2 years due to oral-fecal contamination; exposure to farm animals or reptiles; eating contaminated food; outbreak at a day care centre; and antibiotic use within the past 2 months.

Signs and symptoms: diarrhea that is bloody or contains mucus; tenesmus; persistent high fever (> 40°C); severe abdominal pain

DIET-RELATED CONDITION (E.G., MILK PROTEIN INTOLERANCE)

MILK PROTEIN INTOLERANCE

This includes 2 types of allergic responses: immediate IgE-mediated hypersensitivity and delayed cell-mediated reaction.

It is outgrown in early childhood.

Signs and symptoms: itchy eyes, nose, lips, gums, mouth, throat; blood, mucous in the stool; frequent regurgitation, vomiting; diarrhea; constipation; persistent infantile colic; atopic dermatitis; swollen lips and eyelids; chronic cough, wheezing, runny nose; anaphylaxis (rare); possible umbilical erythema

Investigations: serum IgE antibody test or skin testing; food challenge in controlled environment (this is the gold standard)

ISCHEMIC INTESTINAL DAMAGE (E.G., INTUSSUSCEPTION)

INTUSSUSCEPTION

Signs and symptoms: sudden-onset symptoms (patients usually present within a few hours of onset); bilious vomiting; severe, intermittent abdominal pain; blood, mucous in the stool ("currant jelly" stools); lethargy; fever; Dance sign (palpable mass beneath the right ribs and emptiness in the right lower quadrant on abdominal examination)

Investigations: ultrasound

MALABSORPTION

Lactase deficiency

Signs and symptoms: symptoms that develop shortly after consuming milk products; abdominal pain, bloating, cramping; diarrhea; flatulence; hyperactive bowel sounds; abdominal distension; family history of lactase deficiency; celiac disease; Crohn disease; autoimmune disease; recent treatment with antibiotics, chemotherapy, or radiation

Investigations (it is usually diagnosed clinically): lactose breath hydrogen test

Cystic fibrosis

Signs and symptoms: family history of cystic fibrosis; recurrent pneumonia; shortness of breath; productive cough; failure to thrive; fever; wheezing on lung auscultation

Investigations: positive sweat chloride test

Celiac disease

Signs and symptoms: family history of celiac disease, or signs and symptoms of celiac disease (chronic abdominal pain, rashes)

Investigations: positive serum anti-tTG (with IgA level); duodenal biopsy to detect villous blunting

OTHER CAUSES

Drugs

Examples include antibiotics, ranitidine, and nonsteroidal antiinflammatory drugs (NSAIDs). Herbal tea is also a possible cause.

Laxative abuse

This includes use of laxatives and/or enemas.

Examples of causes include eating disorders and body image dysphoria.

Inflammatory bowel disease

Signs and symptoms: younger than 30 (usually); family history of inflammatory bowel disease; fluctuating symptoms with periods of exacerbation and remission; diarrhea (possibly with nocturnal waking); blood in the stool; abdominal pain; weight loss; fever; fatigue; right lower quadrant and periumbilical pain; extraintestinal manifestations (e.g., uveitis, arthritis)

> Crohn disease: right lower quadrant mass, inflammation of the eyes, arthritis

Investigations: elevated CRP (this suggests active inflammation); fecal calprotectin; colonoscopy with biopsy (this is a standard diagnostic procedure); CT scan or MRI (findings: diagnostic structural changes associated with inflammatory bowel disease)

Strategy for patient encounter

This encounter will likely involve a parent discussing a toddler with diarrhea, which has been present for several months. The child will be absent on some pretext (e.g., someone has taken the child to use the toilet). The specified tasks could engage history, physical exam, investigations, or management.

History

Start with open-ended questions about the duration and severity of the diarrhea: When did it start? How many bowel movements have there been per day? How does this differ from usual? What is the consistency of the bowel movements? Ask about blood or pus in the stools.

Use open-ended inquiry to assess associated symptoms: What other symptoms have you noticed? Listen for evidence consistent with particular entities (e.g., itchiness in milk protein intolerance; recent, sudden-onset diarrhea with severe abdominal pain in intussusception; chronic abdominal pain and rashes in celiac disease; shortness of breath and productive cough in cystic fibrosis).

Check for factors of dehydration: How much is your child drinking? Is your child vomiting? How many times a day is your child urinating?

Check for possible causes, such as infectious contacts, recent travel, recent use of antibiotics, and any chronic illnesses.

Ask about conditions that run in the family, and listen for lactase deficiency, cystic fibrosis, celiac disease, and inflammatory bowel disease.

Ask about the impact of the diarrhea on the child's daily life and activities.

Physical exam

Obtain the patient's vital signs, looking for fever (this is relevant to infection), and tachycardia and/or hypotension (severe dehydration). Compare current weight to previous weight(s) looking for dehydration or failure to thrive (with chronic diarrhea). Assess mental status (lethargy may be a sign of sepsis). Examine mucous membranes (dehydration). In infants, assess for a flat or sunken anterior fontanelle (dehydration). Assess for abdominal skin tenting and capillary refill of longer than 2 seconds (dehydration). Perform a full physical examination, looking for sources of infection. In the abdominal exam, look for masses and peritonitis.

(State that you will examine the child. Since an actual pediatric patient is unlikely, the examiner may interrupt, ask what you are looking for, and provide findings.)

Investigations

Order a complete blood count (CBC) to look for signs of infection and dehydration, and tests for electrolytes and creatinine (relevant to dehydration). Consider stool cultures for febrile children with diarrhea. Order stool examination for ova and parasites in children who have travelled to endemic areas. Consider a urinalysis, because urinary tract infection often coexists with diarrhea. In older children with recent use of antibiotics, consider *Clostridium difficile* stool antigen testing. In suspected intussusception or other intraabdominal process, consider imaging.

Management

Manage any significant dehydration with intravenous fluids. After the patient is stabilized, treat any specific entities identified. Viral gastroenteritis is treated supportively.

Pearls

Acute diarrhea is defined as lasting less than 2 weeks; chronic diarrhea is defined as lasting more than 2 weeks.

38

Diplopia

MCC particular objective

Pay particular attention to whether true binocular diplopia is present (which resolves with occlusion of vision to either eye).

MCC differential diagnosis
with added evidence

MONOCULAR DIPLOPIA (E.G., REFRACTIVE ERROR, CATARACT)

This is double vision in only 1 eye.

Causes include dry eye, refractive error, warped cornea, cataract, macular disorders, and the wrong glasses (monocular diplopia indicates a problem with the eye itself).

BINOCULAR DIPLOPIA

Oculomotor nerve dysfunction

ISCHEMIA

Ischemia of the oculomotor nerve or of the midbrain is the most common cause of palsies that spare the pupil.

The oculomotor nerve (cranial nerve III) controls the movement of 4 of the 6 eye muscles.

Signs and symptoms: diplopia and other focusing impairments; ptosis; paresis of specific eye motions; normal pupil or partial pupil involvement

DIABETES-ASSOCIATED
CRANIAL MONONEUROPATHY III (DIABETIC TYPE)

Signs and symptoms: personal or family history of diabetes; history of diabetic complications and/or inadequate monitoring; polydipsia, polyuria, and/or weight loss

Investigations: fasting glucose or HbA_{1c} test

MULTIPLE SCLEROSIS

Signs and symptoms: variable depending on lesion location

Spinal cord: sensory or motor dysfunction; Lhermitte sign (paresthesias radiating down the extremities or trunk with neck flexion); bowel, bladder or erectile dysfunction

Brainstem: double vision; swallowing, speech difficulties; vertigo; pseudobulbar palsy

Cerebrum: cognitive impairment; depression; upper motor neuron signs; unilateral motor or sensory deficits

Cerebellum: problems with balance and coordination; vertigo

Other symptoms: tonic spasms; fatigue; pain; exercise intolerance; temperature sensitivity; painful unilateral loss of visual acuity

Risk factors: younger than 50, female

Investigations: brain and spinal cord MRI, including advanced MRI techniques, with established occurrence of multiple episodes; CSF fluid analysis

INTRACRANIAL MASS (E.G., ANEURYSM)

ANEURYSM

Pupil involvement is a strong indication for urgent head imaging.

Signs and symptoms: typically asymptomatic if unruptured; dilated pupil that is in a "down and out" position; change in vision; pain, weakness, or numbness in the face or eye region; sudden-onset severe headache (this indicates a more serious situation)

Investigations: CSF analysis to detect blood, CT scan, MRI, CT angiography, cerebral angiography

Myasthenia gravis

Signs and symptoms: ocular weakness (usually just this) with drooping eyelid(s), and blurred vision or double vision; oropharyngeal weakness (dysarthria; hoarseness; chewing and swallowing difficulty); limb weakness with difficulty climbing stairs, working with elevated arms; fluctuating weakness that is asymmetrical and worse with sustained exercise

Investigations: single fibre electromyography, serum anti-AChR antibody

Graves orbitopathy

Signs and symptoms: history of thyroid disease (current or past) or symptoms of hyperthyroidism (enlarged thyroid, tachycardia, palpitations, diarrhea, muscle weakness, tremor, hyperactive reflexes, weight loss, sweating); exposure keratopathy; compressive optic neuropathy; proptosis; red eyes; retracting eyelids

Investigations: MRI of the head; decreased thyrotropin (TSH) (if undiagnosed Graves disease is suspected)

Orbital inflammation, infection, or tumour

ORBITAL CELLULITIS

This condition is an ocular emergency.

Signs and symptoms: fever; malaise; pain with eye movement; reduced vision, diplopia; red eye; swelling and/or redness of the eyelid and surrounding skin; proptosis; relative afferent pupillary defect; mucormycosis (this is a severe and destructive fungal orbital cellulitis): history of diabetes

Risk factors: preseptal cellulitis; sinus, face, or tooth infection; trauma

Investigations: leukocytosis on CBC; elevated CRP, ESR; CT scan or MRI of the head

Fracture of orbital floor or "blow out"

Signs and symptoms: history of facial trauma; facial tenderness; cervical and/or jaw tenderness

Investigations: CT scan of the head (to rule out entrapment of the eye)

Decompensation of childhood phoria (e.g., squint)

Squint (strabismus) is usually identified and treated in childhood.

Signs and symptoms: deviation in eye direction

Risk factors: premature birth; low birth weight; family history of strabismus or amblyopia; developmental disability (e.g., Down syndrome, cerebral palsy); head injury

Investigations: cover test; light reflex test

Strategy for patient encounter

The likely scenario is an older adult with double vision. The specified tasks could engage history, physical exam, investigations, or management.

History

Use open-ended questions to establish the nature of the symptoms: Does the problem involve 1 or both eyes? How constant is the problem? What other symptoms have you noticed? Listen for evidence consistent with particular entities (e.g., intermittent symptoms with muscle weakness in myasthenia gravis; constant diplopia with fever and pain associated with eye movement in orbital cellulitis; intermittent diplopia with neurologic signs such as swallowing difficulty in multiple sclerosis; diplopia with systemic symptoms such as palpitations and heat intolerance in Graves orbitopathy).

Check specifically for symptoms of particular concern if the patient doesn't volunteer them (see the checklist): pain and neurological impairments.

Ask about the patient's medical history. Listen in particular for diabetes and thyroid disease.

Physical exam

Pay particular attention to findings that are red flags (see the checklist).

Obtain the patient's vital signs, looking for fever. Perform a cranial nerve exam. Measure the patient's visual acuity in each eye and both eyes together. Assess whether binocular diplopia is present by covering each eye and checking if the diplopia resolves. Look for bulging of 1 or both eyes, and for pupillary symmetry. Examine the thyroid for enlargement and tenderness. Perform an ophthalmoscopic exam looking for abnormalities of the lens (cataract, displacement) and retina (e.g., detachment).

Investigations

Patients with new onset diplopia should receive a CT scan or MRI and a serum thyrotropin (TSH) test. In patients with intermittent diplopia, consider testing for myasthenia gravis and multiple sclerosis.

Management

Management will depend on the specific entity identified. Red flags (see the checklist) should prompt urgent referral to a neurologist.

39

Dizziness, vertigo

MCC particular objective

Distinguish between vertigo and other causes of dizziness (gait disturbances, orthostatic light-headedness, other disorders).

MCC differential diagnosis
with added evidence

VERTIGO

VERTIGO IN GENERAL
Signs and symptoms: feeling that the world is moving or spinning

Peripheral vestibular dysfunction

BENIGN POSITIONAL VERTIGO
Signs and symptoms: female (more common); middle-aged and older (more common); positive Dix-Hallpike maneuver (this has a positive predictive value of 83% and negative predictive value of 52% for benign positional vertigo)

PERIPHERAL VESTIBULOPATHY
This includes acute labyrinthitis and acute vestibular neuronitis (vestibular neuritis).
Signs and symptoms: vertigo following a recent viral or bacterial infection

MÉNIÈRE DISEASE
Signs and symptoms: recurrent episodes of vertigo, hearing loss, tinnitus, or aural fullness

DRUGS (E.G., AMINOGLYCOSIDES)

ACOUSTIC NEUROMA
Signs and symptoms: unilateral hearing loss; unilateral tinnitus; vertigo; feeling as if the body is tilted; veering towards the side of the affected ear; facial weakness
Investigations: CT scan or MRI of the head

CENTRAL VESTIBULAR DYSFUNCTION

Cerebrovascular disease

CEREBROVASCULAR ACCIDENT

Signs and symptoms: history of stroke, or signs and symptoms consistent with stroke (e.g., unilateral neurologic defects)

Risk factors: hypertension, dyslipidemia, diabetes, coagulopathy

Multiple sclerosis

Signs and symptoms: variable depending on lesion location

> Spinal cord: sensory or motor dysfunction; Lhermitte sign (paresthesias radiating down the extremities or trunk with neck flexion); bowel, bladder or erectile dysfunction

> Brainstem: double vision; swallowing, speech difficulties; vertigo; pseudobulbar palsy

> Cerebrum: cognitive impairment; depression; upper motor neuron signs; unilateral motor or sensory deficits

> Cerebellum: problems with balance and coordination; vertigo

> Other symptoms: tonic spasms; fatigue; pain; exercise intolerance; temperature sensitivity; painful unilateral loss of visual acuity

Risk factors: younger than 50, female

Investigations: brain and spinal cord MRI, including advanced MRI techniques, with established occurrence of multiple episodes; CSF fluid analysis

Drugs (e.g., anticonvulsants, hypnotics, alcohol)

OTHER DIZZINESS

DIZZINESS IN GENERAL

Signs and symptoms: light-headedness (versus the world moving or spinning)

Hyperventilation

Signs and symptoms: episodes of rapid breathing (e.g., accompanying a panic attack)

Disequilibrium (e.g., poor mobility, peripheral neuropathy)

DISEQUILIBRIUM IN GENERAL

Disequilibrium involves proprioceptive impairment (e.g., from peripheral neuropathy, or from dysfunction of the dorsal root ganglia or the posterior columns of the spinal cord).

Examples of causes include diabetes, chronic malnutrition, vitamin B_{12} deficiency, and Parkinson disease.

PERIPHERAL NEUROPATHY

Signs and symptoms:

> Motor: weakness, fatigue, wasting, cramps, twitching, decreased reflexes, myokymia
>
> Sensory: numbness, tingling; burning or stabbing pain; gait and balance difficulty; temperature intolerance; hyperalgesia

Presyncope

Examples of causes include cardiac abnormalities, diabetes, and anemia.

Signs and symptoms: sensation of impending loss of consciousness

Investigations: ECG, serum glucose, CBC

Anxiety or panic disorder[1(pp189-234)]

Examples of anxiety disorders listed in the *Diagnostic and Statistical Manual of Mental Disorders* (*DSM-5*) include generalized anxiety disorder, panic disorder, separation anxiety disorder, social anxiety disorder, and specific phobia. Anxiety disorders can provoke panic attacks (e.g., exposure to a phobic object). In the case of panic disorder, panic attacks occur spontaneously.

Signs and symptoms: history of anxiety disorder and/or symptoms consistent with a panic attack; history of social or emotional triggers for symptoms (possible); lack of evidence for other causes, including hyperthyroidism (anxiety can mimic other conditions and is therefore a diagnosis of exclusion)

> Panic attack: symptoms that peak within minutes; symptoms that can include palpitations, accelerated heart rate, shortness of breath, chest pain, dizziness, numbness or tingling, fear of losing control, fear of dying

Strategy for patient encounter

The likely scenario is a patient with a history of episodic dizziness and hearing loss. The specified tasks could engage history, physical exam, investigations, or management.

History

The first step is to determine if the patient has true vertigo as opposed to a gait disturbance or orthostatic light-headedness. Ask specific questions: Do you feel like the room is spinning? (If yes, this suggests vertigo.) Do you feel unsteady on your feet? (Disequilibrium.) Do you feel light-headed or like you may faint? (Presyncope.)

Use open-ended questions to establish onset, progression, triggers, and accompanying symptoms: When did the symptoms start? How constant are they? What are you doing when you experience the symptoms? What other symptoms do you have? Listen for evidence consistent with particular entities (e.g., onset following an infection or fever in peripheral vestibulopathy; recurring symptoms, including aural symptoms, in Ménière disease; neurological impairments in stroke; symptoms triggered by walking in disequilibrium).

Ask about the patient's medications and whether their medications have changed recently. Listen for aminoglycosides, anticonvulsants, and hypnotics. Ask about alcohol use. Ask about a medical history of diabetes, multiple sclerosis, hypertension, other chronic illness, and anxiety.

Physical exam
Observe the patient walking to assess for a gait disturbance. Perform a neurological exam, with an emphasis on the cranial nerves. Perform the Dix-Hallpike manoeuvre (to diagnose benign positional vertigo). Perform an otoscopic exam. Observe the patient for nystagmus.

Investigations
Note that laboratory tests do not generally provide information useful to diagnosing or managing dizziness or vertigo.

In patients with neurologic signs or symptoms, or progressive unilateral hearing loss (this suggests acoustic neuroma), or risk factors for stroke, order imaging studies (MRI is preferred).

Management
Treatment depends on the specific entity. The Epley manoeuvre usually resolves benign positional vertigo. In suspected peripheral causes, consider referring the patient to an ear, nose, and throat (ENT) specialist. In suspected central causes, consider referral to a neurologist.

Pearls
Some patients with central vertigo require more urgent management. Consider urgent referral to an ENT specialist for patents with vertigo associated with headache, ataxia, loss of consciousness, focal neurological deficits, or prolonged, severe symptoms.

REFERENCE
1 American Psychiatric Association. Diagnostic and statistical manual of mental disorders. 5th ed. Arlington, VA: American Psychiatric Association; 2013. 59–60. 991 p.

40

Dying patient

MCC particular objective

Create a plan for palliative care with attention to human dignity; control of pain and other symptoms; and the importance of family and social support.

MCC differential diagnosis

None stated.

Strategy for patient encounter

The scenario will involve management of a dying patient, including communicating with the patient and their family, plans for end-of-life care and decision making, and symptom management.

Management

BREAKING BAD NEWS TO THE PATIENT AND FAMILY

The patient and family may not be aware of the patient's condition. It's good general preparation for the exam to have a strategy for breaking bad news (see the checklist).

Mnemonics for breaking bad news

A common mnemonic is **ABCDE**:

A — Advance preparation is key. Arrange for adequate time and privacy, confirm medical facts.

B — Build a therapeutic relationship. Identify patient preferences, ensure the right people are present.

C — Communicate. Determine the family's understanding of the situation, proceed at the family's pace, and answer questions.

D — Deal with the family's reactions. Empathize with the family.

E — Encourage and validate emotions.

Another common mnemonic is **SPIKES:**[1]

S — Setting: Choose a private setting where you can sit down and talk to the patient, and their family, if appropriate, in person.

P — Perceptions: Ask the patient for their understanding of their situation.

I — Invitation: Offer to share what you know about their situation. Wait for acceptance of your offer.

K — Knowledge: Describe what you know about the patient's situation and how you came to know it.

E — Empathy: Acknowledge the difficulty of the situation for the patient.

S — Summary, strategy: Summarize and talk about next steps.

End-of-life care

Discuss the patient's wishes regarding end-of-life care. Ask if a personal directive (sometimes called a living will) is in place, which often covers topics such as use of ventilators, cardiopulmonary resuscitation, and artificial feeding; administration of antibiotics, and pain and antinausea medications; continuation of treatments (e.g., chemotherapy or radiation therapy); and organ, tissue or body donation. If the patient has a personal directive, ask for a copy.

Substitute decision makers

Ask if the patient has a substitute decision maker. A personal directive appoints 1 or more substitute decision makers for medical decisions. A power of attorney appoints 1 or more substitute decision makers for financial decisions. Ask if the patient has a will. Encourage the patient to consider appointing substitute decision makers and making a will if they have not done so.

Symptom management

Symptom management in palliative care generally falls into 5 categories.

- **Pain management:** Nonsteroidal antiinflammatory drugs (NSAIDs) may suffice for initial pain management. Manage neuropathic pain syndromes with tricyclic antidepressants. Many patients will require opioids. Start with weak opioids (tramadol, codeine) and move to strong opioids (morphine, hydromorphone, oxycodone, fentanyl, methadone) as needed.
- **Sedation:** This may be a side effect of opioids, but is often multifactorial and may be related to disease progression. If it is related to medication, the patient will often build up a tolerance over time. A main consideration is to balance sedation and pain relief.
- **Respiratory depression:** Like sedation, respiratory depression is often a side effect of opioids. Titration to a dose that balances pain relief and respiratory depression is necessary.
- **Nausea and vomiting:** This is often multifactorial, and may be secondary to medications (steroids, antibiotics,

opioids) or constipation. If secondary to opioids, consider giving haloperidol 0.5 mg every 12 hours or metoclopramide 10 mg 4 times per day. Use dimenhydrinate to treat nausea present with movement. Ensure that constipation is treated.

- **Constipation:** This is a very common symptom, and is often a side effect of opioids and decreased mobility. Start laxatives when opioids are started. Options include oral sennosides, 24 mg 2 times per day; oral polyethylene glycol, 17 g 2 times per day; oral lactulose, 30 mL 2 times per day; bisacodyl 10 mg suppository as needed; and Fleet enema as needed.

Consider referring the patient to a palliative care team or service. Palliative care offers symptom control in the context of holistic care: it provides medical, nursing, psychological, social, and spiritual care in a culturally sensitive manner.

REFERENCE

1 Baile WF, Buckman R, Lenzi R, et al. SPIKES—a six-step protocol for delivering bad news: application to the patient with cancer. Oncologist. 2000;5(4):302–311.

41

Dysphagia

MCC particular objective
Differentiate oropharyngeal causes from esophageal causes.

MCC differential diagnosis
with added evidence

OROPHARYNGEAL DYSPHAGIA
OROPHARYNGEAL DYSPHAGIA IN GENERAL
Signs and symptoms: difficulty with the initiation of swallowing (transferring food from the mouth to the esophagus)

Structural

INFECTION (E.G., PHARYNGITIS, PERITONSILLAR ABSCESS)

Signs and symptoms (in general): recent pharyngitis; fever; hoarse voice; neck pain; difficulty swallowing; peritonsillar swelling

Investigations: elevated WBCs on CBC; lateral neck X-ray to detect pharyngeal swelling; blood culture to detect causative organisms

TUMOUR

Signs and symptoms: onset of dysphagia over months, with or without constitutional symptoms (fever, weight loss, fatigue, night sweats); masses and enlarged lymph nodes on head and neck exam

Risk factors for throat and esophageal cancer: smoking, alcohol use, family history

Investigations: CT scan of the oropharynx, neck, and chest

ZENKER DIVERTICULUM

This is herniation of the esophageal mucosa posteriorly between the cricopharyngeus muscle and the inferior pharyngeal constrictor muscles.

Signs and symptoms: male, elderly (more common); regurgitation of undigested food (common)

Neuromuscular

CENTRAL (E.G., CEREBROVASCULAR ACCIDENT)

CEREBROVASCULAR ACCIDENT

Signs and symptoms: history of stroke, or evidence consistent with stroke (e.g., unilateral neurologic impairments)

Risk factors: hypertension, dyslipidemia, diabetes, coagulopathy

CRANIAL NERVES (E.G., AMYOTROPHIC LATERAL SCLEROSIS)

AMYOTROPHIC LATERAL SCLEROSIS (ALS)

Signs and symptoms: onset in a limb or extremity; weakness, cramps, twitching, muscle wasting (lower motor neuron involvement); walking difficulty due to spasticity (upper motor neuron involvement); general fatigue; reduced exercise tolerance; possible language dysfunction

> Bulbar onset, which may precede limb weakness: swallowing difficulty; slurred speech; jaw jerking; increased gag reflex; tongue twitching (very specific for ALS)

Investigations: EMG, nerve conduction study, MRI

Xerostomia

Signs and symptoms: oral mucosal dryness; use of drugs that cause xerostomia (e.g., tricyclic antidepressants, antipsychotics, antihistamines); history of Sjögren syndrome or evidence consistent with it (dry eyes; dry mouth; history of rheumatoid arthritis, systemic lupus erythematosus)

ESOPHAGEAL DYSPHAGIA

ESOPHAGEAL DYSPHAGIA IN GENERAL

Signs and symptoms: difficulty with swallowing after the transfer of food out of the mouth; sensation of food getting stuck

Mechanical obstruction

INTERMITTENT (E.G., LOWER ESOPHAGEAL RING, WEB)

The oropharyngeal region and esophagus are important for the action of swallowing. Physical anatomical abnormalities can impair their ability to function properly.

Investigations: upper endoscopy of the esophagus, barium X-ray

PROGRESSIVE (E.G., CARCINOMA, PEPTIC STRICTURE)

PROGRESSIVE MECHANICAL OBSTRUCTION IN GENERAL

Signs and symptoms: dysphagia that becomes gradually worse; difficulty with solid foods, and eventually soft foods and liquids

Investigations: endoscopy and biopsy; CT scan

CARCINOMA

Signs and symptoms: often asymptomatic until advanced; pain with swallowing; heartburn-like pain; hoarse cough; nausea, vomiting (sometimes with blood)

Risk factors for throat and esophageal cancer: smoking, alcohol use, family history

PEPTIC STRICTURE

This is the most common benign esophageal stricture (90% of cases).

Signs and symptoms: history of chronic reflux esophagitis

FOREIGN OBJECT

Signs and symptoms: sudden-onset dysphagia that correlates with swallowing an object (e.g., a toothpick) or food (especially chicken and fish)

> "Classic presentation": adult with dentures who chews their food incompletely (e.g., because of alcohol)

Investigations: X-ray of the esophagus to identify location of the object

Neuromuscular disorder

Causes include a central or peripheral nerve disorder or injury, which can alter the control of muscles in the mouth, throat, and esophagus.

Signs and symptoms: neurological impairments (motor, sensory); history of neuromuscular disorder (e.g., amyotrophic lateral sclerosis, muscular dystrophy, multiple sclerosis, Parkinson disease), stroke, spinal cord injury, brain injury

Strategy for patient encounter

The likely scenario is a patient with progressive dysphagia. The specified tasks could engage history, physical exam, investigations, or management.

History

Use open-ended questions to establish the characteristics of the dysphagia and associated symptoms, and to take a medical and medication history.

- **Onset and progression:** When did the difficulty with swallowing start? How constant is it? How has it changed since it started? Onset over months suggests malignancy; gradual onset suggests a progressive cause such as a progressive neuromuscular disorder. Intermittent symptoms suggest dysfunction of the lower esophageal ring or web. Progressive symptoms suggest tumour, peptic stricture, and progressive neuromuscular disorders.

- **Associated symptoms:** What happens when you swallow? Associated symptoms often point to the specific anatomic location of the problem. Listen for coughing, choking, and nasal regurgitation (oropharyngeal localization); or food sticking in the throat or chest (esophageal localization). Associated symptoms can also distinguish neuromuscular motility disorders from mechanical obstruction. Ask if the patient has had progressive difficulty swallowing both solids and liquids (neuromuscular motility disorder). Ask if the patient has had difficulty swallowing solids, but not liquids, with regurgitation of undigested food (mechanical obstruction).

- **Medical and medication history:** What conditions have you been diagnosed with? What medications do you take? Listen for stroke and conditions associated with stroke risk (hypertension, dyslipidemia, diabetes, coagulopathy); Sjögren syndrome or conditions associated with it (rheumatic diseases); gastroesophageal reflux disease; and neuromuscular disorders. Listen for medications that commonly cause dysphagia (nonsteroidal antiinflammatory drugs, anticholinergics, alpha-blockers, ACE inhibitors, doxycycline, tetracycline, clindamycin, trimethoprim-sulfamethoxazole) or xerostomia (tricyclic antidepressants, antipsychotics, antihistamines).

Physical exam
Perform a full neurological examination, including cranial nerves. Assess the patient's gag reflex. Assess the patient's mental status and cognitive functioning.

Investigations
For all patients, order a barium swallow (esophagram). This can both reveal the presence of masses and assess motility. In suspected mucosal abnormalities or masses, order endoscopy (note that this does not assess motility). If no diagnosis is made on barium swallow or endoscopy, order manometry to assess esophageal contractions. In suspected reflux disease, consider 24-hour pH monitoring.

Note that laboratory tests do not usually contribute useful information for diagnosing or managing dysphagia.

Management
Treat any contributing conditions. Refer patients with masses and obstructive lesions to surgery. Refer patients with neuromuscular disorders to neurology. Be aware of the common complications of dysphagia: weight loss, malnutrition, dehydration, and aspiration pneumonia.

Pearls
Dysphagia is a common medical presentation affecting up to 10% of adults older than 50.

42

Dyspnea

MCC particular objective
Identify patients with life-threatening causes of dyspnea.

MCC differential diagnosis
with added evidence

CARDIAC CONDITIONS

Myocardial dysfunction (e.g., ischemic cardiomyopathy)
Signs and symptoms (in general): chest pain (usual), sweating, pallor, abnormal heart sounds, hypotension

Investigations: elevated serum troponin; ECG; chest X-ray to detect cardiac enlargement and pulmonary edema

Valvular heart disease
Signs and symptoms: chest pain; palpitations; dizziness or fainting; fever; rapid weight gain (from fluid retention); lung rales (this suggests heart failure); dependent edema

> History of rheumatic fever, hypertension, myocardial infarction, aortic stenosis, bacterial endocarditis

Investigations: ECG (urgent), chest X-ray, echocardiogram

Pericardial disease (e.g., tamponade)
CARDIAC TAMPONADE
Signs and symptoms: history of invasive heart procedures; chest pain, radiating to the neck and jaw; right upper quadrant pain (due to hepatic venous congestion); tachycardia; elevated jugular venous pressure; pulsus paradoxus

Investigations: ECG (this has findings of abnormalities); chest X-ray (this is normal)

Increased cardiac output (e.g., anemia)
ANEMIA
Signs and symptoms: pallor, chest pain, palpitations, weakness, headache, dizziness, dyspnea

Risk factors: intestinal disorders (Crohn disease, celiac disease), menstruation, pregnancy, chronic disease (e.g., cancer, kidney failure), family history of sickle cell disease

Investigations: CBC; peripheral blood smear (visual examination of RBCs for unusual size, shape, colour)

Arrhythmia

Signs and symptoms: light-headedness, fainting, shortness of breath, tachycardia, bradycardia, hypotension

Investigations: ECG

PULMONARY CONDITIONS

Upper airway (e.g., foreign body, anaphylaxis)

FOREIGN BODY

Foreign body: sudden-onset symptoms correlating with ingestion of food or object; cyanosis; choking; difficulty breathing; loss of consciousness

Investigations: bronchoscopy or laryngoscopy; X-ray of the neck and chest

ANAPHYLAXIS

Signs and symptoms: personal or family history of anaphylaxis; hives; itchiness; peripheral edema; tongue or throat swelling; wheezing; stridor; shortness of breath; tachycardia; cardiovascular collapse; hypotension

Chest wall and pleura (e.g., pleural effusion)

PLEURAL EFFUSION

Some pleural effusions are asymptomatic and discovered incidentally during physical exam or on chest X-ray (they appear as white space at the base of the lung).

Signs and symptoms: pleuritic chest pain; dyspnea; cough (dry or productive); fever; rapid, shallow respiration (this indicates a large-volume effusion)

> Physical exam: absent tactile fremitus; dullness on percussion; decreased breath sounds on the side of the effusion

Investigations: chest X-ray (posteroanterior and lateral), ultrasound, CT scan; thoracentesis and pleural fluid analysis (cell count; pH; protein; LDH; glucose; amylase; cholesterol; triglycerides; NT-proBNP; adenosine deaminase; Gram and AFB stain; bacterial and AFB culture; cytology)

Lower airway (e.g., asthma, chronic obstructive pulmonary disease)

ASTHMA

This is diffuse airway inflammation and narrowing caused by a variety of triggering stimuli that results in bronchoconstriction.

Signs and symptoms: episodic symptoms; episodes that involve dyspnea, tachypnea, tachycardia, chest tightness, cough, wheezing; known triggers for episodes (often); impaired pulmonary function on testing with spirometry

Common triggers: exercise, exposure to workplace irritants (chemicals, dust, smoke), exposure to allergens (e.g., pet dander, pollen), respiratory infections

Risk factors: family history of asthma; other allergic condition (e.g., atopic dermatitis, seasonal allergies); overweight; smoking; chronic exposure to irritants (secondhand smoke, workplace irritants)

CHRONIC OBSTRUCTIVE PULMONARY DISEASE

Signs and symptoms: older than age 40 (usual: symptoms do not appear until significant lung damage has occurred); progressive symptoms; wheezing; chest tightness; chronic productive cough; clubbing of the fingers; cyanosis around the lips and in the extremities; decreased oxygen saturation; impaired pulmonary function on testing with spirometry

Risk factors: smoking, occupational exposure, intrinsic lung disease

Investigations: chest X-ray, CT scan; ABG

Alveolar (e.g., pneumonia)

PNEUMONIA

Signs and symptoms: shortness of breath; cough; purulent sputum; chest pain on coughing or deep breaths; fatigue; tachypnea; tachycardia; decreased oxygen saturation; lung crackles on auscultation; lung dullness on percussion

Children: fever

Elderly: confusion, low body temperature

Risk factors: very old, very young, smoking, immune compromise (e.g., due to chronic illness), hospitalization

Investigations: chest X-ray to detect consolidation

CENTRAL CONDITIONS (E.G., METABOLIC ACIDOSIS, ANXIETY)

METABOLIC ACIDOSIS

Signs and symptoms: chest pain; palpitations; headache; altered mental status; severe anxiety; decreased visual acuity; nausea, vomiting; abdominal pain; altered appetite; weight gain; muscle weakness; bone pain; joint pain; deep, rapid breathing (Kussmaul respiration)

Investigations: ECG, electrolytes, glucose, renal function, CBC, urinalysis, arterial blood sampling

Arterial blood sampling findings: decreased pH; decreased $PaCO_2$; decreased HCO_3; anion gap (> 12–16 mmol/L is high)

ANXIETY[1(pp189-234)]

Examples of anxiety disorders listed in the *Diagnostic and Statistical Manual of Mental Disorders* (*DSM-5*) include generalized anxiety disorder, panic disorder, separation anxiety disorder, social anxiety disorder, and specific phobia. Anxiety disorders can provoke panic attacks (e.g., exposure to a phobic object). In the case of panic disorder, panic attacks occur spontaneously.

Signs and symptoms: history of anxiety disorder and/or symptoms consistent with a panic attack; history of social or emotional triggers for symptoms (possible); lack of evidence for other causes, including hyperthyroidism (anxiety can mimic other conditions and is therefore a diagnosis of exclusion)

> Panic attack: symptoms that peak within minutes; symptoms that can include palpitations, accelerated heart rate, shortness of breath, chest pain, dizziness, numbness or tingling, fear of losing control, fear of dying

Strategy for patient encounter

The likely scenario is a patient in the emergency room with acute shortness of breath. The specified tasks could engage history, physical exam, investigations, or management.

Respiratory distress is possible in this clinical presentation. No matter what tasks the instructions for the encounter specify, start by checking the patient for respiratory distress.

Assessment for respiratory distress

Check the patient's airway, breathing, and circulation (mnemonic: **ABCs**). Provide emergency care to any patient with unstable vital signs.

If the patient is not in distress, proceed to the history and physical exam.

History

Start with open-ended questions about the onset of the dyspnea: How long have you felt short of breath? How has the problem changed since it began? What other symptoms do you have? Listen for acute or episodic shortness of breath versus chronic symptoms (chronic symptoms suggest chronic underlying disease such as chronic obstructive pulmonary disease or heart disease); worsening symptoms (this could indicate an impending emergency); and symptoms consistent with particular entities (e.g., fever in valvular heart disease, pleural effusion, and pneumonia; cough in pulmonary conditions; chest pain with sweating, dizziness, and/or palpitations in cardiac conditions).

Take a medical history, specifically asking about cardiac disease (ischemic heart disease, congestive heart failure) and pulmonary disease (asthma, chronic obstructive pulmonary disease). Ask whether the patient is or was a smoker. Ask about occupational and environmental exposures to dust and pollutants. Ask about a history of gastroesophageal reflux. Ask about a history of anxiety.

Physical exam

Assess the patient for altered mental status (check their orientation to time, place, and person). Auscultate the heart for murmurs or extra heart sounds. Auscultate the lungs for wheeze (relevant to asthma), stridor (upper airway obstruction), rales (pulmonary edema and pneumonia), and absent breath sounds (pneumothorax). Palpate the chest for subcutaneous emphysema (pneumothorax). Palpate the trachea for lateral deviation (pneumothorax). Assess the patient for elevated jugular venous pressure and dependent edema (congestive heart failure). Percuss the chest for dullness (consolidation or effusions). Examine the abdomen looking for organomegaly.

Investigations

Order an electrocardiogram (ECG), a test for arterial blood gases (ABG), a complete blood count (CBC), and a chest X- ray. In possible pulmonary embolism, order a ventilation-perfusion scan and a D-dimer test. If the diagnosis remains uncertain, consider a CT scan of the chest.

Management

Unstable patients (usually presenting with hypotension, altered mental status, hypoxia, or unstable arrhythmia) require immediate resuscitation. Give supplemental oxygen, obtain intravenous (IV) access, and consider intubation.

Further management depends on the diagnosis identified. Tension pneumothorax is treated with needle thoracentesis. Give a nebulized bronchodilator for asthma or chronic obstructive pulmonary disease. Give IV furosemide if pulmonary edema is present.

REFERENCE

1 American Psychiatric Association. Diagnostic and statistical manual of mental disorders. 5th ed. Arlington, VA: American Psychiatric Association; 2013. 991 p.

43

Ear pain

MCC particular objective

Do a careful head and neck exam, especially when the ear canal, tympanic membrane, and middle ear appear normal.

MCC differential diagnosis
with added evidence

EXTERNAL EAR PAIN

Infection

OTITIS EXTERNA (E.G., FUNGAL, BACTERIAL)

The most common cause is bacterial infection (90% of cases).

Signs and symptoms: ear pain; ear pruritus (this can occur with chronic infection; it is more common with fungal infection); discharge; hearing loss; feeling of fullness; pain with jaw movement; erythema of the external ear; pain on traction of the pinna or pressure on the tragus (these typically do not cause pain in acute otitis media); normal tympanic membrane on otoscopy; pain on otoscopy

> Fungal infection: white, flakey debris

Risk factors: water exposure ("swimmer's ear"), use of ear devices (e.g., headphones, hearing aids), trauma (e.g., Q-Tip use), dermatitis

AURICULAR CELLULITIS

Signs and symptoms: rapid-onset painful, red, swollen auricle

Risk factors: laceration, abrasion, insect bite, dermatitis, ear piercing

Trauma (e.g., frostbite, piercings)

FROSTBITE

Signs and symptoms: prolonged exposure to cold and/or exposure to pronounced cold; progressive symptoms; coldness; burning, throbbing pain; skin discolouration; numbness

> Before rewarming: reduced skin sensation; white or grey skin colour; hard or waxy skin to the touch

> After rewarming (depending on the depth of tissue involvement): erythema and mild edema (mild frostbite); bullae and tissue necrosis (severe frostbite)

Other (e.g., foreign body, cerumen impaction)

Signs and symptoms (in general): hearing loss; ear pain; tinnitus; vertigo; feeling of fullness; history of recent mechanical cleaning of ears (e.g., Q-Tip use); possible visible trauma; foreign body or cerumen impaction on otoscopy

MIDDLE AND INNER EAR PAIN

Infection or inflammation

ACUTE OTITIS MEDIA

Signs and symptoms: ear pain; fever; hearing loss; tympanic membrane that is not translucent; ear discharge (this indicates perforation of the tympanic membrane); loss of bony landmarks; middle ear effusion with bulging or reduced mobility of tympanic membrane on pneumatic otoscopy

> Infants and toddlers: ear tugging, irritability, poor feeding, vomiting, diarrhea

Risk factors: upper respiratory tract infection; allergic rhinitis; chronic rhinosinusitis; attendance at a child care facility (for children); contact with infectious illness; exposure to secondhand smoke; age (the condition peaks at age 6 to 24 months)

SEROUS OTITIS MEDIA

Signs and symptoms: ear pain; hearing loss; feeling of fullness; fluid (yellow or clear) behind a retracted tympanic membrane on otoscopy; reduced mobility of tympanic membrane on pneumatic otoscopy

> Children: speech and/or learning difficulties

Risk factors: recurrent acute otitis media, recent upper respiratory tract infection, environmental allergies, recent airplane travel

Investigations: audiogram to detect conductive hearing loss; tympanogram to detect flat configuration

MASTOIDITIS

Signs and symptoms: symptoms that occur 2 weeks after inadequately or untreated acute otitis media (typical); fever; headache; hearing loss; discharge from the ear; protruding ear; tenderness, erythema over the mastoid; retroauricular swelling; otitis media on otoscopy

Investigations: CT scan to detect loss of mastoid air cells

Trauma (e.g., perforation, barotrauma)

TYMPANIC MEMBRANE PERFORATION

Signs and symptoms: ear pain; clear, pus-filled, or bloody discharge from the ear; hearing loss; tinnitus; dizziness

> History of otitis media infection; barotrauma or head trauma; acoustic trauma; foreign object in the ear (e.g., Q-tip)

Investigations: culture of discharge; tympanometry; audiology assessment

Neoplasms

NEOPLASMS IN GENERAL

Signs and symptoms: ear pain that is nonresponsive to treatment for presumed underlying causes; constitutional symptoms (fever, night sweats, weight loss); lymphadenopathy; abnormalities on cranial nerve exam

> Skin cancer lesion: asymmetrical lesion; irregular borders; colour that is not uniform; distinctly different appearance from surrounding skin lesions; recent growth; ulceration

> Head and/or neck cancers: epistaxis, hoarseness, difficulty swallowing, odynophagia, shortness of breath, stridor, hemoptysis

Investigations: ultrasound, MRI, CT scan to detect head and/or neck mass; biopsy (definitive diagnosis)

CHOLESTEATOMA

Signs and symptoms: ear pain; progressive hearing loss; feeling of fullness; fever

> Otoscopy findings: retraction pocket in tympanic membrane (this may contain keratin debris); tympanic membrane perforation; granulation tissue; polyps; discharge from the ear

Risk factors for acquired cholesteatoma: acute otitis media, eustachian tube dysfunction (e.g., tympanostomy tubes, history of ear surgery)

REFERRED PAIN (SINUSITIS, DENTAL, TEMPOROMANDIBULAR JOINT DYSFUNCTION)

SINUSITIS

Signs and symptoms: purulent nasal discharge (or congestion) and facial pain that persists > 10–14 days or is worsening after 5 days; fever; maxillary toothache; facial swelling; tender paranasal sinuses; erythema or swelling of the nasal mucosa; postnasal drip; periorbital swelling

DENTAL DISEASE

Signs and symptoms: toothache, or sensitivity of a tooth to cold; fever and/or chills (this suggests infection); abnormalities on dental exam; deep neck space infection on full head and neck exam

TEMPOROMANDIBULAR JOINT (TMJ) DYSFUNCTION

Signs and symptoms: pain that is worse with jaw motion (chewing, talking), especially in the morning; pain that may radiate to the ear, cheek, temple, neck, or shoulder; headache; TMJ symptoms (pain, tightness, crepitation, clicking, catching sensation); TMJ symptoms on palpation or applied finger pressure (clicking, limited range of motion, subluxation, deviation of jaw, pain)

Strategy for patient encounter

The likely scenario is a patient with ear pain. The specified tasks could engage history, physical exam, investigations, or management.

History

Start with open-ended questions about the ear pain: When did it start? How constant is it? What other symptoms do you have? Listen for evidence consistent with particular entities (e.g., sudden-onset constant pain, fever, and hearing loss in acute otitis media; ear pain with constitutional symptoms in neoplasm; headache, and ear pain made worse with jaw motion, in temporomandibular joint malfunction). Ask about recent or current infections (sinus, throat) and recent viral illnesses. Ask about possible trauma (e.g., Q-Tip use; head trauma; exposure to a loud noise; pressure changes from recent flights or scuba diving). Ask about a history of allergies (this is common in eustachian tube dysfunction).

Physical exam

Perform an examination of the ears, head, and neck. Look for causes such as sinusitis, dental disease, and temporomandibular joint dysfunction (this is especially important when the ear exam is normal, which is likely in a standardized patient). Remember to palpate the mastoid process for tenderness (this is relevant to mastoiditis).

Investigations

Consider a complete blood count (CBC) to look for an elevated white blood cell (WBC) count (relevant to infection). If ear discharge is present, send a sample for culture and sensitivity. Order an audiogram in patients with hearing loss. Order other tests as indicated (see the information this resource lists in the MCC differential diagnosis).

Management

Management is directed at the underlying cause.

Refer patients with tympanic membrane rupture or malignancy to an ear, nose, and throat (ENT) surgeon.

Pearls

Ear pain from a dental problem is both common and commonly missed. In addition, approximately half of all patients with no identifiable cause experience spontaneous resolution.

44

Generalized edema

MCC particular objectives

Differentiate between systemic edema and localized edema.

Categorize the general mechanism of edema, because this can affect management.

MCC differential diagnosis
with added evidence

INCREASED CAPILLARY HYDROSTATIC PRESSURE

Increased plasma volume due to renal sodium retention

HEART FAILURE

The most common causes are coronary artery disease, hypertension, alcohol use, and valve disease.

Common precipitating factors include hypertension; poor medication adherence; dietary indiscretion (eating foods high in salt); anemia (possible symptoms: blood in stool, melena, palpitations, shortness of breath, fatigue); arrhythmia (possible symptoms: palpitations, shortness of breath, syncope, falls); ischemic heart event (possible symptoms: chest pain, sweating); infection (possible symptoms: fever and/or chills); and pulmonary disease (possible signs and symptoms: history of smoking, blood clot, shortness of breath, productive cough, fever, chills, sputum production).

Signs and symptoms: chest pain, shortness of breath, orthopnea, paroxysmal nocturnal dyspnea, cough, syncope, fatigue, peripheral edema

> Left-sided heart failure: hypotension, reduced capillary refill, peripheral cyanosis, pulsus alternans, mitral regurgitation murmur, S3, pulmonary crackles

> Right-sided heart failure: tricuspid regurgitation murmur, S3, peripheral edema, increased jugular venous pressure, Kussmaul sign, hepatosplenomegaly

Investigations: chest X-ray to detect interstitial edema (redistribution of Kerley B lines, bronchiolar-alveolar cuffing), cardiomegaly, or pleural effusion; CBC to detect low hemoglobin or elevated WBCs; electrolytes; elevated thyrotropin (TSH) (thyrotoxicosis can precipitate congestive heart failure); creatinine, BUN to detect renal insufficiency (due to reduced renal blood flow from reduced cardiac output in more severe congestive heart failure); elevated troponin (if cardiac ischemia is present); HbA$_{1c}$; liver function tests; elevated BNP; urinalysis to detect proteinuria; echocardiogram; ECG

REDUCED SYSTEMIC VASCULAR RESISTANCE (E.G., CIRRHOSIS)

CIRRHOSIS

Signs and symptoms: jaundice; easy bruising, bleeding; itching; ascites; spiderlike blood vessels on the skin; systemic symptoms (anorexia, weight loss, weakness, fatigue)

> History of chronic alcohol abuse; chronic infection with hepatitis B virus (HBV) or hepatitis C virus (HCV); hemochromatosis; nonalcoholic fatty liver disease

> HBV and HCV risk factors: unprotected sex, intravenous drug abuse, blood transfusions, tattoos, body piercings, imprisonment, workplace exposure to body fluids

Investigations: liver function tests

PRIMARY SODIUM RETENTION (E.G., RENAL DISEASE, DRUGS)

RENAL DISEASE

Signs and symptoms: history of kidney disease, chronic renal failure, and/or current renal dialysis; bilateral lower limb swelling; shortness of breath; paroxysmal nocturnal dyspnea; orthopnea; elevated jugular venous pressure; pulmonary crackles; peripheral pitting edema

Risk factors: diabetes, diabetic complications, and/or inadequate monitoring; hypertension; smoking

Investigations:

> Markers of renal disease: reduced calcium; elevated phosphate; elevated creatinine; elevated BUN; reduced GFR; reduced vitamin D; elevated albumin:creatinine ratio; red cell casts, proteinuria on urinalysis; hyperkalemia; elevated phosphate; anemia on CBC; elevated PTH

> Cardiac function: normal echocardiogram once fluid around the heart has been removed (this distinguishes renal etiology from congestive heart failure)

DRUGS

These include nonsteroidal antiinflammatory drugs (NSAIDs), glucocorticoids, fludrocortisones, thiazolidinediones (glitazones), insulin, hormone medications (estrogens, progestins, androgens, testosterone, aromatase inhibitors), vasodilators, and calcium channel blockers.

PREGNANCY

Signs and symptoms: amenorrhea, especially during childbearing years (some experience spotting); sexual activity, especially without contraception or with inconsistent use of contraception; nausea or vomiting (common early sign); breast enlargement and tenderness; increased frequency of urination without other urinary symptoms; fatigue

Investigations: blood or urine β-hCG

Decreased arteriolar resistance (e.g., calcium channel blockers, idiopathic)

CALCIUM CHANNEL BLOCKERS

This is usually due to a recent start of calcium channel blockers or an increase in dose.

IDIOPATHIC

Signs and symptoms: bilateral peripheral edema; normal pulmonary exam; normal cardiac exam (including normal jugular venous pressure); **no** evidence of pulmonary edema (shortness of breath, paroxysmal nocturnal dyspnea, orthopnea), hepatic disease, renal disease, cardiac disease, or medications associated with edema

Investigations: normal albumin, liver enzymes, liver function, and renal function

DECREASED ONCOTIC PRESSURE (HYPOALBUMINEMIA)

Protein loss (e.g., nephrotic syndrome)

NEPHROTIC SYNDROME

Signs and symptoms: progressive lower extremity edema (ankles and feet); swelling around the eyes; weight gain (from water retention); foamy urine

Risk factors: conditions that damage the kidneys (e.g., diabetes, systemic lupus erythematosus, amyloidosis); use of nonsteroidal antiinflammatory drugs (NSAIDs), antibiotics; history of HIV, hepatitis B virus infection (HBV), hepatitis C virus infection (HCV), malaria

Investigations: urine (proteinuria, spot urine protein:creatinine ratio, lipuria); hyponatremia with low fractional sodium excretion; low serum albumin; high total cholesterol (hyperlipidemia); elevated BUN

Reduced albumin synthesis (e.g., liver disease, malnutrition)

LIVER DISEASE

Patients with compensated cirrhosis may be asymptomatic.

HCV is often asymptomatic.

Signs and symptoms: jaundice; abdominal pain, swelling; palpable, tender liver; swelling in the legs and ankles; systemic symptoms (anorexia, weight loss, weakness, fatigue); itching; easy bruising

History of chronic alcohol abuse; chronic HBV or HCV; hemochromatosis; autoimmune conditions; α_1-antitrypsin deficiency; primary biliary cirrhosis; congestive heart failure

HBV and HCV risk factors: unprotected sex, intravenous drug abuse, blood transfusions, tattoos, body piercings, imprisonment, workplace exposure to body fluids

Investigations: tests for liver enzymes (elevated AST, ALT) and liver function (elevated bilirubin; possible abnormal PT/INR); viral serologic tests to detect HBV, HCV; Doppler ultrasound; CT scan; MRI; transient elastography; liver biopsy

MALNUTRITION

Signs and symptoms: weight loss, reduced intake

History of alcohol use disorder, malignancy, diabetes, renal disease, protein-losing enteropathy (e.g., inflammatory bowel disease, Crohn disease, ulcerative colitis)

Investigations: low prealbumin; low albumin

INCREASED CAPILLARY PERMEABILITY (E.G., BURNS, INFLAMMATION)

Signs and symptoms: burns, tissue trauma

Systemic inflammatory response syndrome: temperature $< 35°C$ or $> 38°C$; heart rate > 90 beats/minute; respiratory rate > 20 breaths/minute or $PaCO_2 < 32$ mmHg; white blood cell count $< 4 \times 10^9/L$ or $> 12 \times 10^9/L$ or $> 10\%$ bands

Allergic reaction: skin or mucosal symptoms (e.g., urticaria, pruritus, angioedema), shortness of breath, hypotension, nausea, vomiting

INCREASED INTERSTITIAL ONCOTIC PRESSURE (E.G., MYXEDEMA)

MYXEDEMA

This is nonpitting edema due to deposition of glycosaminoglycans and is typically a severe presentation of hypothyroidism.

Signs and symptoms: history of hypothyroidism or symptoms of severe hypothyroidism (hypothermia, bradycardia, decreased reflexes, dry skin, weight gain, impaired cognition); hypotension; hypoventilation; generalized edema

Risk factors: infection, cerebrovascular disease, congestive heart failure, trauma-induced myocardial infarction

Investigations: elevated thyrotropin (TSH); hypoglycemia; hyponatremia

Strategy for patient encounter

The likely scenario is a patient with bilateral ankle edema. The specified tasks could engage history, physical exam, investigations, or management.

History

Start with open-ended questions about the onset and characteristics of the edema: When did it start? Where is the swelling? What makes it better? What makes it worse? Listen for gradual-onset versus sudden-onset edema (gradual onset suggests an underlying chronic condition); unilateral versus bilateral edema (bilateral edema usually indicates a systemic condition); and changes in swelling with changes in body position (edema caused by chronic venous insufficiency often improves with limb elevation; edema associated with decreased oncotic pressure does not).

Take a general medical history, listening for disorders commonly associated with edema (congestive heart failure, renal disease, liver disease, sleep apnea, thyroid disease). In cases of

CHECKLIST

Wells criteria for deep vein thrombosis (DVT)

CRITERIA	SCORE
Paralysis, paresis, or recent orthopedic casting of a lower extremity	1
Recently bedridden for longer than 3 days or major surgery within the past 4 weeks	1
Localized tenderness in the deep vein system	1
Swelling of an entire leg	1
Calf swelling 3 cm greater than the other leg, measured 10 cm below the tibial tuberosity	1
Pitting edema greater in the symptomatic leg	1
Collateral nonvaricose superficial veins	1
Active cancer or cancer treated within 6 months	1
Alternative diagnosis more likely than DVT (e.g., Baker cyst, cellulitis, muscle damage, postphlebitic syndrome, inguinal lymphadenopathy, external venous compression)	−2
Modified score: previously documented DVT	+1
INTERPRETATION	TOTAL SCORE
High probability of DVT	≥ 3
DVT likely	2–3
Moderate probability of DVT	1–2
DVT unlikely	≤ 1
Low probability of DVT	≤ 0

Reprinted from The Lancet, Vol. 350, Wells PS, Anderson DR, Bormanis J, et al, Value of assessment of pretest probability of deep-vein thrombosis in clinical management, pp 1795-8, 1997, with permission from Elsevier.

lower limb edema, deep vein thrombosis (DVT) is a possibility, especially if the swelling is asymmetrical: apply the Wells criteria (see the checklist).

Take a medication history, looking specifically for use of calcium channel blockers.

Physical exam

Perform a full physical exam, assessing affected areas for pitting, tenderness, and skin changes. Look for signs of heart failure (rales, increased jugular venous pressure), liver disease (jaundice, ascites, asterixis), and thyroid disease (hyper- or hypothermia, tachy- or bradycardia, exophthalmos, tremor).

In cases of lower limb edema, apply the Wells criteria (see the checklist).

Investigations

For all patients, order tests for creatinine, liver function (relevant to liver disease), and serum albumin (hypoalbuminemia), and order a urinalysis (renal disease) and a chest X-ray (heart failure). In patients with sleep apnea, consider echocardiography to detect associated pulmonary hypertension (this is common).

In cases of lower limb edema, pursue further investigations based on the Wells criteria:

- **Wells criteria score ≤ 0:** This indicates low risk of DVT. Order a D-dimer test. If this is positive, the patient should receive an ultrasound. A negative ultrasound rules out DVT.
- **Wells criteria score 1–2:** This indicates moderate risk of DVT. Order a high-sensitivity D-dimer (if available). A negative result rules out DVT. Order an ultrasound for patients with positive results.
- **Wells criteria score ≥ 3:** This indicates likely DVT. D-dimer testing is not needed in these patients. Order an immediate ultrasound. In patients with a negative ultrasound, consider a repeat ultrasound in 1 week if symptoms persist.

Management

Treatment is directed toward the underlying etiology. For patients with chronic venous insufficiency, treatment includes emollients, topical steroid creams as needed, and compression stockings.

45

Localized edema

MCC particular objective

Consider deep vein thrombosis.

MCC differential diagnosis
with added evidence

VENOUS INSUFFICIENCY (INCLUDING POSTPHLEBITIC SYNDROME)

Signs and symptoms: history of deep vein thrombosis (DVT) (particularly recurrent DVT; this is a major risk factor for the development of postphlebitic syndrome), pain, leg heaviness, ankle and calf swelling (relieved by elevation), tightness, skin irritation, muscle cramps, itching, varicose veins

> Skin symptoms: overlying skin changes; dry skin; brown hyperpigmentation (hemosiderin deposits); stasis dermatitis; lipodermatosclerosis (fibrosing dermatitis of subcutaneous fat) if the condition is chronic; ulcers (weeping, painless, with irregular borders) above the medial malleolus

Investigations: duplex ultrasound to detect venous reflux (retrograde flow)

DEEP VEIN THROMBOSIS

Signs and symptoms: history of recent stroke or uncontrolled severe hypertension; red, painful, warm, and/or swollen calf (the affected calf is erythematous, tender, swollen; it is > 3 cm larger than the other calf when measured 10 cm distal to the tibial tuberosity)

> Symptoms if concurrent with pulmonary embolism: chest pain, shortness of breath

Risk factors: recent surgery; trauma; malignancy; blood disorders; prolonged immobilization; increased estrogen (e.g., pregnant, oral contraceptive use); antiphospholipid syndrome; congestive heart failure; a score of 2 or 3 on Wells criteria

Investigations: positive D-dimer (this should prompt further diagnostic tests); duplex ultrasonography

> D-dimer testing should only be considered in patients with a low pretest probability (e.g., the patient is young, is presenting with their first episode of DVT, and has few medical comorbidities) and the result is only helpful if it is negative.

TRAUMA

An example is an anterior cruciate ligament (ACL) tear.

LYMPHEDEMA (E.G., MALIGNANCY, PRIMARY)

Signs and symptoms (in general): swelling; reduction in mobility; pain; nonpitting edema

Risk factors: history of malignancy, radiation, surgery, infection

INFECTION (CELLULITIS; INFECTION OF SOFT TISSUE OR BONE)

Symptoms (in general): unilateral erythema, tenderness, and warmth (affected areas have poorly demarcated borders); fever and/or malaise (these are severe symptoms); wet or dry wound (if present, a wet wound has purulent discharge)

Risk factors: recent trauma; instrumentation; surgery; lymphedema; diabetes; peripheral vascular disease

Strategy for patient encounter

The likely scenario is a patient with a swollen calf. The specified tasks could engage history, physical exam, investigations, or management.

History

Determine if the edema is acute or chronic. Acute edema, especially in 1 leg, raises the possibility of deep vein thrombosis (DVT), although chronic edema does not exclude DVT. Apply the Wells criteria to all cases of lower limb edema (see the checklist). Ask about a history of cancer, trauma, pelvic surgery (including inguinal lymphadenectomy), and radiation therapy.

Physical exam

Examine the extremity for signs of a clot (a palpable clot, tenderness), pitting or nonpitting edema, hemosiderin (relevant to venous insufficiency), and ulcers (relevant to venous insufficiency).

Investigations

Assess the patient using the Wells criteria (see the checklist) and order further investigations as follows:

- **Wells criteria score ≤ 0:** This indicates low risk of DVT. Order a D-dimer test. If this is positive, the patient should

CHECKLIST
Wells criteria for deep vein thrombosis (DVT)

CRITERIA	SCORE
Paralysis, paresis, or recent orthopedic casting of a lower extremity	1
Recently bedridden for longer than 3 days or major surgery within the past 4 weeks	1
Localized tenderness in the deep vein system	1
Swelling of an entire leg	1
Calf swelling 3 cm greater than the other leg, measured 10 cm below the tibial tuberosity	1
Pitting edema greater in the symptomatic leg	1
Collateral nonvaricose superficial veins	1
Active cancer or cancer treated within 6 months	1
Alternative diagnosis more likely than DVT (e.g., Baker cyst, cellulitis, muscle damage, postphlebitic syndrome, inguinal lymphadenopathy, external venous compression)	−2
Modified score: previously documented DVT	+1
INTERPRETATION	**TOTAL SCORE**
High probability of DVT	≥ 3
DVT likely	2–3
Moderate probability of DVT	1–2
DVT unlikely	≤ 1
Low probability of DVT	≤ 0

Reprinted from The Lancet, Vol. 350, Wells PS, Anderson DR, Bormanis J, et al, Value of assessment of pretest probability of deep-vein thrombosis in clinical management, pp 1795-8, 1997, with permission from Elsevier.

receive an ultrasound. A negative ultrasound rules out DVT.

- **Wells criteria score 1–2:** This indicates moderate risk of DVT. Order a high-sensitivity D-dimer (if available). A negative result rules out DVT. Order an ultrasound for patients with positive results.
- **Wells criteria score ≥ 3:** This indicates likely DVT. D-dimer testing is not needed in these patients. Order an immediate ultrasound. In patients with a negative ultrasound, consider a repeat ultrasound in 1 week if symptoms persist.

Management

DVT can be managed on an outpatient basis for most patients. Administer low molecular weight heparin and start direct oral anticoagulants (see the checklist on contraindications). Overlap these until the patient's prothrombin time/international normalized ratio (PT/INR) is higher than 2 for at least 24 hours (this usually takes about 5 days).

Treat venous insufficiency (stasis dermatitis) with emollients, topical steroid creams, and compression stockings (rule out peripheral arterial disease before prescribing compression stockings).

Treat any other underlying associated conditions.

CHECKLIST

Contraindications to anticoagulant therapy

ABSOLUTE CONTRAINDICATIONS
Active bleeding

Severe underlying bleeding disorder or platelet count below 20 X 10⁹/L

Intracranial hemorrhage

Neurosurgery or ocular surgery in the previous 10 days

RELATIVE CONTRAINDICATIONS
Mild to moderate bleeding disorder or thrombocytopenia

Brain metastases

Recent trauma

Recent gastrointestinal or genitourinary bleed

Recent abdominal surgery

Endocarditis

46

Eye redness

MCC particular objective

Distinguish benign causes from those that require prompt referral to prevent significant vision loss.

MCC differential diagnosis
with added evidence

LIDS, LASHES, ORBITS, OR LACHRYMAL SYSTEM
BLEPHARITIS
Signs and symptoms: usually bilateral; red, swollen, and/or itchy eyelids; gritty, burning sensation in the eyes; tearing; crusted eyelashes

on wakening; flaky, greasy eyelid skin; loss of eyelashes; eyelashes growing at abnormal angles (misdirected eyelashes); malposition of eyelids from chronic inflammation

> History of seborrheic dermatitis (common), rosacea (common), acne, eczema, smoking, allergies, retinoid use

CONJUNCTIVA, SCLERA

CONJUNCTIVITIS

Signs and symptoms: red eye; eye discharge; gritty, burning sensation in the eye

> Bacterial: unilateral symptoms that progress to bilateral symptoms; purulent discharge; infectious contacts

> Viral: unilateral symptoms that progress to bilateral symptoms; watery discharge; upper respiratory tract infection (usual) or infectious contacts; pruritus

> Allergic: bilateral symptoms; pruritus; mucosal discharge; history of atopy (allergic rhinitis, eczema, asthma)

SUBCONJUNCTIVAL HEMORRHAGE

This may be spontaneous in elderly patients, but always check for traumatic injury.

Signs and symptoms: painless, well-demarcated area of conjunctival erythema with no visual disturbances; use of anticoagulants (possible contributing factor)

Risk factors: trauma; recent coughing, sneezing; recent heavy lifting

EPISCLERITIS

Signs and symptoms: possibly asymptomatic; abrupt-onset redness, tearing, and/or irritation

> History of associated conditions: rheumatoid arthritis, inflammatory bowel disease, vasculitis, systemic lupus erythematosus, infection (e.g., Lyme disease, herpes zoster ophthalmicus), atopy, rosacea

Investigations: blanching of vessels with application of phenylephrine (this differentiates episcleritis from scleritis)

ORBITAL CELLULITIS

This condition is an ocular emergency.

Signs and symptoms: fever; malaise; pain with eye movement; reduced vision, double vision; red eye; swelling and/or redness of the eyelid and surrounding skin; proptosis; relative afferent pupillary defect; mucormycosis (this is a severe and destructive fungal orbital cellulitis); history of diabetes

Risk factors: preseptal cellulitis; sinus, face, or tooth infection; trauma

Investigations: leukocytosis on CBC; elevated CRP, ESR; CT scan or MRI of the head

CORNEA

KERATITIS

This is inflammation of the cornea, commonly caused by infection. Other causes include neurotrophic, interstitial, fungal, and viral keratitis.

Signs and symptoms: use of contact lenses (common), including wearing lenses too long, not cleaning lenses properly, and/or not replacing lenses regularly; redness; eye pain; feeling of something in the eye; excessive tearing; photophobia

> Herpes keratitis: history of herpes infection (e.g., cold sores); branching pattern on fluorescein stain (possible)

DRY EYE

This is due to insufficient tear production or poor quality tears.

Signs and symptoms: redness, scratchy feeling in the eyes, eye pain, eye discharge

CORNEAL ABRASION

Signs and symptoms: unilateral (usually); sensation of a foreign object in the eye; pain; redness

ANTERIOR CHAMBER, IRIS

IRITIS

Signs and symptoms: typically unilateral; photophobia; redness; pain; globe tenderness or ache; ciliary flush; lacrimation; history of connective tissue disease (e.g., reactive arthritis, psoriatic arthritis, inflammatory bowel disease, ankylosing spondylitis, juvenile idiopathic arthritis), infection (herpes simplex virus, toxoplasmosis, HIV, syphilis, tuberculosis, Lyme disease)

Investigations: tonometry (intraocular pressure is usually reduced unless there is severe or infectious etiology that can lead to inflammatory glaucoma); slit-lamp exam (anterior chamber cells are visible)

ACUTE ANGLE-CLOSURE GLAUCOMA

This is an ocular emergency and requires emergency care.

Signs and symptoms: fixed, middilated pupil; exquisitely painful red eye (usually unilateral); reduced, blurry vision; halos seen around lights; nausea, vomiting; photophobia

Investigations: tonometry to detect increased intraocular pressure (> 40 mmHg); slit-lamp exam to detect cloudy cornea, shallow anterior chamber

ENDOPHTHALMITIS

This is an ocular emergency and requires emergency care.

Signs and symptoms: swollen eyelid; pain; redness; photophobia; eye discharge; reduced vision; proptosis; possible globe rupture, hypopyon

Risk factors: immunosuppression, systemic infections (endogenous factors); intraocular surgery, small ocular procedures, penetrating eye injury (exogenous factors)

Investigations: slit-lamp exam (findings: cells in the anterior chamber, corneal edema, hypopyon, reduced red reflex)

HYPOPYON (PUS IN ANTERIOR CHAMBER)

This is an ocular emergency. It requires an urgent ophthalmology consultation because it can be associated with infectious keratitis and endophthalmitis.

Signs and symptoms: history of blunt-force trauma; history of ocular disease (corneal ulcer, iritis, posterior uveitis, endophthalmitis, vitreitis)

Investigations: slit-lamp exam to detect WBCs in the anterior chamber

TRAUMA

Strategy for patient encounter

The likely scenario is a patient with unilateral eye redness. The specified tasks could engage history, physical exam, or management. Laboratory investigations do not generally provide information useful to diagnosing or managing eye redness.

History

Use open-ended questions to establish onset and symptoms: When did the eye redness start? Which eye is involved? What other symptoms do you have? Listen for evidence consistent with ocular emergencies (see the checklist) and particular entities (e.g., eyelash loss or abnormalities in blepharitis; bilateral itchy eyes with discharge in allergic conjunctivitis; recent-onset extreme unilateral eye pain with nausea, impaired vision, photophobia, and perceived halos around lights in acute angle-closure glaucoma). Ask about contact lens use. Ask about eye trauma. Ask about allergies and systemic disease.

Physical exam

Examine the eyes and eyelids. Record pupil sizes and reaction to light. Test visual acuity. Examine the head and neck for lymphadenopathy. In cases of corneal abrasion, check for a retained foreign body under the upper eyelid.

CHECKLIST

Findings that require immediate ophthalmology referral

Severe pain not relieved with topical anesthetics

Vision loss

Traumatic eye injury

Herpes infection

Recent ocular surgery

Corneal involvement

Distorted pupil

Copious purulent discharge

Perform a slit-lamp exam (including fluorescein staining in suspected abrasion or herpes infection). Consider measuring intraocular pressure.

Management
Identify patients who require immediate ophthalmology referral (see the checklist).

Management for common conditions includes:
- **Blepharitis:** eyelid scrubs
- **Allergic conjunctivitis:** topical antihistamines or histamine H_1 receptor antagonist agents
- **Bacterial conjunctivitis:** topical antibiotics
- **Viral conjunctivitis:** supportive therapy, handwashing (viral conjunctivitis is highly contagious)
- **Corneal abrasion:** topical antibiotics
- **Dry eye:** artificial tears
- **Episcleritis:** supportive therapy (episcleritis is self-limiting); in cases of recurrent episodes, referral to an ophthalmologist
- **Subconjunctival hemorrhage:** supportive therapy

47

Frailty in the elderly

MCC particular objectives
Assess the patient's level of function and cognition.

Demonstrate awareness of the importance of a multidisciplinary approach.

MCC differential diagnosis
with added evidence

MEDICATIONS
Signs and symptoms: poor adherence to current medications, recent dose changes, sensitivity to adverse effects of medications

ENVIRONMENTAL OR SOCIAL FACTORS (E.G., ISOLATION, POVERTY, ELDER ABUSE, NEGLECT)

ISOLATION, POVERTY

Signs and symptoms: living alone; lack of family or social supports; restricted income

ELDER ABUSE, NEGLECT

Signs and symptoms: disclosed abuse (physical, sexual, psychological, financial, neglect); resistance by a caregiver to having the patient interviewed alone (usual); fear of the patient towards a caregiver; isolation; depression; unexplained changes in financial situation; bruising, scars, healed fractures; poor hygiene; sudden weight loss, malnutrition

> Note: victims do not always disclose abuse.

Risk factors:

> Victim: female; advanced age (especially older than 80); vulnerability due to a chronic disorder, functional impairment, or cognitive impairment
>
> Perpetrator: substance abuse, psychiatric disorder, history of violence, cohabitation, dependence on the elderly person for support

MEDICAL DISEASE

Always consider illnesses that are more likely to occur at the extremes of age among vulnerable populations. For example, seniors living in isolation and poverty are at risk for hemolytic uremic syndrome, which may be overlooked because it is often considered a pediatric condition.

Common medical conditions associated with frailty include depression, malignancy, rheumatic disease, cardiovascular disease, endocrine disease, renal insufficiency, hematological disease, nutritional deficiency, and neurological disease.

Signs and symptoms (in general): weight loss; fatigue; weakness; reduced physical activity and walking pace; increased burden of symptoms; reduced ability to adapt to or recover from medical interventions

Investigations: CBC, creatinine, electrolytes, ALT, AST, GGT, ALP, PT/INR, bilirubin; albumin, vitamin B_{12}, thyrotropin (TSH), urinalysis

MALNUTRITION (E.G., FROM POOR DENTITION, MALABSORPTION, DYSPHAGIA)

POOR DENTITION

Signs and symptoms: missing teeth, dental caries, swollen gums

MALABSORPTION

Signs and symptoms: diarrhea; steatorrhea; weight loss despite adequate food intake; fatigue; edema; easy bruising, bleeding; pathological fractures; anorexia; flatulence; abdominal distention

> History of peptic ulcer disease, bowel resection, alcohol abuse, autoimmune conditions

Investigations: low electrolytes, calcium, and magnesium; prolonged PT/INR; low triglycerides, cholesterol; low vitamin B_{12}, ferritin, folic acid; hypoalbuminemia; elevated CRP (this suggests an inflammatory condition)

DYSPHAGIA

Several medical conditions at the end of life can contribute to dysphagia (e.g., patients with end-stage chronic obstructive pulmonary disease may have profound weakness, which impairs the coordination of breathing and swallowing).

Symptoms: choking on fluid intake; prolonged mealtime; nasal regurgitation; difficulty initiating swallowing; dry mouth; solids getting stuck in the throat; drooling; regurgitation after swallowing; painful swallowing; recurrent pneumonia; abnormalities of cranial nerves V, VII, IX, X, XII on cranial nerve exam

> History of malignancy of upper gastrointestinal tract and brain; progressive neurological disorders (e.g., amyotrophic lateral sclerosis, Parkinson disease, multiple sclerosis, dementia); cerebrovascular event

Investigations: barium swallow, esophagogastroduodenoscopy

PSYCHIATRIC CONDITION (E.G., MILD COGNITIVE IMPAIRMENT, DEMENTIA, DEPRESSION, PSYCHOSIS)

MAJOR OR MILD NEUROCOGNITIVE DISORDER

Signs and symptoms: gradual impairment of ≥ 1 cognitive area (complex attention; executive function; learning and memory; language; perceptual-motor skills; social interaction); **no** evidence that the cognitive impairment occurs only with delirium; **no** evidence of depression

> Mild cognitive impairment: deficits that **do not** significantly interfere with day-to-day life

> Major cognitive impairment (dementia): deficits that interfere with day-to-day life (e.g., ability to pay bills)

MAJOR DEPRESSIVE DISORDER[1(pp160-161)]

Signs and symptoms: symptoms that are present most of the time for ≥ 2 weeks; symptoms with significant impact on day-to-day life

> Key symptoms: depressed mood and/or loss of interest in usual activities

> Other symptoms: significant weight change; sleep disturbance; slowed or agitated mental processes; loss of concentration; recurrent thoughts of death or suicide

Risk factors: family history of mental health disorders (depression, anxiety, suicide); personal history of other mental health disorders; substance abuse; chronic illness (e.g., cancer, stroke, chronic pain)

PSYCHOSIS

Schizophrenia is the most common primary disorder associated with psychosis, but it is very uncommon as a new disorder in the elderly. Psychotic symptoms in the elderly are more likely caused by delirium, dementia, or drug-induced depression.

CHANGES IN VISUAL ACUITY

CHANGES IN AUDITORY ACUITY

DECREASED MOBILITY

Causes include history of falls; lower extremity weakness; underlying cognitive impairment; balance problems; polypharmacy, particularly psychotropic medication; pain (e.g., osteoarthritis, lumbar radiculopathy); history of stroke; orthostatic symptoms; anemia; and dizziness.

Strategy for patient encounter

The likely scenario is an elderly patient in frail health. The specified tasks could engage history, physical exam, investigations, or management.

History

Use open-ended questions to establish risk factors for frailty (see the checklist).

- **Psychosocial history:** What friends and family do you see regularly? How is your financial situation? How often do you drink alcohol? Listen for evidence of social isolation, poverty, and alcohol abuse. Ask the patient about elder abuse. Ask about activities of daily living: Do you need someone to help you with getting dressed, shopping, cooking, or showering?
- **Medical history:** What conditions have you been diagnosed with? Listen for a history of chronic illness and/or psychiatric conditions. Ask about unintended weight loss. Ask about the patient's usual diet, looking for malnutrition.
- **Medication history:** What medications do you take? Listen for drugs that are associated with an increased risk of falls (antidepressants, sedatives, anticholinergic drugs,

hypoglycemic agents, benzodiazepines, antihypertensive drugs, corticosteroids) and for the presence of poly-pharmacy (more than 4 prescription medications).

Physical exam

Obtain the patient's pulse and blood pressure, looking for any abnormal signs.

Examine the patient's mouth, looking for dental problems such as missing teeth, dental caries, and swollen gums.

Assess the patient's mental status. You could use a mini–mental status exam (see the quick reference), if appropriate (available time may determine your decision, because a typical MMSE takes 5 to 10 minutes). Otherwise, ask the patient for their full name and date of birth. Ask them to state where they are and how they got here.

Consider asking the patient to perform a gait-speed test (the patient walks 4 metres; a completion time longer than 5 seconds suggests frailty), and a chair-stand test (the patient stands up from a chair, walks 3 metres, turns around, walks back to the chair, and sits down; a completion time longer than 10 seconds suggests frailty).

QUICK REFERENCE
Mini–mental status exams (MMSEs)

A mini–mental status exam is a common way to assess for cognitive impairment.

Several versions of MMSEs exist. It's good general preparation for the exam to research MMSEs, and choose or prepare a version for your own use (this isn't the only clinical presentation where an MMSE may be appropriate).

MMSEs generally assess:

- orientation to time and place
- recall (e.g., remembering a short list of words)
- calculation (e.g., spelling a word backwards)
- language comprehension (e.g., naming objects; following a written command, a verbal command, and a complex instruction; repeating back a spoken phrase)

Investigations

Order a complete blood count (CBC). Order tests for electrolytes and creatinine to assess nutritional and renal status.

Order additional tests to assess the status of any acute or chronic conditions. These conditions and tests commonly include:

- **Rheumatological disease:** tests for serum autoantibodies of rheumatoid factors and/or anticitrullinated peptide/ protein antibodies; thrombocytosis; erythrocyte sedimentation rate (note that ESR values increase with increasing age); C-reactive protein
- **Cardiovascular disease:** lipid panel
- **Endocrine disease:** fasting blood glucose or glycated hemoglobin (HbA_{1c}) test, and thyrotropin (TSH) test
- **Hematological disease:** tests for serum ferritin and iron levels, and folate level

Management

Consider referring the patient to home care and community care agencies, if self-care, including nutrition, is an issue. Consider referring the patient for a geriatric medicine evaluation.

Discuss health goals with the patient, including their desire for cardiopulmonary resuscitation (CPR). If this is not desired, provide the patient with a form or letter stating "no CPR (do not resuscitate)," and tell family and caregivers about its location.

Refer the patient for counselling if there are financial concerns. Report abuse to adult protection services or the police.

Consider steps to prevent falls (e.g., modifying medications; recommending proper footwear, walking aids, and grab bars in the bathroom).

Consider referring the patient for a road safety test if driving competency is an issue.

REFERENCE

1 American Psychiatric Association. Diagnostic and statistical manual of mental disorders. 5th ed. Arlington, VA: American Psychiatric Association; 2013. 991 p.

48

Failure to thrive (infant, child)

MCC particular objective

Pay particular attention to psychosocial and environmental factors, and to disease entities, that give rise to poor infant and child maturation.

MCC differential diagnosis
with added evidence

PRENATAL

See clinical presentation 172 on intrauterine growth restriction (IUGR).

POSTNATAL

FAILURE TO THRIVE (INFANT, CHILD) IN GENERAL

This is the inability of an infant or child to grow adequately or to maintain growth, usually based on at least 1 of the following growth-chart measurements:

- weight: < third percentile for age and sex; < 80% of expected weight for height and age
- height: < fifth percentile for age and sex
- major percentile curves: crosses ≥ 2 over time
- body mass index (BMI): < fifth percentile for age

Failure to thrive does **not** apply if a child:

- has normal growth velocity, although apparently underweight (e.g., even < second percentile for weight)
- is genetically small
- is small for other reasons (e.g., constitutional growth delay, prematurity, or intrauterine growth restriction), but has normal weight for length and normal growth velocity

Inadequate calorie intake

CAREGIVER

INADEQUATE FEEDING SKILLS

Examples include giving too much juice or pop; preparing formula improperly (e.g., dilution); not providing enough food; providing an inappropriate diet (e.g., a vegetarian diet that is low in protein and essential vitamins); restricting foods (e.g., because of suspected allergies or cultural views); not establishing proper eating protocols (e.g., propping a bottle instead of holding it; allowing distractions such as TV during meals); not responding to the child's hunger cues (e.g., because disengaged or irritable); and not allowing enough time for feeding.

INAPPROPRIATE FOOD FOR AGE

Examples include delayed introduction of solid foods (e.g., the child is exclusively breast-feeding or exclusively drinking milk or formula after age 6 months); too-early introduction of solid food (at younger than 4 months); and lack of knowledge about the dietary needs of infants (e.g., knowing that it is appropriate to introduce soft foods such as rice cereal at 4 to 6 months).

> Delayed introduction of solid foods can lead to iron deficiency anemia, food aversion, delayed oral motor function, and atopy.

> Too-early introduction of solid foods can lead to new-food intolerance, allergies, and food aspiration.

INSUFFICIENT LACTATION

Causes include maternal stress or fatigue, which decreases milk supply (symptom: poor letdown sensation); history of breast surgery or breast radiation; high androgen or prolactin levels; too-small breasts; medications; decreased frequency of feeds (e.g., due to separation of child and mother); and poor latch.

INFANT

SUCKING OR SWALLOWING DYSFUNCTION

Causes include pain (e.g., dental caries); craniofacial or oral abnormalities (e.g., cleft lip and/or palate; ankyloglossia); and neuromuscular disorder (e.g., dystrophies, hypotonia, cerebral palsy, hydrocephalus).

CHRONIC DISEASE (E.G., INFECTION, METABOLIC DISORDER)

INFECTION

Signs and symptoms: fever (> 38.0°C) or low rectal temperature (< 36.6°C); difficulty feeding; sleepiness; lethargy; irritability; rapid breathing; pallor; jaundice; blue lips or mouth

> History of chronic infection (e.g., urinary tract infections, tuberculosis, HIV), immunodeficiency

METABOLIC DISORDER

Signs and symptoms (these begin a few weeks after birth): lethargy; poor appetite; abdominal pain; vomiting; weight loss; jaundice; developmental delay; seizures; coma; abnormal odour in the urine, breath, sweat, or saliva; chronic renal failure; family history of metabolic disorders (e.g., hypercalcemia, inborn errors of metabolism, storage diseases, diabetes, adrenal insufficiency)

INADEQUATE CALORIC ABSORPTION (E.G., GASTROINTESTINAL REFLUX)

GASTROESOPHAGEAL REFLUX DISEASE

Acid reflux is common in healthy infants aged up to 1 year.

Gastroesophageal reflux disease differs from this and is a serious condition.

Signs and symptoms: nonforceful regurgitation into the oral cavity, especially if it is worsening in infants older than 6 months; excessive vomiting; refusal to feed, or irritability during and after feeding; persistent cough, heartburn, gas, belly pain

Investigations: upper GI series (X-ray); pH probe; upper GI endoscopy; gastric emptying study

Increased caloric requirements (e.g., hyperthyroidism, congenital heart disease)

HYPERTHYROIDISM

Signs and symptoms: enlarged thyroid, tachycardia, palpitations, diarrhea, muscle weakness, tremor, hyperactive reflexes, weight loss, sweating, thinning hair

Investigations: decreased thyrotropin (TSH)

CONGENITAL HEART DISEASE

Symptoms: sweating with feeds; feeding intolerance; rapid breathing; fatigue; heart failure (increased work of breathing; decreased urine output)

Maternal history of diabetes; preeclampsia; older age; multiple gestation; thyroid disorders; congenital heart disease; connective tissue disorder; epilepsy; depression; bipolar disorder; use of drugs, alcohol during pregnancy; rubella exposure during pregnancy

Genetic anomaly (infant): trisomy 21, 18, 13; Turner syndrome; Klinefelter syndrome; DiGeorge syndrome; other single gene mutations (e.g., Noonan syndrome, Marfan syndrome, Ehler-Danlos syndrome)

Investigations: echocardiogram to detect cardiac abnormality

Social determinants (e.g., poverty, societal disorder)

Poverty involves restricted family income and, often, social isolation.

Examples of societal disorder include war zones, refugee camps, and disaster areas.

Signs and symptoms of adverse social determinants in children: depression; symptoms of posttraumatic stress disorder (PTSD) (e.g., flashbacks); anxiety; poor academic performance; abdominal pain, headache, or other physical symptoms

Risk factors for adverse social determinants: parental psychiatric condition; family discord including domestic abuse; young single mother; parental substance use; medically or developmentally challenging child

Strategy for patient encounter

This encounter will likely involve a parent discussing their child. The child will be absent on some pretext (e.g., a nurse is taking the child's growth measurements and vital signs in another room). The specified tasks could engage history, physical exam, investigations, or management.

Failure to thrive is most commonly caused by inadequate caloric intake associated with behavioural or psychosocial issues.

History

Use open-ended questions to obtain a dietary history, psychosocial history, and general medical history.

- **Dietary history:** What foods do you offer your child? How often do you offer food in a typical day? What does your child eat in a typical day? Listen for the presence or absence of appropriate food choices for the child's age, adequately frequent meals, and adequate caloric intake.
- **Psychosocial history:** What is your family income? What is your living situation? What is your family background with traumatic events? What concerns do you have about violence, addiction problems, or child abuse in your home? Ask whether the parents or caregivers have a history of psychiatric disorders. Listen for evidence of social risk factors (poverty; unstable living situation; exposure to disasters or other trauma; child abuse; caregivers with a history of substance abuse and/or psychiatric disorders).
- **Medical history:** What conditions has your child been diagnosed with? What conditions run in your family? Listen for chronic conditions and infections (e.g., neuromuscular disorders, HIV, tuberculosis, congenital heart disease, cystic fibrosis, metabolic disorders).

Physical exam

Measure the child's height, weight, and head circumference and plot these on a growth curve. Perform a full physical examination, staying alert to signs of abuse (e.g., burn marks, ligature marks, bruising) and neglect (e.g., poor hygiene, poor dental care).

(State that you will examine the child. Because an actual pediatric patient is unlikely, the examiner may interrupt, ask what you are looking for, and provide findings. State that you are looking for abnormal growth measurements, and signs of abuse and neglect. If the history suggests an organic cause, state that you are looking for signs of that organic cause.)

Investigations

Consider tests for specific disorders if the history or physical exam reveal relevant signs or risk factors (e.g., sweat testing for cystic fibrosis, HIV testing, stool testing for fecal fat).

In the absence of localizing features, investigations usually have little useful information to contribute in the diagnosis or management of failure to thrive. However, a major role of testing is to rule out underlying organic illness. Consider ordering a complete blood count (CBC; relevant to infection, anemia, immune deficiency), urinalysis (infection), serum electrolytes and creatinine (renal dysfunction), and liver function tests (protein wasting).

Management

Report cases of abuse or neglect to child protection services or police. Apply a multidisciplinary approach including dietary counselling, social services support, and home nursing visits. Consider referral to a pediatrician and hospitalization for severe cases.

Pearls

Failure to thrive is seen in 5% to 10% of children in primary care settings in the United States.

49

Falls

MCC particular objectives

Recognize patients who are at risk of falling.

Identify contributing factors.

Formulate a prevention plan.

MCC differential diagnosis
with added evidence

MEDICAL CONDITIONS (E.G., VERTIGO, GAIT DISTURBANCES, SYNCOPE)

VERTIGO

Signs and symptoms: positive Dix-Hallpike maneuver (this suggests benign positional vertigo); recent viral or bacterial infection (this suggests peripheral vestibulopathy); recurrent episodes of vertigo, hearing loss, tinnitus, or aural fullness (this suggests Ménière disease); use of aminoglycosides; facial weakness, and ear or mastoid pain (this suggests acoustic neuroma)

GAIT DISTURBANCES

Signs and symptoms: poor balance; ataxia; antalgic gait; Trendelenburg sign; waddling; knee failing to lock; toe scuffing with steps; spastic gait; high stepping, stamping; decreased stride length; festinating gait (this is a symptom of Parkinson disease); impaired braking and acceleration (stumbling, lurching, staggering, slow pace, wide base, reeling); veering gait; cautious gait; difficulty initiating or maintaining gait

SYNCOPE

Signs and symptoms: fainting; use of antihypertensives; history of cardiovascular condition (arrhythmia, aortic stenosis, myocardial infarction), carotid artery disease, stroke, hypoglycemia, panic attacks

PSYCHIATRIC CONDITIONS (E.G., COGNITIVE IMPAIRMENT, SUBSTANCE ABUSE)

COGNITIVE IMPAIRMENT

Causes include Parkinson disease, Huntington disease, paraneoplastic syndrome, dementia (Alzheimer disease, fronto-temporal dementia, vascular dementia, Lewy body dementia), depression, delirium, sleep disorders, infection (e.g., prion disease, HIV, chronic meningitis), chronic brain injury, medications (anticholinergics, antihistamines), metabolic conditions (vitamin B_{12} deficiency, hypothyroidism, hypoglycemia), subdural hematoma, tumour, and normal pressure hydrocephalus.

SUBSTANCE ABUSE

Examples include abuse of cocaine, heroin, alcohol, amphetamines, and prescription medications (opioids, sedatives, stimulants).

Signs and symptoms: personal or family history of substance abuse; excessive worry; loss of interest in friends and usual activities; adverse experience (e.g., emotional, physical, or sexual abuse; death of a friend or family member); physical evidence (track marks on the arms, nasal septum perforation); tachycardia; tremor and/or sweating

MEDICATIONS

Examples include antipsychotics, anticonvulsants, benzodiazepines, narcotics, opioids with codeine, tricyclic antidepressants, diuretics, selective serotonin reuptake inhibitors (SSRIs), and antihypertensives.

Polypharmacy (> 4 medications) increases the risk of complications such as falls.

ENVIRONMENTAL OR BEHAVIOURAL FACTORS (E.G., WALKING SURFACES, CHOICE OF FOOTWEAR)

Examples include loose area rugs or frayed carpets; slippery floors; uneven walking surfaces; stairs, especially if steep or shallow; poor lighting; footwear that is too large, unstable, or damaged; walking in stockings or bare feet, instead of in shoes; lack of grab bars or railings; and unfamiliar environments.

OTHER CONTRIBUTORS (E.G., DECREASED VISION, URINARY URGENCY)

DECREASED VISION

Signs and symptoms: falls while walking or doing routine tasks (often); use of multifocal lenses; decreased visual acuity, depth perception, contrast sensitivity

URINARY URGENCY

Signs and symptoms: frequent or urgent urination; difficult or painful urination; hematuria; incontinence; fever (this suggests urinary tract infection)

> History of recurrent or recent urinary tract infection; atrophic urethritis; vaginitis; prostate enlargement; use of pharmaceuticals (diuretics, benzodiazepines, alcohol, caffeine); endocrine disorders (e.g., hypercalcemia, diabetes mellitus); restricted mobility; stool impaction

Investigations: urinalysis to detect WBCs, nitrites; urine culture

Strategy for patient encounter

The likely scenario is an elderly patient with a history of falls, who is accompanied by a family member. The specified tasks could engage history, physical exam, or management. Specific lab and imaging studies do not usually contribute information useful to diagnosing or managing the cause of falls.

History

Use open-ended questions to establish the circumstances of the fall: What specifically were you doing before you fell? Where exactly did the fall occur? What injuries did you have from the fall? How many times have you fallen in the past? How similar were the circumstances of this fall to previous falls? Ask about specific risk factors for falls (see the checklist on risk factors).

If the family member saw the fall (the scenario is likely to include an accompanying family member), ask this person for details.

Take a general medical history to determine the presence of any known chronic or acute illnesses: What conditions have you been diagnosed with?

Take a medication history, noting drugs that are associated with an increased risk of falls (antidepressants, sedatives, anticholinergic drugs, hypoglycemic agents, benzodiazepines, antihypertensive drugs, corticosteroids) and the presence of polypharmacy (more than 4 prescription medications). Ask about alcohol and illicit drug use.

Ask about environmental risk factors for falls at home (e.g., poor lighting; unsafe stairways; loose floor mats; irregular or slippery floor surfaces; lack of grab bars for toilets and tubs).

CHECKLIST
Risk factors for falls in the elderly
Older than 75
Housebound
Cane or walker use
Falling in the past
Polypharmacy
Living alone
Vision impairment
Cognitive impairment
Physical disability
Difficulty rising from a chair

Physical exam

Perform a complete physical, including taking the patient's blood pressure sitting and standing (relevant to postural hypotension), and assessing vision. In the neurological exam, assess for vertigo, balance, and strength. Examine the feet for sensation.

Assess the patient's mental status. You could use a mini-mental status exam (see the quick reference), if appropriate (available time may determine your decision, because a typical MMSE takes 5 to 10 minutes). Otherwise, ask the patient for their full name and date of birth. Ask them to state where they are and how they got here.

QUICK REFERENCE

Mini-mental status exams (MMSEs)

A mini-mental status exam is a common way to assess for cognitive impairment.

Several versions of MMSEs exist. It's good general preparation for the exam to research MMSEs, and choose or prepare a version for your own use (this isn't the only clinical presentation where an MMSE may be appropriate).

MMSEs generally assess:

- orientation to time and place
- recall (e.g., remembering a short list of words)
- calculation (e.g., spelling a word backwards)
- language comprehension (e.g., naming objects; following a written command, a verbal command, and a complex instruction; repeating back a spoken phrase)

Management

Multifactorial interventions are effective in preventing falls.

Treat any identified underlying conditions. Consider scheduling a home visit, which can be helpful in identifying and modifying environmental factors. Consider referring the patient to a falls clinic, if available. Otherwise, consider referring the patient for a geriatric medicine evaluation. Always consider patient safety and the feasibility of the patient continuing in their current living conditions.

Pearls

Recurrent falls are defined as more than 2 falls in a 6-month period.

50

Fatigue

MCC particular objectives

None stated.

MCC differential diagnosis
with added evidence

FATIGUE IN GENERAL

The MCC states that this clinical presentation is about entities where fatigue is the dominant presenting symptom.

IATROGENIC OR PHARMACOLOGIC CONDITIONS

Prescription medications

Examples include sedatives or hypnotics such as barbiturates and benzodiazepines; antidepressants such as monoamine oxidase inhibitors (MAOIs), selective serotonin reuptake inhibitors (SSRIs), serotonin and norepinephrine reuptake inhibitors (SNRIs), and tricyclics; antipsychotics; and antihypertensives.

Drugs of abuse

Examples include cocaine, heroin, alcohol, amphetamines, and sedatives.

IDIOPATHIC

Chronic fatigue syndrome

Signs and symptoms: extreme fatigue unexplainable by any underlying medical condition; symptoms that do not improve with rest; symptoms for ≥ 6 months

> Key symptoms: loss of memory or concentration; sore throat; enlarged lymph nodes (neck, armpits); muscle pain; pain that moves among joints without swelling or redness; headache of a new type, pattern, or severity; unrefreshing sleep; extreme exhaustion lasting > 24 hours after mental or physical exertion

Fibromyalgia

This is a diagnosis of exclusion.

Signs and symptoms: female (more common); chronic, widespread pain for ≥ 3 months; pain that is bilateral, and above and below the waist; aching pain; fatigue; long sleep; restless legs syndrome; sleep apnea;

impaired concentration, memory; dizziness; cramping (e.g., menstrual, abdominal); morning stiffness; numbness, tingling in the extremities; tender points; urinary symptoms (difficult or painful urination, irregular urination); sensitivity to noise, light, temperature

> Coexisting conditions (often): headaches, irritable bowel syndrome, interstitial cystitis

OTHER

Psychiatric condition

Signs and symptoms: personal or family history of psychiatric conditions (e.g., anxiety, major depressive disorder); excessive worry; loss of interest in friends and usual activities; changes in sleep habits; hallucinations or delusions; suicidal thoughts; history of adverse experience (emotional, physical, or sexual abuse; recent stress such as death of a friend or family member), or substance abuse

Endocrine-metabolic condition

DIABETES

Signs and symptoms: personal or family history of diabetes; history of diabetic complications and/or inadequate monitoring; polydipsia, polyuria, and/or weight loss

Investigations: fasting glucose or HbA_{1c} test

HYPOTHYROIDISM

Signs and symptoms: history of hypothyroidism or symptoms of hypothyroidism (cold intolerance, decreased reflexes, dry skin, weight gain, impaired cognition)

Investigations: elevated thyrotropin (TSH)

HYPERCALCEMIA

Signs and symptoms: constipation, polyuria, polydipsia, dehydration, anorexia, nausea, muscle weakness, altered sensory status

> History of sarcoidosis, malignancy, hyperparathyroidism, immobilization, use of diuretics (thiazide)

Investigations: blood test (hypercalcemia is total calcium ≥ 2.63 mmol/L or ionized calcium ≥ 1.4 mmol/L); albumin; PTH

KIDNEY DISEASE

Signs and symptoms: history of kidney disease, chronic renal failure, and/or current renal dialysis; bilateral lower limb swelling; shortness of breath; paroxysmal nocturnal dyspnea; orthopnea

Risk factors: diabetes, diabetic complications, and/or inadequate monitoring; hypertension; smoking

Investigations: renal function tests (reduced calcium; elevated phosphate; elevated creatinine); reduced vitamin D

LIVER DISEASE

Patients with compensated cirrhosis may be asymptomatic.

Hepatitis C virus (HCV) is often asymptomatic.

Signs and symptoms: jaundice; abdominal pain, swelling; palpable, tender liver; swelling in the legs and ankles; systemic symptoms (anorexia, weight loss, weakness, fatigue); itching; easy bruising

> History of chronic alcohol abuse; chronic hepatitis B virus (HBV) or HCV infection; hemochromatosis; autoimmune conditions; α_1-antitrypsin deficiency; primary biliary cirrhosis; congestive heart failure

> HBV and HCV risk factors: unprotected sex, intravenous drug abuse, blood transfusions, tattoos, body piercings, imprisonment, workplace exposure to body fluids

Investigations: tests for liver enzymes (elevated AST, ALT) and liver function (elevated bilirubin; possible abnormal PT/INR); viral serologic tests to detect HBV, HCV; Doppler ultrasound; CT scan; MRI; transient elastography; liver biopsy

Cardiopulmonary condition

CONGESTIVE HEART FAILURE

Signs and symptoms: history of heart disease (or risk factors for heart disease: diabetes, hypertension, hyperlipidemia, and smoking) or hepatic vein thrombosis (Budd-Chiari syndrome); severe shortness of breath; elevated jugular venous pressure; edema in the abdomen and legs; pink phlegm; heart murmurs and extra cardiac sounds

Investigations: chest X-ray to detect pulmonary edema; NT-proBNP level; echocardiogram to distinguish forms of heart failure; cardiac stress testing, either with exercise or pharmacological agent

CHRONIC OBSTRUCTIVE PULMONARY DISEASE

Signs and symptoms: older than age 40 (usual: symptoms do not appear until significant lung damage has occurred); progressive symptoms; wheezing; chest tightness; chronic productive cough; clubbing of the fingers; cyanosis around the lips and in the extremities; decreased oxygen saturation; impaired pulmonary function on testing with spirometry

Risk factors: smoking, occupational exposure, intrinsic lung disease

Investigations: chest X-ray; CT scan; ABG

Infectious condition (e.g., mononucleosis)

MONONUCLEOSIS

Signs and symptoms (classic triad): fever, pharyngitis, lymphadenopathy (usually posterior cervical)

> Additional signs and symptoms: fatigue and malaise; headache; abdominal pain; nausea, vomiting; rash; splenomegaly; palatal exanthems or petechiae

Investigations: CBC, lymphocytosis (> 50%); peripheral blood smear to detect atypical lymphocytes; heterophile antibody test (e.g., Monospot); EBV-specific serology testing (definitive)

Sleep disturbance (e.g., shift work)

Examples of causes include poor sleep environment, irregular work schedule (e.g., shift work), and insomnia.

> Poor sleep environments may have too much light, too much noise, uncomfortable temperatures (too hot or too cold), or cosleepers with sleep disorders (e.g., snoring).

> Insomnia may be due to pain, sleep apnea, snoring, gastroesophageal reflux disease, pregnancy, and postpartum routines.

Neoplastic-hematologic condition

ANEMIA

Risk factors: intestinal disorders (Crohn disease, celiac disease), menstruation, pregnancy, chronic disease (e.g., cancer, kidney failure), family history of sickle cell disease

Investigations: CBC; visual examination of RBCs for unusual size, shape, colour

LEUKEMIA

Signs and symptoms: fever; chills; persistent fatigue and weakness; frequent or severe infections; weight loss; pallor; swollen lymph nodes; enlarged liver or spleen; easy bleeding and bruising; recurrent nosebleeds; petechiae; excessive sweating; bone pain or tenderness

Investigations: CBC; peripheral blood smear; flow cytometry; bone marrow aspiration and biopsy

LYMPHOMA

Signs and symptoms (non-Hodgkin): constitutional symptoms (fatigue, fever, night sweats, weight loss), swollen lymph nodes, chest pain, coughing, shortness of breath

> Hodgkin lymphoma (less common): constitutional symptoms (fatigue, fever, night sweats, weight loss); swollen lymph nodes; itching; pain on drinking alcohol, or increased sensitivity to alcohol

Investigations: blasts or cancer cells on peripheral blood smear; excess blasts or cancer cells on bone marrow examination

MALIGNANCY

Signs and symptoms: history of solid organ cancer (e.g., breast, lung, renal, colon); easy bruising or bleeding; nodules or lumps anywhere on the body; constitutional symptoms (fever, weight loss, night sweats)

Investigations: X-ray, CT scan, MRI; biopsy

Strategy for patient encounter

The likely scenario is a patient with a recent history of fatigue. The specified tasks could engage history, physical exam, investigations, or management.

History

Ask open-ended questions to establish the characteristics of the fatigue and related symptoms, and to take a sleep and drug history. Follow up with focused questions about risk factors for infection and occupational exposures.

- **Fatigue characteristics:** When did the fatigue start? How constant it is? How has it changed since it started? How does rest affect it? How does mental or physical exertion affect it? Listen for evidence consistent with particular entities (e.g., recent-onset fatigue in infection; progressive fatigue in chronic conditions; extreme intermittent fatigue after mental or physical effort that is unrelieved by rest in chronic fatigue syndrome).

- **Related symptoms:** What other symptoms do you have? Listen for constitutional symptoms (these suggest malignancy: weight loss, fever, night sweats); excessive thirst and urination (diabetes); gastrointestinal symptoms, steatorrhea, and weight loss (celiac disease); intolerance to cold (hypothyroidism); shortness of breath (heart failure, chronic obstructive pulmonary disorder); chest pain (coronary artery disease); and anxiety and depression (psychiatric condition).

- **Sleep routines:** How regular is your sleep? How much sleep do you get? Listen for evidence of disrupted sleep.

- **Drug history:** What medications do you take? Pay particular attention to antidepressants, antiepileptics, antihistamines, antihypertensives, neuroleptics, corticosteroids, and diuretics. Ask about recreational drug use and substance abuse.

- **Risk factors for infection:** Screen the patient for a history of immunosuppression (this is relevant to Cytomegalovirus); exposure to unpasteurized dairy products (brucellosis); exposure to areas where Lyme disease is endemic; intravenous drug use and/or unprotected sex (HIV, hepatitis B and C); and contact with cat feces (toxoplasmosis).

- **Occupational exposures:** Ask about possible occupational and recreational exposure to heavy metals such as demolition (lead exposure) and artisanal glass manufacture (arsenic, cadmium).

Ask about the impact of the fatigue on the patient's quality of life and daily functioning.

Physical exam

Perform a physical exam, focusing on cardiovascular and neurologic systems. Check for pallor, tachycardia, and a systolic ejection murmur (relevant to anemia). Remember that normal findings are likely.

Investigations

Consider specific tests if evidence from the history and physical exam suggests a specific disorder (see the information this resource lists in the MCC differential diagnosis).

In the absence of localizing features, investigations may have limited success in diagnosing a specific entity. However, a major role of testing is to rule out underlying organic illness. Consider ordering a complete blood count (CBC), an erythrocyte sedimentation rate (ESR), a fasting blood glucose or glycated hemoglobin (HbA_{1c}) test, liver function tests, and tests to measure electrolytes, creatinine, creatine kinase, calcium, and thyrotropin (TSH). Ensure that age- and sex-appropriate cancer screening is up to date.

Management

Treat any conditions identified. In the absence of an apparent organic cause, strongly consider depression. It is acceptable practice to follow most patients without apparent cause and with negative workups, and to suggest lifestyle modifications (e.g., avoid triggers for fatigue as much as possible).

Pearls

Fatigue in patients older than 60 usually has an organic cause. Fatigue in younger patients (especially younger than 40) is more likely to have an unidentifiable cause.

51

Ataxia (gait)

MCC particular objectives
Distinguish ataxia from other abnormalities.

Establish the localization and cause.

MCC differential diagnosis
with added evidence

CEREBELLAR ATAXIA
CEREBELLAR ATAXIA IN GENERAL
Signs and symptoms: imbalance; head and trunk swaying; impaired ability to control movement in the limbs; vertigo with nausea and vomiting; positive Romberg test; rapid eye movements that occur in irregular episodes, especially nystagmus; dysdiadochokinesia; intention tremor; scanning speech

Tumours
Tumours cause symptoms due to hemorrhage, or compression of the cerebellum and associated structures.

Signs and symptoms: history of cerebellar primary tumours (this is more common in children; examples include meningioma, astrocytoma, hemangioblastoma) or metastatic cancer (this is more common in adults; examples include breast cancer, small cell lung cancer, ovarian cancer, Hodgkin lymphoma)

Investigations: head imaging to detect cerebellar mass

Vascular conditions
Signs and symptoms: history of vascular conditions such as stroke, cerebellar arterial dissection, vasculitis, hemorrhage (burst aneurysm, arteriovenous malformation), hypertension, repeat subarachnoid bleeding

Hereditary conditions
Signs and symptoms: chronic symptoms; family history of hereditary spinocerebellar ataxia, Friedrich ataxia, telangiectasia, mitochondrial disorders, fragile X syndrome, Tay-Sachs disease, Niemann-Pick disease

Multiple sclerosis
Signs and symptoms: variable depending on lesion location
> Spinal cord: sensory or motor dysfunction; Lhermitte sign (paresthesias radiating down the extremities or trunk with neck flexion); bowel, bladder or erectile dysfunction

Brainstem: double vision; swallowing, speech difficulties; vertigo; pseudobulbar palsy

Cerebrum: cognitive impairment; depression; upper motor neuron signs; unilateral motor or sensory deficits

Cerebellum: problems with balance and coordination; vertigo

Other symptoms: tonic spasms; fatigue; pain; exercise intolerance; temperature sensitivity; painful unilateral loss of visual acuity

Risk factors: younger than 50, female

Investigations: brain and spinal cord MRI, including advanced MRI techniques, with established occurrence of multiple episodes; CSF fluid analysis

Drugs

Examples include sedatives, anticonvulsants, benzodiazepines, amiodarone, metronidazole, chemotherapeutic drugs (fluorouracil), solvents, and lithium.

Alcohol

Signs and symptoms: history of alcohol abuse (this is associated with Wernicke encephalopathy); difficulty balancing; ataxia that affects the legs and gait, not the arms

Wernicke encephalopathy: ataxia, confusion, ophthalmoplegia

Investigations: elevated liver enzymes (AST:ALT ratio > 2; elevated GGT)

SENSORY ATAXIA

Vestibular condition

ACOUSTIC NEUROMA

Signs and symptoms: unilateral hearing loss; unilateral tinnitus; vertigo; feeling as if the body is tilted; veering towards the side of the affected ear; facial weakness

Investigations: CT scan or MRI of the head

Proprioceptive condition

Signs and symptoms: clumsiness; high stepping gait with stamping; history of diabetes, spinal myelopathy, brain lesion

Investigations: MRI of spinal cord and head

Visual condition

Signs and symptoms: decreased visual acuity, depth perception, and/or contrast sensitivity

OTHER (E.G., PARKINSON DISEASE)

PARKINSON DISEASE

Signs and symptoms (mnemonic **TRAP**): **t**remor at rest; **r**igidity of the lower limbs; **a**kinesia, bradykinesia; **p**ostural instability

Other symptoms: cognitive impairment; dementia; shuffling gait with stooped posture and loss of arm swing; micrographia; hypophonia; masklike facies, "pill rolling"; lack of blinking; orthostatic hypotension

History of use of antipsychotics, antiemetics; toxin ingestion (e.g., carbon monoxide, cyanide); head trauma; vascular disease; other neurodegenerative disease (e.g., Lewy body dementia, Huntington disease); brain tumour, hydrocephalus; metabolic conditions (e.g., hypoparathyroidism, Wilson disease, chronic liver failure); infections that spread to the brain (HIV/AIDS, syphilis, prion disease, toxoplasmosis, encephalitis lethargica, progressive multifocal leukoencephalopathy)

Strategy for patient encounter

The likely scenario is a patient with cerebellar dysfunction or Parkinson disease. The specified tasks could engage history, physical exam, investigations, or management.

History

The most important information to obtain from the history is the age of onset of the movement disorder, the tempo of disease (acute onset, gradual onset, progressive), and the presence or absence of a family history of the same condition. If there is a positive family history, try to determine the pattern of inheritance (autosomal recessive, autosomal dominant, X-linked). Obtain a drug and alcohol history, looking for possible nutritional deficits and medications that may have movement side effects (neuroleptics). Ask about a history of vertigo, tinnitus, and hearing loss (this suggests a peripheral vestibular problem). Ask about a history of headache, nausea, and vomiting (this suggests increased intracranial pressure). Ask about a history of other neurological problems, including motor weakness and sensory loss (this suggests multiple sclerosis). Take a medical history: What conditions have you been diagnosed with? Listen for relevant entities (e.g., stroke, cancer).

Physical exam

The physical examination starts with an assessment of the patient's speech during the history, looking for difficulty speaking and scanning speech (variation in speech volume). Explicitly mention to the examiner that you have been assessing the patient's speech while taking the history. Perform a full neurological exam. Pay particular attention to observing the patient's gait for ataxia, and assessing for broad-based stance and gait. Test tandem walking. Remember to assess for nystagmus and perform a fundoscopic exam (this is relevant to increased intracranial pressure). Look for limb dysmetria by performing a finger-to-nose test on both sides. Assess for neck stiffness.

Investigations

Consider brain imaging for most patients. CT scan is the usual first choice. This is particularly important in detecting strokes, masses, lesions, and demyelination. Vascular lesions may require evaluation with angiography, CT angiogram, or MR angiogram. In suspected infection, perform a lumbar puncture, except when contraindicated (see the checklist).

CHECKLIST

Contraindications for lumbar puncture

Cellulitis near the site for the lumbar puncture

Increased intracranial pressure

Uncorrected coagulopathy

Acute spinal cord trauma

Management

Consider referring the patient to a neurologist for assistance in diagnosis and management. Note, however, that an obvious diagnosis is likely on a standardized exam. Remember that Wernicke encephalopathy is treated with vitamin B_1 and usually shows rapid improvement.

52

Genetic concerns

MCC particular objective

Recognize when an individual or population is at risk of a genetic or epigenetic condition.

MCC differential diagnosis
with added evidence

CHROMOSOMAL ABNORMALITIES (E.G., ANEUPLOIDY, REARRANGEMENTS)

Autosomal anomalies (e.g., Down syndrome) are more common than sex-linked anomalies (e.g., Klinefelter syndrome, Turner syndrome).

Chromosomal abnormalities are either numerical or structural. Numerical abnormalities involve an extra chromosome (trisomy; e.g., Down syndrome, Klinefelter syndrome) or a missing chromosome (monosomy; e.g., Turner syndrome). Structural abnormalities involve translocations, or deletions and duplications, of genetic material.

Risk factors:

> Down syndrome: older maternal age; other children with Down syndrome
>
> Klinefelter syndrome, Turner syndrome: none known

Investigations: noninvasive prenatal screening; ultrasound; amniocentesis; chorionic villus sampling

SINGLE-GENE ABNORMALITIES

Mendelian (e.g., autosomal dominant)

Examples include Huntington disease, Marfan syndrome, neurofibromatosis type 1, Charcot-Marie-Tooth disease type 1, and familial Mediterranean fever.

Risk factors: family history

> Either parent can transmit the mutation. A parent with an autosomal dominant disease has a 50% chance of transmitting the mutation to their children.
>
> Children of either sex can be affected. Children who do not inherit the disorder do not have the mutation.
>
> Ethnicity is a risk factor for some entities, including familial Mediterranean fever, which is more common among people of Mediterranean descent (e.g., Turkish, Greek, north African, Italian, Arab).

Nonmendelian (e.g., mitochondrial, epigenetic)

MITOCHONDRIAL

Examples include Leber hereditary optic neuropathy; myoclonic epilepsy with ragged red fibres; and mitochondrial myopathy, lactic acidosis, and stroke (MELAS).

Risk factors: mothers with mitochondrial disorders

> Only females can transmit mitochondrial mutations.

> Children of either sex can be affected. Children who inherit the mutation may be phenotypically normal.

EPIGENETIC

These are environmental factors that modify genotype-phenotype correlations in monogenic (single gene mutation) and complex diseases.

Risk factors: smoking; alcohol use; obesity; asbestos exposure; carcinogenic exposures (e.g., sun tanning, radon)

PRENATAL EXPOSURE

Drugs or toxins (e.g., fetal alcohol spectrum disorder)

FETAL ALCOHOL SPECTRUM DISORDER

This results from maternal alcohol consumption during pregnancy. No safe limit of alcohol consumption is known, but it is known that the risk increases with consumption.

Signs and symptoms:

> Pathognomonic dysmorphic features: small eye openings; thin upper lip; smooth philtrum; maxillary hypoplasia; small lower jaw; short upturned nose; flat nasal bridge; abnormal ear position or formation

> Other features: growth deficits before and after birth (at birth: low weight; short length; head circumference ≤ tenth percentile); defects in the heart, kidneys, bones; deformities in the joints, limbs, extremities; neurobehavioural impairments

Infectious exposure (e.g., congenital rubella)

CONGENITAL RUBELLA INFECTION

This is rare in developed countries due to rubella vaccination programs. Cases in North America occur in families who have emigrated from countries without rubella vaccination programs.

Infection risks: fetal death in utero, preterm delivery, congenital defects

> First trimester infection: high incidence of defects

> Infection after 18 to 20 weeks gestation: little to no incidence of defects

> Third trimester infection: fetal growth restriction

Infants with congenital rubella infection are asymptomatic at birth but develop manifestations over time.

> Neonates: fetal growth restriction, meningoencephalitis, microcephaly, deafness or hearing impairment, infantile glaucoma, cataracts, retinopathy, cardiac defects (patent ductus arteriosus, pulmonary artery stenosis), hepatosplenomegaly, radiolucent bones

> Infants and children: deafness (bilateral and sensorineural), cardiac and vascular anomalies, congenital heart disease, eye lesions, cataracts, central nervous system (CNS) abnormalities (microencephaly)

> Late manifestations: permanent hearing loss (bilateral, sensorineural); cataracts; glaucoma; pigmentary retinopathy; endocrine disorders (diabetes, thyroid disease); coronary, cerebral, and peripheral vascular diseases; immune deficiencies (hypogammaglobulinemia); learning disabilities; ataxia

Investigations: antibody titres (rubella-specific IgG and IgM in infants aged 6 to12 months suggests chronic rubella infection); viral cultures (nasopharynx sample; urine; CSF; buffy coat from blood collection; conjunctiva sample)

Maternal disease (e.g., maternal diabetes)

MATERNAL DIABETES

The outcome for an infant (fetal, neonatal, and long-term complications) exposed to maternal diabetes depends on the mother's onset, duration, and severity of glucose intolerance and diabetes during pregnancy.

> Fetal complications from first trimester onset (including time of conception): diabetic embryopathy, congenital malformations (cardiovascular, central nervous system), spontaneous abortions; from second and/or third trimester onset: fetal hyperglycemia, hyperinsulinism, macrosomia

> Neonatal complications: increased risk of prematurity, larger-than-average size, birth injury, respiratory distress, perinatal asphyxia, hypoglycemia, hypocalcemia, hyperbilirubinemia, cardiomyopathy

> Long-term complications: increased risk of postnatal diabetes, obesity, impaired glucose metabolism; increased incidence of neuropsychiatric morbidity

MULTIFACTORIAL CONDITION (E.G., NEURAL TUBE DEFECTS)

NEURAL TUBE DEFECTS

Types of defects include spina bifida (spine), anencephaly (brain), encephalocele (skull), and iniencephaly (neck).

Outcomes for infant: bladder and/or bowel dysfunction; partial or complete paralysis; deformities (weakness in the feet, hips, legs)

Maternal risk factors (gene-environment interaction): folate antimetabolites (e.g., methotrexate); diabetes; obesity; mycotoxins in contaminated cornmeal; arsenic; hyperthermia; radiation; smoking, secondhand smoke

Investigations: prenatal screening for AFP; ultrasound; amniocentesis; postnatal ultrasound, MRI, CT scan

Strategy for patient encounter

The likely scenario is a family with a history of genetic abnormality, now pregnant again. The likely tasks include history, investigations, or management (not physical exam).

History

Use open-ended questions to gather evidence in the following areas:

- **Obstetrical history:** How many times have you been pregnant? How many times have you miscarried? What health issues do your children have? Listen for a history of repeated spontaneous abortions (this suggests genetic factors) and hereditary health issues in existing children.
- **Medical history:** What conditions have you been diagnosed with? Listen for hereditary conditions (e.g., Marfan syndrome), diabetes, and conditions treated with folate antimetabolites (e.g., psoriasis, rheumatoid arthritis). Ask about maternal drug and alcohol use, and smoking (including exposure to secondhand smoke). Ask whether the mother has been vaccinated for rubella.
- **Family history:** Take a 3-generation family history of inherited disorders. Who in your family has had an inherited disorder? Draw a 3-generation pedigree noting affected individuals. Pay particular attention to consanguinity. Also note the ethnic and geographic origin of the family.
- **Social determinants of health:** What is your income? What is your level of education? Who helps you when you need help? Ask about language barriers, where appropriate. Note any determinants with negative impacts (poverty, little education, few family supports, presence of language barriers).

Investigations

Consider genetic testing, karyotype analysis, and imaging studies, to diagnose the specific entities listed in the MCC differential diagnosis.

Management

In the context of a known hereditary disorder, provide genetic counselling and information on reproductive options (in the case of an already pregnant patient, this means evaluating the fetus with the possibility of terminating the pregnancy). In the context of suspected hereditary disorders, consider referral for specialized evaluation and genetic testing. For all patients, consider referral to community resources, and for social and psychological support services.

Pearls

Remember the common genetic disorders that follow different inheritance patterns:

- **Autosomal dominant:** Huntington disease, polycystic kidney disease, Marfan syndrome
- **Autosomal recessive:** cystic fibrosis, sickle cell disease Tay-Sachs disease
- **Multifactorial:** heart disease, diabetes, most cancers, alcoholism, obesity, mental illness, Alzheimer disease
- **Chromosome disorders:** Down syndrome (trisomy 21), Prader-Willi syndrome (absence or nonexpression of a group of genes on chromosome 15), chronic myeloid leukemia (translocation 9;22)

53

Congenital anomalies, dysmorphic features

MCC particular objectives

Determine the severity of the immediate presentation.

Identify patients requiring early referral for specialized care.

Provide supportive counselling for parents.

MCC differential diagnosis
with added evidence

TERATOGENIC DISORDERS (E.G., FETAL ALCOHOL SPECTRUM DISORDER, CONGENITAL CYTOMEGALOVIRUS INFECTIONS)

FETAL ALCOHOL SPECTRUM DISORDER

Signs and symptoms: history of exposure to alcohol in utero

> Pathognomonic dysmorphic features: small eye openings; thin upper lip; smooth philtrum; maxillary hypoplasia; small lower jaw; short upturned nose; flat nasal bridge; abnormal ear position or formation

> Other features: growth deficits before and after birth (at birth: low weight; short length; head circumference ≤ tenth percentile); defects in the heart, kidneys, bones; deformities in the joints, limbs, extremities; neurobehavioural impairments

CONGENITAL CYTOMEGALOVIRUS INFECTIONS

Infection usually occurs by vertical transmission. The mother may not be aware she has Cytomegalovirus if the virus is dormant.

Most neonates infected with Cytomegalovirus do not have symptoms and do not develop symptoms later in life.

Signs and symptoms:

> Neonatal: retinal inflammation; jaundice; large spleen and liver; mineral deposits in the brain; seizures; small head size; rash; low birth weight

> Later life: neurologic abnormalities (difficulty with movement, physical activity; vision impairment, blindness; deafness)

Investigations: antibody titre against Cytomegalovirus (maternal and infant); CBC; liver function tests; urine culture to detect

Cytomegalovirus in the first 2 to 3 weeks of life; TORCH screen; CT scan or ultrasound of the head; chest X-ray; fundoscopy to examine the structures at the back of the eye

GENETIC DISORDERS (E.G., DOWN SYNDROME, FRAGILE X SYNDROME)

DOWN SYNDROME

Signs and symptoms: characteristic dysmorphic features (small head, flattened facial features, protruding tongue, upward slanting eyes, small hands and feet, short fingers, single crease on the palms of the hands)
> Other: ligamentous laxity

Risk factors: older maternal age, siblings with Down syndrome

Investigations: genetic testing, X-rays of target areas to assess development

FRAGILE X SYNDROME

This is the most common type of inherited disability. Fathers pass it on to all their daughters; mothers have a 50% chance of passing it on to all their children.

Signs and symptoms: possibly asymptomatic; learning disabilities; speech and language problems (these are usual in boys and include unclear speech, stuttering, leaving out parts of words; some children are nonverbal); behavioural problems (hyperactivity, anxiety, aggression); sensitivity to bright light, loud noises, texture of clothing
> Physical symptoms (common): onset during puberty; narrow face, large head, prominent forehead, large ears, flexible joints, flat feet

MECHANICAL FORCES (E.G., CONSTRICTION BAND SYNDROME)

CONSTRICTION BAND SYNDROME

This is a group of birth defects that result from strands of detached amniotic sac wrapping around parts of the fetus.

Signs and symptoms: facial cleft; legs and arms that are partially or completely missing; permanent band or indentation around a leg, arm, toe, finger; defects in the abdomen and chest

Strategy for patient encounter

The likely scenario is a consultation by parents of a dysmorphic child. The child will be absent on some pretext (e.g., a nurse is taking the child's vital signs and weight in another room). The specified tasks could engage history, physical exam, investigations, or management.

History

Take a 3-generation family history of congenital anomalies and dysmorphic features. Get details on which family members (including age and sex) were affected, when they were diagnosed, what their symptoms were, and when they died. Be sure to establish if there was consanguinity with the current patient.

Use open-ended inquiry to obtain a prenatal history of the patient: How did the pregnancy for this child go? Listen for evidence of unusual symptoms or circumstances. Ask specifically about possible toxic exposures during the pregnancy.

Physical exam

Perform a full head-to-toe physical exam. Pay particular attention to cardiovascular abnormalities, ambiguous genitalia, and phenotypic patterns suggestive of a particular disorder (e.g., Down syndrome).

(State that you will perform these exams. Because an actual pediatric patient is unlikely, the examiner may interrupt, ask what you are looking for, and provide findings.)

Investigations

Imaging (X-ray for skeletal assessment, CT scan for internal organs) may be necessary to diagnose internal abnormalities. Consider chromosome analysis and genetic testing.

Management

Consult a medical geneticist. The specific diagnosis and pattern of inheritance (either the known pattern for a particular disorder or the observed pattern in the family history) are important for discussion of recurrence risk. Refer the family for genetic counselling, for any specialized medical care needed, and for family support.

Pearls

Dysmorphic features, multiple anomalies, unexplained neurocognitive impairment, and/or a family history of recurrent or unexplained disorders all suggest the presence of genetic conditions. Remember to perform a full examination, including imaging, even if there is an obvious abnormality.

54

Glucose abnormalities

MCC particular objectives

Manage emergent situations.

Prevent complications.

MCC differential diagnosis
with added evidence
GLUCOSE ABNORMALITIES IN GENERAL

The MCC notes that the common clinical problem is diabetes mellitus.

HYPOGLYCEMIA

HYPOGLYCEMIA IN GENERAL

The most common cause is diabetes treatment.

Signs and symptoms: palpitations, pallor, sweating, nightmares, fatigue, hunger

> Severe: confusion, disorientation, blurred vision, seizures, coma

Investigations: low plasma glucose level (symptoms typically develop at concentrations ≤ 3.0 mmol/L)

Postprandial

Signs and symptoms: symptom onset after meals

Fasting

SECONDARY TO MEDICATION (E.G., SULFONYLUREAS)

Sulfonylurea use has a high risk of hypoglycemia (symptomatic within 2 hours of ingestion). Insulin therapy can also lead to hypoglycemia.

SECONDARY TO IMPAIRED GLUCOSE PRODUCTION (E.G., ADRENAL INSUFFICIENCY)

Signs and symptoms: symptoms that develop slowly (often over several months); hyperpigmentation; fatigue; weight loss; dizziness; muscle and/or joint pain; salt craving

Investigations: fasting plasma glucose; serum sodium, potassium, cortisol; ACTH stimulation test (artificial stimulation of the adrenal gland) to determine adrenal gland function; CT scan of the adrenal gland

HYPERGLYCEMIA

HYPERGLYCEMIA IN GENERAL

Signs and symptoms: often asymptomatic

> Mild to moderate: polydipsia, polyuria, weight loss, hunger, blurred vision, fatigue, weakness, unconsciousness

> Severe (e.g., diabetic ketoacidosis): abdominal pain, coma, dehydration, hypokalemia, hypotension, lethargy, metabolic acidosis, Kussmaul respiration, fruity breath

Investigations: high blood glucose levels (> 16.7 mmol/L is a medical emergency); high anion gap, low pH, low bicarbonate, elevated ketones (in diabetic ketoacidosis); high serum osmolality

Diabetes mellitus

Signs and symptoms: personal or family history of diabetes; history of diabetic complications and/or inadequate monitoring; polydipsia, polyuria, and/or weight loss

Presence of diabetes on screening: fasting glucose or HbA_{1c} test

Endocrine condition

DIABETES MELLITUS (COMMON) — SEE ABOVE

HYPERCORTISOLISM (CUSHING DISEASE)

Signs and symptoms: history of glucocorticoid therapy; cushingoid features (round, red face; pronounced abdominal weight; hump on the upper back; thin arms and legs; high blood pressure; stretch marks; acne)

Investigations: high cortisol levels on either a 24-hour urine cortisol test or dexamethasone suppression test

Drug-induced condition (e.g., steroids)

These include medications to reduce cardiovascular risks (thiazide diuretics, beta-blockers, statins); glucocorticoids; antipsychotics (clozapine, olanzapine, risperidone); and protease inhibitors, which are part of highly active antiretroviral therapy (HAART).

Strategy for patient encounter

The likely scenario is a patient with glucose abnormalities confirmed or identified on blood work. The specified tasks could engage history, physical exam, investigations, or management.

History

Begin by asking how the patient knows they have a glucose problem (if they do know). Did they have a glucose test?

Use open-ended inquiry to establish the patient's symptoms. Since the patient may not have been aware of any glucose abnormalities, phrase this in general terms: How has your health been generally? Mild hyperglycemia usually is occult, but symptoms can be present with long-standing diabetes or with high sugars. Autonomic symptoms of hypoglycemia occur below about 3.3 mmol/L and can include sweating, nausea, anxiety, tremulousness, palpitations, hunger, and paresthesias. Neurologic symptoms occur below about 2.8 mmol/L and can include headache, blurred or double vision, confusion, difficulty speaking, seizures, and coma.

Use open-ended questions to take a medical and medication history: What conditions have you been diagnosed with? What medications do you take? Listen for disorders associated with glucose abnormalities (diabetes mellitus, central nervous system tumours, adrenal disease, hepatic failure, chronic infection); and insulin, oral hypoglycemic agents, beta-blockers, disopyramide, and antibiotics. Ask about the timing of hypoglycemic symptoms following meals.

Ask about diet, exercise, family history of diabetes, personal history of gestational diabetes, and ethnicity.

Physical exam
Obtain the patient's vital signs, looking for tachycardia and hypotension (relevant to dehydration). Assess the patient for confusion: ask them to state their full name, date of birth, where they are, and how they got here.

Perform a neurological exam, looking for focal neurologic signs (these may occur in both hyperglycemia and hypoglycemia). Measure the patient's height and weight, and calculate their body mass index (BMI). Measure the patient's waist circumference.

Examine the skin for poor skin turgor (relevant to dehydration), and infections or nonhealing ulcers (these suggest hyperglycemia). Look for signs of insulin resistance (acanthosis nigricans, skin tags).

Investigations
For cases of impaired glucose tolerance, order a glucose tolerance test. If the etiology of hypoglycemia is unclear, order a 48-hour or 72-hour fast (a 48-hour fast is usually sufficient for diagnosis);

measure blood glucose at regular intervals and whenever symptoms occur. Also consider measuring C-peptide and serum insulin to distinguish endogenous (pancreatic production of insulin) from factitious hypoglycemia. In suspected other disorders, order additional tests (see the information this resource lists in the MCC differential diagnosis).

Management

Hyperglycemia is managed the same way as diabetes mellitus. The main task in hypoglycemia is to distinguish between true hypoglycemia, pseudohypoglycemia, artifactual hypoglycemia, and factitious hypoglycemia (see the checklist). Pseudohypoglycemia is demonstrated by a normal blood glucose level during symptoms. Artifactual hypoglycemia can be confirmed by repeating the test. Factitious hypoglycemia secondary to insulin use can be confirmed by looking at C-peptide and serum insulin levels: exogenous insulin use results in a low C-peptide level and a high level of insulin. Symptoms within 2 to 3 hours after eating suggests hyperinsulinemia.

CHECKLIST
Types of hypoglycemia

- **Pseudohypoglycemia:** This involves symptoms of hypoglycemia (e.g., palpitations, sweating, fatigue, hunger) **without** abnormal glucose levels.

- **Artifactual hypoglycemia:** This is a lab error caused by allowing whole blood to stand too long before separation (glucose metabolism continues in the blood tube).

- **Factitious hypoglycemia:** This is hypoglycemia caused by taking insulin or another hypoglycemic drug (this can be intentional or due to improper dosing).

Pearls

Remember that in addition to pseudohypoglycemia, many people with low glucose levels actually have no symptoms.

55

Diabetes mellitus

MCC particular objectives

Pay particular attention to early detection of disease.

Recognize medical emergencies (acute hypoglycemia, diabetic ketoacidosis, hyperosmolar nonketotic coma).

MCC differential diagnosis
with added evidence

TYPE 1 DIABETES MELLITUS

Autoimmunity

Signs and symptoms: family history of type 1 diabetes, autoimmune disease; age 4 to 14 years (peak incidence); polydipsia; polyuria; new-onset bed wetting; extreme hunger; weight loss; blurry vision; vaginal yeast infection

Investigations: blood tests (elevated glucose; HbA_{1c}); urine tests (glucose and ketones)

TYPE 2 DIABETES MELLITUS

Obesity

Signs and symptoms: body mass index (BMI) $\geq$ 30; family history of type 2 diabetes, obesity; polydipsia; polyuria; fatigue

Investigations:

> Blood and urine tests to detect indicators of metabolic disorder associated with obesity (lipid profile, uric acid, liver enzymes); HbA_{1c}

Other (e.g., genetic predisposition, medications)

GENETIC PREDISPOSITION

Signs and symptoms: family history of type 2 diabetes; African, Hispanic, First Nations, Asian descent; personal history of polycystic ovary syndrome

MEDICATIONS

These include medications to reduce cardiovascular risks (thiazide diuretics, beta-blockers, statins); glucocorticoids; antipsychotics (clozapine, olanzapine, risperidone); and protease inhibitors, which are part of highly active antiretroviral therapy (HAART).

GESTATIONAL DIABETES MELLITUS

Gestational diabetes involves the onset of glucose intolerance during pregnancy.

Signs and symptoms: usually asymptomatic (it is detected by routine screening during pregnancy)

Risk factors: age 35 or older; family history of type 2 diabetes; previous gestational diabetes; previous baby > 4.1 kg at birth; history of unexplained stillbirth; obesity; African, Hispanic, First Nations, or Asian descent; history of prediabetes; polycystic ovary syndrome; use of corticosteroids

Investigations: oral glucose challenge, oral glucose tolerance test

Strategy for patient encounter

This encounter could involve screening for, or diagnosing, diabetes, or managing patients with known diabetes. The specified tasks could engage history, physical exam, investigations, or management.

History

For encounters focused on screening for, or diagnosing, diabetes, use the FINDRISC tool to direct the history. (Current screening guidelines for diabetes in Canada require the calculation of patient risk using the FINDRISC tool. This stratifies patients into risk groups and informs the frequency of recommended screening. The website of the Canadian Task Force on Preventive Health Care has a version of this tool under "tools and resources.")

For encounters that deal with derangement in glucose level in known diabetics, ask about sweating, nausea, tremulousness, palpitations, headache, blurred or double vision, anxiety, confusion, seizures, and difficulty speaking (these symptoms indicate hypoglycemia). In type 1 diabetics, ask about concurrent illness (pneumonia, urinary tract infection) and missed insulin treatments (relevant to diabetic ketoacidosis). In type 2 diabetics, ask about acute febrile illness or infection (especially pneumonia and urinary tract infection); and altered consciousness, focal or generalized seizures, and transient hemiplegia (these symptoms suggest nonketotic hyperosmolar syndrome). Obtain a complete medical history and medication history, including compliance with diabetic medications.

Physical exam

Obtain the patient's vital signs (looking for dehydration and fever) and body mass index (BMI). Perform a full physical exam, looking especially for sources of infection and diabetic complications (neuropathy, retinopathy). Remember to look for Kussmaul respirations (rapid and deep breathing to compensate for metabolic acidosis) in patients with possible diabetic ketoacidosis.

Investigations

Testing has 4 purposes: assessing glycemic status via serum glucose or glycated hemoglobin (HbA_{1c}) levels; assessing possible intercurrent disease (infection) via complete blood count (CBC), C-reactive protein (CRP) levels, chest X-ray, and urinalysis; looking for acute complications via arterial blood gas (ABG) measurement, electrolyte levels, serum ketone level, and calculation of serum osmolality; and looking for long-term complications, including nephropathy (via tests for creatinine and urine protein) and cardiovascular risk and damage (via electrocardiogram and serum lipid levels).

Management

Manage any acute conditions (diabetic ketoacidosis, nonketotic hyperosmolar syndrome, hypoglycemia); admit these patients and treat any underlying causes (e.g. infection).

The first-line management for newly diagnosed type 2 diabetes (the likely scenario for this clinical presentation) involves diet modification, regular exercise, and weight reduction. If these steps prove ineffective, or in patients with pronounced lack of glycemic control, consider medical therapy. First-line oral

> **TIP**
>
> ## Tailoring information to individual patients
>
> The MCC identifies providing generic information as a common exam error.
>
> To avoid this error, ask patients about aspects of their lives that might affect their condition. Provide information that targets their situation and engage the patient in figuring out next steps.
>
> For example, diet and exercise changes might be relevant for this case:
>
> - Ask what the patient ate yesterday for breakfast, lunch, and supper. Use this to personalize guidelines on dietary changes they need to make.
>
> - Ask what the patient did for exercise last week. Discuss short-term goals with the patient: What could the patient do next week to exercise every day? (For example, when could the patient fit in a 30-minute walk?)

therapy is metformin; second-line agents depend on the presence of cardiovascular disease. In the event of metabolic decompensation, insulin is the first-line therapy.

Counsel the patient regarding long-term risk and prevention of complications: heart disease, vascular disease, peripheral neuropathy (including erectile dysfunction), nephropathy, eye damage (potentially blindness), infection (e.g., in feet due to poor circulation), and pregnancy complications (eclampsia, pre-eclampsia, birth defects). Discuss management of other risk factors (hypertension, smoking, sedentary lifestyle, hyperlipidemia).

56

Skin and integument conditions

This clinical presentation combines several, formerly separate, clinical presentations into a more logical, but also larger, category.

The creation of the larger category probably signals that only 1 of the entities it lists might appear on the exam, as opposed to potentially more than 1. Of the entities in the larger category, likely possibilities for the exam include any of the macular entities (because easier to simulate with makeup), melanoma (because possible to simulate with makeup), and androgenic alopecia (because common, and therefore possibly present among available standardized patients).

Within the larger category, it should be easy to determine where, among 3 broad possibilities, a patient's problem lies. It will either be a skin problem, a nail problem, or a hair problem.

To create a slightly more detailed discussion of the larger category, this resource treats each of these 3 possibilities separately as:

- 56a Skin rashes, tumours, and ulcers
- 56b Nail presentations
- 56c Hair presentations

56A

Skin rashes, tumours, and ulcers

MCC particular objective

Determine whether a condition is benign, malignant, or associated with an underlying condition.

MCC differential diagnosis
with added evidence

RASHES

Macules

MACULES IN GENERAL
These are flat, abnormally coloured lesions.

VIRALLY CAUSED MACULES
Causes include measles, rubella, and Epstein-Barr virus (EBV).

Signs and symptoms: small, pink-red spots or patches (typical) that appear in 1 area and can spread to others (e.g., they appear on the trunk and then spread to the arms and legs); viral symptoms (e.g., fever, headache)

PHOTO-DISTRIBUTED MACULES
Drugs that commonly cause photosensitivity include phenothiazines and tricyclics (psychiatrics); tetracyclines and sulfonamides (antibiotics); methotrexate (chemotherapy); sulfonylureas (antihyperglycemics); and chlorothiazide (diuretic).

Signs and symptoms: dermatitis-like rash with red macules (more common), or areas of grey-blue hyperpigmentation (less common), on sun-exposed skin

TINEA VERSICOLOR
This is a fungal overgrowth infection.

Signs and symptoms: white, pink, red, or brown spots that spread slowly and do not tan (they become more noticeable on tanning); dry, scaly (possibly); itchy (possibly); located on the trunk and shoulders (common; also on the back, chest, neck, upper arms)

VITILIGO
This involves the death or dysfunction of melanocytes. It is often associated with autoimmune disease processes.

Signs and symptoms: segmental or localized discoloured patches; located anywhere on the body

Papules

PAPULES IN GENERAL

These are raised lesions that may be isolated with distinct borders (e.g., keratoacanthoma) or involved in eruptions (e.g., acne).

KERATOACANTHOMA

These are noncancerous skin growths associated with sun exposure.

Signs and symptoms: round, firm lesions located on sun-exposed skin (face, lips, ears, scalp, neck, back of hands, forearms) that contain characteristic central keratinous material

ACNE VULGARIS

Signs and symptoms: erythema; telangiectasia; presence of whiteheads, blackheads, pustules, nodules, cystic lesions; located on the face, neck, chest, back, shoulders, scalp (usual)

Vesiculobullous

VARICELLA-ZOSTER INFECTION

This causes chickenpox (this is generally a childhood disease, which has become less common because of immunization) and, in adults, shingles. Chickenpox is generally diagnosed clinically.

Signs and symptoms: itchy, red fluid-filled lesions that start on the scalp or trunk (typical) and spread; fever (often)

Investigations: culture of blisters (in suspected shingles)

HERPES SIMPLEX INFECTION (HSV)

HSV-1 causes oral herpes. HSV-2 causes genital herpes.

Signs and symptoms: burning, sore, or itchy skin for 1 or 2 days before the appearance of the rash; rash composed of ≥ 1 painful, fluid-filled sores that break open, ooze, and form crusts

> Oral herpes: sores on the lips and around the mouth (common); also on the face or tongue
>
> Genital herpes: sores on the penis, vagina, buttocks, and/or anus

CONTACT DERMATITIS

Signs and symptoms: red rash with macules, dry scaly skin, and blisters at the site(s) of allergen contact (e.g., hands)

STEVENS-JOHNSON SYNDROME

Less than 10% of body surface is affected in Stevens-Johnson syndrome; if > 30% is affected, the condition is toxic epidermal necrolysis by definition.

Signs and symptoms: first, blisters on the skin and the mucous membranes of the mouth, nose, eyes, and genitals; then, painful red or purplish rash

Pustular

IMPETIGO

This is generally diagnosed clinically.

Signs and symptoms: red sores around the mouth and nose (common) that rupture, ooze, and crust over; mild itching and soreness

Risk factors: age 2 to 5 years (more common); attendance at school or day care (common); summer (more common)

FOLLICULITIS

Causes include bacterial infection (e.g., *Staphylococcus aureus*, *Pseudomonas*) and yeast infection (*Pityrosporum*).

Signs and symptoms: small, raised red- or white-headed lesions around hair follicles that are itchy, burning, and/or tender

> Pseudomonas folliculitis ("hot-tub folliculitis"): onset of symptoms 1 to 2 days after exposure to bacteria in a hot tub or swimming pool (common)

Plaques

INFECTIONS (E.G., FUNGAL, LYME DISEASE)

Infectious plaques grow if left untreated.

Signs and symptoms (in general): raised red patches; circular or ring-shaped; no scales

ACANTHOSIS NIGRICANS

This is caused by a systemic condition and typically occurs in obese or diabetic individuals.

Signs and symptoms: slow-developing dark, thick, "velvety" skin; located in folds and creases (e.g., armpits, groin, and neck folds)

ECZEMA, PSORIASIS

Signs and symptoms (in general): raised, red skin lesions or patches (abundant or few); scaly (sometimes: scales are silvery if present); located anywhere on the body

TUMOURS

Benign

EPIDERMAL INCLUSION CYST

This is the most common cutaneous cyst. It is usually diagnosed clinically.

Signs and symptoms: age 30 to 40 (more common); male (more common); skin-coloured dermal cyst or nodule; visible central punctum; asymptomatic (usually); freely mobile on palpation; located on the face, neck, trunk (common)

> If infected: larger, erythematous, painful

Investigations: histology

Premalignant

ACTINIC KERATOSIS

This may progress to invasive squamous cell carcinoma.

Signs and symptoms: adult male (more common); fair skin, older age (common); solitary or multiple lesions; erythematous, scaly macules or papules, or plaques; ≤ 2 cm in diameter; located on sun-exposed skin (balding scalp; neck; backs of hands; top sides of forearms; lower extremities for women); sun damage on surrounding skin (yellow or pale; spotted hyperpigmentation; telangiectasia; xerosis)

Risk factors: chronic sun exposure

Investigations: biopsy to distinguish between actinic keratosis and squamous cell carcinoma

Malignant (e.g., melanoma)

MELANOMA

Signs and symptoms (mnemonic: **ABCDE**): **a**symmetry; **b**order irregularities; **c**olour variation in the same region (deep coloured: red-purple-blue-brown-black variations); **d**iameter > 6 mm; **e**volution or enlargement of symptoms over time

> Location: sun-exposed skin (common: the face, back, arms, legs), but possible anywhere on the body

Risk factors: personal or family history of melanoma; moles (nevi) that are atypical and numerous; sun or ultraviolet (UV) exposure, especially at a young age; sun-sensitive individuals (light skin; fair hair; high-density freckles; green, blue, or hazel eyes)

Investigations: biopsy

ULCERS

Vascular cause

ARTERIAL INSUFFICIENCY

Signs and symptoms: ischemic ulcers on the feet and ankles; intermittent claudication and atypical pain in the affected muscles

> Ischemic ulcers: minor wounds that do not heal (due to lack of blood supply)

Risk factors: male; African descent; age 70 or older; smoking; diabetes; arteriosclerosis; hypertension; hyperlipidemia

Infectious cause

BACTERIAL INFECTION

Signs and symptoms: erythema; warmth; tenderness; swelling; pus or foul smelling discharge at ulcer site

Autoimmune disorder

VASCULITIS

Signs and symptoms: ulcers that are symmetrically distributed; asymptomatic, or associated with pruritus, burning sensations, pain

> Vasculitis of small dermal vessels: superficial ulcers with regular borders, palpable purpura, hemorrhagic bullae
>
> Vasculitis of muscular arteries (medium-sized vessels): irregularly shaped deep ulcers or gangrene; painful red nodules
>
> Rheumatoid arthritis (patients with this condition have chronic ulcers due to vasculitis): deep ulcers on the lower legs (medium-sized vessels vasculitis); nail-fold lesions; palpable purpura; digital ischemic lesions and gangrene; rheumatoid nodules

Investigations: skin biopsy; immunofluorescence on the most recent lesions of the ulcers (< 48 hours) to detect inflammation in vessels

Pressure ulceration

This commonly occurs in residents of nursing homes, and bed- or wheelchair-bound individuals.

The cause is soft tissue compression, usually between a bony prominence and the overlying skin.

Signs and symptoms: nonblanchable erythema of intact skin, or deep ulcers down to the bone; muscle that is resistant and necrotic before the skin breaks; chronic pain (exacerbated by ulcer exam)

Risk factors: immobility, malnutrition, sensory loss, reduced perfusion

Tumours

INVASIVE CUTANEOUS SQUAMOUS CELL CARCINOMA (SCC)

Signs and symptoms: skin ulcers with papules, plaques, or nodules on the head and neck (common; possible anywhere on the body)

> Oral SCC: ulcers (or indurated plaques) in the oral cavity (common: floor of the mouth and lateral/ventral tongue); history of tobacco or alcohol use
>
> SCC of the lip: ulcers (or nodules, or indurated white plaques) on the lower lip

Investigations: biopsy

Toxic

SPIDER BITES

Spider bites that become problematic are rare.

Signs and symptoms: ulcer (or papule, pustule, welt, plaque, or ecchymotic plaque at site of bite); mild pain, itching; swelling, burning, numbness, or tingling

Strategy for patient encounter

The likely scenario is a patient with a skin lesion. The specified tasks could engage history, physical exam, investigations, or management.

History

Start with open-ended questions to determine the patient's medical and medication history: What conditions have you been diagnosed with? What medications do you take? Listen for diabetes, hypertension, hyperlipidemia, and rheumatoid arthritis (relevant for ulcers); drugs that can cause photosensitivity (phenothiazines, tricyclics, tetracyclines, sulfonamides, methotrexate, sulfonylureas, chlorothiazide); and recent changes in medication (relevant for possible drug eruptions).

Ask open-ended questions to obtain a history of the lesions: Where are the lesions? What have you noticed about them? How have they changed? Listen for details of location (e.g., location on sun-exposed skin suggests malignancy or actinic keratosis); pain, itching, and/or discharge (these suggest ulcer or infection); and growth of an individual mole (looking for features of melanoma). Ask about risk factors for melanoma (sun exposure, family history, fair complexion).

Physical exam

If indicated by the history, take the patient's vital signs, looking for fever (this suggests viral infection) and hypertension (this is relevant for vascular causes). Examine the lesions: their morphology and distribution will considerably narrow the possible entities (see the information this resource lists in the MCC's differential diagnosis).

Investigations

As appropriate, based on the history and physical exam, consider bacterial, fungal, and viral cultures, or investigations for underlying disease. If the diagnosis is in doubt, perform a skin biopsy.

(Biopsies are not performed on standardized patients, so state your intention to pursue this investigation. The examiner will likely interrupt and provide findings.)

Management

Depending on the specific diagnosis, consider topical or systemic therapy, patient education, and changes to the patient's workplace environment or recreation routine. Consider referral to a dermatologist.

56B

Nail presentations

MCC particular objective

Determine whether a condition is benign, malignant, or associated with an underlying condition.

MCC differential diagnosis
with added evidence

NAIL PRESENTATIONS

Local nail problems

PARONYCHIA

Signs and symptoms: tenderness or redness of the nail or surrounding skin; blisters or pustules; detachment of the nail; changes in nail colour, texture, or shape

> History of nail biting; cuticle injury (e.g., aggressive pushing down of cuticles during manicures); hands in water for long periods

Investigations: biopsy to detect nail fungi

HERPETIC WHITLOW

Signs and symptoms: pain and swelling of the terminal phalange of a finger (typical; it may affect > 1 finger; it may affect toes)

Investigations: tests to detect HSV-1 or HSV-2 (Tzanck; viral cultures of vesicle fluid; serum antibody titres; fluorescent antibody testing; DNA PCR hybridization)

INGROWN TOENAIL

Signs and symptoms: redness and swelling of the surrounding skin; overgrowth of skin around the nail; pain; bleeding; oozing pus

> History of chronic infections, diabetes, injury to foot, or new footwear

Associated with an underlying condition

CLUBBING

Signs and symptoms: gradual swelling of the terminal phalanges of the fingers or toes; concave nails (Schamroth sign); **no** associated pain

> History of associated underlying disease: pulmonary disease, cardiovascular disease, neoplastic disease, infection, hepatobiliary disease, endocrine disease, gastrointestinal disease

Investigations: CBC to detect elevated WBCs; imaging to detect abnormalities associated with hypoxia (chest X-ray, cardiovascular imaging)

PSORIASIS

Signs and symptoms: nail pitting; current or prior erythematous scaly rashes; family history of psoriasis or similar skin conditions; history of other autoimmune diseases

Investigations (usually diagnosed clinically): biopsy

SUBUNGUAL MELANOMA

Signs and symptoms: changes to the nail of the thumb or big toe (more common); symptoms that develop over weeks to months; widening of the nail (especially at the cuticle); changes in nail colour (e.g., brown or black streaks) that eventually spread to the nail fold (Hutchison sign)

Risk factors: darker skin

Investigations: biopsy

Strategy for patient encounter

The likely scenario is a patient with long-standing nail changes. The specified tasks could engage history, physical exam, investigations, or management.

History

Use open-ended questions about the nail changes: When did you first notice the nail changes? What characterizes the changes? Listen for recent-onset versus long-standing changes (long-standing changes suggest an underlying condition); and for associated pain (this suggests a local nail problem as opposed to an underlying condition). Ask about a history of trauma to the affected nails.

Obtain a medical history with emphasis on hypoxia (clubbing) and psoriasis.

Physical exam

Examine all the nails and perform a general physical exam.

Investigations

Depending on the evidence from the history and physical exam, perform a biopsy, obtain fungal scrapings, or order lab tests and imaging.

(Biopsies and scrapings are not performed on standardized patients, so state your intention to pursue these investigations. The examiner will likely interrupt and provide findings.)

Management

Treat paronychia with antibiotics, and incision and drainage of any abscess. Onychomycosis is most commonly due to tinea infection, and can be treated with amorolfine nail lacquer, or with oral terbinafine, itraconazole, or fluconazole. Treat ingrown nails with partial or complete nail resection: counsel the patient to avoid tight fitting footwear to prevent recurrence. Psoriatic nail changes do not have a specific treatment other than general psoriasis management. Painful or large subungual hematomas are treated by drilling a hole with a 19-gauge needle, or creating a hole in the nail with a heated paperclip. Suspected subungual melanomas require biopsy, and referral to a dermatologist or plastic surgeon.

56 C

Hair presentations

MCC particular objective

Determine whether a condition is benign, malignant, or associated with an underlying condition.

MCC differential diagnosis
with added evidence

HAIR PRESENTATIONS

Alopecia

SCARRING

CICATRICIAL ALOPECIA IN GENERAL

Common causes include lichen planopilaris, chronic cutaneous lupus erythematosus, central centrifugal cicatricial alopecia, acne keloidalis nuchae, and dissecting cellulitis.

Signs and symptoms: onset during young adulthood (more common); absence of pores within the area of hair loss (sometimes magnification is needed to see this); history of skin disease, systemic lupus erythematosus, or autoimmune disease (possible)

> Lichen planopilaris: itching scalp; lesions showing most inflammation at the centre
>
> Cutaneous lupus erythematosus: lesions showing most inflammation at the edges
>
> Central centrifugal cicatricial alopecia, acne keloidalis nuchae, dissecting cellulitis: African descent

Investigations: microscopic examination of individual hairs for follicle damage; scalp biopsy

NONSCARRING

ANDROGENIC ALOPECIA

This is a common form of alopecia.

Signs and symptoms: gradual-onset hair loss

> Male-pattern hair loss: receding hairline, bald spots
>
> Female-pattern hair loss: thinning hair over the crown of the head

ALOPECIA AREATA

This is a common form of alopecia.

Signs and symptoms: loss of hair in patches on the head or other parts of the body (e.g., beard); "exclamation point" hairs (short, broken-off hairs at the edge of the bald patches); recovery within a year in mild cases; several episodes in a lifetime, with the first episode before age 30 (common); pitting of nails

> Alopecia totalis (this is a type of alopecia areata): loss of all hair of the scalp; loss of eyebrows and eye lashes (often)

Risk factors: family history of alopecia areata

> Cooccuring conditions: vitiligo; thyroiditis; pernicious anemia (due to vitamin B_{12} deficiency)

TELOGEN EFFLUVIUM (LOSS OF MATURE HAIR) DUE TO ACUTE ILLNESS OR SURGERY

Signs and symptoms: hair loss that occurs 3 to 4 months after an acute illness or surgery, and that decreases over 6 to 8 months (this is usually a temporary condition); diffuse hair loss

ANAGEN EFFLUVIUM (LOSS OF GROWING HAIR) DUE TO CHEMOTHERAPY

Chemotherapy drugs target fast-growing cells like cancer and hair.

Hair regrowth starts 3 to 6 months after the cessation of chemotherapy. Regrowing hair may have a different texture or colour at first.

Signs and symptoms: hair loss all over the body (e.g., the scalp, eye lashes, eyebrows, armpit hair, pubic hair) that begins 2 to 4 weeks after chemotherapy

TRICHOTILLOMANIA[1(p251)]

Signs and symptoms: visible hair loss from recurrent plucking or pulling (common sites are the head, eyebrows, eye lashes); repeated attempts to stop the behaviour; symptoms with significant impact on day-to-day life

TINEA CAPITIS

This is a contagious fungal infection of the scalp and hair shafts.

Signs and symptoms: bald patches on the scalp that are itchy and scaly; contagious contacts (the infection is most common in toddlers and schoolchildren)

Investigations: potassium hydroxide wet mount of plucked hairs or scalp scrapings

Hirsutism

HIRSUTISM IN GENERAL

Signs and symptoms:

> Women (more common than men): male-pattern hair growth of terminal body hair in androgen-stimulated areas (i.e., the face, chest, areolae)

> Men: excessive growth of terminal body hair in androgen-stimulated areas

FAMILIAL CONDITION (NO ENDOCRINE DISORDER)

Signs and symptoms: women of South Asian or Mediterranean descent (more common); symptom onset in puberty; normal rate of hair growth; **no** evidence of irregular menstruation or elevated serum testosterone

ANDROGEN EXCESS

ANDROGEN EXCESS IN GENERAL

Signs and symptoms: voice changes, increased libido, irregular menstruation, odorous perspiration, acne, clitoromegaly, increased muscle mass, temporal hair recession and balding, loss of normal female body shape

Investigations: elevated DHEA-S levels, elevated serum testosterone

POLYCYSTIC OVARY SYNDROME

Signs and symptoms: symptom onset after puberty, with increased rate of hair growth and male-pattern hair growth; irregular menstruation; infertility; obesity; acne

Investigations: elevated LH:FSH ratio (2:1 or 3:1) (usual); elevated testosterone; ultrasound to detect ovarian cysts; normal prolactin levels; normal thyroid function

OVARIAN TUMOUR (ARRHENOBLASTOMA)

Signs and symptoms: abrupt-onset symptoms (often); hirsutism; virilization (e.g., clitoromegaly, increased muscle mass, temporal hair recession and balding, loss of normal female body shape); palpable ovarian mass

Investigations: suppressed LH and FSH levels; elevated androgen levels; CT scan or ultrasound of the pelvis

Hypertrichosis

HYPERTRICHOSIS IN GENERAL

Signs and symptoms (in men and women): excessive hair growth in nonandrogen-stimulated areas

IDIOPATHIC

Signs and symptoms: diffuse increase in vellus hair growth

Investigations: normal serum androgen levels

DRUGS (E.G., PHENYTOIN, MINOXIDIL)

Examples include phenytoin, minoxidil, cyclosporine hydrocortisone, and psoralens.

SYSTEMIC ILLNESS

HYPOTHYROIDISM

Signs and symptoms: history of hypothyroidism or symptoms of hypothyroidism (cold intolerance, decreased reflexes, dry skin, weight gain, impaired cognition)

Investigations: elevated thyrotropin (TSH)

ANOREXIA NERVOSA[1(pp338–339)]
Signs and symptoms: significantly low body weight; intense fear of gaining weight or persistent behaviour that interferes with gaining weight; excessive focus on body weight or shape in self-evaluation, or persistent lack of recognition of current low body weight

Strategy for patient encounter

The likely scenario is a male patient with male-pattern baldness. The specified tasks could engage history, physical exam, investigations, or management.

History

Start with open-ended questions about the hair loss or growth: When did it start? What characterizes it? Listen for evidence consistent with particular entities (e.g., gradual-onset thinning with receding hairline in men with androgenic alopecia; recent-onset patchy loss of head or beard hair in alopecia areata; bald, itchy spots on the scalp in tinea capitis; sudden-onset male-pattern hair growth in women with ovarian tumour).

Take a medical and medication history. Listen for relevant conditions (see the information this resource lists in the MCC differential diagnosis), and for common drugs of concern (cortisone, penicillamine, psoralens, phenytoin, diazoxide, minoxidil, and cyclosporine).

In women, ask about menstrual irregularities and amenorrhea (these suggest androgen excess, including polycystic ovary syndrome).

Ask about a family history of hair loss (this is common in androgenic alopecia). Ask about recent extreme stresses (surgery, severe illness, emotional crisis, pregnancy) that might precipitate telogen effluvium.

Physical exam

Examine the skin looking for the pattern of hair growth or loss. Note if it is localized or generalized. Perform a general physical exam.

Investigations

Order a test for thyrotropin (TSH) in cases of hypertrichosis and female hair loss. In women with hair loss, consider ordering a complete blood count (looking for anemia) and a test for vitamin D (looking for low levels), because these have been implicated in female hair loss. In hirsute women, order tests for polycystic ovarian syndrome and congenital adrenal hyperplasia. In cases of localized hair loss, perform a skin biopsy.

(Biopsies are not performed on standardized patients, so state your intention to pursue this investigation. The examiner will likely interrupt and provide findings.)

Management

Treatment of hypertrichosis and hirsutism is directed at the underlying cause. Hyperandrogenic hirsutism may be treated with cyproterone acetate and spironolactone. Other options include bleaching agents, depilatory creams, shaving, waxing, and electrolysis.

Treatments for androgenic alopecia include hair transplantation, and topical minoxidil or oral finasteride.

Reassure patients with telogen effluvium that spontaneous regrowth will occur over a period of 2 to 3 months.

In cases of scarring alopecia or where the diagnosis is uncertain, refer the patient to a dermatologist.

Pearls

Remember that medications for androgenic alopecia are only effective during the time the patient is taking the medication.

REFERENCE

1 American Psychiatric Association. Diagnostic and statistical manual of mental disorders. 5th ed. Arlington, VA: American Psychiatric Association; 2013. 991 p.

57

Headache

MCC particular objective

Differentiate benign from potentially serious causes.

MCC differential diagnosis
with added evidence

PRIMARY HEADACHE (E.G., MIGRAINE, CHRONIC DAILY HEADACHE WITH MEDICATION OVERUSE)

MIGRAINE

Signs and symptoms: symptom onset in childhood or adolescence; known triggers for symptoms (e.g., light, weather changes, certain foods)

> Prodrome: irritability, hyperactivity, depression, food craving
>
> Aura: visual disturbances, vision loss, pins-and-needles sensations, aphasia, limb weakness
>
> Attack: light-headedness; nausea, vomiting; light sensitivity; bilateral or unilateral pulsating or throbbing head pain

CHRONIC DAILY HEADACHE WITH MEDICATION OVERUSE

Definition, chronic daily headache: headaches for ≥ 15 days a month for ≥ 3 months

Signs and symptoms: history of headaches; regular, daily, or clustered headaches, including headaches with migraine symptoms; routinely taking analgesics ≥ 2 days per week or ≥ 9 days per month

SECONDARY HEADACHE

Associated with vascular disorders (e.g., severe arterial hypertension)

SEVERE ARTERIAL HYPERTENSION

Signs and symptoms (hypertensive crisis): systolic blood pressure ≥ 180 mmHg and/or diastolic blood pressure ≥ 120 mmHg; family history of hypertension; renal conditions; diabetes; adrenal or thyroid conditions; vascular conditions; catecholamine excess; obstructive sleep apnea

Risk factors: lack of exercise, high-sodium diet, obesity

Associated with nonvascular disorders (e.g., intracranial infection)

INTRACRANIAL INFECTION

Signs and symptoms: triad of fever, neck stiffness, and altered mental status

> History of infectious contacts (viral, bacterial, or fungal meningitis; or viral, bacterial, or fungal encephalitis); HIV or immunosuppression (this suggests abscesses, toxoplasmosis)

Investigations: MRI, CT scan; CSF analysis to detect abnormal cells or infection

Other (e.g., systemic viral infection, carbon monoxide exposure)

SYSTEMIC VIRAL INFECTION

Signs and symptoms: fever; malaise; myalgia or diffuse pain; respiratory symptoms; joint pain; dehydration on physical examination (skin turgor, sunken eyes, sunken fontanelle in babies); **no** focal neurological symptoms

Investigations: CBC, viral serology, systemic inflammatory markers, endotoxin testing

CARBON MONOXIDE EXPOSURE

Signs and symptoms: dull headache, weakness, dizziness, nausea, vomiting, shortness of breath, confusion, blurred vision, loss of consciousness

> History of indoor chemical or charcoal heater use; indoor portable generator use

Investigations: elevated serum carboxyhemoglobin

Strategy for patient encounter

The likely scenario is a patient with recurrent headaches. The specified tasks could engage history, physical exam, investigations, or management.

History

Use open-ended questions to assess the symptoms of the current headache, the presence of a headache pattern, and medical conditions and medications as secondary causes.

- **Current headache:** When did your current headache start? How severe it is? How does it compare to previous headaches? What other symptoms do you have? Listen for evidence of a sudden-onset first or worst headache (these symptoms suggest hypertensive crisis or intracranial infection); and for evidence consistent with particular entities (e.g., neck stiffness in intracranial infection; fever and myalgia in viral infection; nausea and shortness of breath in carbon monoxide exposure).

- **Headache pattern:** How often do you get headaches? When did you start getting headaches? What triggers have you noticed? What symptoms characterize your headaches? What changes have you noticed in your headaches? Listen for patterns consistent with particular entities (e.g., childhood-onset recurrent headaches with prodromal symptoms and triggers in migraine; recent-onset daily headaches in medication-overuse headaches); and for recent increases in the frequency or severity of headaches.

- **Medical conditions and medications:** What conditions have you been diagnosed with? Listen for a history of hypertension, renal conditions, diabetes, adrenal conditions, thyroid conditions, vascular conditions, or obstructive sleep apnea (relevant to hypertensive crisis), or conditions associated with immunosuppression (relevant to intracranial infection). Ask about recent head trauma, and medical and dental procedures. Ask about the use of analgesics, looking for overuse.

Pay particular attention to evidence of red flags (see the checklist), which indicate the need for neuroimaging or urgent referral.

CHECKLIST

Red flags for acute headache

Sudden onset of headache

New onset of headaches after age 50

Increased frequency or severity of headaches

Focal neurologic symptoms

Papilledema

Headache subsequent to head trauma

Physical exam

Obtain the patient's vital signs, looking for hypertension and fever. Perform a thorough neurological exam. Examine the retinas for papilledema.

Investigations

Patients with sudden-onset severe headache, new headaches after age 50, increased frequency or severity of headaches, abnormal findings on neurological exam, and headaches associated with systemic illness or head trauma should have neuroimaging. First-line imaging is a noncontrast CT scan.

Management

Patients with red flags and a normal CT scan should receive a lumbar puncture, except where contraindicated (see the checklist on contraindications). Refer patients without a diagnosis, or who do not respond to management, to a neurologist or headache clinic.

Treat tension headaches occurring fewer than 15 times per month with as-needed analgesics: acetylsalicylic acid (ASA), acetaminophen, or nonsteroidal antiinflammatory drugs (NSAIDs). Opioids should generally be avoided. Patients with more frequent headaches may respond to daily tricyclic antidepressants, avoidance of triggers, and lifestyle modifications (adequate sleep, exercise, and limiting alcohol and caffeine).

Medication-overuse headaches are treated by the supervised withdrawal of the overused medication and lifestyle changes. Cluster headaches are treated acutely with 100% oxygen. Triptans are the mainstay of treatment for migraine headaches, and may also be used for cluster headaches. Preventive treatment for cluster headaches may include verapamil or prednisone.

CHECKLIST
Contraindications for lumbar puncture

Cellulitis near the site of the lumbar puncture

Increased intracranial pressure

Uncorrected coagulopathy

Acute spinal cord trauma

TIP
Tailoring information to individual patients

The MCC identifies providing generic information as a common exam error.

To avoid this error, ask patients about aspects of their lives that might affect their condition. Provide information that targets their situation and engage the patient in figuring out next steps.

For example, changes in sleep and exercise routines might be relevant for this case:

- Ask what sleep-hygiene routines the patient practises (e.g., limiting screen time, caffeine, and alcohol in the evening; maintaining a cool, quiet, dark sleep environment). What could the patient do tonight to improve their sleep hygiene?

- Ask what the patient did for exercise last week. Discuss short-term goals with the patient: What could the patient do next week to exercise every day? (For example, when could the patient fit in a 30-minute walk?)

58

Hearing loss

MCC particular objectives

Differentiate conductive from sensory-neural hearing loss.

Counsel patients about preventing further hearing loss.

Identify hearing loss in infants as early as possible to prevent developmental delay.

MCC differential diagnosis
with added evidence

CONDUCTIVE HEARING LOSS

External ear pathology

CONGENITAL DISORDER (E.G., ATRESIA)
CONGENITAL AURAL ATRESIA

Causes include prenatal infections; prenatal environmental exposure to ototoxic agents, including aminoglycoside medications; and maternal drug abuse.

Signs and symptoms: absence of auricle and partial external auditory meatus; recurrent otitis media, mastoiditis, or cholesteatoma

> Associated abnormalities: other ear, nose, and throat congenital abnormalities, including the following syndromes: Goldenhar, Treacher, Down, Nager, CHARGE (CHARGE is a mnemonic for a collection of congenital abnormalities: coloboma, heart defects, atresia choanae, growth retardation, genital abnormalities, and ear abnormalities)

Risk factors: family history of congenital abnormalities

INFLAMMATION OR INFECTION (E.G., OTITIS EXTERNA)
OTITIS EXTERNA

The most common cause is bacterial infection (90% of cases).

Signs and symptoms: ear pain; ear pruritus (this can occur with chronic infection; it is more common with fungal infection); discharge; hearing loss; feeling of fullness; pain with jaw movement; erythema of the external ear; pain on traction of the pinna or pressure on the tragus (these typically do not cause pain in acute otitis media); normal tympanic membrane on otoscopy; pain on otoscopy

> Fungal infection: white, flakey debris

Risk factors: water exposure ("swimmer's ear"); use of ear devices (e.g., headphones, hearing aids); trauma (e.g., Q-Tip use); dermatitis

OBSTRUCTION OF CANAL (E.G., WAX, FOREIGN BODY)

Signs and symptoms: hearing loss; ear pain; tinnitus; vertigo; feeling of fullness; history of recent mechanical cleaning of the ears (e.g., Q-Tip use); possible visible trauma; foreign body or cerumen impaction on otoscopy

Middle ear pathology

CONGENITAL DISORDER (E.G., ATRESIA)

Signs and symptoms (in general): recurrent otitis interna; tympanic membrane abnormalities; inner ear ossicular or cochleosaccular abnormalities

> Associated abnormalities: other ear, nose, and throat congenital abnormalities such as congenital rubella syndrome and VACTERL association (VACTERL is a mnemonic for a collection of associated congenital abnormalities: vertebrae, anus, cardiac, trachea, esophageal, renal, limb); vascular abnormalities (e.g., internal carotid artery aneurysms, jugular bulb abnormalities)

Investigations: CT scan, MRI; audiology assessment

INFECTION (E.G., OTITIS MEDIA)

OTITIS MEDIA

Signs and symptoms; ear pain; fever; hearing loss; tympanic membrane that is erythematous and may be opaque, white, yellow, or green (typically; this demonstrates pus behind the tympanic membrane); ear discharge (this indicates perforation of the tympanic membrane); loss of bony landmarks; middle ear effusion with bulging or reduced mobility of the tympanic membrane on pneumatic otoscopy

> Infants and toddlers: ear tugging, irritability, poor feeding, vomiting, diarrhea

Risk factors: upper respiratory tract infection; allergic rhinitis; chronic rhinosinusitis; attendance at a day care facility (for children); contact with infectious illness; exposure to secondhand smoke; age (the condition peaks age 6 to 24 months)

OSSICULAR PATHOLOGY (E.G., OTOSCLEROSIS)

This is diagnosed via investigations (not clinically).

Investigations: CT scan, MRI (findings: complete or partial absence of ossicular bones; intratympanic muscle changes; facial nerve aberrant course); abnormalities on audiology assessment

TRAUMA (E.G., TYMPANIC MEMBRANE PERFORATION)

TYMPANIC MEMBRANE PERFORATION

Signs and symptoms: ear pain; clear, pus-filled, or bloody discharge from the ear; hearing loss; tinnitus; dizziness

> History of otitis media infection; barotrauma or head trauma; acoustic trauma; foreign object in the ear (e.g., cotton swab)

Investigations: culture of discharge; tympanometry; audiology assessment

TUMOUR (E.G., GLOMUS, ADENOMA)

Signs and symptoms (in general): gradual hearing loss; tinnitus; problems with balance, vertigo; facial numbness, tingling, and weakness; changes in taste perception; difficulty swallowing; hoarseness; headaches; clumsiness; confusion; family history of neurofibromatosis (type II); personal history of vascular malformations and/or hemangiomas

Investigations: CT scan, MRI; biopsy; audiology assessment

SENSORY-NEURAL HEARING LOSS

Acquired disorder (e.g., presbycusis, noise-induced hearing loss)

PRESBYCUSIS

Signs and symptoms: gradual bilateral hearing loss; loss of ability to hear high-pitched sounds; loss of ability to discern sounds or voices in noisy areas; tinnitus; dizziness

Risk factors: older than 50 (most common); chronic noise exposure; family history of presbycusis; use of ototoxic medication (e.g., high-dose aspirin); genetic syndrome; prenatal infection (toxoplasmosis, rubella, herpes); history of meningitis, mumps, measles, scarlet fever; Ménière disease

Investigations: positive Rinne and Weber tests for sensory-neural hearing loss

NOISE-INDUCED HEARING LOSS

Signs and symptoms: unilateral or bilateral hearing loss that is gradual or sudden (depending on the cause); tinnitus

> Sudden loss: history of exposure to a sudden, loud noise (e.g., explosion, gunshots, jet engine)

> Gradual loss: history of chronic exposure to loud noise from an occupation (e.g., machinery noise in construction, factory work, farming) or recreation (e.g., listening to loud music; snowmobiling; woodworking)

Investigations: positive Rinne and Weber tests for sensory-neural hearing loss

Congenital disorder (e.g., Alport syndrome)

Signs and symptoms (in general): hearing loss at birth or in childhood (often bilateral); no startle response to loud noise; speech delay; family history of hearing loss; hematuria; renal failure

Investigations: genetic testing

Strategy for patient encounter

The likely scenario is an older man discussing hearing loss on urging from his spouse. The specified tasks could engage history, physical exam, investigations, or management.

History

Use open-ended questions to establish the history of the hearing loss and related evidence: When did the hearing loss begin? Which ear is affected? What other symptoms do you have? What medications do you take? Listen for gradual-onset versus sudden-onset hearing loss (sudden onset suggests infection or trauma; gradual onset suggests tumour or presbycusis); bilateral versus unilateral loss (bilateral loss suggests presbycusis or a congenital disorder); other symptoms consistent with particular entities (e.g., ear pain, redness, itchiness, and discharge in otitis externa; ear pain and discharge with fever in otitis media; neurologic symptoms and headache in tumour); and medications such as aminoglycosides and high-dose aspirin. Ask about a family history of hearing loss. Ask about trauma to the ear or head, and exposure to a sudden loud noise (e.g., an explosion). Ask about occupational and recreational exposure to noise; in cases of chronic noise exposure, ask whether the patient wears ear protection.

Stay alert to evidence of unilateral, unexplained sensory-neural hearing loss that has occurred within the last 72 hours, because this is a medical emergency.

Physical exam

Perform an otoscopic exam looking for wax, obstructions, tumour, infection, effusion, discharge, and tympanic perforation. Perform an exam of the cranial nerves. Perform Rinne and Weber tests to assess for sensory-neural hearing loss.

Investigations

In all patients, order an audiogram. In suspected vestibular neuroma (symptoms: vertigo, neurologic symptoms, headache), order a CT scan.

Management

Treat reversible causes. Consider referral to an ear, nose, and throat (ENT) specialist. Counsel the patient about preventing further hearing loss.

Sudden sensory-neural hearing loss (acute unexplained hearing loss, nearly always unilateral, that occurs over less than a 72-hour period) is a medical emergency. These cases may have viral or autoimmune causes. Some evidence supports administering prednisolone 1 mg/kg/day to a maximum of 60 mg/day for 7 to 14 days. No evidence supports the use of antivirals in this context. In general, offer the patient steroid treatment and discuss the case with an ENT specialist.

TIP

Tailoring information to individual patients

The MCC identifies providing generic information as a common exam error.

To avoid this error, ask patients about aspects of their lives that might affect their condition. Provide information that targets their situation and engage the patient in figuring out next steps.

For example, hearing protection in the context of presbycusis may be relevant for this case.

- Explain that hearing loss from presbycusis cannot be stopped, but that hearing protection is still important and useful.
- Ask about the loudest noise the patient routinely experiences (e.g., noise from household appliances or tools; traffic noise; noise in recreation facilities).
- Ask what would help the patient make earplug use routine in those situations.

59

Cerebrovascular accident (CVA) and transient ischemic attack (TIA)

MCC particular objectives

Take action in the case of CVA or TIA.

Reduce the risk of CVA and TIA through preventive health care.

MCC differential diagnosis
with added evidence

ISCHEMIC STROKE

Thrombotic

Signs and symptoms (these depend on the affected blood vessel): hemiparesis, monoparesis, or (rarely) quadriparesis; hemisensory deficits; vision loss in 1 or both eyes; visual field deficits; double vision; difficulty speaking; facial droop; ataxia; vertigo; aphasia; fever; sudden decrease in level of consciousness

> History of hypertension, diabetes, smoking, high cholesterol, coronary artery disease, coagulopathies, illicit drug use (especially cocaine), migraines, oral contraceptive use

Investigations: CT scan, MRI; ECG to detect atrial fibrillation; presence of cardiac markers (troponins, CKMB); abnormalities on PTT and/or PT/INR

Embolic

Signs and symptoms: symptoms similar to thrombosis (see above)

> History of atrial fibrillation, cardiac defects, hypertension, coronary artery disease

Investigations: abnormal ECG; presence of cardiac markers (troponins, CKMB); abnormalities on PTT, and/or PT/INR

HEMORRHAGIC STROKE

Intracerebral and cerebellar

Signs and symptoms: symptoms with sudden onset that gradually become worse (e.g., over hours); symptoms that include neurologic deficits (e.g., weakness or hemiparalysis in the face, arms, or legs), headache, impaired vision, aphasia, dysphasia, nausea, vomiting, sleepiness, loss of consciousness, confusion, delirium, fever

> History of head injury or trauma; known cerebral aneurysm or arteriovenous malformation; bleeding disorders or use of blood thinners; bleeding tumours; cocaine use (this can cause severe hypertension)

Investigations: CT scan, cerebral angiogram

Subarachnoid

Signs and symptoms: sudden-onset severe symptoms; symptoms that include severe headache (this is the most common symptom; it is sometimes called a "thunderclap" headache), neck or shoulder pain, meningismus with nuchal rigidity, photophobia, pain with eye movements, nausea, vomiting, seizures, confusion, fever, syncope (prolonged or atypical), abnormalities on neurological exam

> History of congenital berry aneurysm; bleeding from an

arteriovenous malformation; bleeding disorders or use of
blood thinners

Investigations: CT scan, MRI; cerebral angiogram; transcranial
ultrasound

Strategy for patient encounter

The likely scenario is a patient with acute neurological deficits.
The specified tasks could engage history, physical exam, investigations, or management.

History

In the case of acute stroke, the patient will likely be unable to give
a history. Seek information from an accompanying caregiver.

Ask about risk factors for stroke including hypertension, diabetes, smoking, high cholesterol, coronary artery disease, coagulopathies, illicit drug use (especially cocaine), migraines, oral
contraceptive use, and a history of TIA or stroke.

Physical exam

Obtain the patient's vital signs, including temperature. Perform
a full neurological exam, looking for deficits. Examine the heart
and lungs. Listen for bruits over the carotid arteries and abdominal aorta.

Investigations

In all cases of suspected stroke, immediately perform a point-of-care glucose measure and order an emergent CT scan of the head.
Usual blood work includes complete blood count (CBC) and tests
for electrolytes, creatinine, prothrombin time/international normalized ratio (PT/INR), activated partial thromboplastin time
(aPTT), troponin (to rule out concurrent or recent heart attack),
and blood glucose level. Order an electrocardiogram (ECG) (to
detect atrial fibrillation and/or recent myocardial infarction).

Management

Obtain an emergent referral to a stroke team or acute stroke unit.

Treat ischemic stroke patients presenting within 4.5 hours (or
within 3 hours for patients older than 80) with fibrinolytic therapy
(see the checklist for inclusion criteria and absolute contraindications). Order patients to have nothing by mouth. Before allowing
oral food, liquids, or pills, perform a swallowing assessment.

For patients with a fever > 38°C, administer acetaminophen rectally.

For all patients, consider supplemental oxygen and order a cardiac monitor to assess for ischemic changes and atrial fibrillation.

Treat patients with antihypertensives *only* if systolic pressure is > 220 mmHg or if diastolic pressure is > 120 mmHg, *except* in the administration of fibrinolytic therapy (where systolic blood pressure > 185 mmHg or diastolic pressure > 110 mmHg is a contraindication and so requires treatment). First-line antihypertensive medications include:

- **Labetalol:** 10–20 mg administered intravenously every 10 to 20 minutes
- **Nicardipine:** 5 mg/hour; titrate by 2.5 mg/hour every 5 to 15 minutes; maximum 15 mg/hour

When target blood pressure is reached, lower the dose of labetalol or nicardipine to 3 mg/hour, or administer enalapril 1.25 mg by intravenous (IV) push.

In patients who do not respond to fibrinolytic therapy or who are not candidates, refer emergently for endovascular therapy (stent placement).

CHECKLIST
Criteria for fibrinolysis with tissue plasminogen activator (tPA)
Note: additional relative contraindications also exist, but are unlikely to form part of a standardized exam.

INCLUSION CRITERIA	ABSOLUTE CONTRAINDICATIONS
Age 18 or older	Intracranial hemorrhage (usually diagnosed on CT scan) or history of intracranial hemorrhage
Clinical diagnosis of ischemic stroke causing neurologic deficit(s)	Subarachnoid hemorrhage
	Neurosurgery, head trauma, or stroke in past 3 months
Symptom onset over less than 4.5 hours	Uncontrolled hypertension (> 185 mmHg systolic blood pressure or > 110 mmHg diastolic blood pressure)
	Intracranial arteriovenous malformation, neoplasm, or aneurysm
	Active internal bleeding
	Suspected or confirmed endocarditis
	Known bleeding diathesis
	Abnormal blood glucose (especially hypoglycemia, which can mimic stroke): correct with intravenous dextrose 50% solution (D50 IV)

In patients with TIAs, start low-dose acetylsalicylic acid (ASA) and evaluate for treatable risk factors (hypertension, smoking, diabetes, high cholesterol, carotid stenosis). TIAs confer a 10% risk of stroke in the next 30 days. When stroke occurs after a TIA, 50% occur within the next 48 hours.

Following acute treatment, refer the patient to an occupational therapist and for rehabilitation therapy.

Pearls

Stroke is the number 3 cause of death in Canada. Ischemic strokes make up 85% of cases and hemorrhagic strokes the remaining 15%.

60

Anemia

MCC particular objectives

Pay particular attention to:

- red cell morphology
- common causes of anemia in specific populations
- risk factors for serious underlying conditions

MCC differential diagnosis
with added evidence

NORMOCYTIC ANEMIA

Red blood cell loss

OBVIOUS (E.G., TRAUMA, METRO- OR MENORRHAGIA)

OCCULT BLOOD LOSS

Signs and symptoms: abdominal pain; black or tarry stools; blood in vomit; fatigue; dizziness

History of peptic ulcer disease; liver disease; abnormal coagulation or bleeding disorder; gastrointestinal bleeding; alcoholism

Investigations: endoscopy; colonoscopy; CBC; peripheral blood smear; CT scan

Decreased red blood cell production

MARROW PRODUCTION (E.G., STEM CELL DISORDER, BONE MARROW REPLACEMENT)

STEM CELL DISORDER

Signs and symptoms: fatigue; tachycardia or tachypnea; bone pain; headaches; frequent infections; mucosal or joint bleeding

Investigations: CBC; peripheral blood smear; bone marrow biopsy; flow cytometry; chromosomal analysis; genetic testing to detect *JAK2* or *BCR-ABL* mutation

Increased red blood cell destruction (e.g., sickle cell anemia, immune-mediated conditions, mechanical conditions)

SICKLE CELL DISEASE

Signs and symptoms: family history of sickle cell disease; painful swelling of the hands and feet

Investigations: CBC to detect anemia, sickle cells; positive sickle cell screen; abnormalities on peripheral blood smear; abnormalities on hemoglobin electrophoresis

IMMUNE-MEDIATED CONDITIONS

Signs and symptoms: fatigue, weakness, fever, hepatosplenomegaly, jaundice, dark urine

> History of recent transfusion; recent infections (Epstein-Barr virus, hepatitis, *Streptococcus*, *Escherichia coli*); autoimmune disorders (systemic lupus erythematosus, Wiskott-Aldrich syndrome); new medications (e.g., antibiotics); leukemia or lymphoma; HELLP syndrome (HELLP is a mnemonic for hemolysis, elevated liver enzymes, low platelet count)

Investigations: DAT, IAT, CBC, peripheral blood smear, kidney function tests

MECHANICAL CONDITIONS

Signs and symptoms: fatigue, dizziness, tachycardia, tachypnea

> History of heart valve replacement; recent rapid transfusion or blood warmer use; arteriovenous malformations; genetic conditions or syndromes

Investigations: CT scan, MRI, ultrasound, ECG

Anemia of chronic disease

Signs and symptoms: fatigue, dizziness, tachycardia, tachypnea

> History of chronic systemic disease: autoimmune disorders, chronic kidney disease, chronic infections, cancer

Investigations: normal to high serum ferritin, low iron, low reticulocyte count, low hemoglobin

MICROCYTIC ANEMIA (E.G., IRON DEFICIENCY, HEMOGLOBINOPATHIES)

IRON DEFICIENCY

Signs and symptoms: fatigue, dizziness, tachycardia, tachypnea, enlarged tongue

> History of menorrhagia, dietary restriction (e.g., anorexia, starvation, poverty), pregnancy, melena

Investigations: low serum ferritin, low iron, low reticulocyte count, low hemoglobin, colonoscopy

HEMOGLOBINOPATHIES

Causes include sickle cell disease (see above), thalassemia, and chronic blood transfusions.

THALASSEMIA

Signs and symptoms: fatigue, dizziness, tachycardia, tachypnea

Risk factors: family history of thalassemia; African, Middle Eastern, or South Asian descent

Investigations: abnormalities on CBC; low serum ferritin; low iron; low reticulocyte count; low hemoglobin; abnormalities on hemoglobin electrophoresis; abnormalities on hemoglobin HPLC

MACROCYTIC ANEMIA (E.G., VITAMIN B_{12} OR FOLATE DEFICIENCY, ALCOHOL USE)

Signs and symptoms (in general): fatigue; dizziness; tachycardia; tachypnea; ataxia; burning or prickling sensations

> History of chemotherapy medication use; folate or vitamin B_{12} deficiency (pernicious anemia); alcoholism; poor diet

Investigations: abnormalities on CBC; abnormalities on peripheral blood smear; low vitamin B_{12} and folate levels; Schilling test to detect low vitamin B_{12} absorption

Strategy for patient encounter

The likely scenario is a patient with anemia found on routine blood work. The specified tasks could engage history, physical exam, investigations, or management. See figures 1 through 3, which present diagnostic algorithms for normocytic, microcytic, and macrocytic anemia.[1]

History

Ask open-ended questions to take a medical history: What conditions have you been diagnosed with? Listen for malignancy and chronic disease. Ask about family history of anemia and clarify the ethnic background of the patient (hemoglobinopathies are prevalent in patients of African, Middle Eastern, or South Asian descent).

Physical exam

Obtain the patient's vital signs, looking for hypotension and tachycardia.

Examine the skin, looking for pallor, purpura, petechiae, and jaundice. Examine the sclera for icterus. Auscultate the heart for a systolic ejection (flow) murmur at the left sternal border. Examine the abdomen for hepatosplenomegaly. Perform a rectal exam for masses and to check for fecal occult blood.

(State that you will perform a rectal exam. Since this exam is not performed on standardized patients, the examiner will likely interrupt, ask what you are looking for, and provide findings.)

Investigations

Order a complete blood count (CBC), peripheral blood smear, and tests for serum ferritin and iron levels. For cases of macrocytosis, order tests for serum vitamin B_{12} and folate. Consider referring the patient for a bone marrow biopsy.

Management

Optimize the management of any underlying disorders and correct any nutritional deficiencies. Consider referring the patient to a hematologist. For patients with refractory anemia, consider blood transfusion.

Pearls

History (including family history) may give clues to the cause of anemia. However, red cell indices and findings on peripheral blood smear are key to making a diagnosis.

REFERENCE

1 Faulkner L. Lab literacy for Canadian doctors. Edmonton, Canada: Brush Education Inc.; 2014. Chapter 8, Hematology; 133–171 (Figures 6–8, 159–163).

Figure 1 Diagnostic algorithm for normocytic anemia

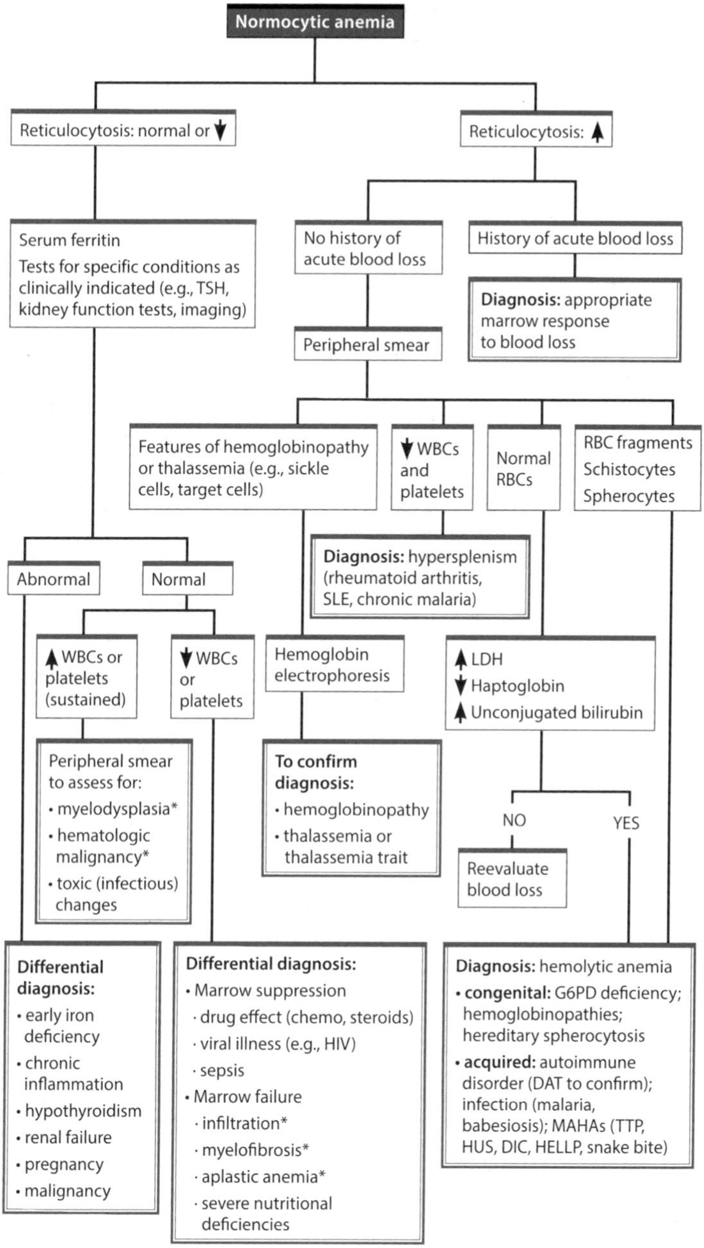

*Requires bone marrow biopsy or special tests to confirm.

Figure 2   Diagnostic algorithm for microcytic anemia

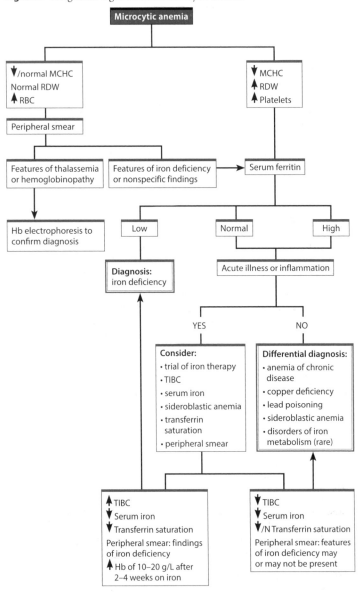

Figure 3 Diagnositic algorithm for macrocytic anemia

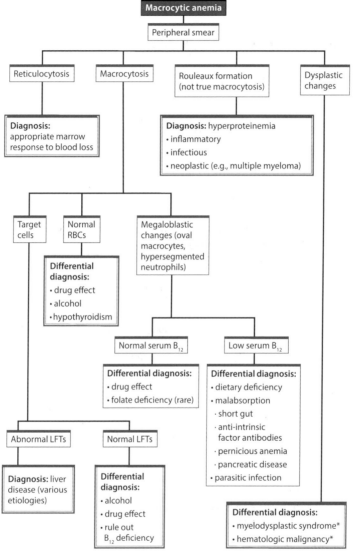

*Requires bone marrow biopsy or special tests to confirm.

61

Elevated hemoglobin

MCC particular objectives
None stated.

MCC differential diagnosis
with added evidence

INCREASED RED CELL MASS

Polycythemia vera: low or normal erythropoietin (EPO)
Signs and symptoms: possibly asymptomatic, pruritus (this is worse after warm baths), burning sensations in distal extremities, fatigue, dizziness, headache, gouty nodules, hepatomegaly, splenomegaly

Investigations:

> Blood tests: elevated findings (platelets, hemoglobin, hematocrit, RBCs, WBCs); low EPO
>
> Bone marrow biopsy: increased cellularity, panmyelosis (erythroid, granulocytic, megakaryocytic lines)

Secondary erythrocytosis: elevated EPO

APPROPRIATE EPO ELEVATION (E.G., HYPOXEMIA)
HYPOXEMIA
Causes include living in high altitudes, lung disease (e.g., chronic obstructive pulmonary disease), smoking, and heart disease (e.g., congenital heart disease, arteriovenous malformations).

Signs and symptoms: cyanosis

INAPPROPRIATE EPO ELEVATION (E.G., EPO-EXCRETING TUMOUR)
INAPPROPRIATE EPO ELEVATION IN GENERAL
Causes include renal tumour, blood doping, and use of steroids.

RENAL TUMOUR
Signs and symptoms: possible palpable abdominal mass

Investigations: CT scan, ultrasound

RELATIVE POLYCYTHEMIA (DEHYDRATION)

Causes of dehydration include vomiting, diarrhea, sweating, and burns.

Signs and symptoms: low jugular venous pressure, low blood pressure, decreased skin turgor, dry mouth, sunken eyes, tachycardia

Investigations: elevated creatinine

Strategy for patient encounter

The likely scenario is a patient with elevated hemoglobin on routine blood work. The specified tasks could engage history, physical exam, investigations, or management.

History

The primary goal is to distinguish primary from secondary erythrocytosis. Ask about secondary causes of elevated hemoglobin including heart disease, respiratory disease, smoking, congenital heart disease, and causes of dehydration.

Physical exam

Examine the heart and lungs, looking for signs of cardiovascular and respiratory disease. Examine the abdomen looking for an enlarged liver and/or spleen.

Investigations

In suspected dehydration, order a test for serum creatinine. The upper limit of normal for hemoglobin is 160 g/L for adult women and 180 g/L for adult men. If common secondary causes have been ruled out, and especially if there are elevations in other blood cells (platelets and neutrophils), order blood testing for the *JAK2* mutation (*JAK2* V617F). This is present in 95% of patients with polycythemia vera. In suspected polycythemia vera, or in cases of unknown cause, consider referring the patient for a bone marrow biopsy.

Management

Manage any secondary causes identified. Refer patients with polycythemia vera to a hematologist. Complications of polycythemia vera (stroke, blood clots) are managed with regular phlebotomy and low-dose acetylsalicylic acid (ASA). Hematologists may also treat polycythemia vera with chemotherapy.

62

Language and speech disorders

MCC particular objective

Differentiate speech from language abnormalities:

- **Speech disorder:** impaired articulation, fluency, voice
- **Language disorder:** impaired comprehension and/or use of the form, content, or function of language

MCC differential diagnosis
with added evidence

LANGUAGE DISORDER

Delayed and developmental language impairment (e.g., hearing impairment, autism spectrum disorder, neglect, abuse)

DELAYED AND DEVELOPMENTAL LANGUAGE IMPAIRMENT IN GENERAL (PEDIATRIC)

Signs and symptoms: differences in language development compared to other children of the same age; problems with social interactions with other children

HEARING IMPAIRMENT

Signs and symptoms: problems identifying the sources of sounds; complications during gestation (e.g., toxin exposure such as alcohol) and/or delivery; blocked (from impacted wax or mass) or nonmobile (from chronic effusion) tympanic membranes

Investigations: hearing test

AUTISM SPECTRUM DISORDER[1(pp50-51)]

Signs and symptoms: deficits in social interaction and communication; repetitive, stereotyped behaviours (motor and/or vocal); restricted interests; sensory problems; presence of symptoms in all contexts (e.g., home, school); presence of symptoms from early childhood

NEGLECT

Neglect involves failure to provide all or some basic physical, emotional, educational, and medical needs. Examples include rejecting a child and not giving love; not feeding a child; not dressing a child in proper clothing; not giving needed medical or dental care; and abandonment by leaving a child alone for a long time.

Signs and symptoms: not attending school regularly; poor hygiene, dental care; malnutrition; reports by the child suggesting lack of physical and/or emotional care at home

ABUSE

Signs and symptoms: disclosed abuse (victims do not always disclose abuse); resistance by the parent or caregiver to having the patient interviewed alone (usual)

Physical abuse: inconsistency between an injury and the explanation for the injury and/or the developmental stage of the child; facial contusions; marks on the neck or limbs; burn marks; ligature marks on the wrists or ankles; bite marks; lash marks; bruises or broken bones unexplainable by usual activities

Sexual abuse: behaviour and knowledge that is inappropriate for the child's age; pregnancy or sexually transmitted infection (STI); blood in the child's underwear; trouble walking or sitting, or complaints of genital pain; sexual abuse of other children by victim

Psychological abuse: problems in school; eating disorders leading to weight loss or poor weight gain; emotional issues (anxiety, low self-esteem); depression; extreme behaviour (e.g., acting out to seek attention); trouble sleeping

No evidence of medical conditions that could mimic abuse (e.g., malabsorption; developmental delay due to complications during gestation or delivery; genetic or metabolic disorders)

Risk factors: history of substance abuse by the parents or caregivers; unstable living situation of the parents or caregivers

Degenerative, vascular, or other central nervous system disorders (e.g., stroke)

Signs and symptoms (in general): older age (more common); personal or family history of cardiovascular or cerebrovascular disease; obesity; smoking; diabetes; hypertension; dyslipidemia; lack of physical activity; poor diet

Head injury

Signs and symptoms: history of trauma or assault (high-risk mechanisms include pedestrian-vehicle accidents; accidents where people are ejected from vehicles; and falls from heights ≥ 1 metre, or down ≥ 5 stairs); motor or sensory deficits on neurological exam

Investigations: CT scan of the head

SPEECH DISORDER

Articulation disorder (e.g., dysarthria)

DYSARTHRIA

Causes include trauma, neurological injury, stroke, cerebral palsy, muscular dystrophy, amyotrophic lateral sclerosis, and multiple sclerosis.

Signs and symptoms: drooling and/or difficulty swallowing; incomprehensible speech; limited movement of the tongue, lip, or jaw on speaking; abnormalities in voice rate, quality, pitch, nasality, or rhythm; motor or sensory deficits on neurological exam

Fluency (e.g., stuttering, Parkinson disease)

FLUENCY IN GENERAL

Signs and symptoms: involuntary repetition of sounds (initial consonants usually); prolongation of sounds or syllables; involuntary silent pauses

STUTTERING

Signs and symptoms: childhood onset

PARKINSON DISEASE

Signs and symptoms (mnemonic **TRAP**): **t**remor at rest; **r**igidity of the lower limbs; **a**kinesia, bradykinesia; **p**ostural instability

> Other symptoms: cognitive impairment; dementia; shuffling gait with stooped posture and loss of arm swing; micrographia; hypophonia; masklike facies, "pill rolling"; lack of blinking; orthostatic hypotension

> History of use of antipsychotics, antiemetics; toxin ingestion (e.g., carbon monoxide, cyanide); head trauma; vascular disease; other neurodegenerative disease (e.g., Lewy body dementia, Huntington disease); brain tumour, hydrocephalus; metabolic conditions (e.g., hypoparathyroidism, Wilson disease, chronic liver failure); infections that spread to the brain (HIV/AIDS, syphilis, prion disease, toxoplasmosis, encephalitis lethargica, progressive multifocal leukoencephalopathy)

Speech apparatus lesions (e.g., cleft palate, head and neck neoplasm)

CLEFT PALATE

This is usually diagnosed at birth. When it affects only the muscles of the palate (submucous cleft palate), it may not be detected until later.

Signs and symptoms (submucous cleft palate): difficulty swallowing, hypernasal voice resonance, auditory issues, frequent ear infections

HEAD AND NECK CANCER

Signs and symptoms: symptoms for > 3 weeks; persistent unilateral throat discomfort

> Lesion in the oral cavity: persistent red and/or white patches on the oral mucosa; ulceration and/or swelling of the oropharynx or mucosa; persistent mass; tongue pain; tongue deviation; hoarseness; unexplained tooth mobility and/or looseness; earache; difficulty swallowing; bleeding in the oral cavity; stridor; facial pain or numbness

Lesion in the nasopharynx: neck lump; bloody nasal discharge; nasal blockage; unilateral hearing loss; ringing in the ear; recurrent otitis media; headache; facial pain or numbness; double vision; persistent cough

Investigations: endoscopic visualization; fine needle aspiration or core biopsy of mass

Strategy for patient encounter

This encounter will likely involve a parent discussing a child who has speech delay. The child will be absent on some pretext (e.g., someone has taken the child to use the toilet). The specified tasks could engage history, physical exam, investigations, or management.

The distinction between language disorders and speech disorders is key for this patient encounter. Language disorders involve difficulty understanding speech or sharing thoughts. Speech disorders involve difficulty producing speech sounds correctly.

History

Ask the parent about the child's speech and language milestones (see the checklist). Ask whether the family can understand what the child says. Ask about a family history of attention deficit hyperactivity disorder and autism spectrum disorder. Ask about a history of head injury.

Physical exam

Observe the child speaking or interacting with an adult. Examine the ears, nose and throat, including otoscopy. Perform a neurological exam.

CHECKLIST
Simplified speech and language milestones

- **12 months:** babbles and uses gestures
- **15 months:** says a few words and correctly points to objects or pictures
- **18 months:** understands simple commands and has more than 20 words
- **24 months:** has 50 to 100 words, joins 2 words together
- **36 months:** has more than 300 words, asks questions, makes simple grammatically correct sentences
- **4 years:** is able to tell a simple story

(State that you will observe and examine the child. Because an actual pediatric patient is unlikely, the examiner may interrupt you, ask what you are looking for, and provide findings. State that you are looking for lesions, masses, blocked abnormal tympanic membranes, and neurological abnormalities.)

Investigations
Order a hearing test. In the presence of trauma or neurologic symptoms, order a CT scan of the head.

Management
Refer pediatric patients for speech therapy. Consider referral to an ear, nose, and throat (ENT) surgeon or neurologist, as appropriate.

REFERENCE

1 American Psychiatric Association. Diagnostic and statistical manual of mental disorders. 5th ed. Arlington, VA: American Psychiatric Association; 2013. 59–60. 991 p.

63

Acid-base abnormalities, hydrogen

MCC particular objective
Initiate an appropriate management plan for high anion gap metabolic acidosis.

MCC differential diagnosis
with added evidence

METABOLIC ACIDOSIS
METABOLIC ACIDOSIS IN GENERAL
Investigations: decreased pH; decreased $PaCO_2$; decreased HCO_3^-

High anion gap
Definition: > 12–16 mmol/L
Calculation: Anion Gap = (Sodium) − (Chloride + Bicarbonate)

INCREASED ACID PRODUCTION
EXOGENOUS (E.G., METHANOL)
Signs and symptoms (in general): vision changes, abdominal pain,

confusion, fever, jaundice, tachycardia, altered level of consciousness, dilated pupils

History of ingesting methanol, acetaminophen, isoniazid, iron, ethanol, ethylene glycol, propylene glycol, salicylate

Investigations: toxin screen to detect particular toxins; elevated urine or serum ketones (possible); elevated lactate (possible); elevated osmolar gap (possible); creatinine

ENDOGENOUS (E.G., KETOACIDOSIS)

KETOACIDOSIS

Common causes of ketoacidosis include type 1 diabetes, alcohol abuse, and starvation.

Symptoms: polydipsia; polyuria; nausea, vomiting; weakness; lethargy; dehydration (tachycardia, hypotension); deep respirations; fruity odour on the breath (ketone breath); altered mental status; hypertension and bradycardia (these indicate cerebral edema)

History of new-onset type 1 diabetes, signs of infection (e.g., fever), reduced insulin intake, atherosclerotic disease, change in diet, alcohol use, drug use, pregnancy

Investigations: serum glucose (elevated in diabetes; normal–low in alcohol abuse, starvation); acidosis (bicarbonate < 18 mmol/L; blood pH < 7.3); serum ketones (present); electrolytes (anion gap > 10); CBC with differential; blood gas; urine dipstick to detect ketones; urinalysis; renal and liver function tests; urine culture; blood culture; ECG; chest X-ray

DECREASED RENAL ACID EXCRETION (KIDNEY INJURY)

KIDNEY INJURY

Signs and symptoms: history of kidney disease, chronic renal failure, and/or current renal dialysis; bilateral lower limb swelling; shortness of breath; paroxysmal nocturnal dyspnea; orthopnea

Risk factors: diabetes, diabetic complications, and/or inadequate monitoring; hypertension; smoking

Investigations: renal function tests (reduced calcium; elevated phosphate; elevated creatinine); reduced vitamin D

Normal anion gap

GASTROINTESTINAL BICARBONATE LOSS (E.G., DIARRHEA)

RENAL BICARBONATE LOSS (E.G., RENAL TUBULAR ACIDOSIS, INTERSTITIAL NEPHRITIS)

RENAL TUBULAR ACIDOSIS (PROXIMAL)

Causes include Fanconi syndrome; multiple myeloma; amyloidosis; use of medications such as acetazolamide; renal transplant; autoimmune disease; and low aldosterone.

Investigations: blood tests (reduced bicarbonate; reduced phosphate; reduced glucose; reduced vitamin D; hyper- or hypokalemia)

INTERSTITIAL NEPHRITIS

Signs and symptoms: fever; rash; arthralgia; use of diuretics, antibiotics, analgesics (usual); history of autoimmune disorders

Investigations: urine eosinophils (their presence is suggestive); urinalysis (normal findings for RBCs, proteinuria, and red cell casts); blood tests (normal creatinine; normal complement level); renal biopsy (definitive)

METABOLIC ALKALOSIS

METABOLIC ALKALOSIS IN GENERAL

Investigations: elevated pH; elevated $PaCO_2$; elevated HCO_3^-

Expanded effective arterial blood volume (e.g., mineralocorticoid excess)

Causes include primary hyperaldosteronism (Conn syndrome), secondary hyperaldosteronism (e.g., renovascular disease, renin-secreting tumour), and hypertension.

Investigations: elevated urine chloride levels

Contracted effective arterial blood volume

GASTROINTESTINAL LOSS (E.G., VOMITING)

RENAL LOSS (E.G., DIURETICS)

Exogenous ingestion

Causes include bicarbonate use (e.g., sodium bicarbonate antacid, intravenous infusion).

RESPIRATORY ACIDOSIS

RESPIRATORY ACIDOSIS IN GENERAL

Investigations: decreased pH; elevated $PaCO_2$; elevated HCO_3^-

Neuromuscular causes (e.g., medications, illicit drugs)

A common cause is use of sedatives (e.g., opioids, barbiturates, benzodiazepines).

Pulmonary causes of decreased alveolar ventilation (e.g., chronic obstructive pulmonary disease)

CHRONIC OBSTRUCTIVE PULMONARY DISEASE

Signs and symptoms: older than 40 (usual: symptoms do not appear until significant lung damage has occurred); progressive symptoms; wheezing; chest tightness; chronic productive cough; clubbing of fingers; cyanosis around the lips and in the extremities; decreased oxygen saturation; impaired pulmonary function on testing with spirometry

Risk factors: smoking; occupational exposure; intrinsic lung disease

Investigations: chest X-ray; CT scan; ABG

Kyphoscoliosis

Signs and symptoms: poor posture; uneven limb length; abnormal gait; shortness of breath or difficulty breathing

Investigations: X-ray, CT scan of the spine and chest

Hypoventilation (e.g., due to obesity)

Signs and symptoms (in general): excess body weight; snoring; shallow breathing; daytime fatigue; sleep disturbances

RESPIRATORY ALKALOSIS

RESPIRATORY ALKALOSIS IN GENERAL

Investigations: elevated pH; decreased $PaCO_2$; decreased HCO_3^-

Hypoxemia

Causes include living in high altitudes, lung disease (e.g., chronic obstructive pulmonary disease), and heart disease (e.g., congenital heart disease, arteriovenous malformations).

Signs and symptoms: cyanosis

Metabolic disorder (e.g., hepatic failure)

HEPATIC FAILURE

Signs and symptoms: history of liver disease; jaundice; abdominal pain, swelling; palpable, tender liver; swelling in the legs and ankles; systemic symptoms (anorexia, weight loss, weakness, fatigue); itching; easy bruising

> History of chronic alcohol abuse; chronic infection from hepatitis B virus (HBV) or hepatitis C virus (HCV) (HCV is often asymptomatic); hemochromatosis; autoimmune conditions; α_1-antitrypsin deficiency; primary biliary cirrhosis; congestive heart failure

> HBV and HCV risk factors: unprotected sex, intravenous drug abuse, blood transfusions, tattoos, body piercings, imprisonment, workplace exposure to body fluids

Investigations: tests for liver enzymes (elevated AST, ALT) and liver function (elevated bilirubin; possible abnormal PT/INR); viral serologic tests to detect HBV, HCV

Cardiopulmonary disorder (e.g., pneumonia, embolism)

PNEUMONIA

Signs and symptoms: shortness of breath; cough; purulent sputum; chest pain on coughing or deep breaths; fatigue; tachypnea; tachycardia; decreased oxygen saturation; lung crackles on auscultation; lung dullness on percussion

> Children: fever

> Elderly: confusion, low body temperature

Risk factors: very old, very young, smoking, immune compromise
(e.g., due to chronic illness), hospitalization

Investigations: chest X-ray to detect consolidation

PULMONARY EMBOLISM

Signs and symptoms: sharp chest pain; shortness of breath; cough
(possibly with blood); hypoxia; possible unilateral swelling of the
lower limbs (this indicates deep vein thrombosis); elevated pulse and
respiratory rate; arrhythmias; lung rales on auscultation; lower-lung
dullness on percussion; motor or sensory deficits

Risk factors: heart failure; cancer; surgery; prolonged immobility
(e.g., long plane trips); smoking; estrogen replacement therapy; oral
contraceptives; current pregnancy; previous deep vein thrombosis,
embolism, or stroke; family history of embolism

Investigations: elevated D-dimer level; area of reduced pulmonary
perfusion on V/Q scan; CT angiography to detect blocked vessel

Central nervous system disorder (e.g., subarachnoid hemorrhage)

SUBARACHNOID HEMORRHAGE

Signs and symptoms: sudden-onset severe symptoms; symptoms
that include severe headache (this is the most common symptom;
it is sometimes called a "thunderclap" headache), neck or shoulder
pain, meningismus with nuchal rigidity, photophobia, pain with eye
movements, nausea, vomiting, seizures, confusion, fever, syncope
(prolonged or atypical), abnormalities on neurological exam

> History of congenital berry aneurysm; bleeding from an
> arteriovenous malformation; bleeding disorders or use of
> blood thinners

Investigations: CT scan, MRI; cerebral angiogram; transcranial
ultrasound

Drugs (e.g., salicylate)

SALICYLATE POISONING

Signs and symptoms: history of using skin products that contain
salicylates, such as over-the-counter acne remedies; abdominal pain;
tinnitus; nausea, vomiting (blood in the vomit); hyperthermia; mental
status changes (agitation and seizures; or lethargy, central nervous
system depression, and coma)

Other (e.g., fever, pain, pregnancy)

Strategy for patient encounter

The likely scenario is a patient with metabolic acidosis. The specified tasks could engage history, physical exam, investigations, or
management.

This patient encounter will likely start with the interpretation of blood work, or will involve a classic presentation from the MCC differential diagnosis that strongly suggests the presence of an acid-base abnormality.

History

Ask about medication and drug use, medical history (especially type 1 diabetes and renal failure), and a history of recent illness (vomiting, diarrhea).

Physical exam

Obtain the patient's vital signs, looking for fever and tachypnea. Examine the skin for jaundice and the sclera for icterus, and observe the patient for decreased level of consciousness.

Investigations

Order a test for arterial blood gases (ABG). Order a "Chem 7" blood panel: blood urea nitrogen (BUN); carbon dioxide (CO_2) or bicarbonate (HCO_3^-); creatinine; glucose; chloride; potassium; and sodium.

Steps 1 to 5, which follow, outline how to evaluate acid-base status.

STEP 1

Look at the pH to determine if the patient has acidemia (decreased pH) or alkalemia (elevated pH). The important principle here is that, while there will be metabolic or respiratory compensation for the primary disorder, the acidemia or alkalemia will never be overcorrected.

STEP 2

Use the following table to classify the primary acid-base abnormality.

TYPE OF DISORDER	pH	$PaCO_2$	HCO_3^-
Metabolic acidosis	Decreased	Decreased	Decreased
Metabolic alkalosis	Increased	Increased	Increased
Respiratory acidosis	Decreased	Increased	Increased
Respiratory alkalosis	Increased	Decreased	Decreased

STEP 3

Evaluate for compensation for the primary disturbance:

- **Metabolic acidosis:** For every decrease of HCO_3^- by 10, $PaCO_2$ is expected to decrease by 12.
- **Metabolic alkalosis:** For every increase in HCO_3^- by 10, the $PaCO_2$ is expected to increase by 6.
- **Acute respiratory acidosis:** For every increase in $PaCO_2$ by 10, the HCO_3^- is expected to increase by 1.
- **Chronic respiratory acidosis:** For every increase in $PaCO_2$ by 10, the HCO_3^- is expected to increase by 4.
- **Acute respiratory alkalosis:** For every decrease in $PaCO_2$ by 10, the HCO_3^- is expected to decrease by 2.
- **Chronic respiratory alkalosis:** For every decrease in $PaCO_2$ by 10, the HCO_3^- is expected to decrease by 5.

STEP 4

If the patient has acidemia, determine if there is an anion gap:

$$\text{Anion Gap} = (\text{Sodium}) - (\text{Chloride} + \text{Bicarbonate})$$

See the checklist for causes of high anion gap metabolic acidosis.

STEP 5

In cases of high anion gap metabolic acidosis, check for a secondary acid-base disturbance (in addition to compensation) by calculating the ratio of the increase in anion gap (AG) to the decrease in HCO_3^- as follows:

$$\frac{(\text{Calculated AG} - \text{Expected AG})}{24 - \text{Measured HCO}_3^-}$$

This is called the delta:delta ratio. A delta:delta ratio less than 0.4 usually indicates a pure normal anion gap metabolic acidosis; a ratio of 0.4 to 0.8 indicates a mixed normal and high anion gap metabolic acidosis; a ratio of 0.8 to 2.0 indicates a pure high anion gap metabolic acidosis; and a ratio greater than 2 indicates a mixed high anion gap metabolic acidosis and a metabolic alkalosis.

Management
This will depend on the specific entity identified. All patients should be admitted and observed. Consider referral to an internist.

64

Infertility

MCC particular objectives
Diagnose the cause and complications.

Explain therapeutic options.

MCC differential diagnosis
with added evidence

FEMALE

Ovulatory dysfunction (e.g., hypogonadotropic hypogonadism, polycystic ovary syndrome)
HYPOGONADOTROPIC HYPOGONADISM
Signs and symptoms: abnormal puberty; low libido and sexual function; absence or delay of normal Tanner stage for age

History of primary congenital syndrome (e.g., Kallmann syndrome, gonadotropin-releasing hormone sensitivity); secondary acquired syndrome (e.g., tumour; trauma; use of medications such as opioids, gonadotropin-releasing hormone analogs, gonadal analogs, glucocorticoids)

Investigations: decreased FSH; decreased LH; decreased estrogen; thyrotropin (TSH) (elevated in prolactinoma); prolactin (elevated in prolactinoma); decreased serum progesterone 1 week before expected onset of menstruation

POLYCYSTIC OVARY SYNDROME

Signs and symptoms: symptom onset after puberty, with increased rate of hair growth and male-pattern hair growth; irregular menstruation; infertility; obesity; acne

Investigations: LH:FSH ratio (elevated: 2:1 or 3:1) (usual); elevated testosterone; ultrasound to detect ovarian cysts; normal prolactin levels; normal thyroid function

Tubal and peritoneal abnormalities (e.g., pelvic inflammatory disease)

PELVIC INFLAMMATORY DISEASE

Signs and symptoms: lower abdominal and pelvic pain; pain during intercourse; fever; urinary symptoms; vaginal discharge; irregular menstruation; pelvic tenderness and pain associated with 1 or both adnexa

> History of gonorrhea, chlamydia, or risk factors for them (multiple partners, unprotected sex); intrauterine device (IUD); childbirth; gynecologic procedure

Investigations: cultures for gonorrhea and chlamydia; ultrasound (this has normal findings); hysterosalpingography to detect tubal abnormalities

Uterine and cervical factors (e.g., fibroids)

FIBROID (LEIOMYOMA)

Signs and symptoms: commonly asymptomatic; premenopausal (usual); heavy or prolonged menstrual bleeding; pelvic, abdominal pressure; painful intercourse; urinary symptoms (incontinence; frequent urination; difficulty emptying the bladder); constipation; pelvic mass or enlarged, irregular uterus on bimanual palpation

Risk factors: family history of leiomyoma; African descent

Investigations: ultrasound to detect mass ≥ 1 cm in diameter

MALE

Testicular dysfunction (e.g., hypogonadotropic hypogonadism, viral orchitis)

Signs and symptoms (in general): loss of libido, fever, testicular pain

> History of medications (e.g., chemotherapy, anabolic steroids), chromosomal abnormality (e.g., Klinefelter syndrome), trauma, mumps, malaria, neoplasm, radiation, testicular surgery

Investigations: semen analysis (decreased quantity or quality of semen); abnormal FSH (elevated in primary hypogonadism, decreased in secondary hypogonadism); decreased serum testosterone; pelvic ultrasound to detect mass

Strategy for patient encounter

The likely scenario is a couple who are unable to conceive. The specified tasks could engage history, physical exam, investigations, or management.

History

Infertility is usually described as inability to conceive after 1 year of regular intercourse without contraception (6 months for women older than 35 years).

Ask if the woman has ever become pregnant and if the man has ever fathered a child. Use open-ended questions about the frequency and timing of intercourse: How often do you have sex? When do you have sex in terms of the menstrual cycle?

Use open-ended questions about the timing and regularity of the woman's menstrual cycles: How often do you menstruate? How regular is your cycle? Ask about a history of endometriosis, pelvic infections, and ectopic pregnancies.

Ask the man about a history of chemotherapy or radiation, testicular surgery or trauma, anabolic steroid use, chromosomal abnormalities, mumps, and malaria.

Physical exam

Examine the man for testicular abnormalities. Perform a pelvic exam on the woman, looking for masses and tenderness.

(State that you will perform these exams. Since these exams are not performed on standardized patients, the examiner will likely interrupt you, ask what you are looking for, and provide findings.)

Investigations

An important first step is to determine if the problem is with the man, woman, or both. For every man, order a semen analysis. For every woman, order a serum progesterone test at cycle day 21 (or 7 days before expected menstruation if the cycle is not 28 days) to confirm ovulation, and order tests for serum prolactin and thyrotropin (TSH). Evaluation of anatomic abnormalities of the female reproductive tract may be done via a hysterosalpingography in previously healthy women, or by a hysteroscopy or laparoscopy in women with a history of endometriosis, pelvic infections, or ectopic pregnancy.

Management

Sperm abnormalities may be treated with gonadotropin therapy, intrauterine insemination, or in vitro fertilization. Anovulation may be treated with aromatase inhibitors. In cases of polycystic ovary syndrome or obesity, the first line of treatment is weight loss (with or without metformin in polycystic ovary syndrome). Consider referral to a fertility clinic or to a gynecologist for treatment of female reproductive tract obstruction. Consider referral for intrauterine insemination or in vitro fertilization.

Pearls

Remember to counsel all women contemplating pregnancy on the preconceptual use of folic acid and the need for up-to-date immunizations.

65

Fecal incontinence

MCC particular objective

Recognize that incontinence may be multifactorial (e.g., patients may have a disease that affects mobility or cognition, which leads to incontinence in cases of fecal urgency or diarrhea; or they may have a defect in the pelvic floor that is overwhelmed by diarrhea).

MCC differential diagnosis
with added evidence

PELVIC FLOOR INTACT

Neurologic conditions

Causes include diabetes, multiple sclerosis, amyotrophic lateral sclerosis, spinal cord injury, acute brain injury, stroke, spina bifida, peripheral neuropathy, Parkinson disease, Huntington disease, Alzheimer disease, and dementia.

Overflow (e.g., impaction)

Causes include physical inactivity, malnutrition (especially lack of fibre), not drinking enough water, medications (opioids, sedatives, iron supplements), gastrointestinal disorders (e.g., irritable bowel syndrome), neurological disorders, diabetes, autoimmune diseases (amyloidosis, celiac disease, systemic lupus erythematosus, scleroderma), hypothyroidism, spinal cord injury, and pelvic or colorectal surgery.

Signs and symptoms: chronic constipation; abdominal pain, bloating; leaking of liquid stool; nausea, vomiting; headache; weight loss; loss of appetite; necrosis and ulcers of rectal tissue

>   Severe: rapid heart rate, hyperventilation, dehydration, fever, confusion, agitation

PELVIC FLOOR AFFECTED

Acquired condition (e.g., traumatic birth)

TRAUMATIC BIRTH

The most common cause is obstetric anal sphincter injury.

It is underreported: it could occur in up to 25% of women following vaginal birth.

Signs and symptoms: history of forceps delivery and/or third and fourth degree perineal tears

Congenital

HIRSCHSPRUNG DISEASE

This is caused by nerves in the colon that do not fully develop.

The condition is usually diagnosed in neonates (rarely in adults).

Risk factors: family history of Hirschsprung disease; other congenital conditions (e.g., Down syndrome, congenital heart disease)

Strategy for patient encounter

The likely scenario is an adult with recent-onset fecal incontinence. The specified tasks could engage history, physical exam, investigations, or management.

Given the MCC's particular objective for this clinical presentation, stay alert for evidence that several disorders are contributing to the patient's fecal incontinence (e.g., gastrointestinal infection together with cognitive impairment).

History

Use open-ended questions to obtain a history of the incontinence and a medical history: When did the incontinence start? What makes it better or worse? What symptoms go with it? What conditions have you been diagnosed with? Listen for recent-on-set versus chronic incontinence (recent onset suggests a new problem contributing to an underlying problem); incontinence made better or worse with diet or exercise (this suggests overflow incontinence); gastrointestinal symptoms such as diarrhea, constipation, gas, or bloating (these suggest overflow incontinence, or a gastrointestinal infection contributing to an underlying problem); and relevant comorbid conditions (e.g., ulcerative colitis, Crohn disease, diabetes, multiple sclerosis, chronic constipation, Alzheimer disease). Ask about the patient's mobility: Are you able to get to the toilet quickly when you need to? Ask about a history of radiation therapy to the pelvic area.

In women, ask about a history of traumatic childbirth involving forceps or episiotomy.

Physical exam

Perform a digital rectal exam to evaluate sphincter strength, detect any rectal abnormalities, and evaluate for the presence of stool in the rectum. Ask the patient to bear down and observe for rectal prolapse.

(State that you will perform these exams. Since these exams are not performed on standardized patients, the examiner will likely interrupt, ask what you are looking for, and provide findings.)

Investigations

Refer the patient for anal manometry to measure the strength of the anal sphincter and the functioning of the rectum. Refer the patient for colonoscopy or sigmoidoscopy to look for abnormalities of the colon. Consider an MRI to assess the anatomy of the anal sphincter.

Management

Kegel exercises, biofeedback, and maintenance of a regular defecation schedule may help reduce incontinence. Manage constipation by increasing exercise, fibre, and fluids; consider bulk laxatives (methylcellulose or psyllium). For diarrhea, consider treatment with loperamide hydrochloride, or diphenoxylate hydrochloride and atropine sulfate. Consider referring the patient to a gastroenterologist. Refer patients with rectal prolapse or damaged anal sphincters to a surgeon.

66

Incontinence, urine, adult

MCC particular objective

Address the 2 most common causes: stress and urgency.

MCC differential diagnosis
with added evidence

TRANSIENT CONDITION

Polyuria

Signs and symptoms: history of uncontrolled diabetes mellitus (this is the most common cause), primary polydipsia, central diabetes insipidus (DI), and/or nephrogenic DI

Investigations: water restriction test; plasma sodium concentration; urine osmolality (except in suspected nephrogenic DI)

> Urine output > 3 L/day in adults
>
> Urine osmolality < 250 mmol/kg

Drugs, alcohol

Examples include alcohol, caffeine, and loop diuretics (these increase urine production); antidepressants, antihistamines, and calcium channel blockers (these interfere with bladder contraction, which can lead to overflow incontinence); and antipsychotics and sedatives (these slow mobility and increase the urge to urinate).

NEUROLOGIC CONDITION (E.G., CAUDA EQUINA SYNDROME)

CAUDA EQUINA SYNDROME

This occurs when the spinal cord is compressed in the lumbar spine.

Common causes include herniated disk, spinal stenosis, infection, and trauma.

Signs and symptoms: leg pain, numbness, weakness; urinary symptoms (incontinence, retention, frequent urination); fecal incontinence; loss of rectal tone; abnormal bulbocavernosus and anal wink reflexes; erectile dysfunction; decreased muscle tone and deep tendon reflexes in the legs; saddle anesthesia (loss of sensation in the inner thighs, back of the legs, around the rectum)

Investigations: X-ray, CT scan, MRI, myelography

ANATOMIC CONDITION

Stress incontinence

Signs and symptoms: female, aged 45 or older (more common); no bladder contractions during episodes of incontinence; incontinence during coughing, sneezing, running, heavy lifting, laughing, standing up, exercise, sexual intercourse

Risk factors: childbirth, especially vaginal deliveries; obesity; illnesses that cause sneezing or coughing; smoking (coughing); use of alcohol or caffeine; hormonal deficiency or hormone replacement therapy; hysterectomy; prostatectomy

Urgency incontinence (e.g., cystitis)

CYSTITIS

Signs and symptoms: bladder contractions during episodes; increased frequency of urination; painful urination; pelvic pain and/or flank pain; fever; tenderness over the bladder

Investigations: urinalysis, urine culture

Overflow incontinence (e.g., prostate enlargement, multiple sclerosis)

ENLARGED PROSTATE

Signs and symptoms: older male; urinary frequency, urgency, hesitancy, intermittency; nocturia; dribbling, incomplete bladder emptying; bladder distention (sometimes); nontender, enlarged prostate with rubbery consistency and lack of median furrow on digital rectal exam

Investigations: transrectal ultrasound of the prostate; PSA blood test

MULTIPLE SCLEROSIS

Signs and symptoms: variable depending on lesion location

Spinal cord: sensory or motor dysfunction; Lhermitte sign (paresthesias radiating down the extremities or trunk with neck flexion); bowel, bladder or erectile dysfunction

Brainstem: double vision; swallowing, speech difficulties; vertigo; pseudobulbar palsy

Cerebrum: cognitive impairment; depression; upper motor neuron signs; unilateral motor or sensory deficits

Cerebellum: problems with balance and coordination; vertigo

Other symptoms: tonic spasms; fatigue; pain; exercise intolerance; temperature sensitivity; painful unilateral loss of visual acuity

Risk factors: younger than 50, female

Investigations: brain and spinal cord MRI, including advanced MRI techniques, with established occurrence of multiple episodes; CSF fluid analysis

Strategy for patient encounter

The likely scenario is an elderly woman with stress incontinence. The specified tasks could engage history, physical exam, investigations, or management.

History

Use open-ended questions to obtain a medical, surgical, and obstetric history: What conditions have you been diagnosed with? What surgeries have you had? How many children do you have? What was the method of delivery? Listen for diabetes, disorders in the lumbar spine, and multiple sclerosis; surgeries on the lumbar spine; and multiple vaginal deliveries.

Ask the patient about circumstances associated with incontinence, looking for evidence to separate stress from urge incontinence, and to identify comorbid conditions (e.g., neurologic symptoms in cauda equina). Consider asking the patient to complete a voiding diary at home. Take a medication history and ask about alcohol use.

Physical exam

Perform pelvic, rectal, and neurological exams. Perform a cough stress test by asking the patient to stand with a full bladder. Ask the patient to cough and observe for leakage of urine. Perform a cotton swab test to look for bladder hypermobility (see the checklist). In males, perform a prostate exam.

(State that you will perform these exams and tests. Since these exams and tests are not performed on standardized patients, the examiner will likely interrupt you, ask what you are looking for, and provide findings.)

Investigations

Order a urinalysis and culture to look for infection and hematuria. If hematuria is present, order urine cytology. Order a test for serum

> **CHECKLIST**
> ## Cotton swab test for bladder hypermotility
> Insert an anesthetic-lubricated swab into either the urethra or vagina (the vagina is better tolerated).
>
> Ask the patient to perform a Valsalva maneuver (this involves the action of exhaling, but with the mouth closed and nose pinched shut, which increases pressure in the chest and abdomen).
>
> Hypermobility (weak pelvic floor and urethral connective tissue) is demonstrated by a deviation of > 30° from horizontal during straining or a change in angle of > 30° during straining.

creatinine to assess renal function, and a fasting glucose or gly-cated hemoglobin (HbA_{1c}) test to rule out diabetes. Order a pros-tate-specific antigen (PSA) test in men. Order an ultrasound to measure postvoid residual urine (normal is < 50 mL), and eval-uate for hydronephrosis, hydroureter, and urinary tract stones. Consider urodynamic testing in patients with an unclear etiol-ogy. Refer women to urology or gynecology for consideration of surgery or insertion of a pessary.

Management

Several behavioural techniques can be useful for incontinence, including bladder training (delaying urination when the urge is felt), double voiding (urinating, then going again a few minutes later), scheduling toilet trips every 2 to 4 hours, weight loss, Kegel exercises, and reduced fluid intake. If these are ineffective, con-sider medications (anticholinergics, Mirabegron, alpha-blockers, or topical estrogen for women). Consider referral to an inconti-nence program, or to a urologist (men) or gynecologist (women) for surgical options.

67

Incontinence, urine, pediatric (enuresis)

MCC particular objective

Determine whether a physical abnormality is causing inconti-nence in a child aged 5 years or older.

MCC differential diagnosis
with added evidence

PRIMARY ENURESIS (E.G., FAMILY HISTORY)

This is bedwetting that occurs during sleep in children 5 years or older. It is the most common type of enuresis.

Signs and symptoms: family history of nocturnal enuresis

Common contributing factors: nocturnal polyuria, detrusor overactivity, disturbed sleep

SECONDARY ENURESIS (E.G., URINARY TRACT INFECTION, VESICOURETERAL REFLUX)

URINARY TRACT INFECTION

Signs and symptoms: frequent urination; painful urination; pelvic pain and/or flank pain; fever; tenderness over the bladder

Investigations: urinalysis, urine culture

VESICOURETERAL REFLUX

The most common form (primary vesicoureteral reflux) resolves spontaneously as the child grows.

Signs and symptoms:

> Prenatal: fetal hydronephrosis on prenatal ultrasound
>
> Postnatal: recent urinary tract infection (this has a higher risk of vesicoureteral reflux if accompanied by fever)

Risk factors: family history, male (prenatal vesicoureteral reflux), female (postnatal vesicoureteral reflux), Caucasian descent

Investigations: contrast voiding cystourethrogram or radionuclide cystogram

Strategy for patient encounter

This encounter will likely involve a parent discussing a child who has nocturnal enuresis. The child will be absent on some pretext (e.g., a nurse is taking the child's vital signs and weight in another room). The specified tasks could engage history, physical exam, investigations, or management.

History

Take a thorough history of the enuresis: When did it start? A key question is whether the child has never had nighttime bladder control (which indicates primary nocturnal enuresis) or has lost nighttime bladder control (which indicates secondary nocturnal enuresis). Ask about a family history of enuresis. Ask about coexisting symptoms, and listen for evidence consistent with urinary tract infection (e.g., fever, painful urination). Take a psychosocial history, specifically looking for new or significant social stressors.

Physical exam

Perform a physical exam including palpation of the abdomen for tenderness and masses, and examination of the genitals for rashes and physical abnormalities.

(State that you will perform these exams. Because an actual pediatric patient is unlikely, the examiner may interrupt, ask what you are looking for, and provide findings.)

Investigations

In patients with a reassuring history and physical exam, investigations may not be necessary. Consider ordering a urinalysis and urine culture to rule out urinary tract infection.

Management

Maintenance of the child's self-esteem is paramount. For primary nocturnal enuresis, educate and reassure the parents. Treatment should only be considered when enuresis poses a significant problem for the child. Behavioural modifications include avoidance of caffeine-containing foods and excessive fluids before bedtime, waking the child at night to urinate, and having the child urinate before bedtime. Treatment with alarm devices may be useful, especially in older children. Desmopressin acetate may also be useful, especially on an as-needed basis for sleepovers and camps.

68

Erectile dysfunction

MCC particular objectives

None stated.

MCC differential diagnosis
with added evidence

ERECTILE DYSFUNCTION IN GENERAL

Definition: inability for ≥ 3 months to have or maintain an erection adequate for intercourse

NEUROLOGIC CONDITION (E.G., DIABETES MELLITUS)

DIABETES

Signs and symptoms: personal or family history of diabetes; history of diabetic complications and/or inadequate monitoring; polydipsia, polyuria, and/or weight loss

Investigations: fasting glucose or HbA_{1c} test

CARDIOVASCULAR DISORDER

Signs and symptoms: history of atherosclerosis, hyperlipidemia, hypertension, venoocclusive dysfunction

PHARMACOLOGIC-CAUSED DISORDER (E.G., ALCOHOL)

DRUGS

These include antidepressants and other psychiatric medications; antihistamines; antihypertensives; diuretics, beta-blockers; medications for Parkinson disease; chemotherapy medications; opiate analgesics; and recreational drugs (alcohol, amphetamines, barbiturates, cocaine, marijuana, methadone, nicotine, opiates).

HORMONAL DISORDER (E.G., TESTOSTERONE DEFICIENCY)

TESTOSTERONE DEFICIENCY

This is reversible with testosterone treatment.

Signs and symptoms: older age (more common), poor morning erection, decreased sexual libido

> Other symptoms: irritability; mood changes; fatigue; decreased muscle bulk and strength; decline in cognitive function; hot flashes

Investigations: serum testosterone concentration < 8 nmol/L

PSYCHOLOGICAL OR EMOTIONAL CONDITION (E.G., PERFORMANCE ANXIETY)

PSYCHOLOGICAL CONDITION IN GENERAL

Signs and symptoms: personal or family history of psychiatric conditions (e.g., anxiety, major depressive disorder); excessive worry; loss of interest in friends and usual activities; changes in sleep habits; hallucinations or delusions; suicidal thoughts; history of adverse experience (emotional, physical, or sexual abuse; recent stress such as death of a friend or family member), or substance abuse

PERFORMANCE ANXIETY

Signs and symptoms: maintenance of erections during masturbation or sleep; inability to maintain erections during intercourse

Strategy for patient encounter

The likely scenario is a middle-aged man with erectile dysfunction. The specified tasks could engage history, physical exam, investigations, or management.

History

Take a sexual history: Do you have a new sexual partner? How often are you sexually active? When did the erectile dysfunction begin? Does it happen every time you have sex? Do you have nighttime erections?

Use open-ended questions to obtain a medical and medication history: What conditions have you been diagnosed with? What medications do you take? Listen for heart disease, diabetes, peripheral vascular disease, and hypertension; and hypertension medications, antihistamines, sedatives, and antidepressants. Ask about smoking and alcohol use.

Physical exam

Take the patient's blood pressure, and document his body mass index (BMI). Perform penile, testicular, and digital rectal exams.

(State that you will perform these exams. Since these exams are not performed on standardized patients, the examiner will likely interrupt, ask what you are looking for, and provide findings. State that you are looking for abnormalities such as masses, tenderness, hypogonadism, and testicular atrophy.)

> **TIP**
>
> **Tailoring information to individual patients**
>
> The MCC identifies providing generic information as a common exam error.
>
> To avoid this error, ask patients about aspects of their lives that might affect their condition. Provide information that targets their situation and engage the patient in figuring out next steps.
>
> For example, diet and exercise changes, and smoking cessation, might be relevant for this case:
>
> - Ask what the patient ate yesterday for breakfast, lunch, and supper. Use this to personalize guidelines on dietary changes they need to make.
> - Ask what the patient did for exercise last week. Discuss short-term goals with the patient: What could the patient do next week to exercise every day? (For example, when could the patient fit in a 30-minute walk?)
> - In a patient who smokes, express your concern with their continued smoking. Ask what experience they have had with methods to quit. Provide information about other methods, as appropriate. Ask if there is a method they would like to pursue now, and describe the support you can offer them.

Investigations

There is no diagnostic test for erectile dysfunction. Testing is directed toward identifying comorbidities: order a test for morning serum testosterone, a fasting blood glucose or HbA_{1c} test, a lipid panel, and a test for thyrotropin (TSH).

Management

If applicable, counsel the patient on lifestyle changes (weight loss, exercise, smoking cessation). Optimize diabetes management. Consider stopping or substituting contributing medications. Inhibitors of phosphodiesterase type V are the first-line treatment. The primary contraindication is concurrent treatment with nitrates. Second-line therapy is intraurethral or intracavernosal alprostadil and vacuum pump devices.

Pearls

Erectile dysfunction is very common, affecting a third of men over their lifetimes.

69

Jaundice

MCC particular objective

Identify life-threatening conditions.

MCC differential diagnosis
with added evidence

UNCONJUGATED HYPERBILIRUBINEMIA (PREHEPATIC)

Overproduction (e.g., hemolysis)

HEMOLYTIC ANEMIA

Signs and symptoms: fatigue, shortness of breath, decreased exercise tolerance, dark urine

Severe: jaundice

Investigations: peripheral blood smear to detect schistocytes, spherocytes, and/or bite cells; blood tests (hemoglobin, WBCs, platelet count, RBCs, mean corpuscular volume, hematocrit, bilirubin, lactate dehydrogenase, haptoglobin, reticulocyte indices)

Decreased hepatic uptake (e.g., congestive heart failure)

CONGESTIVE HEART FAILURE

Signs and symptoms: history of heart disease (or risk factors for heart disease: diabetes, hypertension, hyperlipidemia, and smoking) or hepatic vein thrombosis (Budd-Chiari syndrome); severe shortness of breath; elevated jugular venous pressure; edema in the abdomen and legs; pink phlegm; heart murmurs and extra cardiac sounds

Investigations: chest X-ray to detect pulmonary edema; NT-proBNP level; echocardiogram to distinguish forms of heart failure; cardiac stress testing, either with exercise or pharmacological agent

Decreased bilirubin conjugation (e.g., Gilbert syndrome)

GILBERT SYNDROME

This inherited disorder does not impair health and requires no treatment.

Signs and symptoms: usually asymptomatic, jaundice

> Triggers for jaundice in Gilbert syndrome: current illness (e.g., flu, cold) or menstruation; recent fasting; certain medications (e.g., acetaminophen, irinotecan)

Risk factors: family history of Gilbert syndrome (to inherit the disorder, both parents must carry the gene)

Investigations: elevated unconjugated bilirubin, normal CBC

CONJUGATED HYPERBILIRUBINEMIA (HEPATIC)

Intrahepatic cholestasis (e.g., drugs, cirrhosis)

DRUGS

These include antibiotics (e.g., penicillin, tetracycline, amoxicillin-clavulanate, macrolide), anabolic steroids, estrogen (e.g., estradiol), chlorpromazine, cimetidine, imipramine, prochlorperazine, terbinafine, and tolbutamide.

CIRRHOSIS

Signs and symptoms: jaundice; easy bruising, bleeding; itching; ascites; spiderlike blood vessels on the skin; systemic symptoms (anorexia, weight loss, weakness, fatigue)

> History of chronic alcohol abuse; chronic viral hepatitis B (HBV) or hepatitis C (HCV), or risk factors for them (unprotected sex, intravenous drug abuse, blood

transfusions, tattoos, body piercings, imprisonment, workplace exposure to body fluids); hemochromatosis; nonalcoholic fatty liver disease

Investigations: liver function tests

Extrahepatic cholestasis (e.g., cholelithiasis)

CHOLELITHIASIS (GALLSTONES)

Symptoms: right upper quadrant abdominal pain, under the ribs; pain that prevents normal or deep breathing; Murphy sign (while palpating near the gallbladder, severe pain on taking a breath); vomiting

> Pain characteristics: 15 minutes to 24 hours in duration; radiating to the right upper back or shoulder blade; no relief with moving or changing position; onset at night, on waking, or after eating
>
> Symptoms of bile duct blocked by gallstone: jaundice, dark urine, light-coloured stools, fever, chills

Risk factors: high body mass index (BMI) or obesity; high-fat diet; diabetes; older than 60; estrogen medications; family history of gallstones; female

Investigations: ultrasound, abdominal X-ray, CT scan, hepatobiliary scan, MRCP, ERCP

Hepatocellular injury (e.g., sepsis, hypoperfusion)

SEPSIS

Definition: infection with systemic inflammatory response, dysfunction of ≥ 1 organ system

Signs and symptoms: fever or hypothermia; tachycardia; tachypnea; infection (most common: pneumonia, abdominal infection, kidney infection, bacteremia)

> Severe: oliguria; mental status changes; shortness of breath; extreme hypotension, unresponsive to fluid replacement (this indicates septic shock)

Risk factors: very young or very old; compromised immune system; wounds, burns; catheterization, intubation

Investigations: CBC with differential; cultures (blood, CSF, urine) to detect causative organism; ABG to detect acidosis; elevated creatinine; chest X-ray to detect pulmonary edema

HYPOPERFUSION (ISCHEMIC HEPATITIS)

Signs and symptoms: weakness, fatigue, mental confusion, low urine production, jaundice, loss of liver function (rare and transient)

Investigations: AST, ALT (both > 1000 U/L); ALP; GGT; bilirubin (direct, total, indirect); albumin; PT/INR

Other (e.g., infiltrative states, fatty liver)

INFILTRATIVE STATES

Examples of causes include hepatocellular carcinoma, sarcoidosis, pancreatic cancer, cholangiocarcinoma, and lymphoma.

Signs and symptoms: nausea, abdominal pain, anorexia, malaise, fever, chills, jaundice, dark urine, light stools, pruritus

> Malignancy: recent weight loss

Investigations: liver function tests, MRI, biopsy

> AST, ALT: normal or mildly elevated (30–40 U/L, < 300 U/L); AST:ALT ratio < 1
>
> ALP: > 4 times upper normal limit
>
> Conjugated hyperbilirubinemia: direct bilirubin fraction > 20%

NONALCOHOLIC FATTY LIVER DISEASE

This is the most common form of chronic liver disease.

Signs and symptoms: usually asymptomatic, fatigue, right upper quadrant abdominal pain, enlarged liver, muscle weakness

> More severe: jaundice, gynecomastia, enlarged spleen, red palms

Risk factors: high cholesterol; high serum triglycerides; obesity; type 2 diabetes; metabolic syndrome; polycystic ovary syndrome; hypothyroidism; hypopituitarism; recent weight gain or loss

Investigations: blood tests (CBC, liver enzymes, lipid profile); abdominal ultrasound, CT scan, MRI; transient elastography

Strategy for patient encounter

The likely scenario is an adult patient with jaundice and right upper abdominal pain. The specified tasks could engage history, physical exam, investigations, or management.

History

Use open-ended questions to establish onset and related symptoms: When did the jaundice start? What other symptoms do you have? Listen for evidence consistent with particular entities (e.g., shortness of breath in hemolytic anemia and congestive heart failure; right upper quadrant abdominal pain in cholelithiasis and fatty liver disease). Specifically ask about systemic symptoms that may indicate the presence of malignancy or infection (fever, weight loss, fatigue, night sweats). Ask about risk factors for infectious hepatitis (unprotected sex, intravenous drug abuse, blood transfusions, tattoos, body piercings, imprisonment, workplace exposure to body fluids), and about possible occupational exposures to toxic substances. Ask about a history of gall bladder disease.

Use open-ended questions to take a medication and alcohol-use history: What medications do you take? How many alcoholic drinks do you have in a week? Listen for hepatotoxic drugs and alcohol abuse.

Physical exam

Obtain the patient's vital signs, looking for fever. Examine the skin for jaundice and the sclera for icterus. Examine the abdomen for masses and tenderness, and the extremities for edema (edema suggests congestive heart failure). Auscultate the heart for murmurs, and the lungs for rales.

Investigations

Order tests for total and direct bilirubin levels to distinguish conjugated (direct) from unconjugated (indirect) hyperbilirubinemia. A direct bilirubin level of ≥ 10 μmol/L, with an elevated total bilirubin level, indicates conjugated hyperbilirubinemia. For all patients, order a complete blood count (CBC) (this is relevant for hemolysis); tests for aspartate aminotransferase (AST) and alanine aminotransferase (ALT); and serologic tests for infectious hepatitis, including hepatitis C (HCV) antibody, hepatitis B surface antigen (HBsAg), anti–hepatitis B core antibody (anti-HBcAb), HIV antibodies, and heterophile antibody (Monospot test). Order a test for serum lipase to rule out pancreatic disease and/ or obstruction. In suspected biliary obstruction, order tests for alkaline phosphatase (ALP) and γ-glutamyltransferase (GGT).

If a diagnosis is not made, consider more specialized studies, including blood alcohol level, acetaminophen level, iron studies, antimitochondrial antibody, ceruloplasmin level, and antinuclear antibodies (ANA). Order a liver ultrasound to exclude biliary obstruction and to look for fatty liver, tumour, and cirrhosis. In cases of tumour, cirrhosis, or biliary atresia, refer the patient for liver biopsy.

Management

Management depends on the specific diagnosis. Remove any offending medications or drugs. In mechanical obstruction or tumour, refer the patient to surgery. In hemolysis, refer the patient to hematology. If indicated, consider referral to a hepatologist for diagnosis and treatment.

70

Neonatal jaundice

MCC particular objective
Pay particular attention to jaundice within the first 3 days of birth or that has rapid onset.

MCC differential diagnosis
with added evidence

UNCONJUGATED HYPERBILIRUBINEMIA

Increased bilirubin production

HEMOLYTIC CAUSE
This is sometimes diagnosed and treated before birth.

Signs and symptoms: jaundice that develops quickly after birth; Rh-negative mother and Rh-positive baby

Investigations: direct antibody test of cord blood (Coombs test) and blood type if the mother is Rh-negative; serum bilirubin; transcutaneous bilirubin; bilirubin:albumin (B:A) ratio; total and conjugated bilirubin

Decreased bilirubin conjugation

METABOLIC OR GENETIC CAUSE (E.G., GILBERT SYNDROME, HYPOTHYROIDISM)

GILBERT SYNDROME
This inherited disorder does not impair health and requires no treatment.

Signs and symptoms: usually asymptomatic, jaundice

> Triggers for jaundice in Gilbert syndrome: current illness (e.g., flu, cold), recent fasting, certain medications (e.g., acetaminophen, irinotecan)

Risk factors: family history of Gilbert syndrome (to inherit the disorder, both parents must carry the gene)

Investigations: elevated unconjugated bilirubin, normal CBC

HYPOTHYROIDISM

Signs and symptoms: history of hypothyroidism or symptoms of hypothyroidism (decreased reflexes, dry skin)

Investigations: elevated thyrotropin (TSH)

PHYSIOLOGIC CAUSE (E.G., BREAST MILK JAUNDICE)

JAUNDICE ASSOCIATED WITH BREAST-FEEDING IN GENERAL

Two types of neonatal jaundice are associated with breast-feeding: breast-feeding jaundice and breast milk jaundice.

Breast-feeding jaundice is very common, and develops during the period after birth when breast-feeding is becoming established. It is due to inadequate milk intake (because mother's milk is not established, or baby's latch is not established), which leads to jaundice through dehydration and delayed passage of meconium.

Breast milk jaundice generally occurs later (e.g., second week of life) and persists longer (e.g., 3 to 6 weeks). It is generally a diagnosis of exclusion.

Gastrointestinal (e.g., sequestered blood)

Examples of causes include anal fissure (most common); esophageal, gastric, or duodenal erosions; and stress gastritis.

Signs and symptoms: blood in the stool (bright red, dark red, black); blood in vomit; maternal use of acetylsalicylic acid (ASA), cephalothin, phenobarbital during pregnancy; prematurity; history of neonatal distress, mechanical ventilation

CONJUGATED HYPERBILIRUBINEMIA

Decreased bilirubin uptake

INFECTION (E.G., SEPSIS, NEONATAL HEPATITIS)

NEONATAL SEPSIS

Definition: infection with systemic inflammatory response, dysfunction of ≥ 1 organ system

Infection usually occurs by vertical transmission. Examples include group B streptococci, *Escherichia coli*, *Staphylococcus aureus*, *Listeria monocytogenes*, *Streptococcus viridans*, *Haemophilus influenzae*, Cytomegalovirus, respiratory syncytial virus, human metapneumovirus, parainfluenza virus, human coronavirus, herpes simplex virus (HSV), HIV, *Candida albicans*, *Candida parapsilosis*, and *Aspergillus*.

Signs and symptoms: fever, tachycardia, tachypnea, poor muscle tone, poor feeding, vomiting, jaundice, abdominal distention, poor perfusion

Severe: oliguria; mental status changes; shortness of breath; extreme hypotension, unresponsive to fluid replacement (this indicates septic shock)

Risk factors: compromised immune system; wounds, burns; catheterization, intubation

Maternal factors: chorioamnionitis (intrauterine onset of infection); intrapartum maternal temperature $\geq 38°$ C; < 37 weeks gestation; membrane rupture > 18 hours before delivery

Investigations: CBC with differential (elevated neutrophils is a common finding); CRP; blood culture; cultures of other fluids (CSF, urine)

NEONATAL HEPATITIS

Note that neonates are generally asymptomatic: symptoms generally appear 1 to 2 months after birth.

Signs and symptoms: maternal history of viral hepatitis, Cytomegalovirus, rubella; jaundice; enlarged liver and spleen; poor weight gain and growth

CHOLESTASIS (E.G., TOTAL PARENTERAL NUTRITION)

PARENTERAL NUTRITION–ASSOCIATED CHOLESTASIS

This is usually associated with long-term parenteral nutrition. It is chronic and irreversible, and leads to liver failure.

Signs and symptoms: poor feeding; vomiting; diarrhea; lethargy, hypotonia; symptoms of advanced liver failure (e.g., tarry or bloody stools; bleeding from the umbilical stump; bruising or purpura); hepatomegaly, possible splenomegaly, or ascites

Investigations: elevated direct/conjugated bilirubin (either > 20% of total serum bilirubin or at minimum > 17.1 μmol/L); abdominal ultrasound; liver biopsy

Other tests for liver enzymes and liver function: AST, ALT, ALP, PT/INR, PTT, albumin, glucose, ammonia

METABOLIC CAUSE

GALACTOSEMIA, HEREDITARY FRUCTOSE INTOLERANCE, GLYCOGEN STORAGE DISEASES

Signs and symptoms: hypoglycemia, lethargy, vomiting, failure to thrive, diarrhea, jaundice, renal insufficiency

NIEMANN-PICK DISEASE, GAUCHER DISEASE, TYROSINEMIA

Signs and symptoms: hepatomegaly, splenomegaly, central nervous system dysfunction

Gaucher disease: bruising, anemia, low platelet count

$α_1$-ANTITRYPSIN DEFICIENCY

Signs and symptoms: liver symptoms with asthma-like symptoms (shortness of breath, wheezing, rhonchi, rales)

Investigations: newborn screening (enzyme function tests, DNA analysis); enzyme tests from blood or liver biopsy

GENETIC CAUSE

DUBIN-JOHNSON AND ROTOR SYNDROMES

These are generally benign disorders showing mild, nonitching jaundice with elevated conjugated bilirubin.

Obstructive cause (e.g., biliary atresia)

BILIARY ATRESIA

This is a rare disease of the bile ducts that occurs in infants.

Signs and symptoms: jaundice that develops 2 to 3 weeks after birth; dark urine; light stools; full term baby; low birth weight (often)

> Associated disorders (10% to 15% of cases): cardiac anomalies (murmurs), polysplenia, blood vessel abnormalities (inferior vena cava, preduodenal portal vein), intestine abnormalities (situs inversus or malrotation)

> Investigations: blood tests for liver function, liver biopsy

Strategy for patient encounter

The likely scenario is a parent concerned about a newborn with high bilirubin 2 days after birth (an actual newborn patient is unlikely). The newborn will be absent on some pretext (e.g., a nurse is taking the infant's vital signs and weight in another room). The specified tasks could engage history, physical exam, investigations, or management.

History

Use open-ended questions to obtain a general history and an obstetrical history.

- **General history:** How often does your baby have a wet diaper? What are your baby's stools like? What medical conditions run in the family? Listen for evidence of dehydration (this suggests infrequent feeding); tarry or bloody stools (this suggests a gastrointestinal cause); and a family history of Gilbert syndrome, Dubin-Johnson syndrome, and Rotor syndrome. Ask if the baby is breastfed and how often. Ask about risk factors for neonatal jaundice (see the checklist).

CHECKLIST

Risk factors for neonatal hyperbilirubinemia

High-risk bilirubin level

Jaundice < 24 hours after delivery or while still in hospital

ABO incompatibility and positive Coombs test

Glucose-6-phosphate dehydrogenase (G6PD) deficiency

Premature delivery (< 36 weeks gestation)

History of sibling jaundice or phototherapy

Significant neonatal bruising

Exclusively breastfed

East Asian descent

- **Obstetrical history:** What complications did you have during this pregnancy? What complications were there during the delivery? Listen for evidence of neonatal distress and risk factors for infection (e.g., premature birth, intrapartum maternal fever, early membrane rupture in labour). Ask about the infant's birth weight.

Physical exam

Examine the neonate for jaundice, scleral icterus, and bruising. Take the infant's weight and compare this to the infant's birth weight (a loss of more than 10% of birth weight suggests inadequate milk intake).

(State that you will perform a physical exam. Because an actual pediatric patient is unlikely, the examiner may interrupt, ask what you are looking for, and provide findings.)

Investigations

The total serum bilirubin or transcutaneous bilirubin level should be plotted on a nomogram against the infant's age in hours. This will indicate the need for treatment, further investigations, or further testing. Ask for a copy of the nomogram, which the patient or examiner may provide (it may also be part of the written instructions for this patient encounter).

In infants requiring phototherapy or in those with rapidly rising bilirubin, order tests for total and direct serum bilirubin to help distinguish between conjugated (direct) and unconjugated (indirect) hyperbilirubinemia (see the information this resource lists in the MCC differential diagnosis). Direct bilirubin is considered elevated when it exceeds 20% of the total bilirubin level. In infants with elevated direct bilirubin, order a urinalysis and urine culture. In infants receiving phototherapy, order a blood type and Coombs test. In infants with prolonged jaundice (weeks), review the neonatal tests for hypothyroidism and galactosemia.

Management

Admit all neonates requiring treatment according to the nomogram. The nomogram will indicate the need for phototherapy or exchange transfusion. In neonates with mild jaundice not requiring phototherapy, increasing the frequency of feedings will help lower the bilirubin level. Provide intravenous (IV) fluids if the infant is dehydrated. Retest bilirubin levels according to advice given in the nomogram.

All newborns should have frequent clinical assessments for jaundice in the first 24 hours after birth, and a follow-up assessment within 48 hours after birth. Infants with risk factors for hyperbilirubinemia should have their total serum bilirubin level (or transcutaneous bilirubin level) measured 24 to 72 hours after discharge.

Pearls

Breastfed neonates are less likely to develop jaundice if fed 8 to 12 times per 24 hours, as opposed to less frequently.

It is unconjugated (indirect) bilirubin that is toxic to the central nervous system.

71

Oligoarthralgia (pain in 1 to 4 joints)

MCC particular objectives

Differentiate joint disease from other anatomic causes.

Identify patients who need immediate, definitive management or referral.

MCC differential diagnosis
with added evidence

ACUTE JOINT PAIN

Injury (e.g., meniscal tear)
JOINT INJURY IN GENERAL

Signs and symptoms: history of trauma (e.g., sports injury, bicycle accident); joint pain made worse by activity and relieved by rest (as opposed to resting joint pain in inflammatory conditions); joint swelling, redness, warmth, bruising; movement difficulty around the joint

Investigations: X-ray, MRI, CT scan

MENISCAL TEAR

Signs and symptoms: knee pain, effusion; history of changing speed and direction at the same time; mechanical symptoms (locking, popping, catching, buckling); persistent focal joint line tenderness

Infection

Common pathogens in joint infections include *Staphylococcus aureus* and streptococci.

Infants and younger children may be asymptomatic.

Signs and symptoms: symptoms in 1 joint (usual); acute joint pain, tenderness, warmth, redness; restricted joint motion; loss of joint function; fever; sweating; rigor; abscesses; hemorrhagic pustules; symptoms of endocarditis (e.g., fatigue, new heart murmur, night sweats, shortness of breath, petechiae)

> Locations: knee (most common: ~50 % of cases), hip, shoulder, elbow

Risk factors: advanced age; intravenous (IV) drug use; underlying joint injury; prosthetic joint; skin conditions (e.g., psoriasis, eczema); immunocompromised (e.g., diabetes, kidney disease, liver disease, use of immunosuppressants)

Investigations: synovial fluid analysis (cell counts, Gram stain, culture, WBCs); blood cultures

Crystal

PSEUDOGOUT (CALCIUM PYROPHOSPHATE DIHYDRATE DEPOSITION DISEASE)

Signs and symptoms: older than 65 (usual); severe joint pain with stiffness, tenderness, swelling, erythema that peaks in 6 to 24 hours

> Location: knee, wrist, hand, pelvis, hip (common)

> History of illness, surgery, medication (bisphosphonates, intraarticular hyaluronic injections, granulocyte colony-stimulating factor)

Investigations: analysis of synovial fluid or biopsy specimen to detect calcium pyrophosphate dihydrate crystals; X-ray, ultrasound to detect chondrocalcinosis

GOUT

Chronic gout is characterized by recurrent severe acute attacks from monosodium urate crystals in joints.

Signs and symptoms: severe joint pain, erythema, warmth, swelling that peaks in 24 to 48 hours

> Locations: first metatarsophalangeal joint (most common), midfoot, ankles, knees (gout is uncommon in axial joints)

> Progressing chronic gout: possible persistent arthritis and white-yellow intradermal deposits

Risk factors: obesity, hypertension, alcohol use, high purine diet (e.g., high in meat and seafood), use of antihypertensives (e.g., diuretics, beta-blockers)

Investigations: urate crystal detection (e.g., synovial fluid analysis; ultrasound of joint or tophus); blood tests (CBC, BUN, creatinine)

Hemarthrosis (e.g., clotting disorder)

Hemarthrosis occurs in patients with hemophilia and other clotting disorders.

Signs and symptoms: personal or family history of hemophilia; joint tingling, tightness followed by joint swelling, warmth, pain

> Locations: ankles, knees, elbows (most common); shoulders, wrists, hips (less common)

> Late symptoms: pain at rest; extreme loss of motion

Investigations: coagulation profile (PT/INR, aPTT, platelet count, von Willebrand factor assay)

> Diagnosis of clotting disorder: factor IX inhibitor (hemophilia B), factor VIII activity (hemophilia A), gene mutation testing

Acute reactive arthritis

Symptoms: acute, asymmetric pain in 1 to 4 joints; inflammation of ligaments or tendons; tendonitis; swollen toes, fingers; recent or current mild, bilateral conjunctivitis; recent gastrointestinal, genitourinary, or respiratory infection; fever; malaise; weight loss; morning stiffness lasting > 1 hour

> Locations: knee, ankle, and/or heel (usual) (it is uncommon in the upper limbs)

Investigations: positive HLA-B27; elevated acute phase reactants; serology, urinalysis, stool cultures to detect recent infection

CHRONIC JOINT PAIN

Osteoarthritis

This is breakdown of joint cartilage and underlying bone.

Signs and symptoms: joint pain and stiffness following exercise initially and progressing to permanence (over years)

> Joint symptoms: often asymmetrical; swelling; impaired function; instability; buckling; bone tenderness and/or enlargement; crepitus

> Locations: ends of the fingers; bases of the thumbs; the neck, lower back, knees, hips

Risk factors: older age; female; obesity; joint injuries; abnormal joint or limb development; family history of osteoarthritis

Investigations: X-ray

Periarticular disease (e.g., bursitis, tendinosis)

BURSITIS

This is inflammation of the bursae, which are sacs that cushion bones and the structures surrounding joints.

The most common cause is repetitive pressure on bursae (e.g., kneeling, leaning on the elbows, sitting for long periods on hard surfaces).

Investigations: X-rays, ultrasound, or MRI to rule out other causes; blood tests or analysis of fluid from inflamed bursae to identify the cause

TENDINOSIS

This is cellular-level damage to tendons that results from chronic overuse, and involves the generation of new blood vessels to the injury. It can develop from untreated tendonitis.

Signs and symptoms: tendon pain that persists for weeks or months; history of chronic repetitive low-grade trauma or overuse (common); history of sports injury (common); pain on palpation of the affected tendon; pain with tendon loading

> Achilles tendon: heel pain (this is common in runners)
>
> Biceps: anterior shoulder pain in the bicipital groove that is worse on flexing the shoulder or supination of the forearm
>
> Lateral epicondylitis ("tennis elbow"): pain of the lateral elbow that is worse on grasping and twisting
>
> Medial epicondylitis ("golfer's elbow"): pain of the medial elbow
>
> Patellar ("jumper's knee"): male (more common); history of sports involving jumping and running (common); pain on standing up from sitting, and climbing stairs or hills
>
> Rotator cuff, shoulder: dull, aching shoulder pain that is difficult to localize and radiates into the upper arm toward the chest; painful range of motion; pain that is worse at night

Pediatric disorder (e.g., slipped epiphysis, Osgood-Schlatter disease)

SLIPPED CAPITAL FEMORAL EPIPHYSIS

This is the most common hip disorder in adolescents.

It requires accurate diagnosis and immediate treatment.

Symptoms: hip pain (sometimes groin, thigh, or knee pain) that becomes worse with physical activity; altered gait (limping; walking with a leg turned outward; waddling walk)

Risk factors: obesity, hypothyroidism, growth hormone deficiency, Down syndrome, prior radiation therapy

Investigations: X-ray (anteroposterior and lateral views of the bilateral hips)

> Anteroposterior view shows a blurry junction between the metaphysis and the growth plate.
>
> Both views show the line of Klein passing outside the epiphysis (instead of intersecting it) or passing just at its superior edge.

OSGOOD-SCHLATTER DISEASE

This is a common cause of anterior knee pain in adolescents.

Signs and symptoms: gradual-onset knee pain with swelling in nearby tibial tuberosity, which is tender on palpation; unilateral (usual); stiffness in the hamstring, rectus femoris; symptoms exacerbated by running, jumping, and direct pressure (e.g., kneeling); fluctuating symptoms for 12 to 24 months

Investigations: X-ray to exclude other causes

Strategy for patient encounter

The likely scenario is an adult patient with isolated joint pain. The specified tasks could engage history, physical exam, investigations, or management.

A major goal of the encounter is to determine the source of pain (joint or other tissues), and identify patients who need immediate management.

History

Use open-ended questions to obtain a pain history: Which joints are painful? When did the pain start? How constant is the pain? What other symptoms do you have? Listen for evidence consistent with entities that require immediate management (e.g., recent-onset knee pain with fever in infection); and evidence consistent with particular entities (e.g., recurrent episodes of severe pain at the base of a toe in gout; recent trauma).

Use open-ended questions to obtain a medical and medication history: What conditions have you been diagnosed with? What medications do you take? Listen for skin diseases, diabetes, kidney disease, and liver disease (relevant to infection); clotting disorders (relevant to hemarthrosis); and use of immunosuppressant drugs.

Ask about the patient's occupation and recreation routines, listening for evidence of repetitive stress or pressure (relevant to tendinopathy and bursitis). Ask how the pain affects function, including work and recreation.

Physical exam

Obtain the patient's vital signs, looking for fever. Examine the affected joints, looking for joint swelling, redness, warmth, and bruising. Palpate the surrounding soft tissues. Test the active and passive range of motion of the joint. Auscultate the heart looking for murmurs (relevant to endocarditis in infection).

Investigations

Consider imaging (X-ray, MRI). In suspected infection or gout, perform a joint aspiration for culture, cell count, and crystals. Consider tests for serum uric acid (gout) and C-reactive protein (CRP) (inflammation). Consider a complete blood count (CBC) (infection).

Management

Management depends on the probable entity. Be aware of red flags for immediate management of acute joint pain: joint pain in addition to fever, tachycardia, and/or signs of endocarditis.

Pearls

Remember that there are 3 main underlying causes of joint pain: trauma, inflammation, and mechanical disorders.

72

Polyarthralgia (pain in more than 4 joints)

MCC particular objectives

Differentiate joint disease from other causes of pain.

Differentiate inflammatory from mechanical causes.

MCC differential diagnosis
with added evidence

INFLAMMATORY JOINT PAIN (E.G., RHEUMATOID ARTHRITIS, JUVENILE POLYARTHRITIS)

RHEUMATOID ARTHRITIS

This is a chronic, systemic, inflammatory disease that involves synovial joints.

Signs and symptoms: symmetrical symptoms; pain, stiffness (morning stiffness); swelling in multiple joints that improves with movement; symptoms that progress from the periphery to proximal joints; decreased grip strength; fatigue; fever; weight loss; impaired activities of daily living; joint deformities and locomotor disability (later disease); rheumatoid nodules in the fingers, knuckles, elbows, forearms, knees, backs of heels (in about 25% of patients)

> Commonly affected joints: metacarpophalangeal and proximal interphalangeal joints of the fingers; interphalangeal joints of the thumbs and wrists; metatarsophalangeal joints of the toes

> Other joints: synovial joints of the upper and lower limbs (elbows, shoulders, ankles, knees)

Investigations: blood tests (to detect autoantibodies of rheumatoid factors and/or anticitrullinated peptide/protein antibodies; anemia; thrombocytosis; elevated ESR; elevated CRP); tests of synovial joint fluid (leukocyte count of 1500–25,000/mm^3 with predominance of polymorphonuclear cells); X-rays of the hands and feet to detect narrowing joint spaces, and erosions of bone and cartilage

JUVENILE POLYARTHRITIS

Signs and symptoms: symptoms for > 6 weeks; symptoms in ≥ 5 joints within 6 months; joint pain, tenderness; reduced range of motion; refusal to walk or use affected joints; guarding of affected joints; limping; irritability; malaise; fatigue; diffuse pain; low-grade fever

> Rheumatoid factor–positive subtype: similar symptoms to adult rheumatoid arthritis; involvement of small joints; symmetrical symptoms; rheumatoid nodules

> Rheumatoid factor–negative subtype: asymmetrical symptoms; involvement of fewer joints (knees, wrists, ankles); fewer rheumatoid nodules

Diagnosis: blood tests (IgM rheumatoid factor; CBC, to rule out septic arthritis or acute lymphoblastic leukemia; ESR; ANA; CRP); imaging (ultrasound, MRI, X-ray)

MECHANICAL JOINT PAIN (E.G., OSTEOARTHRITIS)

OSTEOARTHRITIS

This is breakdown of joint cartilage and underlying bone.

Signs and symptoms: joint pain and stiffness following exercise initially and progressing to permanence (over years)

> Joint symptoms: often asymmetrical; swelling; impaired function; instability; buckling; bone tenderness and/or enlargement; crepitus

> Locations: ends of the fingers; bases of the thumbs; the neck, lower back, knees, hips

Risk factors: older age; female; obesity; joint injuries; abnormal joint or limb development; family history of osteoarthritis

Investigations: X-ray

NONARTICULAR DISEASE (E.G., FIBROMYALGIA, POLYMYALGIA RHEUMATICA)

FIBROMYALGIA

This is a diagnosis of exclusion.

Signs and symptoms: female (more common); chronic, widespread pain for ≥ 3 months; pain that is bilateral, and above and below the waist; aching pain; fatigue; long sleep; restless legs syndrome; sleep apnea; impaired concentration, memory; dizziness; cramping (e.g., menstrual, abdominal); morning stiffness; numbness, tingling in the extremities; tender points; urinary symptoms (difficult or painful urination; irregular urination); sensitivity to noise, light, temperature

> Coexisting conditions (often): headaches, irritable bowel syndrome, interstitial cystitis

POLYMYALGIA RHEUMATICA

Signs and symptoms: older than 50 (always); female (more common); northern European descent (higher incidence); history of giant cell temporal arteritis (many patients have this, but it may not be active at the same time as polymyalgia rheumatica); symmetrical symptoms (usual); shoulder pain (more common), hip pain, neck pain; stiffness (morning stiffness usually lasts ≥ 30 minutes, with inability to abduct shoulders past 90 degrees); pain that is worse with movement; synovitis and bursitis (many patients have distal musculoskeletal manifestations)

Investigations: elevated ESR (≥ 50 mm/h); elevated serum CRP

Strategy for patient encounter

The likely scenario is a patient with generalized joint pain. The specified tasks could engage history, physical exam, investigations, or management.

History

Use open-ended questions to obtain a pain history: When did the pain start? Where is the pain? Listen for joint pain versus nonarticular pain. In joint pain, determine what joints are involved (the symmetrical involvement of many joints suggests rheumatoid arthritis) and whether the pain is always in the same joints (polyarthralgia that migrates suggests an inflammatory arthritis, such as rheumatoid arthritis). Ask about factors that make the pain better and worse (pain that is better with movement suggests an inflammatory cause; pain that is worse with movement or use suggests a mechanical cause). Ask about a daily pattern of pain or stiffness (morning pain and stiffness suggests an inflammatory cause). Ask about associated symptoms and listen for evidence consistent with specific entities (e.g., fatigue, fever, and weight loss in rheumatoid arthritis; joint swelling in osteoarthritis). Ask how the pain affects function, including work and recreation.

Physical exam

Examine the affected joints looking for warmth, erythema, swelling, and range of motion. Look for rheumatoid nodules.

Investigations

For all patients, order a test for erythrocyte sedimentation rate (ESR) or C-reactive protein (CRP). Order X-rays of affected joints. Order additional tests depending on the likely diagnosis (see the information this resource lists in the MCC differential diagnosis).

Management

Refer patients with inflammatory arthritis to a rheumatologist. Treat patients with osteoarthritis with analgesics (acetaminophen or nonsteroidal antiinflammatory drugs), and counsel exercise and weight control.

TIP

Tailoring information to individual patients

The MCC identifies providing generic information as a common exam error.

To avoid this error, ask patients about aspects of their lives that might affect their condition. Provide information that targets their situation and engage the patient in figuring out next steps.

For example, diet and exercise changes might be relevant for this case:

- Ask what the patient ate yesterday for breakfast, lunch, and supper. Use this to personalize guidelines on dietary changes they need to make.

- Ask what the patient did for exercise last week. Discuss short-term goals with the patient: What could the patient do next week to exercise every day? (For example, when could the patient fit in a 30-minute walk?)

73

Nonarticular musculoskeletal pain

MCC particular objectives

Differentiate symptoms from the following sources: bone, muscle, nerve, blood vessels.

Determine if urgent action is required.

MCC differential diagnosis
with added evidence

GENERALIZED PAIN

Acute pain (e.g., viral infections)

VIRAL INFECTIONS

Myalgia without trauma is often due to viral infections (e.g., influenza).

Signs and symptoms: fever, headache, malaise, nonproductive cough

Investigations: blood culture and testing to detect infectious agents

Chronic pain (e.g., fibromyalgia, polymyalgia rheumatica)

FIBROMYALGIA

This is a diagnosis of exclusion.

Signs and symptoms: female (more common); chronic, widespread pain for ≥ 3 months; pain that is bilateral, and above and below the waist; aching pain; fatigue; long sleep; restless legs syndrome; sleep apnea; impaired concentration, memory; dizziness; cramping (e.g., menstrual, abdominal); morning stiffness; numbness, tingling in the extremities; tender points; urinary symptoms (difficult or painful urination; irregular urination); sensitivity to noise, light, temperature

> Coexisting conditions (often): headaches, irritable bowel syndrome, interstitial cystitis

POLYMYALGIA RHEUMATICA

Signs and symptoms: older than 50 (always); female (more common); northern European descent (higher incidence); history of giant cell temporal arteritis (many patients have this, but it may not be active at the same time as polymyalgia rheumatica); symmetrical symptoms (usual); shoulder pain (more common), hip pain, neck pain; stiffness (morning stiffness usually lasts ≥ 30 minutes, with inability to abduct shoulders past 90 degrees); pain that is worse with movement;

synovitis and bursitis (many patients have distal musculoskeletal manifestations)

Investigations: elevated ESR ($\geq$ 50 mm/h); elevated serum CRP

LOCALIZED PAIN

Acute pain

TRAUMA

Trauma is the most common cause of nonarticular musculoskeletal pain.

Signs and symptoms: history of trauma; pain with active movement or stretches, or with movement in specific planes; pain localized to an extraarticular structure; superficial tenderness; limited range of motion

> Trauma to muscle: deep, penetrating, or dull pain (but not as intense as bone pain); possible muscle cramp or spasm

> Trauma to tendon or ligament: sharp pain that is worse on stretching or movement, and better with rest

Investigations: X-ray (this may show soft tissue calcifications)

INFECTION (E.G., OSTEOMYELITIS, NECROTIZING FASCIITIS)

OSTEOMYELITIS

Signs and symptoms: fever; lethargy; irritability; site-specific pain; bone instability and tenderness; erythema; swelling; delayed wound healing; exposed bone (highly specific for osteomyelitis)

> Children: acute osteomyelitis (more common) in the long bones of the legs and upper arms (more common)

> Adults: chronic osteomyelitis (more common) in vertebrae (more common); motor and/or sensory dysfunction in the limbs

Risk factors: diabetes; peripheral vascular disease; trauma; intravenous (IV) drugs or catheters

Investigations: CBC to detect inflammation markers; bone biopsy (definitive)

NECROTIZING FASCIITIS

This is an emergency requiring immediate surgery.

Signs and symptoms:

> Early symptoms: severe disproportionate pain (this precedes skin changes by 1 to 2 days); influenza-like symptoms; gastroenteritis-like symptoms

> In-course symptoms (day 3 or 4): erythema, swelling, blisters, bullae, ulcers, black-blue skin, loss of sensation, severe worsening pain, symptoms of systemic toxicity (fever, tachycardia, hypotension, delirium)

Risk factors: damage to skin from trauma, injury, lesions, skin infections, ulcers; immune-suppressing comorbidities (e.g., diabetes, cancer, alcohol abuse)

Investigations: biopsy

VASCULAR (E.G., COMPARTMENT SYNDROME, SICKLE CELL ANEMIA)

COMPARTMENT SYNDROME

Signs and symptoms: history of trauma or hemorrhagic event; symptoms in the limbs (usual: the lower leg is the most common site); palpable swelling; tenderness; escalating pain disproportionate to the injury; pain on passive stretch; paresthesia; paresis; pallor overlying compartment; absence of distal pulses

Investigations: limb intracompartment pressure measurement

SICKLE CELL ANEMIA

Signs and symptoms: family history of sickle cell disease; painful swelling of the hands and feet; jaundice (if concomitant liver disease)

Investigations: CBC to detect anemia, sickle cells; positive sickle cell screen

Chronic pain

MECHANICAL (E.G., TENDINOPATHY, BURSITIS)

TENDINOPATHY

Signs and symptoms: history of chronic repetitive low-grade trauma or overuse (common); history of sports injury (common); pain on palpation of the affected tendon; pain with tendon loading

> Achilles tendon: heel pain (this is common in runners)
>
> Biceps: anterior shoulder pain in the bicipital groove that is worse on flexing the shoulder or supination of the forearm
>
> Lateral epicondylitis ("tennis elbow"): pain of the lateral elbow that is worse on grasping and twisting
>
> Medial epicondylitis ("golfer's elbow"): pain of the medial elbow
>
> Patellar ("jumper's knee"): male (more common); history of sports involving jumping and running (common); pain on standing up from sitting, and climbing stairs or hills
>
> Rotator cuff, shoulder: dull, aching shoulder pain that is difficult to localize and radiates into the upper arm toward the chest; painful range of motion; pain that is worse at night

BURSITIS

This is inflammation of the bursae, which are sacs that cushion bones and the structures surrounding joints.

The most common cause is repetitive pressure on bursae (e.g., kneeling, leaning on the elbows, sitting for long periods on hard surfaces).

Investigations: X-rays, ultrasound, or MRI to rule out other causes; blood tests or analysis of fluid from inflamed bursae to identify the cause

VASCULAR (E.G., INTERMITTENT CLAUDICATION)

INTERMITTENT CLAUDICATION

Signs and symptoms: muscle pain, cramps, numbness, fatigue;

calf-muscle symptoms (usual); symptoms worse with muscle use, better with rest; acute limb ischemia (paresthesia, paralysis, pallor, pulselessness, urgent pain); positive Buerger test (redness on returning a limb to a dependent position)

> Severe: cyanosis, hair loss, shiny skin, decreased temperature, bradycardia

Investigations: magnetic resonance angiography; duplex ultrasonography

NEOPLASTIC

Signs and symptoms: history of cancer

Types of pain and their causes:

> Acute pain: recent treatment or procedures
>
> Chronic pain: usually caused by the condition; possible impaired memory, attention
>
> Somatic pain: tissue, tendon, or bone injury from surgery, trauma, inflammation, tumour
>
> Visceral pain: organ damage or tumour infiltration
>
> Neuropathic pain: tumour infiltration of peripheral nerves, roots, spinal cord; treatment side effects

NEUROPATHIC

Signs and symptoms:

> Motor: weakness, fatigue, wasting, cramps, twitching, decreased reflexes, myokymia
>
> Sensory: numbness, tingling; burning or stabbing pain; gait and balance difficulty; temperature intolerance; hyperalgesia
>
> Other: skin, hair, or nail changes; foot and leg ulcers, infections

Investigations: nerve conduction studies; EMG

COMPLEX REGIONAL PAIN SYNDROME

Signs and symptoms: chronic unilateral pain in an arm or leg; history of trauma to the limb (most cases involve trauma; others may involve surgery, stroke, heart attack, or diabetes); pain out of proportion to the initial injury

> Early symptoms in the affected limb: pain; swelling; redness; changes in skin temperature (from sweaty and hot to cold); cold, touch sensitivity
>
> Later symptoms in the affected limb: changes in skin colour (pallor), texture (thin, shiny, tender), hair growth, and nail growth; muscle spasms

Investigations: sympathetic nervous system tests to detect disturbances; bone scan to detect possible bone changes; X-rays for later stage bone-mineral assessment

Strategy for patient encounter

The likely scenario is a patient with chronic regional pain. The specified tasks could engage history, physical exam, investigations, or management.

This clinical presentation has a wide differential diagnosis. To narrow the possible diagnosis, determine whether the pain is localized or diffuse, and acute or chronic, and note specific findings on physical exam.

History

Take a pain history: Where is the pain? When did it start? How constant is it? What triggers the pain? What other symptoms do you have? Ask about a history of trauma. Ask about the patient's occupation and recreation routines, listening for evidence of repetitive stress or pressure (relevant to tendinopathy and bursitis). Ask how the pain affects function, including work and recreation.

Physical exam

Examine the area of the pain, looking for tenderness, masses, erythema, and swelling.

Investigations

Order an X-ray of the affected region. Order further specific tests depending on the probable diagnosis (see the information this resource lists in the MCC differential diagnosis).

Management

Urgent intervention is required for patients with obvious fractures or dislocations, and with signs and symptoms consistent with necrotizing fasciitis or compartment syndrome.

74

Back pain and related symptoms (e.g., sciatica)

MCC particular objective

Determine if the patient requires urgent intervention.

MCC differential diagnosis
with added evidence

MECHANICAL PROBLEM

Common back pain

Causes include muscle or ligament damage; bulging or ruptured disks; arthritis; skeletal irregularities; and osteoporosis.

Signs and symptoms: symptoms that last ≥ 6 weeks in the acute form (usual); muscle aches; shooting or stabbing pain; pain radiating down the leg; limited range of motion of the back; **no** bowel or bladder changes, fever, or history of trauma (e.g., a fall)

Acute, discogenic nerve root entrapment

Lumbar radiculopathy arises from a compressed nerve root in the lower back, which often results in inflammation of the nerve root. It is commonly called *sciatica*, because nerve roots comprising the sciatic nerve are often involved in this condition.

Causes include changes in the tissues surrounding the nerve root (typically); herniation of a spinal disc between vertebrae; bone spurs; and ossification of spinal ligaments.

Signs and symptoms: numbness, paresthesia, sharp pain in the back or legs; weakness or loss of reflexes in the legs; sciatic pain on straight leg raise

Investigations: nerve conduction studies, EMG, MRI

Spinal stenosis and/or cauda equina syndrome

SPINAL STENOSIS

This is narrowing of the intraspinal canal, commonly caused by osteoarthritis.

Signs and symptoms: lower back pain (usual); symptoms that develop over months to years; motor weakness; pain or claudication in the buttocks, thighs, calves when the patient is active (standing, walking, running, climbing stairs); **no** pain when sitting, lying down, squatting, or bending forward

Risk factors: older than 50; history of spinal surgery

Investigations: X-ray, CT scan, or MRI of the spine

CAUDA EQUINA SYNDROME

This occurs when the spinal cord is compressed in the lumbar spine. Common causes include herniated disk, spinal stenosis, infection, and trauma.

Signs and symptoms: leg pain, numbness, weakness; urinary symptoms (incontinence, retention, frequent urination); fecal incontinence; loss of rectal tone; abnormal bulbocavernosus and anal wink reflexes; erectile dysfunction; decreased muscle tone and deep tendon reflexes in the legs; saddle anesthesia (loss of sensation in the inner thighs, back of the legs, around the rectum)

Investigations: X-ray; CT scan; MRI (this is preferred for suspected spinal cord compression); myelography

INFLAMMATORY ARTHRITIS (E.G., ANKYLOSING SPONDYLITIS)

ANKYLOSING SPONDYLITIS

Signs and symptoms: unilateral or bilateral pain in the buttocks that spreads to the upper thighs, chest, hips, peripheral joints; back pain or stiffness that is worse on waking, lasts ≥ 30 minutes, and improves with activity; loss of mobility; anterior uveitis (unilateral eye symptoms including pain, photophobia, redness, watering, irregularly shaped pupil, slow-reacting pupil); diffuse swelling in the fingers, toes; large joint arthritis; stooped posture with cautious gait

Investigations: X-ray

RHEUMATOID ARTHRITIS

This is a chronic, systemic, inflammatory disease that involves synovial joints.

Signs and symptoms: symmetrical symptoms; pain, stiffness (morning stiffness); swelling in multiple joints that improves with movement; symptoms that progress from the periphery to proximal joints; decreased grip strength; fatigue; fever; weight loss; impaired activities of daily living; joint deformities and locomotor disability (later disease); rheumatoid nodules in the fingers, knuckles, elbows, forearms, knees, backs of heels (in about 25% of patients)

> Commonly affected joints: metacarpophalangeal and proximal interphalangeal joints of the fingers; interphalangeal joints of the thumbs and wrists; metatarsophalangeal joints of the toes

> Other joints: synovial joints of the upper and lower limbs (elbows, shoulders, ankles, knees)

Investigations: blood tests (to detect autoantibodies of rheumatoid factors and/or anticitrullinated peptide/protein antibodies; anemia; thrombocytosis; elevated ESR; elevated CRP); tests of synovial joint fluid (leukocyte count of 1500–25,000/mm^3 with predominance of polymorphonuclear cells); X-rays of the hands and feet to detect narrowing joint spaces, and erosions of bone and cartilage

PSORIATIC ARTHRITIS

Signs and symptoms: symptoms of psoriasis (chronic plaque psoriasis is the most common form); joint pain, stiffness, swelling; pain and stiffness in the morning or after inactivity (pain lasts > 30–45 minutes); symptoms that affect ≥ 5 joints with asymmetric distribution and distal interphalangeal joint involvement; finger and/or toe swelling (sausage-like dactylitis); inflammation at sites of tendon insertion; nail lesions

> Chronic plaque psoriasis: symmetrically distributed cutaneous lesions that are erythematous, raised above normal skin, 1–10 cm in diameter, with clearly defined margins, and a thick, coarse, silvery scale; located on the scalp, elbows, knees, back (most common sites)

Investigations: X-ray

INFECTION

Factors that suggest infection include immunosuppression, intravenous (IV) drug use, unexplained fever, chronic steroid use, infection at another site, and progressive, disabling symptoms.

Investigations (infection detection): blood tests (glucose, WBCs, protein, culture); antigen and antibody tests (blood, urinalysis); imaging

FRACTURE

Signs of spinal fracture: history of trauma (e.g., a fall from a height; car accident; strenuous lifting, especially with osteoporosis); sudden-onset severe pain in the spine; point tenderness over vertebrae; structural spine deformity

> Pain is made better by lying down or reclining.

> Pain is made worse by prolonged sitting; activities where the arms are elevated or used away from the body (e.g., vacuuming); and bending forward.

Investigations: X-ray of the lumbar spine; CT scan to detect stress fractures; MRI to detect disk lesions

NEOPLASM

SPINAL CORD TUMOUR

Tumours can be malignant or benign (e.g., osteoblastoma, neurofibroma).

Signs and symptoms: chronic pain for > 1 month that is unimproved by bed rest or therapy; focal spine pain that is tender on palpation; possible neurologic effects (weak or numb limbs; lack of coordination; bladder or bowel dysfunction); constitutional symptoms (weight loss, vomiting, fever, chills)

Risk factors: history of cancer (especially lung, prostate, breast, multiple myeloma)

Investigations: spinal X-ray, MRI, CSF analysis

Strategy for patient encounter

The likely scenario is a patient with chronic lower back pain. The specified tasks could engage history, physical exam, investigations, or management.

History

Use open-ended questions to obtain a pain history: When did the pain start? What were you doing when the pain started? How constant is the pain? What other symptoms do you have? Listen for evidence of sudden onset and trauma (this suggests common back pain or fracture); chronic pain (this suggests neoplasm or an inflammatory condition); symptoms of infection (e.g., fever); and neurological symptoms (e.g., associated leg pain and/ or incontinence in cauda equina syndrome). Determine the presence of any red flags (see the checklist). Ask how the pain affects function, including work and recreation.

Physical exam

Obtain vital signs, looking for fever. Examine the patient for gait and range of motion. Perform a neurological exam. Perform a straight-leg-raise test to assess for herniated lower lumbar disc.

Investigations

Order imaging (X-ray, CT scan, or MRI) for patients whose pain has lasted more than 4 to 6 weeks despite conservative treatment, and for

CHECKLIST

Red flags for urgent intervention in back pain

Back pain concurrent with any of the following findings suggests a serious cause (e.g., aortic aneurysm, cancer, gastrointestinal bleed, or infection) with the possible need for urgent intervention.

- abdominal aorta > 5 cm
- lower extremity pulse deficit
- acute, tearing midback pain
- cancer, either diagnosed or suspected
- duration of pain longer than 6 weeks
- fever
- gastrointestinal findings (e.g., localized abdominal tenderness)
- infection risk factors
- meningismus
- neurologic deficits
- severe nocturnal or disabling pain
- unexplained pain after age 55
- unexplained weight loss

patients with red flags. In patients with fever or suspected infection, order a complete blood count (CBC) and a test for C-reactive protein (CRP).

Management

In the absence of red flags, treat patients conservatively with acetaminophen, nonsteroidal antiinflammatory drugs (NSAIDs), muscle relaxants, heat, and/or physical therapy. Advise patients to stay active. Refer patients with neurological symptoms, fracture, infection, or malignancy to an orthopedic surgeon or neurosurgeon.

Pearls

In patients without red flags, delay imaging for 4 to 6 weeks. The pain usually resolves, avoiding the need for imaging.

75

Neck pain

MCC particular objective

Determine if the patient requires urgent intervention.

MCC differential diagnosis
with added evidence

MECHANICAL PROBLEM

Neck strain

Signs and symptoms: history of neck injury (a common cause is whiplash from an automobile accident or sports injury; pain may have delayed onset after injury); stiffness, numbness, tingling, weakness in the arms, face, scalp; loss of range of motion; pain that is worse with movement; headaches that start at the base of the skull; fatigue; dizziness

> Other: shortness of breath, hoarse voice, difficulty swallowing, blurred vision, tinnitus, irritability

Investigations: CT scan, MRI

Spondylosis

Cervical spondylosis is difficult to distinguish from other causes of neck pain.

Signs and symptoms: older adult (often: aging is an important factor in disc degeneration); pain that originates in the lower cervical spine (common); pain and/or stiffness that is chronic or intermittent in the neck and shoulders; **no** associated neurologic signs (often)

> Other symptoms (less common): headache; suboccipital and arm pain; tingling and weakness

Acute, discogenic nerve root entrapment

Cervical radiculopathy arises from a compressed nerve root in the neck, which often results in inflammation of the nerve root.

Causes include changes in the tissues surrounding the nerve root (typically); herniation of a spinal disc between vertebrae; bone spurs; and ossifications of spinal ligaments.

Signs and symptoms: numbness, paresthesia, sharp pain, or weakness in the shoulders and arms (nerves in the neck primarily control sensation in the arms and hands)

Investigations: nerve conduction studies, EMG, MRI

Spinal stenosis and/or cord compression

CERVICAL SPINAL STENOSIS (CHRONIC CORD COMPRESSION)

This is narrowing of the intraspinal canal, commonly caused by osteoarthritis.

Signs and symptoms: male, older than 55 (more common); symptoms that develop over months to years; numbness, weakness, or tingling in the limbs and extremities (tingling in the hand is the most common symptom); subtle loss of hand dexterity; positive Hoffman or Babinski sign; hyperreflexia; clonus

Investigations: X-ray, CT scan, or MRI of the cervical spine

ACUTE AND SUBACUTE CORD COMPRESSION

The usual cause is extramedullary lesions (in subacute compression; another common cause of subacute compression is herniated disk).

Signs and symptoms: localized neck pain with radicular pain

> Acute compression: symptoms that develop over minutes to hours; history of trauma (often)

> Subacute compression: symptoms that develop over days to weeks; history of cancer (metastatic cancer is a common cause)

Investigations: immediate MRI

INFLAMMATORY ARTHRITIS (E.G., ANKYLOSING SPONDYLITIS)

ANKYLOSING SPONDYLITIS

Signs and symptoms: unilateral or bilateral pain in the buttocks that spreads to the upper thighs, chest, hips, peripheral joints; back pain or stiffness that is worse on waking, lasts ≥ 30 minutes, and improves with activity; loss of mobility; anterior uveitis (unilateral eye symptoms including pain, photophobia, redness, watering, irregularly shaped pupil, slow-reacting pupil); diffuse swelling in the fingers, toes; large joint arthritis; stooped posture with cautious gait

Investigations: X-ray

RHEUMATOID ARTHRITIS

This is a chronic, systemic, inflammatory disease that involves synovial joints.

Signs and symptoms: symmetrical symptoms; pain, stiffness (morning stiffness); swelling in multiple joints that improves with movement; symptoms that progress from the periphery to proximal joints; decreased grip strength; fatigue; fever; weight loss; impaired activities of daily living; joint deformities and locomotor disability (later disease); rheumatoid nodules in the fingers, knuckles, elbows, forearms, knees, backs of heels (in about 25% of patients)

> Commonly affected joints: metacarpophalangeal and proximal interphalangeal joints of the fingers; interphalangeal joints of the thumbs and wrists; metatarsophalangeal joints of the toes

> Other joints: synovial joints of the upper and lower limbs (elbows, shoulders, ankles, knees)

Investigations: blood tests (to detect autoantibodies of rheumatoid factors and/or anticitrullinated peptide/protein antibodies; anemia; thrombocytosis; elevated ESR; elevated CRP); tests of synovial joint fluid (leukocyte count of 1500–25,000/mm^3 with predominance of polymorphonuclear cells); X-rays of the hands and feet to detect narrowing joint spaces, and erosions of bone and cartilage

PSORIATIC ARTHRITIS

Signs and symptoms: symptoms of psoriasis (chronic plaque psoriasis is the most common form); joint pain, stiffness, swelling; pain and stiffness in the morning or after inactivity (pain lasts > 30–45 minutes); symptoms that affect ≥ 5 joints with asymmetric distribution and distal interphalangeal joint involvement; finger and/or toe swelling (sausage-like dactylitis); inflammation at sites of tendon insertion; nail lesions

> Chronic plaque psoriasis: symmetrically distributed cutaneous lesions that are erythematous, raised above normal skin, 1–10 cm in diameter, with clearly defined margins, and a thick, coarse, silvery scale; located on the scalp, elbows, knees, back (most common sites)

Investigations: X-ray

INFECTION

INFECTION IN GENERAL

Factors that suggest infection include immunosuppression; intravenous (IV) drug use; unexplained fever; chronic steroid use; infection at another site; and progressive, disabling symptoms.

Infections particularly associated with neck pain include meningitis and retropharyngeal abscess. Other infections may also cause neck pain (e.g., strep throat, mononucleosis, tuberculosis, catscratch disease, HIV, Cytomegalovirus, toxoplasmosis).

Investigations (infection detection in general): CSF glucose, WBCs, protein, culture; throat culture; antigen and antibody tests (blood, urinalysis); imaging

MENINGITIS

Signs and symptoms: fever; stiff neck; headache; Kernig sign (flexing the patient's hip 90 degrees, then extending the knee, causes pain); Brudzinski neck sign (flexing the patient's neck causes flexion of the hips and knees)

Investigations: positive culture in CSF; meningeal inflammation (increased pleocytosis, low glucose in CSF); CSF absolute neutrophil count ≥ 1000/µL; CSF protein level ≥ 80 mg/dL; peripheral blood absolute neutrophil count ≥ 10,000/µL; CT, MRI

RETROPHARYNGEAL ABSCESS

Signs and symptoms: pain on swallowing; fever; enlarged lymph nodes in the neck; noisy breathing; stridor (in children); severe neck pain (in adults)

Investigations: neck X-ray, CT scan

FRACTURE

Signs and symptoms: history of trauma; neck symptoms (pain, tenderness, tightness, inability to move, swelling, muscle spasms); numbness, pain, tingling at the base of the head; difficulty swallowing; loss of feeling or pinprick pain in the arms and legs; double vision; loss of consciousness

Investigations: C-spine X-ray, CT scan, MRI

> Range of motion test: if the patient can rotate their neck 45 degrees left and right, imaging is not required (perform range of motion testing only in low-risk neck injury)

NEOPLASM

SPINAL CORD TUMOUR

Tumours can be malignant or benign (e.g., osteoblastoma, neurofibroma).

Signs and symptoms: chronic pain for > 1 month that is unimproved by bed rest or therapy; focal spine pain that is tender on palpation; possible neurologic effects (weak or numb limbs; lack of coordination;

bladder or bowel dysfunction); constitutional symptoms (weight loss, vomiting, fever, chills)

Risk factors: history of cancer (especially lung, prostate, breast, multiple myeloma)

Investigations: spinal X-ray, MRI, CSF analysis

THYROID CANCER

Signs and symptoms: female (more common); asymptomatic early in disease (symptoms present once the tumour is large enough); palpable lump on the anterior neck, resulting from swollen lymph nodes; voice change; difficulty speaking; increased hoarseness; difficulty swallowing; shortness of breath; pain in the neck and throat

> Papillary carcinoma (slowest growing): most common type of thyroid cancer; well differentiated; patient aged 30 to 50 (common)

> Follicular thyroid cancer: well differentiated; patient older than 50 (common)

> Medullary thyroid cancer: elevated serum calcitonin

> Anaplastic thyroid cancer (fastest growing, rare): undifferentiated; highly aggressive and metastatic; patient older than 60 (common)

Risk factors: exposure to radiation; family history of thyroid cancer or goiters; residence in an iodine-deficient area of the world

Investigations: thyroid ultrasound

HEAD AND NECK CANCER

Signs and symptoms: symptoms for > 3 weeks; persistent unilateral throat discomfort

> Lesion in oral cavity: persistent red and/or white patches on the oral mucosa; ulceration and/or swelling of the oropharynx or mucosa; persistent mass; tongue pain; tongue deviation; hoarseness; unexplained tooth mobility and/or looseness; earache; difficulty swallowing; bleeding in the oral cavity; stridor; facial pain or numbness

> Lesion in nasopharynx: neck lump; bloody nasal discharge; nasal blockage; unilateral hearing loss; ringing in the ear; recurrent otitis media; headache; facial pain or numbness; double vision; persistent cough

Investigations: endoscopic visualization; fine needle aspiration or core biopsy of mass

PAIN FROM SOFT TISSUE STRUCTURES (E.G., THYROID, PHARYNX)

THYROIDITIS

Causes of thyroiditis include suppurative thyroiditis, Hashimoto thyroiditis, fibrous thyroiditis, thyroid cancer (see above), and use of amiodarone and lithium.

Signs and symptoms: swollen, tender thyroid; neck pain that is worse on swallowing and that may radiate locally; difficulty swallowing; voice changes; fever

Investigations: blood tests to assess thyroid function (thyrotropin, T_4, T_3, anti-TPO antibodies); CBC with differential; thyroid ultrasound or CT scan; radioactive iodine uptake; endoscopic laryngoscopy

PHARYNGITIS
Signs and symptoms: history of upper respiratory tract infection (usual); sore throat; fever; runny nose; cough; headache; hoarse voice

Strategy for patient encounter

The likely scenario is a patient with acute severe neck pain. The specified tasks could engage history, physical exam, investigations, or management.

History

Use open-ended questions to obtain a pain history: When did the pain start? How constant is it? What makes it better? What makes it worse? How bad is the pain on a scale of 1 to 10? What other symptoms do you have? Listen for evidence consistent with particular entities (e.g., pain that is worse with movement in neck strain; pain, numbness, or weakness in the shoulders and hands in discogenic nerve root entrapment; slow-developing tingling in the hand in cervical spinal stenosis; pain that improves with movement in inflammatory arthritis; severe pain, fever, and pain on swallowing in retropharyngeal abscess; difficulty swallowing in thyroid, head, and neck cancer). Ask about a history of trauma and cancer. Ask how the pain affects function, including work and recreation.

Physical exam

Examine the neck, assessing for tenderness, masses, and range of motion. Perform a neurological exam. Obtain the patient's vital signs, looking for fever. Look for signs of meningitis (Kernig sign, Brudzinski neck sign). Examine the oropharynx, looking for a retropharyngeal abscess.

Investigations

If the patient has a fever, order a complete blood count (CBC) and a test for C-reactive protein (CRP). Order imaging (X-ray, CT scan, or MRI depending on most likely diagnosis). In suspected meningitis, perform a lumbar puncture.

Management

For all fractures and cases with neurologic symptoms, refer the patient to a neurosurgeon. Manage other conditions as outlined by this resource in the MCC differential diagnosis. Prescribe pain control as necessary: the first-line analgesics are nonsteroidal antiinflammatory drugs (NSAIDs). Counsel the patient about returning to work and recreation.

76

Abnormal serum lipids

MCC particular objectives

Identify patients who will benefit from serum cholesterol reduction, as well as primary and secondary prevention.

MCC differential diagnosis
with added evidence

HYPERCHOLESTEROLEMIA

Primary (familial)

Signs and symptoms: extreme hypercholesterolemia (low-density lipoproteins) without secondary causes; corneal arcus at younger than 45; xanthomas in the tendons of the feet, hands, elbows, knees (the Achilles tendon is the most common site), and around the eyes (xanthelasma)

> Family history: elevated low-density lipoprotein (LDL); early onset (younger than 50) coronary heart disease (especially premature myocardial infarction)
>
> Personal history: premature coronary heart disease, cardiovascular disease

Secondary

ENDOCRINE DISORDER (E.G., DIABETES MELLITUS, HYPOTHYROIDISM)

DIABETES

Signs and symptoms: personal or family history of diabetes; history of diabetic complications and/or inadequate monitoring; polydipsia, polyuria, and/or weight loss

Investigations: fasting glucose or HbA$_{1c}$ test

HYPOTHYROIDISM

Signs and symptoms: history of hypothyroidism or symptoms of hypothyroidism (cold intolerance, decreased reflexes, dry skin, weight gain, impaired cognition)

Investigations: elevated thyrotropin (TSH)

CHOLESTATIC LIVER DISEASE

Signs and symptoms: abdominal pain; nausea, vomiting; jaundice; itchiness; palpable, tender liver and/or gallbladder; history of liver disease, gallstones, cancer; current pregnancy

Investigations: abnormal liver enzyme tests, elevated bilirubin, abdominal ultrasound

NEPHROTIC SYNDROME OR CHRONIC KIDNEY INJURY

NEPHROTIC SYNDROME

Signs and symptoms: progressive lower extremity edema (ankles and feet); swelling around the eyes; weight gain (from water retention); foamy urine

Risk factors: conditions that damage the kidneys (e.g., diabetes, systemic lupus erythematosus, amyloidosis); use of nonsteroidal antiinflammatory drugs (NSAIDs), antibiotics; history of HIV, hepatitis B virus (HBV), hepatitis C virus (HCV), malaria

Investigations: urine (proteinuria, spot urine protein:creatinine ratio, lipuria); hyponatremia with low fractional sodium excretion; low serum albumin; high total cholesterol (hyperlipidemia); elevated BUN

CHRONIC KIDNEY INJURY

Signs and symptoms: history of kidney disease, chronic renal failure, and/or current renal dialysis; bilateral lower limb swelling; shortness of breath; paroxysmal nocturnal dyspnea; orthopnea

Risk factors: diabetes, diabetic complications, and/or inadequate monitoring; hypertension; smoking

OTHER

OBESITY

Signs and symptoms: body mass index (BMI) of ≥ 30.0

DRUGS (E.G., STEROIDS)

STEROIDS

Examples of steroids include corticosteroids, anabolic steroids, and progestins.

> Glucocorticoids and estrogens elevate triglycerides and raise high-density lipoproteins (HDL).
>
> Oral anabolic steroids reduce HDL.
>
> Injectable testosterone does not affect the LDL:HDL ratio.
>
> Progestins have different effects on HDL, LDL, and triglycerides.

HYPERTRIGLYCERIDEMIA

Primary (familial)

Signs and symptoms: family history of hypertriglyceridemia; personal or family history of coronary heart disease; pancreatitis; elevated blood pressure; xanthomas

> Xanthomas: palmar (yellow creases on the palms); tuberous (red/orange, shiny nodules on the elbows and knees); or eruptive (small yellow papules on the back, chest, proximal extremities)

Secondary

OBESITY—SEE ABOVE

DIABETES MELLITUS—SEE ABOVE

NEPHROTIC SYNDROME OR CHRONIC KIDNEY INJURY—SEE ABOVE

DRUGS (E.G., ESTROGEN)

Examples of drugs associated with hypertriglyceridemia include oral contraceptives, beta-blockers, and thiazide-type diuretics.

ALCOHOL

LOW HIGH-DENSITY LIPOPROTEIN

Primary

Signs and symptoms: personal or family history of premature atherosclerosis, coronary heart disease, stroke

Secondary

OBESITY—SEE ABOVE

DRUGS

Examples of drugs associated with low HDL include progesterone, anabolic steroids, and beta-blockers.

METABOLIC SYNDROME

Signs and symptoms: obesity, elevated blood pressure, elevated serum glucose, dyslipidemia

> Diagnostic criteria (at least 3): increased waist circumference ($\geq$ 102 cm for men and $\geq$ 88 cm for women); systolic blood pressure $\geq$ 130 mmHg, diastolic $\geq$ 85 mmHg; fasting glucose $\geq$ 6.1 mmol/L; triglycerides $\geq$ 1.7 mmol/L; HDL < 1.03 mmol/L (men), < 1.3 mmol/L (women)

Strategy for patient encounter

The likely scenario is a patient with elevated lipids on routine screening. The specified tasks could engage history, physical exam, investigations, or management.

History

Ask about a family history of high cholesterol, premature heart disease, and stroke. Ask about a personal history of heart disease, diabetes, kidney disease, and stroke. Ask about the patient's diet and exercise routines.

Physical exam

Obtain the patients vital signs, height, and weight, and calculate the patient's body mass index (BMI). Measure the patient's waist circumference. Listen to the heart and lungs. Examine the eyes for corneal arcus and the skin for xanthomas.

Investigations

If not already done, order a lipid panel, and tests for creatinine, glycated hemoglobin (HbA$_{1c}$), thyrotropin (TSH), liver enzymes, and serum albumin. Order a urinalysis. Estimate the patient's risk of cardiovascular disease with a Framingham risk score (FRS) calculation (see the quick reference).

QUICK REFERENCE
Framingham risk score

It's good general preparation for the exam to know how to calculate Framingham risk scores (this isn't the only clinical presentation that calls for this calculation).

The website of the Canadian Cardiovascular Society includes the Framingham risk score under "calculators and forms," which is a section of "guideline resources."

TIP
Tailoring information to individual patients

The MCC identifies providing generic information as a common exam error.

To avoid this error, ask patients about aspects of their lives that might affect their condition. Provide information that targets their situation and engage the patient in figuring out next steps.

For example, diet and exercise changes might be relevant for this case:

- Ask what the patient ate yesterday for breakfast, lunch, and supper. Use this to personalize guidelines on dietary changes they need to make.

- Ask what the patient did for exercise last week. Discuss short-term goals with the patient: What could the patient do next week to exercise every day? (For example, when could the patient fit in a 30-minute walk?)

Management

For all patients, recommend lifestyle changes (diet, exercise, weight reduction). Discuss the risks and benefits of lipid-lowering drugs.

Prescribe lipid-lowering drugs in the following cases:

- high FRS (higher than 20%) or intermediate FRS (10% to 19%) with LDL ≥ 3.5 mmol/L or non-HDL ≥ 4.3 mmol/L
- men aged 50 or older, and women aged 60 or older, with 1 additional risk factor (low HDL, smoking, hypertension, impaired fasting glucose, large waist circumference)
- presence of clinical atherosclerosis (acute coronary syndrome, stable angina, stoke, transient ischemic attack, peripheral arterial disease), abdominal aortic aneurysm, diabetes mellitus (in patients 40 years or older, or 30 years or older with diabetes for at least 15 years; or with micro-vascular complications), chronic kidney disease, LDL ≥ 5.0 mmol/L

Pearls

Fasting is no longer required in screening for lipid levels.

77

Abnormal liver function tests

MCC particular objective

Assess for underlying liver disorder or systemic disease.

MCC differential diagnosis
with added evidence

HEPATOCELLULAR CAUSE

Acute condition (e.g., infection, medication)

Infectious causes include hepatitis A, B, and E viruses (HAV, HBV, HEV), Cytomegalovirus, herpes simplex virus (HSV), Epstein-Barr virus (EBV), and yellow fever.

Medication causes include acetaminophen (most common), antibiotics, nonsteroidal antiinflammatory drugs (NSAIDs), antiepileptics, statins, antihypertensives, and antivirals (also herbs and supplements: kava kava, Herbalife, Hydroxycut).

Signs and symptoms: viral-like illness; right upper quadrant abdominal pain; jaundice; intracranial hypertension; progression to encephalopathy over weeks

> Viral hepatitis: skin lesions, enlarged liver

> Intracranial hypertension: posturing, peripheral reflex changes, systemic hypertension, bradycardia

> Encephalopathy: behavioural change, disorientation, drowsiness, confusion, incoherent speech, coma, unresponsiveness to pain

Investigations: blood tests (electrolytes, phosphate, glucose); liver enzyme and function tests (PT/INR, AST, ALT, ALP, GGT, bilirubin, albumin); toxicology screen, viral hepatitis serologies

> AST > 3500 units/L suggests acetaminophen toxicity.

Chronic condition (e.g., infection, medication)

CHRONIC LIVER DISEASE IN GENERAL

Patients with compensated cirrhosis may be asymptomatic.

Common causes include viral hepatitis, nonalcoholic fatty liver disease, and alcohol abuse. Medication-induced chronic liver disease is less common.

Signs and symptoms: jaundice; abdominal pain, swelling; swelling in the legs and ankles; systemic symptoms (anorexia, weight loss, weakness, fatigue); itching; easy bruising

Investigations: CBC (decreased platelets); liver enzyme and function tests (e.g., PT/INR, PTT, AST, ALT, bilirubin total, direct and indirect); liver biopsy; Doppler ultrasound; CT scan; MRI; transient elastography

CHRONIC VIRAL HEPATITIS B (HBV) OR HEPATITIS C (HCV) INFECTION

HCV is often asymptomatic.

Risk factors: autoimmune conditions, unprotected sex, intravenous drug abuse, blood transfusions, tattoos, body piercings, imprisonment, workplace exposure to body fluids

NONALCOHOLIC FATTY LIVER DISEASE

This is the most common form of chronic liver disease.

Signs and symptoms: usually asymptomatic, fatigue, right upper quadrant abdominal pain, enlarged liver, muscle weakness

> More severe: jaundice, gynecomastia, enlarged spleen, red palms

Risk factors: high cholesterol; high serum triglycerides, obesity, type 2 diabetes, metabolic syndrome, polycystic ovary syndrome, hypothyroidism, hypopituitarism, recent weight gain or loss

CHOLESTATIC CAUSE

Intrahepatic condition (e.g., pregnancy)

PREGNANCY

Signs and symptoms: amenorrhea; sexual activity, especially without contraception or with inconsistent use of contraception; nausea, vomiting (common early sign); breast enlargement and tenderness; increased frequency of urination without pain or difficulty; fatigue

Investigations: blood or urine β-hCG

Extrahepatic condition (e.g., gallstones)

GALLSTONES

Symptoms: right upper quadrant abdominal pain, under the ribs; pain that prevents normal or deep breathing; Murphy sign (while palpating near the gallbladder, severe pain on taking a breath); vomiting

> Pain characteristics: 15 minutes to 24 hours in duration; radiating to the right upper back or shoulder blade area; no relief with movement or changing position; onset at night, on waking, or after eating

> Symptoms of bile duct blocked by gallstone: jaundice, dark urine, light-coloured stools, fever, chills

Risk factors: high body mass index (BMI) or obesity; high-fat diet; diabetes; older than 60; estrogen medications; family history of gallstones; female

Investigations: ultrasound, abdominal X-ray, CT scan, hepatobiliary scan, MRCP, ERCP

CONGENITAL ABNORMALITIES (E.G., GILBERT SYNDROME)

GILBERT SYNDROME

This inherited disorder does not impair health and requires no treatment.

Signs and symptoms: usually asymptomatic, jaundice

> Triggers for jaundice in Gilbert syndrome: current illness (e.g., flu, cold) or menstruation; recent fasting; certain medications (e.g., acetaminophen, cancer drug irinotecan)

Risk factors: family history of Gilbert syndrome (to inherit the disorder, both parents must carry the gene)

Investigations: elevated unconjugated bilirubin, normal CBC

OTHER (E.G., CELIAC DISEASE)

CELIAC DISEASE

Signs and symptoms: family history of celiac disease, or signs and symptoms of celiac disease (chronic abdominal pain, rashes)

Investigations: positive serum anti-tTG (with IgA level); duodenal biopsy to detect villous blunting

Strategy for patient encounter

The likely scenario is a patient who is feeling systemically unwell, with blood work that shows abnormal liver function. Note that abnormal liver function may be discovered incidentally, as part of the workup for systemic disease, abdominal pain, or jaundice. The specified tasks could engage history, physical exam, investigations, or management.

History

Start with open-ended questions about the abnormality: How was it discovered? What other symptoms do you have? Listen for incidental discovery associated with a specific workup; and symptoms associated with particular entities (e.g., missed menstrual periods in pregnancy; sudden-onset abdominal pain that is worse with deep breaths in gallstones; rash and chronic abdominal pain in celiac disease). Ask about a family history of liver disease. Ask about alcohol and drug use. Ask about risk factors for viral hepatitis (unprotected sex, intravenous drug abuse, blood transfusions, tattoos, body piercings, imprisonment, workplace exposure to body fluids) and about immunizations for hepatitis A and B viruses (HAV, HBV).

Physical exam

Obtain the patient's vital signs, looking for fever. Examine the skin and sclera for jaundice. Examine the abdomen, looking for an enlarged and/or tender liver and spleen, and for ascites. Check for stigmata of chronic liver disease (e.g., palmar erythema, spider angioma, gynecomastia). Note the presence of lymphadenopathy (posterior cervical in infectious mononucleosis).

Investigations

In all patients, order:

- a complete blood count (CBC)
- liver function tests: bilirubin, total and direct; alanine aminotransferase (ALT); alkaline phosphatase (ALP); γ-glutamyltransferase (GGT); and prothrombin time/ international normalized ratio (PT/INR)
- a creatinine test
- serology for infectious causes
- an ultrasound or CT scan of the abdomen

Consider other tests depending on the likely entity (see the information this resource lists in the MCC differential diagnosis).

Management

Treat the underlying condition. Identify complications from the presence of liver disease (e.g., bleeding, ascites). Consider referring the patient to a hepatologist or general surgeon.

78

Lump or mass, musculoskeletal

MCC particular objective

Distinguish benign from malignant disease.

MCC differential diagnosis
with added evidence

NEOPLASTIC CONDITIONS

Soft tissue

BENIGN (E.G., LIPOMA)

LIPOMA

This is a subcutaneous lesion made of adipose tissue.

Signs and symptoms: age 40 to 60 years (more common); family history of lipoma (often); smooth, soft, movable, painless, mass; usually small (< 5 cm in diameter); slow growing; located on the upper extremities, neck, trunk, axillae (common)

Investigations: ultrasound; MRI

MALIGNANT (E.G., LEIOMYOSARCOMA)

LEIOMYOSARCOMA

This is a smooth muscle tumour.

Symptoms: postmenopausal bleeding; vaginal discharge; pelvic pain (in uterine leiomyosarcoma); abdominal pain; bloating

> Common locations: uterus, stomach, small intestine, retroperitoneum

Investigations: biopsy to detect microscopic features (tumour cell necrosis, atypia, high mitotic activity)

Bone

BENIGN (E.G., CYST)

CYST

This is a fluid-filled hole inside a bone.

It can clinically or radiologically mimic solitary bone tumour.

Signs and symptoms: child, young adult (more common); generally asymptomatic; pain; swelling

Investigations: X-ray

MALIGNANT (E.G., EWING SARCOMA)

EWING SARCOMA

This is a rare cancer. It can occur in any bone.

Signs and symptoms: child, young adult (typically); pain and swelling at the site of the tumour

> Common location: in and around the bone

Investigations: bone scan, X-ray, or CT scan to locate the primary tumour and detect possible metastasis; biopsy

NONNEOPLASTIC

Infection (e.g., osteomyelitis)

OSTEOMYELITIS

Signs and symptoms: fever; lethargy; irritability; site-specific pain; bone instability and tenderness; erythema; swelling; delayed wound healing; exposed bone (highly specific for osteomyelitis)

> Children: acute osteomyelitis (more common) in the long bones of the legs and upper arms (more common)

> Adults: chronic osteomyelitis (more common) in the vertebrae (more common); motor and/or sensory dysfunction in the limbs

Risk factors: diabetes mellitus; peripheral vascular disease; trauma; intravenous (IV) drugs or catheters

Investigations: CBC to detect inflammation markers; bone biopsy (definitive)

Trauma (e.g., hematoma)

HEMATOMA

Hematomas may reduce the mobility of an affected limb and present with symptoms similar to a fracture.

Signs and symptoms: history of trauma; painful lump or mass that is initially firm, and purple/blue in colour (later: spongy, flattening, and yellow/brown)

Investigations (the diagnosis is usually clinical): blood tests (CBC, hemoglobin, hematocrit, PT/INR)

Inflammatory condition (e.g., rheumatoid nodules, tendonitis)

RHEUMATOID ARTHRITIS

This is a chronic, systemic, inflammatory disease that involves synovial joints.

Signs and symptoms: symmetrical symptoms; pain, stiffness (morning stiffness); swelling in multiple joints that improves with movement; symptoms that progress from the periphery to proximal joints; decreased grip strength; fatigue; fever; weight loss; impaired activities of daily living; joint deformities and locomotor disability (in later disease); rheumatoid nodules in the fingers, knuckles, elbows, forearms, knees, backs of heels (in about 25% of cases)

> Common locations: metacarpophalangeal and proximal interphalangeal joints of the fingers; interphalangeal joints of the thumbs and wrists; metatarsophalangeal joints of the toes
>
> Other locations: synovial joints of the upper and lower limbs (elbows, shoulders, ankles, knees)

Investigations: blood tests (to detect autoantibodies of rheumatoid factors and/or anti–citrullinated peptide or protein antibodies; anemia; thrombocytosis; elevated ESR; elevated CRP); tests of synovial fluid (leukocyte count of 1500–25,000/mm^3 with predominance of polymorphonuclear cells); X-rays of the hands and feet to detect narrowing joint spaces, and erosions of bone and cartilage

TENDINITIS

Signs and symptoms: history of chronic repetitive low-grade trauma or overuse (common); history of sports injury (common); pain on palpation of the affected tendon; pain with tendon loading

> Achilles tendon: heel pain (this is common in runners)
>
> Biceps: anterior shoulder pain in the bicipital groove that is worse on flexing the shoulder or supination of the forearm
>
> Lateral epicondylitis ("tennis elbow"): pain of the lateral elbow that is worse on grasping and twisting
>
> Medial epicondylitis ("golfer's elbow"): pain of the medial elbow
>
> Patellar ("jumper's knee"): male (more common); history of sports involving jumping and running (common); pain on standing up from sitting, and climbing stairs or hills
>
> Rotator cuff, shoulder: dull, aching shoulder pain that is difficult to localize and radiates into the upper arm toward the chest; painful range of motion

Strategy for patient encounter

The likely scenario is a patient with a musculoskeletal mass, discovered incidentally. The specified tasks could engage history, physical exam, investigations, or management.

History

Start with open-ended questions about the mass: How did you discover it? How has it changed since you discovered it? What other symptoms do you have? Listen for evidence consistent with particular entities (e.g., a history of trauma; pelvic or abdominal pain in leiomyosarcoma; worsening pain with use in tendinitis; morning stiffness in rheumatoid arthritis; systemic symptoms in osteomyelitis and rheumatoid arthritis). Ask about a family history of sarcoma. Ask about a history of genetic disorders that predispose to sarcoma (neurofibromatosis, Gardner syndrome, retinoblastoma, Li-Fraumeni syndrome). Ask about exposure to radiation (e.g., a history of cancer treatment).

Physical exam

Examine the mass (or surrounding area if it was discovered by radiology). Look for skin changes and enlarged regional lymph nodes. The main goal is to determine the need for imaging and biopsy.

Investigations

Order imaging as indicated (see the information this resource lists in the MCC differential diagnosis). Have a low threshold for performing a tissue biopsy, especially in an exam situation. Features that argue in favour of biopsy include a mass of large size and/or a firm, painless mass.

Management

In malignant masses, refer the patient to a surgeon or oncologist.

Pearls

Remember that a tissue specimen for histology is often necessary for diagnosis: "tissue is the issue."

79

Lymphadenopathy

MCC particular objectives
Determine the need for biopsy.

MCC differential diagnosis
with added evidence

LOCALIZED

Reactive condition (e.g., tonsillitis)
TONSILLITIS

Signs and symptoms: sore throat; difficulty swallowing; fever; scratchy voice; bad breath; stiff neck; intense erythema of tonsils and pharynx; swollen tonsils that may be coated in pus; swollen, tender regional lymph glands

Investigations: throat swab

Neoplastic (e.g., metastatic cancer)
METASTATIC CANCER

Signs and symptoms: history of cancer; constitutional symptoms (weight loss, fever, night sweats)

Investigations: blood tests (CBC with differential; platelet count; ESR); CT scan; tissue biopsy or fine needle aspiration biopsy for histology/ cytology and immunophenotyping

DIFFUSE

DIFFUSE LYMPHADENOPATHY IN GENERAL

Signs and symptoms: swollen lymph nodes in multiple locations, fever, fatigue, nausea, vomiting, loss of appetite, headaches, joint pain, sore throat

Infection (e.g., viral)
Signs and symptoms:

Mononucleosis: classic triad of fever, pharyngitis, lymphadenopathy (usually posterior cervical); fatigue and malaise; headache; abdominal pain; nausea, vomiting; rash; splenomegaly; palatal exanthems or petechiae

Hepatitis: viral-like illness; abdominal pain; jaundice; palpable, tender liver; history of hepatitis A, B, or C virus (HAV, HBV, HCV) or risk factors for them (autoimmune conditions, unprotected sex, intravenous drug abuse, blood transfusions, tattoos, body piercings, imprisonment, workplace exposure to body fluids)

HCV: often asymptomatic

HIV: flu-like symptoms in the first, acute phase; leukopenia in the second, latent, asymptomatic stage (200–499 CD4 cells/μL); lymphadenopathy

Cytomegalovirus: muscle aches, rash

Dengue: pain behind the eyes; rash that appears 2 to 5 days after fever onset

Investigations: blood antigen or antibody tests; urinalysis; throat culture (in suspected strep throat)

Inflammatory condition (e.g., sarcoidosis)

SARCOIDOSIS

Signs and symptoms: lymphadenopathy (a mass in the middle of the mediastinum is the most common lesion), fever, fatigue, weight loss, lung symptoms (dry cough, shortness of breath, wheezing, chest pain)

Risk factors: age 20 to 40, African descent, family history of sarcoidosis

Investigations: chest X-ray to detect enlarged hilar and mediastinal lymph nodes; biopsy to detect granulomas

Neoplastic condition (e.g., lymphoma)

LYMPHOMA

Signs and symptoms (non-Hodgkin): constitutional symptoms (fatigue, fever, night sweats, weight loss), enlarged lymph nodes, chest pain, coughing, shortness of breath

Hodgkin lymphoma (less common): constitutional symptoms (fatigue, fever, night sweats, weight loss); enlarged lymph nodes; itching or pain on drinking alcohol, or increased sensitivity to alcohol

Investigations: blasts or cancer cells on peripheral blood smear; excess blasts or cancer cells on bone marrow examination

Strategy for patient encounter

The likely scenario is a patient with enlarged lymph nodes in the neck. The specified tasks could engage history, physical exam, investigations, or management.

History

Use open-ended questions to establish the duration of the lymphadenopathy and the accompanying symptoms: How long have you had swollen glands? What other symptoms do you have? Listen for recent swelling versus long-standing, more insidious swelling (long-standing swelling suggests a noninfectious condition); and for constitutional symptoms (fever, weight loss, fatigue, and/or night sweats, which also suggest a noninfectious condition). Ask about a personal or family history of cancer and sarcoidosis.

Physical exam

Examine the submandibular, axillary, inguinal, and supraclavicular regions for enlarged nodes. Examine any enlarged nodes noted by the patient. If you identify localized lymphadenopathy, look for an adjacent precipitating lesion (e.g., local infection). Ask the patient if identified enlarged lymph nodes are tender (nontender nodes are more likely in malignant conditions). Examine the spleen for enlargement. In the case of cervical lymphadenopathy, perform a full exam of the head and neck, including the oral cavity, looking for infections and tumours. In the case of axillary lymphadenopathy, perform a breast exam. Examine the skin for rashes.

Investigations

In cases of generalized lymphadenopathy, or where lymphadenopathy has been present for more than 3 to 4 weeks, perform a lymph node biopsy. Order a complete blood count (CBC). Consider specific tests for infection (see the information this resource lists in the MCC's differential diagnosis). Order a CT scan or MRI scan of the affected area(s) to look for internal masses and additional lymphadenopathy.

Management

Most patients with localized lymphadenopathy have a benign infectious cause. Further management will be based on imaging and biopsy results.

Pearls

As a general rule, lymph nodes > 1 cm in diameter are considered abnormal.

80

Mediastinal mass

MCC particular objective
Differentiate among causes based on compartment location.

MCC differential diagnosis
with added evidence

ANTERIOR

Tumour (e.g., thymoma, lymphoma)
THYMOMA

This is the most common neoplasm of the thymus in adults, and the most common anterior mediastinal mass.

It is usually found incidentally during imaging.

It is benign unless it invades through the capsule.

Signs and symptoms: age 40 to 60 (more common); asymptomatic (usual); thoracic symptoms in large tumours (chest pain, shortness of breath, cough, phrenic nerve palsy); paraneoplastic syndrome (myasthenia gravis is the most common: weakness of voluntary skeletal muscles, fatigue, double vision, drooping eyelids, difficulty swallowing)

> Metastasized thymoma: pleural or pericardial effusion, thoracic symptoms

Investigations: CT scan or MRI of mass; resection of mass

LYMPHOMA

Signs and symptoms (non-Hodgkin): constitutional symptoms (fatigue, fever, night sweats, weight loss), enlarged lymph nodes, chest pain, coughing, shortness of breath

> Hodgkin lymphoma (less common): constitutional symptoms (fatigue, fever, night sweats, weight loss); enlarged lymph nodes; itching or pain on drinking alcohol, or increased sensitivity to alcohol

Investigations: blasts or cancer cells on peripheral blood smear; excess blasts or cancer cells on bone marrow examination

Other (e.g., aneurysm)
ANEURYSM

Examples include thoracic aortic aneurysm in the chest cavity and abdominal aortic aneurysm.

Signs and symptoms: pain in the chest or abdomen; back pain

Investigations: echocardiogram or transesophageal ultrasound (in thoracic aneurysm) or abdominal ultrasound (in abdominal aneurysm); chest X-ray to detect masses; CT scan for detailed images; MRI to characterize for size and location

MIDDLE

Tumour (e.g., bronchogenic cancer)

BRONCHOGENIC CANCER (LUNG CANCER)

Signs and symptoms: asymptomatic (usual in early disease); changes in a chronic cough; hemoptysis; shortness of breath; wheezing; hoarseness; weight loss; bone pain; headache

Risk factors: smoking or secondhand-smoke exposure; family history of lung cancer

Investigations: X-ray, CT scan to detect masses and lesions; biopsy

Other (e.g., sarcoidosis)

SARCOIDOSIS

This involves growth of tiny granulomas, most commonly in the lungs, lymph nodes, and skin.

It is usually detected incidentally through X-rays for another reason.

Signs and symptoms: lymphadenopathy (a mass in the middle of the mediastinum is the most common lesion), fever, fatigue, weight loss, lung symptoms (dry cough, shortness of breath, wheezing, chest pain)

Risk factors: age 20 to 40, African descent, family history of sarcoidosis

Investigations: chest X-ray to detect enlarged hilar and mediastinal lymph nodes; biopsy to detect granulomas

POSTERIOR

Tumour (e.g., esophageal cancer)

ESOPHAGEAL CANCER

Signs and symptoms: asymptomatic (often in early disease); pain with swallowing; heartburn-like pain; hoarse cough; nausea, vomiting (sometimes with blood)

Risk factors: smoking, alcohol use, family history

Other (e.g., hiatal hernia)

HIATAL HERNIA

Signs and symptoms: asymptomatic (sometimes); symptoms of gastroesophageal reflux (burning chest pain radiating into the throat with bitter taste in mouth; pain that is worse with lying down and certain foods, better with standing up or antacids; acid damage to teeth)

> Larger hernias: syncope (swallow syncope syndrome); shortness of breath; edema; reduced exercise tolerance with heart failure

Investigations: esophageal X-ray (barium swallow); upper
gastrointestinal endoscopy; manometry; ECG (if cardiac involvement
is suspected)

Strategy for patient encounter

The likely scenario is a patient who has difficulty swallowing, and
with radiology that shows mediastinal mass. The specified tasks
could engage history, physical exam, investigations, or management.

History

Use open-ended inquiry to confirm the patient's mediastinal
mass symptoms: Please tell me about the symptoms you've been
experiencing. Listen for cough, stridor, hemoptysis, shortness of
breath, chest pain, difficulty swallowing, and vocal hoarseness.

Physical exam

Obtain the patient's vital signs (hypotension may be present due
to tamponade or cardiac compression). Examine the face and
upper limbs for swelling (relevant to superior vena cava syndrome). Auscultate the lungs listening for stridor. Examine the
eyes looking for Horner syndrome (unilateral decreased pupil
size and drooping eyelid).

Investigations

Order a CT scan or MRI scan of the chest. Consider other tests
as indicated (see the information this resource lists in the MCC
differential diagnosis).

Management

Refer to thoracic surgery for tissue biopsy and further management.

81

Amenorrhea, oligomenorrhea

MCC particular objectives

Rule out pregnancy first.

In amenorrhea, differentiate between primary and secondary conditions.

MCC differential diagnosis
with added evidence

PRIMARY

Definition: absence of menstruation (i.e., menstruation has not started) in girls age 15 or older, with or without the appearance of other signs of puberty

Central

HYPOTHALAMUS (E.G., FUNCTIONAL)

FUNCTIONAL HYPOTHALAMIC AMENORRHEA

Causes include stress; weight loss (e.g., dieting) or being underweight (e.g., anorexia nervosa); and excessive exercise (e.g., training for a sport).

PITUITARY

PROLACTINOMA

This is the most common type of functioning pituitary tumour.

Signs and symptoms (microprolactinoma):

> General: galactorrhea; clinical signs of estrogen deficiency (vaginal dryness, painful intercourse, decreased bone density in the lower spine and forearm)

> Reproductive-age women: menstrual disturbance (oligomenorrhea, amenorrhea, irregularity) and/or infertility

> Younger women: delayed menarche

> Prepubertal females: hyperprolactinemia

Signs and symptoms (macroprolactinoma): headaches when stretching; vision problems (bitemporal hemianopsia)

Investigations: elevated serum prolactin (> 20 ng/mL); MRI of the head to detect mass in the sella turcica

Ovary (e.g., ovarian dysgenesis, polycystic ovary syndrome)

OVARIAN DYSGENESIS

An example is congenital lack of ovaries.

POLYCYSTIC OVARY SYNDROME

Signs and symptoms: symptom onset after puberty, with increased rate of hair growth and male-pattern hair growth; irregular menstruation; infertility; obesity; acne

Investigations: LH:FSH ratio (elevated: 2:1 or 3:1) (usual); elevated testosterone; ultrasound to detect ovarian cysts; normal prolactin levels; normal thyroid function

Vaginal, outflow tract (e.g., imperforate hymen)

IMPERFORATE HYMEN

This is a structural abnormality of the vagina preventing visible menstrual bleeding by blocking the outflow of blood, without changes in hormone levels or impairment in the development of sexual characteristics.

Signs and symptoms: feeling of fullness in the lower abdomen; pelvic, abdominal, back pain

Investigations: pelvic ultrasound

SECONDARY

Definition: absence of menstruation (sudden cessation) for ≥ 6 months in women who have otherwise experienced normal menstrual cycles

Pregnancy

This is the most common cause.

Signs and symptoms: amenorrhea, especially during childbearing years (some experience spotting); sexual activity, especially without contraception or with inconsistent use of contraception; nausea, vomiting (common early sign); breast enlargement and tenderness; increased frequency of urination without pain or difficulty; fatigue

Investigations: blood or urine β-hCG

Central

HYPOTHALAMUS (E.G., FUNCTIONAL, EXOGENOUS HORMONES)

FUNCTIONAL HYPOTHALAMIC AMENORRHEA—SEE ABOVE

EXOGENOUS HORMONES

An example is glucocorticoid therapy.

PITUITARY (E.G., PROLACTINOMA)

PROLACTINOMA—SEE ABOVE

Other endocrine condition (e.g., thyroid disorders)

THYROID DISORDERS

HYPOTHYROIDISM

Signs and symptoms: history of hypothyroidism or symptoms of hypothyroidism (cold intolerance, decreased reflexes, dry skin, weight gain, impaired cognition)

Investigations: elevated thyrotropin (TSH)

HYPERTHYROIDISM

Signs and symptoms: history of hyperthyroidism or symptoms of hyperthyroidism (changes in menstrual patterns, enlarged thyroid, tachycardia, palpitations, diarrhea, muscle weakness, tremor, hyperactive reflexes, weight loss, sweating, thinning hair)

Investigations: decreased thyrotropin (TSH)

Ovary (e.g., oophorectomy, chemotherapy)

Uterus (e.g., Asherman syndrome)

ASHERMAN SYNDROME

This is scarring of the endometrial or myometrial layers of the uterine wall, preventing the normal buildup and shedding of the uterine lining.

Signs and symptoms: history of uterine surgery (e.g., dilation and curettage; cesarean section; treatment for uterine fibroids)

Investigations: ultrasound of the pelvis; hysteroscopy

Strategy for patient encounter

The likely scenario is an adult patient with amenorrhea. The specified tasks could engage history, physical exam, investigations, or management.

History

Use open-ended questions to obtain a menstrual and gynecological history: When was your last period? How regular is your usual cycle? What gynecological procedures or surgeries have you had (e.g., dilation and curettage, cesarean section, treatment for uterine fibroids, oophorectomy)? Ask about other symptoms the patient is experiencing and listen for evidence of thyroid disease (e.g., dry skin, weight gain, and impaired cognition in hypothyroidism; enlarged thyroid, weight loss, and palpitations in hyperthyroidism) and prolactinoma (e.g., vaginal dryness, galactorrhea). Take a medication history, listening for glucocorticoid therapy and chemotherapy. Ask about recent weight changes (unless the patient has already volunteered this) and changes in exercise routines.

Physical exam

Measure the patient's height and weight, and calculate their body mass index (BMI). Examine the patient for hirsutism, acne, and acanthosis nigricans (hyperpigmentation that is often found in the armpits, groin, and folds of the neck). Perform a pelvic exam to exclude abnormalities such as uterine masses.

(State that you will perform a pelvic exam. Since pelvic exams are not performed on standardized patients, the examiner will likely interrupt, ask what you are looking for, and provide findings.)

Investigations

For all patients, order a pregnancy test. In nonpregnant patients, order tests for thyrotropin (TSH), luteinizing hormone (LH), follicle-stimulating hormone (FSH), estradiol, and testosterone. Consider a test for serum prolactin and an MRI of the head to evaluate the pituitary gland. Consider a pelvic ultrasound or CT scan.

Management

Manage any underlying conditions. Consider referral to an endocrinologist or gynecologist. The approach to treatment of functional hypothalamic amenorrhea includes medical, dietary, and mental health support.

82

Dysmenorrhea

MCC particular objective

Differentiate primary from secondary dysmenorrhea.

MCC differential diagnosis
with added evidence

PRIMARY/IDIOPATHIC (NO PELVIC ABNORMALITY)

Primary dysmenorrhea involves no underlying medical condition, and no identifiable uterine or pelvic cause.

Signs and symptoms: constant, throbbing, dull or intense pain in the lower abdomen that radiates to the back and thighs, usually just before or during menstruation

SECONDARY (ACQUIRED) (E.G., INFECTION, ENDOMETRIOSIS, ADNEXAL ABNORMALITIES)

INFECTION (PELVIC INFLAMMATORY DISEASE)

Signs and symptoms: lower abdominal and pelvic pain; pain during intercourse; fever; urinary symptoms; vaginal discharge; irregular menstruation; pelvic tenderness and pain associated with 1 or both adnexa

> History of gonorrhea, chlamydia, or risk factors for them (multiple partners, unprotected sex); intrauterine device (IUD); childbirth; gynecologic procedure

Investigations: cultures for gonorrhea and chlamydia; ultrasound (this has normal findings)

ENDOMETRIOSIS

Signs and symptoms: pelvic pain associated with menstruation (very common); excessive bleeding during menstruation; pain during intercourse; pain during urination or bowel movement; tenderness on pelvic exam; normal findings on abdominal exam (common)

Risk factors: family history of endometriosis; nulliparity; personal history of pelvic inflammatory disease

Investigations: ultrasound to detect ovarian cysts (common finding); laparoscopy with biopsy

ADNEXAL ABNORMALITIES

OVARIAN CANCER

Signs and symptoms: postmenopausal female (more common); asymptomatic in early stage (usual); abdominal bloating, discomfort, distention (ascites); ovarian or pelvic mass; frequent urination and

urge to urinate; abnormal vaginal bleeding; fatigue; gastrointestinal
symptoms (nausea, heartburn, diarrhea, constipation, early satiety);
shortness of breath
Investigations: transvaginal and abdominal ultrasound; CA 125 blood
test; pelvic or abdominal CT scan; analysis of ascitic fluid; biopsy

Strategy for patient encounter

The likely scenario is a perimenopausal woman with dysmenorrhea. The specified tasks could engage history, physical exam,
investigations, or management.

History

Start with open-ended questions about the timing and quality of
pelvic pain, and other symptoms: How closely does the pain coin-
cide with menstruation or bleeding? What is the pain like? What
other symptoms do you have? Listen for symptoms consistent
with particular entities (e.g., pain that radiates to the thighs in primary dysmenorrhea; heavy menstruation in endometriosis; fever
and/or vaginal discharge in infection; gastrointestinal symptoms
in ovarian cancer). Ask whether the woman has given birth (this
is relevant to endometriosis). Ask about risk factors for pelvic inflammatory disease (history of sexually transmitted infections,
use of an intrauterine device, multiple sexual partners, gynecological procedures). Ask about a family history of endometriosis.

Physical exam

Perform a pelvic exam, looking for pelvic tenderness and pelvic
masses, to exclude possible causes of secondary dysmenorrhea.

(State that you will perform a pelvic exam. Since pelvic exams
are not performed on standardized patients, the examiner will
likely interrupt, ask what you are looking for, and provide findings.)

Investigations

For all patients, order a pregnancy test. Perform a pap smear, cultures for gonorrhea and chlamydia, and an endometrial biopsy.
Order a pelvic ultrasound to exclude uterine and ovarian masses.

Management

Consider referral to a gynecologist. Start management with analgesics and nonsteroidal antiinflammatory drugs (NSAIDs),

which are effective in up to 70% of women. Consider prescribing oral contraceptives. Some alternative therapies (heat, thiamine, magnesium, vitamin E) may be beneficial for some women.

Pearls

Dysmenorrhea is the most common gynecological disorder, regardless of age or ethnicity. It affects up to 95% of women.

83

Premenstrual dysphoric disorder (premenstrual syndrome)

MCC particular objective

Differentiate premenstrual dysphoric disorder from normal premenstrual symptoms, or from other causes of physical and mood changes.

MCC differential diagnosis
with added evidence

PREMENSTRUAL DYSPHORIC DISORDER[1(pp171–172)]

Signs and symptoms: symptoms synchronous with the menstrual cycle (present in the week before menstruation, improving during menstruation, resolved in the week after menstruation); symptoms during most menstrual cycles for ≥ 1 year; symptoms with significant impact on day-to-day life

> Key symptoms: mood swings, irritability, depressed mood, and anxiety
>
> Other symptoms: loss of interest in usual activities; loss of concentration; fatigue; changes in eating and sleeping routines; a sense of loss of control; physical symptoms (e.g., breast tenderness, joint or muscle pain, "bloating," or weight gain)
>
> **No** evidence of thyroid disorder, anemia, or exacerbation of a preexisting mental disorder (e.g., major depressive disorder)

Strategy for patient encounter

The likely scenario is a patient with anger and mood swings

before her period. The specified tasks could engage history, investigations, or management. Physical exam does not usually contribute useful information for diagnosing or managing premenstrual dysphoric disorder.

History

Obtain a history of the patient's symptoms to determine if the symptoms are cyclical. Ask the patient to complete a symptom diary if there is uncertainty about the timing of symptoms. Ask about symptoms of major depressive disorder (e.g., mood symptoms that persist for 2 or more weeks, significant weight change, recurrent thoughts of death or suicide) and risk factors for major depressive disorder (e.g., family history of depression, anxiety, and/or suicide; personal history of substance abuse).

Investigations

In cases of uncertain diagnosis, order a complete blood count (CBC) to rule out anemia, and a thyrotropin test (TSH) to rule out hypothyroidism.

Management

Counsel the patient on lifestyle modifications (diet, exercise, stress reduction). Consider prescribing oral contraceptives to suppress ovulation. Consider the prescription of a selective serotonin reuptake inhibitor (SSRI) to help manage symptoms.

Pearls

Hypothyroidism and anemia may have similar symptoms to premenstrual dysphoric disorder. Exclusion of these conditions is key.

TIP

Tailoring information to individual patients

The MCC identifies providing generic information as a common exam error.

To avoid this error, ask patients about aspects of their lives that might affect their condition. Provide information that targets their situation and engage the patient in figuring out next steps.

For example, better management of stress might be relevant for this case:

- Ask the patient for an example of a stressful situation they encountered last week. What steps could help relieve that situation?

REFERENCE

1 American Psychiatric Association. Diagnostic and statistical manual of mental disorders. 5th ed. Arlington, VA: American Psychiatric Association; 2013. 59–60. 991 p.

84

Menopause

MCC particular objective

Explain and prevent the undesirable effects of menopause.

MCC differential diagnosis

None stated. The MCC defines the focus of this clinical presentation as physiological menopause only.

Strategy for patient encounter

The likely scenario is a menopausal woman with hot flashes. The specified tasks could engage history, investigations, or management. Physical exam does not usually contribute useful information for diagnosing or managing menopause.

History

Take a menstrual history: When was your last period? How old are you? Menopause usually occurs around age 50. It is marked by the last period a woman has: 1 year after the last period the woman is considered "postmenopausal." Ask about the patient's symptoms. Listen for typical symptoms of menopause (e.g., vaginal dryness, chills, hot flashes, night sweats, sleep disturbance, weight gain, irritability). Ask about possible symptoms of hypothyroidism, which can mimic menopause (e.g., dry skin, weight gain, impaired cognition). Ask about age of menopause in the patient's mother and sisters.

TIP

Tailoring information to individual patients

The MCC identifies providing generic information as a common exam error.

To avoid this error, ask patients about aspects of their lives that might affect their condition. Provide information that targets their situation and engage the patient in figuring out next steps.

For example, in the case of hot flashes:

- Ask where the woman works and lives. A woman who works in an office and/or lives in an apartment building may have little control over ambient temperature. Could she install a fan?

- Consider how the woman is dressed today. To what extent has she dressed in layers? How could she make different clothing choices to enhance layering?

Investigations

Investigations are usually not indicated. In cases where the diagnosis of menopause is uncertain, consider tests for follicle-stimulating hormone (FSH), estrogen (estradiol), and thyrotropin (TSH).

Management

Discuss how to manage the patient's symptoms. For vaginal dryness, suggest water- or silicone-based lubricants. For hot flashes, suggest dressing in layers and maintaining cool ambient temperatures. Maintaining a good diet and exercising regularly may also help. Consider treatment of vasomotor symptoms with a selective serotonin reuptake inhibitor (SSRI, in this case paroxetine). Consider hormone replacement therapy (HRT) in patients with severe symptoms or in those with menopause at an early age. Counsel the patient about adequate dietary calcium and vitamin D supplementation to prevent accelerated loss of bone mineral density.

85

Coma

MCC particular objective

Pay particular attention to emergent and urgent conditions.

MCC differential diagnosis
with added evidence

COMA IN GENERAL

Definition: severe impairment of consciousness or alertness, and decreased responsiveness to external stimuli; lack of arousal to any stimulation

FOCAL DISEASE (E.G., TUMOUR, STROKE)

BRAIN TUMOUR

Types of brain tumour include meningioma, astrocytoma, oligodendroglioma, glioblastoma, and Schwannoma.

Signs and symptoms: acute-onset headaches; older than 50; change in chronic headache pattern; increasing intensity and frequency of headaches; headaches that disturb sleep; unilateral headache pain, always on the same side; position-evoked crescendo headache; impaired vision; light-headedness

> Other symptoms: focal seizures, confusion, memory loss, personality change

Investigations: imaging for intracranial masses (MRI with contrast enhancement is best for tumours and abscesses); biopsy

ACUTE STROKE

Coma can ensue from extensive cerebrovascular accident.

Signs and symptoms: speech difficulty and hemiparesis (most common symptoms); weakness or paralysis in the extremities or face; arm or leg numbness; confusion; headache; nonorthostatic dizziness; fever

DIFFUSE DISEASE

Vascular disorder (e.g., hypertensive encephalopathy)

HYPERTENSIVE ENCEPHALOPATHY

This occurs during a hypertensive crisis and requires immediate intervention to reduce blood pressure.

Signs and symptoms: history of hypertension (usual), or use of medications (e.g., epinephrine, Ritalin) or drugs (e.g., cocaine, methamphetamine) that can cause hypertension; headache; confusion; blurred vision; seizure; nausea, vomiting; symptoms of end-organ damage (cardiovascular symptoms, hematuria, or renal failure)

Infection (e.g., meningitis, encephalitis)

MENINGITIS

Signs and symptoms: fever, headache, Kernig sign (flexing the patient's hip 90 degrees, then extending the knee, causes pain), Brudzinski neck sign (flexing the patient's neck causes flexion of hips and knees)

> Neonates: poor feeding, lethargy, irritability, apnea, listlessness, apathy, hypothermia, seizures, jaundice, bulging fontanelle, pallor, shock, hypotonia, hypoglycemia

> Infants and children: nuchal rigidity, opisthotonos, convulsions, photophobia, alterations of the sensorium, irritability, lethargy, anorexia, nausea, vomiting, coma

Investigations: positive culture in CSF; meningeal inflammation (increased pleocytosis, low glucose in CSF); CSF absolute neutrophil count $\geq 1000/\mu L$; CSF protein level ≥ 80 mg/dL; peripheral blood absolute neutrophil count $\geq 10,000/\mu L$; CT scan, MRI

ENCEPHALITIS

Viral infection is the most common cause: herpes simplex virus, type 1 and type 2 (HSV-1, HSV-2); Epstein-Barr virus (EBV); varicella-zoster virus; Enterovirus (e.g., Coxsackievirus); and insect-borne viruses (e.g., West Nile disease, Lyme disease).

Signs and symptoms: seizures, altered mental status (e.g., decreased level of consciousness, lethargy, personality change, behaviour change), fever, headache, nausea, vomiting

> Infants and neonates: poor feeding, irritability, lethargy
>
> Children and adolescents: irritability, movement disorder, ataxia, stupor, coma, hemiparesis, cranial nerve defect, status epilepticus (severe symptom)
>
> Adults: motor or sensory deficits; speech or movement impairment; flaccid paralysis

Investigations: blood tests (CBC, differential, platelets, electrolytes, glucose, BUN, creatinine, aminotransferases, coagulation); MRI (to detect brain edema; inflammation of the cerebral cortex, gray-white matter junction, thalamus, basal ganglia); CSF tests (perform lumbar puncture after results of MRI; order CSF protein, glucose, cell count, differential, Gram stain, bacterial culture); EEG (usually abnormal) to differentiate from nonconvulsive seizure activity

Trauma

Investigations: CT scan to detect hematomas, contusions, skull fractures; MRI to detect subtler findings

Metabolic condition (e.g., uremia, hypercalcemia, hypoglycemia)

UREMIA

Signs and symptoms: history of chronic kidney disease or injury; itchiness

Investigations: blood tests (creatinine, eGFR, potassium, phosphate, calcium, sodium)

HYPERCALCEMIA

Signs and symptoms: constipation, polyuria, polydipsia, dehydration, anorexia, nausea, muscle weakness, altered sensory status

> History of sarcoidosis, malignancy, hyperparathyroidism, immobilization

Investigations: blood test (hypercalcemia is total calcium ≥ 2.63 mmol/L or ionized calcium ≥ 1.4 mmol/L); albumin; PTH

HYPOGLYCEMIA

The most common cause is diabetes treatment.

Signs and symptoms: palpitations, pallor, sweating, nightmares, fatigue, hunger

> Severe: confusion, disorientation, blurred vision, seizures, coma

Investigations: low plasma glucose level (symptoms typically develop at concentrations ≤ 3.0 mmol/L)

Substance use and overdose

Examples of common overdose substances include acetylsalicylic acid (ASA), acetaminophen, anticholinergics (e.g., tricyclics), sympathomimetics (e.g., amphetamines, cocaine), depressants (e.g., alcohol, opiates, sedatives, hypnotics), hallucinogens (e.g., amphetamines), and serotonergics (e.g., selective serotonin reuptake inhibitors).

Signs and symptoms: personal or family history of substance abuse; excessive worry; loss of interest in friends and usual activities; adverse experience (e.g., abuse, death of a friend or family member); physical evidence (track marks on the arms, nasal septum perforation); tachycardia; tremor and/or sweating

> Acetaminophen poisoning: nausea, vomiting; lethargy; pallor; liver enlargement and tenderness

> Salicylate poisoning: abdominal pain, tinnitus, nausea, vomiting (blood in the vomit), hyperthermia, mental status changes (e.g., agitation and seizures; or lethargy, central nervous system depression, and coma)

Investigations: toxicology screen for suspected substance

SEIZURES

Signs and symptoms: history of seizures (e.g., epilepsy)

Investigations: brain and head imaging to detect injury or abnormal brain anatomy; EEG

Strategy for patient encounter

The likely scenario is a patient in the emergency room with decreased level of consciousness. The specified tasks could engage history, physical exam, investigations, or management.

History

The patient will be unable to give a history, so seek collateral information from accompanying caregivers.

Start with open-ended questions about the circumstances surrounding the coma: Where was the patient found? What relevant evidence was found with the patient (e.g., drug paraphernalia)? Ask about medical conditions, medications, trauma, and drug use. Obtain any available medical records.

Physical exam

Use the Glasgow coma scale to document the degree of the patient's unresponsiveness (see the checklist). Perform a neurological exam. Examine the patient's arms for evidence of injection drug use. Obtain the patient's vital signs, looking particularly for fever (this suggests infection or stroke).

CHECKLIST
Glasgow coma scale

ASSESSMENT FOCUS	FINDING	SCORE
Eyes	Do not open to any stimulus	1
	Open in response to pain	2
	Open in response to speech	3
	Open spontaneously	4
Limbs	Do not respond to any stimulus	1
	Extend in response to pain	2
	Flex abnormally in response to pain	3
	Withdraw in response to pain	4
	Exhibit localized pain (patient can point to area)	5
	Respond to commands	6
Speech	Patient does not speak	1
	Makes incomprehensible sounds	2
	Uses inappropriate words	3
	Makes confused conversation	4
	Communicates well	5

Interpretation
Score < 9 severely reduced consciousness; score 9–12 moderately reduced consciousness; score 13–14 mildly reduced consciousness; score 15 normal consciousness

Reprinted from The Lancet, Vol. 2, Teasdale G and Jennett B, Assessment of coma and impaired consciousness: a practical scale, pages 81–84, 1974, with permission from Elsevier.

Investigations
On all comatose patients, perform a point-of-care glucose test (hypoglycemia is a relatively common and reversible cause of coma). Order a CT scan of the head. Order a complete blood count (CBC), urine drug screen, and tests for serum electrolytes, calcium, creatinine, glucose, liver enzymes, and thyrotropin (TSH). Consider a trial of naloxone for possible opioid overdose.

Management
Admit the patient to the intensive care unit (ICU) and consult a critical medicine physician.

86

Delirium

MCC particular objective

Pay particular attention to urgent and emergent conditions.

MCC differential diagnosis
with added evidence

DELIRIUM IN GENERAL

In addition to the disorders listed here (which come from the MCC's objectives for the exam), common causes of delirium include sensory deprivation (e.g., a patient in hospital might not have their glasses or hearing aids), urinary retention, fecaloma, and constipation.

Signs and symptoms: sudden-onset (hours to days), fluctuating symptoms that resolve on treatment of the underlying cause; changes in level of consciousness (hypoactivity, hyperactivity, or alternating states); impaired focus (e.g., confusion, disorientation); visual hallucinations

MEDICATIONS (E.G., SEDATIVE, ANTICHOLINERGIC)

Examples of sedatives include benzodiazepines (e.g., alprazolam, clorazepate, diazepam).

Examples of medications with anticholinergic properties include antihistamines, antidepressants (e.g., amitriptyline), cardiovascular medications (e.g., digoxin), antidiarrheals, gastrointestinal antispasmodics, and antiulcer medications.

The risk of delirium increases with the use of multiple medications, especially psychiatric drugs and sedatives in combination.

METABOLIC CONDITION (E.G., FLUID AND ELECTROLYTE DISTURBANCE)

Metabolic disorders can lead to hormone regulation dysfunction, which can trigger malfunction in brain activity.

Investigations: blood and urine tests to measure electrolyte and hormone levels

HYPOXIA (E.G., ANEMIA, HYPOPERFUSION)

Signs and symptoms (in general): shortness of breath; headache; confusion; history of anemia, heart disease, lung disease, pulmonary embolism

Investigations: CBC, ABG, chest X-ray, echocardiogram

INFECTION

Examples of infections that can cause delirium include urinary tract infection, pneumonia, meningitis, and encephalitis.

Investigations: blood tests to analyze immune function; blood and urine cultures; chest X-ray to detect pneumonia; lumbar puncture (CSF analysis) to detect pathogens

ENDOCRINE CONDITION (E.G., HYPOTHYROIDISM)

HYPOTHYROIDISM

Signs and symptoms: history of hypothyroidism or symptoms of hypothyroidism (cold intolerance, decreased reflexes, dry skin, weight gain, impaired cognition)

Investigations: elevated thyrotropin (TSH)

NEUROLOGICAL CONDITION (E.G., STROKE, DEMENTIA)

ACUTE STROKE

Signs and symptoms: speech difficulty and hemiparesis (most common symptoms); weakness or paralysis in the extremities or face; arm or leg numbness; confusion; headache; nonorthostatic dizziness; fever

DEMENTIA

Signs and symptoms: gradual impairment of ≥ 1 cognitive area (complex attention; executive function; learning and memory; language; perceptual-motor skills; social interaction); deficits that interfere with day-to-day life (e.g., ability to pay bills); **no** evidence that the cognitive impairment occurs only with delirium; **no** evidence of depression

POSTSURGICAL CONDITION

Postsurgical delirium is common, especially in the elderly.

Causes may include pain, pain medications, anesthesia, infection, or deep vein thrombosis.

Investigations: EEG to detect brain disturbances associated with pain

WITHDRAWAL (E.G., ALCOHOL, BENZODIAZEPINE)

ALCOHOL WITHDRAWAL

Signs and symptoms:

Mild withdrawal (symptoms start within 24 hours after cessation): tremulousness, insomnia, anxiety, hyperreflexia, sweating, gastrointestinal upset, mild autonomic hyperactivity

Moderate withdrawal (symptoms start within 24 to 48 hours after cessation): tremors, insomnia, excessive adrenergic symptoms, intense anxiety

Severe withdrawal (symptoms start > 48 hours after cessation): disorientation, agitation, hallucinations, tremulousness, tachycardia, tachypnea, hyperthermia, sweating

BENZODIAZEPINE WITHDRAWAL

Signs and symptoms (symptoms start within 6 to 48 hours after cessation): insomnia, irritability, sweating, dizziness, headache, anxiety, panic attacks, impaired cognition, hallucinations, seizures, nausea

TRAUMA

Investigations: EEG; brain CT scan or MRI

Strategy for patient encounter

The likely scenario is an elderly patient with confusion, whose caregiver is present. The specified tasks could engage history, physical exam, investigations, or management.

History

The patient will be unable to give a coherent history, so seek collateral information from accompanying caregivers.

Use open-ended questions about the onset of the delirium: When did the delirium begin? What other symptoms has the patient had? Listen for triggering events such as change in medication, surgery, substance withdrawal, or trauma; and for accompanying symptoms such as fever (this suggests infection) and speech difficulty (this suggests stroke).

Use open-ended questions to take a medical and medication history: What conditions has the patient been diagnosed with? What medications does the patient take? Listen for a history of hypothyroidism, dementia, and conditions related to hypoxia (e.g., anemia, heart disease, lung disease); and drugs associated with delirium (see the information this resource lists in the MCC's differential diagnosis).

Ask about the patient's age, and about a history of alcohol or drug abuse.

Physical exam

Obtain the patient's vital signs, looking for fever (this suggests infection).

Assess the patient's mental status with a mini–mental status exam, if appropriate (see the quick reference).

Investigations

Order a complete blood count (CBC), and tests for creatinine, thyrotropin (TSH), and arterial blood gases (ABG). In suspected infection, order a blood culture, urine culture, and, if symptoms warrant, a cerebrospinal fluid (CSF) culture. Consider a CT scan of the head.

Management

Treat any underlying conditions and discontinue any potentially causative medications. Admit the patient for observation and to ensure their safety. Consider referral to a geriatrician.

Pearls

An important aspect of management in this clinical presentation is to clarify proxy decision making. Does the patient have an advance directive, or have they named a person to make decisions on their behalf? If the patient has not taken these steps, they may have made "transmitted decisions"—decisions about their care of which they have informed others. In the absence of an advance directive, named proxy decision makers, or transmitted decisions, individuals who know the patient well may make "hypothetical judgements."

QUICK REFERENCE

Mini–mental status exams (MMSEs)

A mini–mental status exam is a common way to assess for cognitive impairment.

Several versions of MMSEs exist. It's good general preparation for the exam to research MMSEs, and choose or prepare a version for your own use (this isn't the only clinical presentation where an MMSE may be appropriate).

MMSEs generally assess:

- orientation to time and place
- recall (e.g., remembering a short list of words)
- calculation (e.g., spelling a word backwards)
- language comprehension (e.g., naming objects; following a written command, a verbal command, and a complex instruction; repeating back a spoken phrase)

87

Major or mild neurocognitive disorders (dementia)

MCC particular objectives

Identify deterioration in cognitive function.

Look for reversible risk factors.

Differentiate early Alzheimer disease from other causes.

MCC differential diagnosis
with added evidence

MAJOR OR MILD NEUROCOGNITIVE DISORDER IN GENERAL

Signs and symptoms: gradual impairment of ≥ 1 cognitive area (complex attention; executive function; learning and memory; language; perceptual-motor skills; social interaction); **no** evidence that the cognitive impairment occurs only with delirium; **no** evidence of depression

> Mild cognitive impairment: deficits that **do not** significantly interfere with day-to-day life

> Major cognitive impairment (dementia): deficits that interfere with day-to-day life (e.g., ability to pay bills)

ALZHEIMER DISEASE

Alzheimer disease is generally diagnosed clinically: the goal of imaging studies, when pursued, is to rule out other causes.

Signs and symptoms: older age (rare onset before age 60; prevalence doubles every 5 years after age 65); insidious onset of impairment (key characteristic); memory impairment (most common initial symptom); executive dysfunction and visuospatial impairment (often relatively early symptoms); language deficits and behavioural changes (often later symptoms)

VASCULAR DEMENTIA (E.G., MULTIINFARCT, LACUNAR INFARCT)

MULTIINFARCT DEMENTIA

Deficits manifest after multiple infarcts over time, or suddenly after a stroke.

Signs and symptoms: age 60 to 70 (more common); male (more common); memory loss; confusion (e.g., getting lost in familiar places); difficulty with short-term memory, performing routine tasks (e.g., paying bills), remembering words; misplacing items; personality and mood changes (depression, poor judgement, social withdrawal); sleep disruption; hallucinations, delusions

Risk factors: previous strokes; vascular factors (heart failure, hypertension, atherosclerosis, atrial fibrillation), smoking, alcohol use, obesity, poor diet, sedentary lifestyle

Investigations: MRI or CT scan

LACUNAR INFARCT

Signs and symptoms: unilateral weakness (face, arm, leg); "dysarthria-clumsy hand syndrome" (facial weakness, difficulty speaking, difficulty swallowing, and slight weakness and clumsiness of 1 hand); ataxic hemiparesis (ipsilateral weakness with limb ataxia); **no** monoplegia, stupor, coma, loss of consciousness, or seizures

> Pure motor hemiparesis (most common): **no** sensory deficit
>
> Pure sensory stroke: **no** motor deficit
>
> Sensorimotor stroke: **no** aphasia, agnosia, neglect, apraxia, hemianopia

Risk factors: systemic hypertension; diabetes; smoking; older age; high low-density lipoprotein (LDL)

Investigations: MRI or CT scan

BRAIN TRAUMA (E.G., POSTCONCUSSIVE CONDITION, ANOXIA)

BRAIN TRAUMA IN GENERAL

This is injury to brain tissue that likely results in functional impairment.

Investigations: EEG depending on symptom severity; CT scan or MRI if swelling or bleeding is suspected

POSTCONCUSSIVE CONDITION

This is a less severe type of brain injury.

Signs and symptoms: history of concussion; headache; impaired alertness; loss of consciousness; memory loss; confusion; drowsiness

ANOXIA

Examples of causes include severe asthma attack, heart attack, carbon monoxide poisoning, and near drowning.

DRUGS (E.G., ALCOHOL, SUBSTANCE ABUSE)

TOXINS (E.G., HEAVY METALS, ORGANIC TOXINS)

Sources of heavy metal exposure include lead (lead paint, lead in water pipes), mercury (eating fish contaminated with mercury), and arsenic (pesticides).

Sources of organic toxin exposure include organophosphate pesticides.

Signs and symptoms: sudden weight loss or gain; changes in skin and hair condition; anemia (fatigue, pallor, dizziness, shortness of breath, tachycardia); abdominal pain; diarrhea

Investigations: blood and urine testing to detect markers of heavy metal or toxin poisoning (e.g., liver function, blood chemistry, urinalysis)

NEURODEGENERATIVE DISORDERS (E.G., PARKINSON DISEASE, LEWY BODY DEMENTIA, HUNTINGTON DISEASE)

PARKINSON DISEASE

Signs and symptoms (mnemonic **TRAP**): **t**remor at rest; **r**igidity of the lower limbs; **a**kinesia, bradykinesia; **p**ostural instability

> Other symptoms: cognitive impairment; dementia; shuffling gait with stooped posture and loss of arm swing; micrographia; hypophonia; masklike facies, "pill rolling"; lack of blinking; orthostatic hypotension

> History of use of antipsychotics, antiemetics; toxin ingestion (e.g., carbon monoxide, cyanide); head trauma; vascular disease; other neurodegenerative disease (e.g., Lewy body dementia, Huntington disease); brain tumour, hydrocephalus; metabolic conditions (e.g., hypoparathyroidism, Wilson disease, chronic liver failure); infections that spread to brain (HIV/AIDS, syphilis, prion disease, toxoplasmosis, encephalitis lethargica, progressive multifocal leukoencephalopathy)

LEWY BODY DEMENTIA

Signs and symptoms: visual hallucinations, movement disorder (slowed movement, rigid muscles, tremor, shuffling walk), dizziness, constipation, sleep difficulties

Risk factors: family history of Lewy body dementia or Parkinson disease; male; older than 60

HUNTINGTON DISEASE

Signs and symptoms: family history of Huntington disease; abnormal eye movements; tics (uncontrolled movement in the fingers, feet, face, trunk); myoclonus; chorea (progressive chorea in late-onset Huntington disease; older than 50); psychiatric symptoms (depression; apathy; anxiety; obsessions, compulsions; irritability; psychosis; paranoid and acoustic hallucinations; hypersexuality); cognitive symptoms (impaired executive function; loss of mental flexibility, concentration, judgement, memory, awareness); motor symptoms (bradykinesia, dystonia, muscle weakness); profuse sweating from autonomic disturbance

Investigations: DNA analysis (PCR or Southern blot); neuroimaging (MRI, CT scan, SPECT, PET scan) for progression monitoring

NORMAL PRESSURE HYDROCEPHALUS

Signs and symptoms (classic triad):

> Gait disturbance (most common and earliest symptom): dizziness; balance and walking difficulty (e.g., tripping, wide stance, short shuffling steps)
>
> Cognitive impairment: organization and concentration difficulty; daytime sleepiness; psychomotor slowing; loss of precise fine movement; short-term memory problems; apathy; reduced speech; dementia
>
> Urinary symptoms: frequent urination, especially at night; urgency; permanent incontinence

Investigations: MRI to detect ventricular enlargement with no macroscopic CSF obstruction; normal or mildly elevated lumbar puncture opening pressure

INTRACRANIAL MASS (E.G., TUMOUR, SUBDURAL MASS, BRAIN ABSCESS)

BRAIN TUMOUR

Types of brain tumour include meningioma, astrocytoma, oligodendroglioma, glioblastoma, and Schwannoma.

Signs and symptoms: acute-onset headaches; older than 50; change in chronic headache pattern; increasing intensity and frequency of headaches; headaches that disturb sleep; unilateral headache pain, always on the same side; position-evoked crescendo headache; impaired vision; light-headedness

> Other symptoms: focal seizures, confusion, memory loss, personality change

Investigations: imaging for intracranial masses (MRI with contrast enhancement is best for tumours and abscesses); biopsy

SUBDURAL HEMATOMA

Signs and symptoms: history of head trauma or use of anticoagulants; local neurological findings (cranial nerve abnormalities; mono- or hemiparesis or hemiplegia); global neurologic findings (confusion, coma); pupil abnormalities; retinal hemorrhage

Investigations: imaging for intracranial masses (CT scan with contrast enhancement is best for hematomas)

BRAIN ABSCESS

This is caused by bacteria (most common), fungi, or parasites.

Signs and symptoms: headache (most common); fever; focal neurologic deficits (vision or hearing loss; tingling; weakness; behaviour or cognitive change); seizures; nausea, vomiting; recent or current infections, or recent trauma or surgery; signs of infection on the skin, or in the sinuses, oral cavity, eye fundus, ears, or other locations (e.g., lung)

Investigations: blood cultures; culture of brain lesion; imaging for intracranial masses (MRI with contrast enhancement is best for tumours and abscesses)

INFECTION (E.G., HIV, NEUROSYPHILIS)

HIV

HIV develops into AIDS when the CD4 cell count is < 200 cells/mm^3 (reference range of CD4: 500–2000 cells/mm^3).

Signs and symptoms: flu-like symptoms in the first, acute phase; leukopenia in the second, latent, asymptomatic stage (200–499 CD4 cells/mm^3); lymphadenopathy

> Neurocognitive symptoms: behavioural changes; difficulty in making decisions; difficulties with attention, concentration, memory; tremors; loss of coordination
>
> AIDS: recurrent, severe opportunistic infections or malignancies

Risk factors: unprotected sex; intravenous (IV) drug use

Investigations: positive HIV-1 p24 antigen in the blood followed by HIV antibody testing (positive ELISA result); PCR to determine HIV RNA level or viral load

NEUROSYPHILIS

Symptoms can present within weeks or years of infection. Some patients are asymptomatic.

Signs and symptoms: headache; stiff neck; nausea, vomiting; loss of vision or hearing; general paresis (changes in personality, mood)

Risk factors: unprotected sex, HIV

Investigations: positive test for syphilis

ENDOCRINE, METABOLIC, OR NUTRITIONAL DISORDER (E.G., HYPOTHYROIDISM, VITAMIN B$_{12}$ DEFICIENCY)

HYPOTHYROIDISM

Signs and symptoms: history of hypothyroidism or symptoms of hypothyroidism (cold intolerance, decreased reflexes, dry skin, weight gain, impaired cognition)

Investigations: elevated thyrotropin (TSH)

VITAMIN B$_{12}$ DEFICIENCY

Signs and symptoms: neuropsychiatric symptoms including memory or cognitive impairment, dementia, depression; anemia (fatigue, pallor, dizziness, shortness of breath, tachycardia), peripheral neuropathy

Investigations: low serum vitamin B$_{12}$ (or cobalamin); CBC with peripheral smear (low hemoglobin, macrocytosis)

Strategy for patient encounter

The likely scenario is an elderly patient with long-standing memory problems. The specified tasks could engage history, physical exam, investigations, or management. The encounter will likely involve administering a mini-mental status exam.

History

Obtain collateral information on the patient's behaviour (e.g., from an accompanying caregiver), if possible.

Start with open-ended questions about the patient's memory problems (a patient with memory problems is the likely scenario): How long have you had memory problems? What other symptoms have you had? Listen for evidence of insidious onset (this is a hallmark of Alzheimer disease); and features consistent with particular entities (e.g., weakness in lacunar infarct; gastrointestinal symptoms in toxic exposure and neurosyphilis; movement abnormalities in neurodegenerative disorders). Screen for symptoms of depression: depressed mood, loss of interest in usual activities, psychomotor changes (agitated or slowed, as observed by others), significant weight change, sleep disturbance, fatigue, indecisiveness, and recurrent thoughts of death or suicide.

Use open-ended inquiry to obtain a medical history: What conditions have you been diagnosed with? Listen for a history of stroke, vascular disorders, hypertension, diabetes, dyslipidemia, heart disease, and HIV. Ask about a history of head trauma or concussions. Ask about drug and alcohol abuse.

QUICK REFERENCE

Mini-mental status exams (MMSEs)

A mini–mental status exam is a common way to assess for cognitive impairment.

Several versions of MMSEs exist. It's good general preparation for the exam to research MMSEs, and choose or prepare a version for your own use (this isn't the only clinical presentation where an MMSE may be appropriate).

MMSEs generally assess:

- orientation to time and place
- recall (e.g., remembering a short list of words)
- calculation (e.g., spelling a word backwards)
- language comprehension (e.g., naming objects; following a written command, a verbal command, and a complex instruction; repeating back a spoken phrase)

Physical exam

Assess the patient's mental status. You could use a mini–mental status exam (see the quick reference), if appropriate (available time may determine your decision, because a typical MMSE takes 5 to 10 minutes). Otherwise, ask the patient for their full name and date of birth. Ask them to state where they are and how they got here.

Perform a full neurological exam.

Investigations

Perform brain imaging on all patients (MRI or CT scan) to diagnose any masses or infarcts. Order tests for thyrotropin (TSH) and vitamin B_{12}, and a VDRL (or other syphilis test).

Management

Management depends on the specific diagnosis. Consider referral to a neurologist, psychiatrist, or geriatrician.

88

Depressed mood

MCC particular objective

Assess suicide risk and the potential need for urgent care.

MCC differential diagnosis
with added evidence

MAJOR DEPRESSIVE DISORDER[1(pp160–161)]

Major depressive disorder is characterized by a persistent "down" mood, with no manic or hypomanic episodes (the presence of these episodes indicates bipolar disorder, by definition—see *bipolar disorder*, below).

Signs and symptoms: symptoms that are present most of the time for ≥ 2 weeks; symptoms with significant impact on day-to-day life

> Key symptoms: depressed mood and/or loss of interest in usual activities

> Other symptoms: significant weight change; sleep disturbance; slowed or agitated mental processes; loss of concentration; recurrent thoughts of death or suicide

Risk factors: family history of mental health disorders (depression, anxiety, suicide); personal history of other mental health disorders; substance abuse; chronic illness (e.g., cancer, stroke, chronic pain)

BIPOLAR DISORDER (TYPE I, TYPE II)[1(pp123–134)]

BIPOLAR DISORDER IN GENERAL

Bipolar I disorder *always* involves at least 1 manic episode, and *may* involve hypomanic and/or major depressive episodes.

Bipolar II disorder *never* involves manic episodes, and *always* involves swings between hypomanic and major depressive episodes.

Family history of bipolar disorder is a risk factor for bipolar disorder.

MANIC EPISODE

Signs and symptoms: symptoms that are present most of the time for ≥ 1 week; symptoms with significant impact on day-to-day life, and that may pose a risk of harm to self and others

> Key symptoms: abnormally elevated (and/or irritable) mood, and goal-directed activity

> Other symptoms: increased self-importance, increased talking, racing thoughts, decreased need for sleep, risky pursuits (e.g., that could damage finances or relationships), psychosis (e.g., delusions, hallucinations)

HYPOMANIC EPISODE

Signs and symptoms: symptoms resembling a manic episode in presentation and duration, except:

> **No** significant impact on day-to-day life

> **No** risk of harm to self or others

> **No** psychosis (e.g., delusions, hallucinations)

MAJOR DEPRESSIVE EPISODE

Signs and symptoms: symptoms that are present most of the time for ≥ 2 weeks; symptoms with significant impact on day-to-day life

> Key symptoms: depressed mood and/or loss of interest in usual activities

> Other symptoms: significant weight change; sleep disturbance; slowed or agitated mental processes; loss of concentration; recurrent thoughts of death or suicide

PERSISTENT DEPRESSIVE DISORDER (DYSTHYMIA)[1(p168)]

Signs and symptoms: symptoms with significant impact on day-to-day life; presence of symptoms for most of the time for ≥ 2 years (children and adolescents: ≥ 1 year), with no break from symptoms for ≥ 2 months; **no** manic or hypomanic episodes

> Key symptoms: depressed mood (or, possibly, irritability in children and adolescents)

Other symptoms: change in eating and sleeping routines; fatigue; low self-esteem; loss of concentration; feelings of hopelessness

CYCLOTHYMIC DISORDER[1(pp139–140)]

Cyclothymic disorder resembles bipolar II disorder, but the mood swings are not as severe.

Signs and symptoms: mood swings, with symptoms that **do not** represent hypomanic or major depressive episodes; symptoms with significant impact on day-to-day life; presence of symptoms for most of the time for ≥ 2 years (children and adolescents: ≥ 1 year), with no break from symptoms for ≥ 2 months

Risk factors: family history of cyclothymic disorder, substance abuse disorders, bipolar disorders

NORMAL GRIEF[1(pp125–126)]

Signs and symptoms: history of a significant personal loss (e.g., death of a family member or friend, financial ruin, serious medical diagnosis); symptoms that resemble a major depressive episode **except**:

Positive feelings or humour often occur.

Symptoms become less intense over time.

Symptoms are triggered by specific reminders of the personal loss.

SUBSTANCE-INDUCED MOOD DISORDER

Examples of drugs that can provoke mood disturbances include stimulants, steroids, levodopa, antibiotics, central nervous system drugs, dermatological agents, chemotherapeutic drugs, immunological agents, and oral contraceptives.

MOOD DISORDER DUE TO A MEDICAL CONDITION

Examples of medical conditions that can provoke mood disturbances include Parkinson disease, Huntington disease, stroke, brain injury from trauma, Cushing disease, hypothyroidism, and multiple sclerosis.

ADJUSTMENT DISORDER[1(pp286–287)]

Signs and symptoms: onset of emotional or behavioural symptoms in response to an identifiable stressor and within 3 months of the stressor; distress out of proportion to the stressor; symptoms with significant impact on day-to-day life; abatement of symptoms within 6 months of cessation of the stressor

Strategy for patient encounter

The likely scenario is a young person feeling down. The specified tasks could engage history, investigations, or management (physical exam is unlikely in this clinical presentation). Suicide risk assessment is crucial in this patient encounter, so include it even if it's not specified.

History

Start with open-ended questions about the patient's symptoms: What symptoms are you experiencing? What impact do they have on your usual routines and relationships? Listen for features consistent with particular entities (e.g., cycling up and down moods in bipolar II disorder; enduring symptoms in persistent depressive disorder and cyclothymic disorder), and the presence of significant impairment and/or distress (this is the hallmark of a mental health disorder). Take a medical and medication history, looking for Parkinson disease, Huntington disease, and other entities associated with mood disorder (e.g., stroke, head trauma, multiple sclerosis). Ask about medications and use of street drugs, looking for drugs associated with mood disorders (e.g., cocaine, antibiotics, oral contraceptives). Ask about current life stressors (this is relevant for normal grief and adjustment disorder). Ask about a family history of mental illness.

Risk assessment

Assess the patient's risk of suicide (see the checklist). Ask if they have specific suicidal plans and intent, and if they have the means to carry out their suicide plan. Ask about previous psychiatric history and previous suicide attempts.

Investigations

Order a urine drug screen if drug abuse cannot be ruled

> **CHECKLIST**
> ## Indicators of suicide risk
> Patients are at risk of suicide if they have suicidal thoughts, a plan, and intent.
>
> The following additional factors put them at high risk of suicide:
> - a history of suicide attempts
> - access to firearms
> - a psychiatric disorder or disorders (e.g., depression, bipolar disorder, schizophrenia, alcohol or substance abuse, personality disorder, anxiety disorder)
> - current substance abuse
> - male
> - lack of social support (e.g., they live alone)
> - for children and adolescents: exposure to abuse, violence, victimization, or bullying; family history of suicides; member of a minority in sexual orientation

out. Order a test for thyrotropin (TSH) to rule out thyroid disorder.

Management

A patient with specific and immediate plans for suicide requires admission to hospital for psychiatric assessment and monitoring. If a patient at risk of suicide refuses admission, consider involuntary admission. The regulations for involuntary admission vary by jurisdiction, but generally require a written order by 2 physicians.

If the patient is not at immediate risk, consider referring the patient to psychiatry. Start pharmacotherapy in the case of major depressive disorder (with an antidepressant medication) or bipolar disorder (with a mood-stabilizing agent such as lithium carbonate or valproic acid). Consider the need for patient and/or family support resources.

REFERENCE

1 American Psychiatric Association. Diagnostic and statistical manual of mental disorders. 5th ed. Arlington, VA: American Psychiatric Association; 2013. 59–60. 991 p.

89

Mania or hypomania

MCC particular objective

Pay particular attention to assessment of risk and the potential need for urgent care.

MCC differential diagnosis
with added evidence

BIPOLAR DISORDER (TYPE I, TYPE II)[1(pp123–134)]

BIPOLAR DISORDER IN GENERAL

Bipolar I disorder *always* involves at least 1 manic episode, and *may* involve hypomanic and/or major depressive episodes.

Bipolar II disorder *never* involves manic episodes, and *always* involves swings between hypomanic and major depressive episodes.

Family history of bipolar disorder is a risk factor for bipolar disorder.

MANIC EPISODE

Signs and symptoms: symptoms that are present most of the time for ≥ 1 week; symptoms with significant impact on day-to-day life, and that may pose a risk of harm to self and others

> Key symptoms: abnormally elevated (and/or irritable) mood, and goal-directed activity

> Other symptoms: increased self-importance, increased talking, racing thoughts, decreased need for sleep, risky pursuits (e.g., that could damage finances or relationships), psychosis (e.g., delusions, hallucinations)

HYPOMANIC EPISODE

Signs and symptoms: symptoms resembling a manic episode in presentation and duration, except:

> **No** significant impact on day-to-day life

> **No** risk of harm to self or others

> **No** psychosis (e.g., delusions, hallucinations)

MAJOR DEPRESSIVE EPISODE

Signs and symptoms: symptoms that are present most of the time for ≥ 2 weeks; symptoms with significant impact on day-to-day life

> Key symptoms: depressed mood and/or loss of interest in usual activities

> Other symptoms: significant weight change; sleep disturbance; slowed or agitated mental processes; loss of concentration; recurrent thoughts of death or suicide

SUBSTANCE-INDUCED MOOD DISORDER

Examples of drugs that can provoke mood disturbances include stimulants, steroids, levodopa, antibiotics, central nervous system drugs, dermatological agents, chemotherapeutic drugs, immunological agents, and oral contraceptives.

MOOD DISORDER DUE TO A MEDICAL CONDITION

Examples of medical conditions that can provoke mood disturbances include Parkinson disease, Huntington disease (diagnostic if present); stroke; brain injury from trauma; Cushing disease; hypothyroidism; and multiple sclerosis.

CYCLOTHYMIC DISORDER[1(pp139–140)]

Cyclothymic disorder resembles bipolar II disorder, but the mood swings are not as severe.

Signs and symptoms: mood swings, with symptoms that **do not** represent hypomanic or major depressive episodes (see *bipolar disorder*, above); symptoms with significant impact on day-to-day life; presence of symptoms for most of the time for ≥ 2 years (children and adolescents: ≥ 1 year), with no break from symptoms for ≥ 2 months

Risk factors: family history of cyclothymic disorder, substance abuse disorders, bipolar disorder

Strategy for patient encounter

The likely scenario is a young person feeling down. The specified tasks could engage history, investigations, or management (physical exam is unlikely in this clinical presentation). Risk assessment is crucial in this patient encounter, so include it even if it's not specified.

History

Obtain collateral information on the patient's behaviour (e.g., from an accompanying caregiver), if possible.

Start with open-ended inquiry: Please tell me about your symptoms. Listen for features consistent with particular entities (e.g., delusions, hallucinations, homicidal thoughts in bipolar I disorder; cycling up and down moods in bipolar II disorder; enduring symptoms in cyclothymic disorder). Take a medical and medication history, looking for Parkinson disease, Huntington disease, and other entities associated with mood disorder (e.g., stroke, head trauma, multiple sclerosis). Ask about medications and use of street drugs, looking for drugs associated with mood disorders (e.g., cocaine, antibiotics, oral contraceptives). Ask about a family history of mental illness.

QUICK REFERENCE

Mental status exams (MSEs)

Many versions of MSEs exist. It's good general preparation for the exam to research MSEs, and choose or prepare a version for your own use (this is not the only clinical presentation where an MSE is relevant). Your MSE could contain a series of ready-made descriptors that you check off, or it could be a framework for taking notes.

Note that MSEs use both observation and direct questioning to make assessments.

Generally, they assess:

- general appearance and behaviour
- mood
- speech: rate, tone, volume
- thought content: obsessions, preoccupations, hallucinations, delusions, suicidal ideation, homicidal ideation
- thought process: circumstantial, tangential, flight of ideas, loosening of associations
- orientation to time and place
- attention and concentration
- patient insight into their present condition

Risk assessment

Perform a mental status exam to assess the patient's capacity, and to identify risk factors for self-harm or harming others (see the quick reference).

Investigations

Order a urine drug screen if drug abuse cannot be ruled out. Order a test for thyrotropin (TSH) to rule out thyroid disorder.

Management

Ensure the immediate safety of the patient and others.

A patient with specific and immediate plans for suicide or homicide requires admission to hospital for psychiatric assessment and monitoring. If a patient at risk of committing suicide or homicide refuses admission, consider involuntary admission. The regulations for involuntary admission vary by jurisdiction, but generally require a written order by 2 physicians.

If the patient is not at immediate risk, consider referring the patient to psychiatry. In patients experiencing a manic phase of bipolar disorder (the likely scenario), start pharmacotherapy with an antipsychotic medication. Consider the need for patient and/or family support resources.

REFERENCE

1 American Psychiatric Association. Diagnostic and statistical manual of mental disorders. 5th ed. Arlington, VA: American Psychiatric Association; 2013. 991 p.

90

Oral conditions

MCC particular objective

Determine if the patient requires specialized care.

MCC differential diagnosis
with added evidence

MOUTH PROBLEMS IN GENERAL

The MCC notes that dental caries and peridontal infections are common.

CONGENITAL CONDITION (E.G., CLEFT PALATE)

CLEFT PALATE

Signs and symptoms: drooling; difficulty swallowing; hypernasal voice resonance; difficulty hearing; frequent ear infections; visible congenital facial or oral malformation

ACQUIRED CONDITION

Infection (e.g., candidiasis)

CANDIDIASIS

This is a fungal infection (*Candida*) that is usually diagnosed clinically.

Signs and symptoms: white plaques in the mouth and throat; feeling of "cotton in the mouth"

Risk factors: dentures; use of inhaled corticosteroids; immunosuppression

Malignancy (e.g., adenocarcinoma, leukoplakia)

ADENOCARCINOMA

Signs and symptoms: mass on the side of the face, below the jaw, or in the mouth; pain; swallowing difficulty; fluid draining from an ear

Risk factors: male (more common); older age; exposure to radiation (e.g., radiation treatment to the head and neck)

LEUKOPLAKIA

This is usually benign (but see risk factors for progression to malignancy, below).

Signs and symptoms: white lesions of the oral mucosa (surface texture and colour may be homogeneous); tobacco use, including smoking, but especially chewing tobacco (common); asymptomatic (usual); discomfort, pain

Risk factors for lesions to become malignant: verrucous type; association with erosion or ulceration; presence of nodule in the lesion; texture that is hard, or lesion with a hard periphery; located in the anterior floor of the mouth, on the undersurface of the tongue

Poor oral hygiene (e.g., caries, periodontal disease)

Signs and symptoms: obvious dental caries

Gingivitis: gingival redness, swelling; gingival bleeding on brushing, flossing, or examination with periodontal probe

Periodontitis: attachment loss; loose teeth; alveolar bone loss

Trauma (e.g., abuse)

The oral cavity may be a central focus for physical abuse due to its significance in communication and nutrition.

Signs and symptoms: contusions, burns, lacerations in the mouth (lips most common); fractured, displaced, avulsed teeth; facial bone and jaw fractures; injury from gags at the corners of the mouth (bruises, lichenification, scarring)

Toxic ingestion

Common toxins causing oral ulcers include methotrexate and other cytotoxic chemotherapy agents; bisphosphonates; nicorandil; propylthiouracil; nonsteroidal antiinflammatory drugs (NSAIDs); and recreational drugs such as cocaine.

Xerostomia (e.g., age, medications)

Signs and symptoms: oral mucosal dryness; use of drugs that cause xerostomia (e.g., tricyclic antidepressants, antipsychotics, antihistamines)

Systemic disease (e.g., lichen planus, Behçet disease)

LICHEN PLANUS

This is a common, chronic inflammatory condition of the skin (common locations: inner wrists, forearms, lower legs, lower back) and mucous membranes (locations: mouth, vagina).

Signs and symptoms (mouth): lacy white lines (Wickham striae) on the inner cheeks; tender red patches in the mouth, which can cause burning sensations, food sensitivity (hot, acidic, spicy), and chewing or swallowing difficulty; recurrent ulcers (rare)

Investigations: biopsy

BEHÇET DISEASE

This is a rare entity that causes inflammation of the body's blood vessels. It is diagnosed clinically.

Signs and symptoms: mouth sores that recur at least 3 times over 12 months (most common symptom); recurring genital sores; uveitis; skin rash

Risk factors: age 20 to 30 (more common); male (more severe); Middle Eastern or Asian descent

Strategy for patient encounter

The likely scenario is a patient with a mouth complaint. The specified tasks could engage history, physical exam, investigations, or management.

History

Start with open-ended inquiry to establish the patient's symptoms: Please tell me about the mouth problem you're experiencing. When did the symptoms start? How often do the symptoms happen? Listen for symptoms consistent with particular entities (e.g., "cotton in the mouth" in candidiasis, gum bleeding in gingivitis, loose teeth in periodontitis, dry mouth in xerostomia, oral ulcers in toxic ingestion), and for constant versus intermittent symptoms (intermittent symptoms suggest Behçet disease).

Take a medical and medication history: What conditions have you been diagnosed with? What medications do you take? What recreational drugs do you take? Listen for cancers of the head and neck (these are relevant for radiation exposure), cleft palate, lichen planus, and Behçet disease; and for medications and drugs associated with particular entities (e.g., corticosteroids in candidiasis; chemotherapy and cocaine in toxic ingestions; tricyclic antidepressants in xerostomia).

Physical exam

Examine the oral cavity looking for masses and mucosal abnormalities. Examine the teeth looking for decay or signs of trauma. Examine the neck looking for masses and enlarged lymph nodes.

Investigations

Consider the need to investigate for potential systemic diseases. Take a tissue sample of any visible lesions.

Management

Management depends on the specific entity diagnosed. Consider the need for referral to a dentist or oral surgeon.

91

Movement disorders, and involuntary or tic disorders

MCC particular objectives
None stated.

MCC differential diagnosis
with added evidence

HYPERKINETIC MOVEMENT

Tics

PRIMARY

TOURETTE SYNDROME

Signs and symptoms: symptom onset during childhood or adolescence (symptoms are commonly present by age 12); presence of motor and vocal tics (not necessarily concurrently); presence of tics for ≥ 1 year

> Motor tics (examples): eye blinking, facial grimacing, head jerking
>
> Vocal tics (examples): grunting, repeating what others say, repeating particular words or phrases

Risk factors: male (3 to 4 times more common); family history of Tourette syndrome or other tic disorder (chronic motor or tic disorder, provisional tic disorder)

HUNTINGTON DISEASE

Signs and symptoms: family history of Huntington disease; abnormal eye movements; tics (uncontrolled movement in the fingers, feet, face, trunk); myoclonus; chorea (progressive chorea in late-onset Huntington disease; older than 50); psychiatric symptoms (depression; apathy; anxiety; obsessions, compulsions; irritability; psychosis; paranoid and acoustic hallucinations; hypersexuality); cognitive symptoms (impaired executive function; loss of mental flexibility, concentration, judgement, memory, awareness); motor symptoms (bradykinesia, dystonia, muscle weakness); profuse sweating from autonomic disturbance

Investigations: DNA analysis (PCR or Southern blot); neuroimaging (MRI, CT scan, SPECT, PET scan) for progression monitoring

SECONDARY

INFECTION (E.G., ENCEPHALITIS, CREUTZFELDT-JAKOB DISEASE)

ENCEPHALITIS

Signs and symptoms: seizures; fever; headache; nausea, vomiting; altered mental status, behaviour, personality; abrupt-onset tic disorder; repetitive, uncontrollable muscle contractions; movements or sounds that occur intermittently and unpredictably outside of normal motor activity

CREUTZFELDT-JAKOB DISEASE

This is the most common form of prion disease (most commonly sporadic), but still rare.

Signs and symptoms: mental deterioration; dementia; myoclonus; personality changes; impaired memory, judgement, cognition, and/or vision; tics and myoclonus that are triggered on startling (common)

> Brain atrophy (common): ventricular enlargement; deep gray structures (caudate, putamen, thalamus); **no** alteration of hippocampus

DRUGS (E.G., STIMULANTS, LEVODOPA)

Dystonia

DYSTONIA IN GENERAL

The diagnosis is primarily clinical.

PRIMARY (SPORADIC AND INHERITED)

Signs and symptoms: sustained involuntary muscle contractions, typically of antagonistic muscle groups in the same body part (the contractions resemble abnormal twisting, spasm, or tremor) and that are generalized, focal, or segmental (depending on body distribution); variable onset

> Inherited: symptom onset in childhood; positive response to low-dose levodopa

Investigations: neurological testing of nerve and muscle function

DYSTONIA-PLUS SYNDROMES (E.G., MEDICATION)

MEDICATIONS

Dystonia-plus syndromes, in general, are nondegenerative neurochemical disorders associated with other neurological conditions.

Causative medications include antipsychotics (e.g., phenothiazines, thioxanthenes, butyrophenones) and antiemetics (e.g., metoclopramide, prochlorperazine).

Signs and symptoms: uncontrollable, sometimes painful muscle spasms; symptoms that develop after weeks (sometimes years) of medication use

Investigations: neurological testing of nerve and muscle function

Stereotypies (typically with mental retardation or autism)

Signs and symptoms: skin picking; mouth opening; facial grimacing; involuntary noises; head nodding or banging; body rocking (this may cause self-injury in severe cases); absence of movements during sleep and on distraction (e.g., calling the child's name)

> Triggers for movements: excitement, happiness, concentration, tiredness, anxiety

> In autistic children: movements > 1 minute in duration that occur multiple times a day

Chorea, athetosis, ballism

CHOREA

This is found in many diseases, for example Huntington disease, chorea gravidarum, Sydenham chorea, Creutzfeldt-Jakob disease, drug-induced chorea, and metabolic and endocrine-related chorea.

Signs and symptoms: nonrepetitive, nonperiodic, involuntary jerking movements of the face, trunk, or limbs that are often enhanced during voluntary movement

> Progressive chorea: increased movements with stress; absence of movements during sleep; movements that cause walking and balance problems

ATHETOSIS

Causes include brain lesions and cerebral palsy.

Signs and symptoms: slow, writhing, continuous movements in the fingers, hands, toes, feet (occasionally in the limbs, neck, tongue); unbalanced, involuntary movements; difficulty maintaining a symmetrical posture

BALLISM

This is a rare type of chorea.

Causes include stroke, traumatic brain injury, and amyotrophic lateral sclerosis.

Signs and symptoms: repetitive, but constantly varying, large amplitude involuntary movement of the proximal parts of the limbs; almost ceaseless activity, often complex and combined

Essential tremor

Essential tremor is the most common form of tremor.

Signs and symptoms (highly variable): tremors in the hands (usual), head (horizontal or vertical movement), voice; tremors on holding out the hands; tremors made worse with movement (usual) and better with alcohol

Risk factors: family history of tremor (autosomal dominant); older age

Myoclonus

This may indicate a nervous system disorder such as multiple sclerosis, Parkinson disease, dystonia, Alzheimer disease, Gaucher disease, Creutzfeldt-Jakob disease, serotonin toxicity, Huntington disease, epilepsy, or intracranial hypotension.

Signs and symptoms:

> Positive myoclonus: sudden muscle contractions (twitches; jerks; seizures; hypnic jerk while falling asleep)
>
> Negative myoclonus: brief lapses of contraction

Investigations: EMG, EEG

BRADYKINETIC MOVEMENT

Parkinson disease

Signs and symptoms (mnemonic **TRAP**): **t**remor at rest; **r**igidity of the lower limbs; **a**kinesia, bradykinesia; **p**ostural instability

> Other symptoms: cognitive impairment; dementia; shuffling gait with stooped posture and loss of arm swing; micrographia; hypophonia; masklike facies, "pill rolling"; lack of blinking; orthostatic hypotension
>
> History of use of antipsychotics, antiemetics; toxin ingestion (e.g., carbon monoxide, cyanide); head trauma; vascular disease; other neurodegenerative disease (e.g., Lewy body dementia, Huntington disease); brain tumour, hydrocephalus; metabolic conditions (e.g., hypoparathyroidism, Wilson disease, chronic liver failure); infections that spread to the brain (HIV/AIDS, syphilis, prion disease, toxoplasmosis, encephalitis lethargica, progressive multifocal leukoencephalopathy)

Wilson disease

This causes accumulation of copper in the body and can be fatal.

Signs and symptoms:

> Neurologic: asymmetric tremor; dysphasia; ataxia; drooling; clumsiness; Fleischer rings in the cornea; masklike facies
>
> Hepatic: liver dysfunction (cirrhosis, acute hepatitis, chronic active hepatitis), jaundice, abdominal pain
>
> Musculoskeletal: osteopenia on radiological exam; joint inflammation that resembles premature osteoarthritis (this is symptomatic after age 20 and occurs in the spine, hips, knees, wrists)
>
> Neuropsychiatric (not as common; usually coexistent with cirrhosis): personality changes, irritability, impaired cognition

Investigations: serum ceruloplasmin < 200 mg/L; urinary copper excretion rate > 100 mcg/day

Huntington disease—see above

TREMOR

Resting tremor (e.g., Parkinson disease, severe essential tremor)

PARKINSON DISEASE—SEE ABOVE

ESSENTIAL TREMOR—SEE ABOVE

Intention tremor (e.g., cerebellar disease, multiple sclerosis)

INTENTION TREMOR IN GENERAL

This is sometimes difficult to distinguish from cerebellar ataxia.

Signs and symptoms: large amplitude tremor whose severity typically increases on approaching a target (e.g., finger to nose, heel to shin)

CEREBELLAR DISEASE

Signs and symptoms: variable depending on etiology

> Common symptoms: ataxia; other motor dysfunction (dysmetria, decomposition of movement, dysdiadochokinesia, nystagmus); speech dysfunction (difficulty speaking, scanning speech); hypotonia

MULTIPLE SCLEROSIS

Signs and symptoms: variable depending on lesion location

> Spinal cord: sensory or motor dysfunction; Lhermitte sign (paresthesias radiating down the extremities or trunk with neck flexion); bowel, bladder or erectile dysfunction
>
> Brainstem: double vision; swallowing, speech difficulties; vertigo; pseudobulbar palsy
>
> Cerebrum: cognitive impairment; depression; upper motor neuron signs; unilateral motor or sensory deficits
>
> Cerebellum: problems with balance and coordination; vertigo
>
> Other symptoms: tonic spasms; fatigue; pain; exercise intolerance; temperature sensitivity; painful unilateral loss of visual acuity

Risk factors: younger than 50, female

Investigations: brain and spinal cord MRI, including advanced MRI techniques, with established occurrence of multiple episodes; CSF fluid analysis

Postural/action tremor (e.g., enhanced physiologic tremor, essential tremor)

POSTURAL TREMOR IN GENERAL

Signs and symptoms: tremor on maintaining a position against gravity (e.g., holding the arms outstretched)

ENHANCED PHYSIOLOGIC TREMOR

Enhanced physiologic tremor is the most common type of postural or action tremor.

Signs and symptoms: tremor with stress, after strenuous exertion, and/or after ingesting substances (drugs, medications, chemicals); **no** neurologic symptoms

> Substances: amphetamines, selective serotonin reuptake inhibitors (SSRIs), tricyclic antidepressants, nicotine, caffeine, corti costeroids, sodium valproate, mercury, lead, arsenic

ESSENTIAL TREMOR—SEE ABOVE

Strategy for patient encounter

The likely scenario is a patient with Parkinson disease. The specified tasks could engage history, physical exam, investigations, or management.

A main goal of this patient encounter is to look for treatable symptoms and causes (e.g., in Parkinson disease, Wilson disease) and reversible causes (medication side effects).

History

Use open-ended questions to determine the patient's family history and medication history: What conditions run in your family? What medications do you take? Listen for any of the entities listed in the MCC differential diagnosis, and for antiemetics and, in particular, antipsychotics. If the patient doesn't volunteer this information, ask specifically about these entities and medications. Ask about street drug use.

Physical exam

Carefully observe the clinical features of the movement disorder. Are the movements hyperkinetic or bradykinetic? Perform a full neurological exam.

Investigations

Order a brain CT scan or MRI for all patients. In suspected Huntington disease, order genetic studies. In suspected Wilson disease, order a serum ceruloplasmin test.

Management

Consider referral to a neurologist. Parkinson disease is treated with levodopa. Wilson disease is treated with chelating agents (e.g., D-penicillamine, trientine).

92

Abnormal heart sounds and murmurs

MCC particular objectives
None stated.

MCC differential diagnosis
with added evidence

ABNORMAL HEART SOUNDS AND MURMURS IN GENERAL
The MCC notes that systolic murmurs are often innocent, but diastolic murmurs are almost always pathological.

ABNORMAL HEART SOUNDS

S1 (e.g., mitral stenosis, atrial fibrillation)

MITRAL STENOSIS
Signs and symptoms: chest pain; shortness of breath (on exertion or when lying down); fatigue; swollen feet or legs; dizziness or fainting; heavy coughing; severe headache and other stroke symptoms; pulmonary edema; arrhythmia

Risk factors: history of rheumatic fever, untreated *Streptococcus* infections

ATRIAL FIBRILLATION
Signs and symptoms: chest pain, shortness of breath, palpitations, weakness, fatigue, dizziness

Risk factors: older age; personal or family history of heart disease; hypertension; chronic disease (thyroid disease, obstructive sleep apnea, diabetes, kidney disease, lung disease); obesity; alcohol use

S2 (e.g., hypertension, aortic stenosis)

HYPERTENSION
Signs and symptoms: systolic blood pressure ≥140 mmHg and/or diastolic blood pressure ≥ 90 mmHg

History of renal conditions; diabetes; adrenal or thyroid conditions; vascular conditions; catecholamine excess; obstructive sleep apnea; family history of hypertension

Risk factors: lack of exercise, high-sodium diet, obesity

AORTIC STENOSIS

Signs and symptoms: chest pain; feeling faint, fainting with exertion; shortness of breath, especially on exertion; fatigue, especially during and after exertion; palpitations

Risk factors: bicuspid aortic valve; older age; history of rheumatic fever

Investigations: echocardiogram; chest X-ray; cardiac catheterization with contrast dye, CT scan, MRI; ECG to measure electrical impulses from the heart muscle; exercise testing

S3 (e.g., congestive heart failure)

CONGESTIVE HEART FAILURE

Signs and symptoms: history of heart disease (or risk factors for heart disease: diabetes, hypertension, hyperlipidemia, and smoking) or hepatic vein thrombosis (Budd-Chiari syndrome); severe shortness of breath; elevated jugular venous pressure; edema in the abdomen and legs; pink phlegm; heart murmurs and extra cardiac sounds

Investigations: chest X-ray to detect pulmonary edema; NT-proBNP level; echocardiogram to distinguish forms of heart failure; cardiac stress testing, either with exercise or pharmacological agent

S4 (e.g., hypertension—see above)

Abnormal splitting (e.g., atrial septal defect)

ATRIAL SEPTAL DEFECT

Signs and symptoms: shortness of breath; fatigue; swelling of the feet, legs, or abdomen; palpitations or skipped beats; frequent lung infections; stroke symptoms

Risk factors: history of rubella infection; history of in-utero exposure to tobacco, alcohol, cocaine; maternal history of diabetes, systemic lupus erythematosus, phenylketonuria, obesity

SYSTOLIC MURMURS

Ejection murmurs (e.g., physiologic, aortic stenosis)

PHYSIOLOGIC (FUNCTIONAL) MURMUR

An example cause is high cardiac output (because of, for example, athletic training, anemia, or pregnancy).

AORTIC STENOSIS—SEE ABOVE

PANSYSTOLIC MURMURS (E.G., MITRAL REGURGITATION)

MITRAL REGURGITATION

Signs and symptoms: shortness of breath; fatigue; palpitations; swollen feet or ankles

Risk factors: personal or family history of valve disease; history of heart attack or heart disease; use of ergotamine, cabergoline; history of endocarditis, rheumatic fever; older age

DIASTOLIC MURMURS

DIASTOLIC MURMURS IN GENERAL

Diastolic heart murmurs are generally low-pitched sounds of softer intensity and longer duration than other heart sounds.

Other sounds or murmurs are generally higher pitched and louder, with a possible click or thrill, and heard in either the systole phase alone or continuously throughout the cardiac cycle.

Early (e.g., aortic regurgitation)

AORTIC REGURGITATION

Signs and symptoms: fatigue; shortness of breath; swollen ankles and feet; chest pain that increases with exercise; light-headedness or fainting; arrhythmia; palpitations

Risk factors: history of endocarditis, rheumatic fever; aortic stenosis; congenital heart disease; hypertension; Marfan syndrome; ankylosing spondylitis; older age

Middiastolic (e.g., mitral stenosis—see above)

PERICARDIAL FRICTION RUBS

PERICARDIAL FRICTION RUBS IN GENERAL

This is caused by movement of inflammatory adhesions between pericardial layers, which results in systolic or multiphase high-pitched squeaking.

ACUTE PERICARDITIS

Signs and symptoms: sudden-onset, stabbing chest pain; pain made worse with inhalation or lying down, made better with sitting up or leaning forward (usual); radiation of pain to the neck, arms, left shoulder, and especially to the trapezius muscle

> History of viral illness (recent), infection (e.g., tuberculosis), autoimmune disease (e.g., systemic lupus erythematosus, rheumatoid arthritis, scleroderma), uremia, myocardial infarction, aortic dissection, chest wall trauma, thoracic surgery

Diagnosis: ECG; chest X-ray to detect pericardial effusion

CARDIAC TAMPONADE

Signs and symptoms: history of invasive heart procedures; chest pain, radiating to the neck and jaw; right upper quadrant abdominal pain (due to hepatic venous congestion); tachycardia; elevated jugular venous pressure; pulsus paradoxus

Investigations: ECG (findings: abnormalities); chest X-ray (findings: normal)

Strategy for patient encounter

The likely scenario is a young athletic patient with systolic murmur. The specified tasks could engage history, physical exam, investigations, or management.

History

Use open-ended questions to determine if the patient is experiencing cardiac symptoms: How has your health been lately? Listen for chest pain, shortness of breath, and exercise intolerance. Ask specifically about these symptoms if the patient doesn't volunteer them. Ask about a personal or family history of heart disease. Ask about risk factors for heart disease: hyperlipidemia, smoking, and diabetes.

Physical exam

Auscultate the lungs and heart, paying particular attention to the features of murmurs that this resource lists in the MCC differential diagnosis. Examine the extremities for edema.

Investigations

Order an electrocardiogram (ECG) and echocardiography.

Management

Refer the patient to cardiology. Consider the need for endocarditis prophylaxis.

Pearls

The recommendations for endocarditis prophylaxis have recently changed. The current recommendation limits routine antibiotic prophylaxis (e.g., for dental procedures) to patients with a prosthetic cardiac valve; a history of infective endocarditis; unrepaired or incompletely repaired cyanotic congenital heart disease; a recently repaired (within the past 6 months) congenital heart defect; and a limited number of additional indications.

93

Neck mass, goiter, thyroid disease

MCC particular objective
Exclude malignancy.

MCC differential diagnosis
with added evidence

BENIGN

Congenital condition (e.g., thyroglossal duct cyst)
THYROGLOSSAL DUCT CYST

This is the most common form of congenital cyst in the neck.

Bacterial infection is a common complication.

Signs and symptoms: child aged 2 to 10 years (most common); midline upper cystic neck mass that is at or below the hyoid bone; cyst that moves up when swallowing or when patient sticks out their tongue; possible cyst tenderness; ectopic thyroid glands (usual); history of recent upper respiratory tract infection (often)

Investigations: CT scan to confirm size, extent, and location of cyst

Inflammatory condition (e.g., reactive lymph nodes)
REACTIVE LYMPH NODES

Signs and symptoms: history of infections, immune system disorders (e.g., systemic lupus erythematosus, rheumatoid arthritis), other inflammatory conditions; nodes that may initially appear as simple palpable enlargements, with possible progression to red, painful, and tender lumps on the neck

Investigations: blood tests to detect infection response and any thyroid condition

Neoplasm (e.g., lipomas)
LIPOMA

This is a subcutaneous lesion made of adipose tissue.

Signs and symptoms: age 40 to 60 (more common); family history of lipoma (often); smooth, soft, movable, painless mass; mass that is small (< 5 cm in diameter, usually), slow growing, and commonly located on the upper extremities, neck, trunk, axillae

Investigations: ultrasound, MRI

Goiter

Goiter involves abnormal growth of the thyroid gland, and may be associated with normal, decreased, or increased thyroid hormone production.

Signs and symptoms: diffuse or nodular neck enlargement; compressive symptoms in large goiters (hoarse voice, difficulty swallowing, dyspnea)

Investigations: thyrotropin (TSH), thyroid ultrasound

MALIGNANT

MALIGNANT NECK MASSES IN GENERAL

Signs and symptoms of malignancy: nodes that are fixed, large, firm; voice changes; difficulty swallowing; shortness of breath; hemoptysis; high thyrotropin (TSH); systemic symptoms (e.g., pulmonary symptoms, neurologic symptoms)

Thyroid cancer

Signs and symptoms: female (more common); asymptomatic early in disease (symptoms present once the tumour is large enough); palpable lump on the anterior neck due to swollen lymph nodes or thyroid nodule; voice change; difficulty speaking; increased hoarseness; difficulty swallowing; shortness of breath; pain in the neck and throat

> Papillary carcinoma (slowest growing): most common type of thyroid cancer; well differentiated; patient age commonly 30 to 50
>
> Follicular thyroid cancer: well differentiated; patient age commonly older than 50
>
> Medullary thyroid cancer: elevated calcitonin in blood
>
> Anaplastic thyroid cancer (fastest growing, rare): undifferentiated; highly aggressive and metastatic; patient age commonly older than 60

Risk factors: exposure to radiation; family history of thyroid cancer or goiters; abnormal amount of iodine in diet

Nonthyroid head and neck cancers

Signs and symptoms: symptoms for > 3 weeks; persistent unilateral throat discomfort

> Lesion in oral cavity: persistent red and/or white patches on the oral mucosa; ulceration and/or swelling of the oropharynx or mucosa; persistent mass; tongue pain; tongue deviation; hoarseness; unexplained tooth mobility and/or looseness; earache; difficulty swallowing; bleeding in the oral cavity; stridor; facial pain or numbness
>
> Lesion in nasopharynx: neck lump; bloody nasal discharge; nasal blockage; unilateral hearing loss; ringing in the ear; recurrent otitis media; headache; facial pain or numbness; double vision; persistent cough

Investigations: endoscopy; fine needle aspiration or core biopsy of mass

Lymphoma

Signs and symptoms: neck or thyroid nodules or lesions that are asymptomatic (often); firm, painless, fixed, persistent, or rapidly enlarging lesions that are "rubbery"; constitutional symptoms (fatigue, weight loss, night sweats)

> Non-Hodgkin lymphoma: constitutional symptoms (fatigue, fever, night sweats, weight loss), enlarged lymph nodes, chest pain, coughing, shortness of breath

> Hodgkin lymphoma (less common): constitutional symptoms (fatigue, fever, night sweats, weight loss); enlarged lymph nodes; itching or pain on drinking alcohol, or increased sensitivity to alcohol

Investigations: CBC with differential, platelet count; CT scan; excisional biopsy for immunophenotyping; fine needle aspiration biopsy for cytologic classification, cytogenetics

Strategy for patient encounter

The likely scenario is a patient with symptoms of hyper- or hypothyroidism. The specified tasks could engage history, physical exam, investigations, or management.

History

Start with open-ended inquiry: Tell me about the symptoms you have been experiencing. Listen for evidence of thyroid dysfunction (e.g., weight gain, cold intolerance, impaired cognition in hypothyroidism; weight loss, tremor, diarrhea in hyperthyroidism), and difficulty swallowing and/or constitutional symptoms (these suggest malignancy). Ask about risk factors for malignancy (smoking, family history, radiation exposure).

Physical exam

Obtain the patient's vital signs, looking for signs of thyroid dysfunction (tachycardia in hyperthyroidism, diastolic hypertension in hypothyroidism). Perform a head and neck exam. Palpate the thyroid and assess for the presence of a goiter or nodules. Assess for the presence of enlarged lymph nodes.

Investigations

If malignancy is possible, order an ultrasound or CT scan. In suspected thyroid disorder or mass, order thyroid function tests.

Management

Management depends on the entity identified. Consider referral to an ear, nose, and throat (ENT) surgeon and/or endocrinologist.

94

Neonatal distress

MCC particular objectives

Assess the need for, and initiate, resuscitation.

Identify causal and ongoing pathologies.

Determine if the infant needs level 2 or 3 neonatal intensive care.

MCC differential diagnosis
with added evidence

PREMATURITY

This section lists conditions related to prematurity that may present with distress.

RESPIRATORY DISTRESS SYNDROME

This is common in premature neonates due to deficiency of pulmonary surfactant.

Signs and symptoms: tachypnea, grunting, chest retractions, nasal flaring, cyanosis, apnea

Investigations: chest X-ray to detect ground-glass appearance, air bronchograms, low lung volume, absence of thymus

APNEA

This may be preceded by squirming, crying, and eye opening.

Signs and symptoms: possible airway obstruction; bradycardia; cyanosis, blood pressure fluctuation

PERSISTENT PULMONARY HYPERTENSION

Signs and symptoms (labile hypoxemia): large variations in peripheral capillary oxygen saturation and arterial partial oxygen pressure; single loud S2 and systolic murmur on auscultation

Investigations: chest X-ray, ECG

PATENT DUCTUS ARTERIOSUS

Signs and symptoms: nonspecific signs (pulmonary edema, loss of lung compliance); systolic or systolic-diastolic murmur at the upper left sternal border; "machinery murmur" (continuous heart murmur louder in the left upper chest or infraclavicular area)

BRONCHOPULMONARY DYSPLASIA

Signs and symptoms: paradoxical breathing pattern (diaphragm dysfunction); rales, coarse rhonchi, wheezing on auscultation

Investigations: chest X-ray or CT scan

NEONATAL HYPOXIC-ISCHEMIC ENCEPHALOPATHY

Signs and symptoms: depressed tone, reflexes, respiration; fetal umbilical artery acidemia

PULMONARY CONDITION (E.G., MECONIUM ASPIRATION, PNEUMOTHORAX)

MECONIUM ASPIRATION SYNDROME

Signs and symptoms: symptoms that develop within 15 minutes of birth; respiratory distress (tachypnea, grunting, chest retractions, nasal flaring, cyanosis, apnea); neonatal depression (bradycardia; decreased respiratory effort and muscle tone); presence of meconium below the vocal cords, or heavy meconium staining in amniotic fluid

Maternal risk factors for meconium-stained amniotic fluid: diabetes, chronic respiratory or cardiovascular disease, preeclampsia, heavy smoking, postterm delivery, cesarean delivery

Investigations: chest X-ray, pulse oximetry

PNEUMOTHORAX

Signs and symptoms: respiratory distress (tachypnea, grunting, chest retractions, nasal flaring, cyanosis, apnea), absence of breath sounds on auscultation

Investigations: chest X-ray; transillumination of the chest to detect pockets of air

DECREASED RESPIRATORY DRIVE (E.G., MATERNAL MEDICATIONS, ASPHYXIA)

MATERNAL MEDICATIONS

Examples of medications include depressants, narcotics (abused or prescribed), barbiturates, local anesthesia, alcohol, and magnesium.

NEONATAL ASPHYXIA

Hypoxic damage can happen to most organs. Brain damage is of most concern.

Signs and symptoms: bradycardia; cyanosis; low perfusion, responsiveness, muscle tone, reflexes; respiratory effort; possible meconium aspiration (see above); acidosis; seizures

CARDIOVASCULAR CONDITION (E.G., ANEMIA, CONGENITAL HEART DISEASE)

ANEMIA

Causes of anemia in neonates include hemolytic anemia, autoimmune hemolytic anemia, transfusion reaction, and alpha-thalassemia.

Signs and symptoms: jaundice, generalized edema, hepatomegaly, splenomegaly, tachycardia, tachypnea

Investigations: fetal hematocrit or hemoglobin via umbilical cord blood sampling, or direct neonatal blood tests; RBCs; peripheral blood smear; blood antigen typing for incompatibility with maternal IgG

CONGENITAL HEART DISEASE

Types of defects include hole in the heart, obstructed flow, blood vessel abnormalities, valve abnormalities, underdeveloped heart, and possibly a combination of defects.

Signs and symptoms: failure to thrive; feeding intolerance; tachypnea; sweating, especially with feeding; cyanosis; slow capillary refill; regional swelling; uneven blood pressure in all 4 limbs

Heart: characteristic gallop rhythm, pathologic murmurs

Investigations: echocardiogram, ECG

INFECTION

Infection usually occurs by vertical transmission. Examples include group B streptococci, *Escherichia coli*, *Staphylococcus aureus*, *Listeria monocytogenes*, *Streptococcus viridans*, *Haemophilus influenzae*, Cytomegalovirus, respiratory syncytial virus, human metapneumovirus, parainfluenza virus, human coronavirus, herpes simplex virus (HSV), HIV, *Candida albicans*, *Candida parapsilosis*, and *Aspergillus*.

Signs and symptoms: chest retractions; tachycardia or bradycardia; nasal flaring; grunting; apnea; rash; lethargy; hypothermia or fever; irritability; poor perfusion; hypotension; acidosis; diarrhea; poor feeding; bulging fontanelle; seizures; disseminated intravascular coagulation; jaundice

Risk factors for sepsis (from mother): chorioamnionitis (intrauterine onset of infection); intrapartum maternal temperature ≥ 38° C; < 37 weeks gestation at delivery; membrane rupture > 18 hours before delivery

Investigations: CBC; CRP; culture or antigen tests (urine, CSF, throat swab, other fluids)

Strategy for patient encounter

This clinical presentation will likely involve a simulated neonate in distress. The likely task is emergency management.

Emergency management

AIRWAY AND HEMODYNAMIC STATUS

The first task is to determine if the child is in respiratory distress. Start by assessing the patient's airway, breathing, and circulation (mnemonic: **ABCs**). Note the presence of tachypnea (respiration rate higher than 60 breaths per minute) and/or tachycardia (heart rate higher than 160 beats per minute). Initiate resuscitation as necessary (see the quick reference).

HISTORY

Perform a history and physical exam at the same time.

Ask focused questions about onset, current symptoms, maternal and obstetric history, and family history.

- **Onset and current symptoms:** Was the onset sudden or gradual? Is the baby's respiration improving or deteriorating? Are there associated symptoms of cough, feeding difficulties, and/or regurgitation?

- **Maternal and obstetric history:** What was your (the mother's) group B streptococcus status? Were there problems during labour and delivery (e.g., prolonged rupture of membranes, maternal fever, birth trauma, meconium aspiration, asphyxia)? What was the baby's Apgar score?

TIP

Working with nurses to provide emergency care

This scenario is likely to involve nurses. The MCC identifies unclear directions to nurses as a common exam error.

To avoid this error, work out some standard directions for nurses in emergency scenarios. Emergency scenarios are likely to involve nurses, and likely to involve similar procedures to stabilize the patient. For example, if 1 nurse is present:

- Ask the nurse to take the patient's vital signs and obtain intravenous access.
- You start ventilation.

If 2 nurses are present:

- Ask for the first name of each nurse present.
- Ask a specific nurse by name to start ventilation.
- Ask a specific nurse by name to take the patient's vital signs and obtain intravenous access.

QUICK REFERENCE

Neonatal resuscitation

The Canadian Paediatric Society released the latest, seventh edition of its Neonatal Resuscitation Program in 2016. Information about the seventh edition is available on the society's website (use the search term *Canadian Paediatric Society 7th edition NRP information* in your browser).

- **Family history:** Is there a family history of lung disorders or congenital heart disease? Is there a family history of early childhood deaths?

PHYSICAL EXAM

Measure the baby's oxygen saturation with a pulse oximeter. Observe the baby for cyanosis, pallor, and asymmetric chest wall movement (relevant for tension pneumothorax). Palpate the trachea (displacement may indicate tension pneumothorax). Auscultate the lungs and heart.

INVESTIGATIONS

Order an arterial blood gas test (or a cord blood gas test, if the baby is postdelivery), complete blood count (CBC), blood cultures, a blood glucose test, and a C-reactive protein (CRP) test (this may be elevated in sepsis). Order a chest X-ray, and consider an echocardiogram or electrocardiogram (ECG), if indicated.

MANAGEMENT

In addition to resuscitation, if necessary, obtain an emergent referral to a neonatologist and provide ongoing supportive care. Specialized neonatal care for ill newborns is categorized as level 2 (newborns of 32 weeks gestational age or older who are expected to improve rapidly) or level 3 (newborns younger than 32 weeks gestational age who are expected to require subspecialty care). Following stabilization, arrange to transfer the neonate to a facility that provides the appropriate level of care.

95

Numbness, tingling, altered sensation

MCC particular objectives
None stated.

MCC differential diagnosis
with added evidence

PERIPHERAL NEUROPATHY (E.G., DIABETIC NEUROPATHY, CARPAL TUNNEL SYNDROME, RADICULOPATHY)

PERIPHERAL NEUROPATHIES IN GENERAL

Signs and symptoms:

> Motor: weakness, fatigue, wasting, cramps, twitching, myokymia, decreased reflexes

> Sensory: numbness, tingling; burning or stabbing pain; gait and balance difficulty; temperature intolerance; hyperalgesia

DIABETIC NEUROPATHY

Signs and symptoms: polydipsia, polyuria, and/or weight loss; autonomic neuropathy effects (in addition to general motor and sensory symptoms, listed above) including indigestion, nausea, diarrhea, constipation, dizziness, difficulty urinating, erectile dysfunction, vaginal dryness

CARPAL TUNNEL SYNDROME

This is caused by compression or irritation of the median nerve within the carpal tunnel.

Signs and symptoms: numbness, tingling, weakness in the arm and hand

Risk factors: previous wrist injury or surgery; female; history of inflammatory conditions (e.g., rheumatoid arthritis); fluid retention from pregnancy (this resolves after delivery) or menopause; workplace factors such as working with vibrating tools, work that requires prolonged or repetitive flexing (e.g., assembly-line work), and working in cold temperatures

Investigations: X-ray (wrist, arm, or hand); EMG; nerve conduction study of the median nerve

RADICULOPATHY

ACUTE LUMBOSACRAL (LOWER BACK) RADICULOPATHY

Signs and symptoms:

> L5 radiculopathy: back pain that radiates down the lateral side of the leg into the foot; reduced strength on flexing the foot in any direction (up, down, in, out); reduced sensation on the lateral side of the lower leg and upper foot (when testing sharp sensation in the web space between the first and second digits)

> S1 radiculopathy: pain that radiates from the back down the posterior side of the leg into the foot; weakness on flexing the foot down, extending the leg, flexing the knee; reduced sensation on the posterior side of the leg and lateral edge of the foot; loss of ankle reflex

CERVICAL (NECK) RADICULOPATHY

Signs and symptoms: pain in the neck (acute or chronic), upper limbs, shoulders, interscapular region, chest, breast, face; possible mild sensory loss

CENTRAL NERVOUS SYSTEM (E.G., MULTIPLE SCLEROSIS)

MULTIPLE SCLEROSIS

Signs and symptoms: variable depending on lesion location

> Spinal cord: sensory or motor dysfunction; Lhermitte sign (paresthesias radiating down the extremities or trunk with neck flexion); bowel, bladder or erectile dysfunction

> Brainstem: double vision; swallowing, speech difficulties; vertigo; pseudobulbar palsy

> Cerebrum: cognitive impairment; depression; upper motor neuron signs; unilateral motor or sensory deficits

> Cerebellum: problems with balance and coordination; vertigo

> Other symptoms: tonic spasms; fatigue; pain; exercise intolerance; temperature sensitivity; painful unilateral loss of visual acuity

Risk factors: younger than 50, female

Investigations: brain and spinal cord MRI, including advanced MRI techniques, with established occurrence of multiple episodes; CSF fluid analysis

DERMATOLOGICAL CONDITION (E.G., HERPES ZOSTER, ANGIOEDEMA)

HERPES ZOSTER (CUTANEOUS)

Signs and symptoms: unilateral dermatomal rash that does not cross the midline (i.e., reaction from a single nerve root or ganglion);

involvement of thoracic, trigeminal, lumbar, and cervical dermatomes (common); rash that is often preceded by prodromal pain, itching, tingling, intense pain to light touch; continuous or episodic symptoms

> Rash progression: red macules to papules to clear vesicles (1 to 5 days) to pustules (1 week) to lesion ulceration and crusting (second week) to lesion healing (2 to 4 weeks)

ANGIOEDEMA

Common triggers include allergies and environmental factors (heat, cold, sunlight, water, pressure on the skin, emotional stress, and exercise).

Signs and symptoms: symptoms that can be chronic (frequent, unpredictable recurrence); involvement of the dermis, subcutaneous tissue, mucosa, submucosa; swelling with pain or burning that can affect the eyes, cheeks, lips, hands, feet, genitals, inside the throat

Investigations: CBC with differential, liver function tests, CRP, ESR, complement protein C4

MENTAL DISORDER (E.G., PANIC ATTACKS)

PANIC ATTACKS[1(pp189-234)]

Panic attacks can arise from anxiety disorders, such as generalized anxiety disorder, panic disorder, separation anxiety disorder, social anxiety disorder, and specific phobia. In panic disorder, panic attacks occur spontaneously. In other anxiety disorders, panic attacks can have specific triggers (e.g., phobic objects in specific phobia).

Signs and symptoms: history of anxiety disorder and/or symptoms consistent with a panic attack; history of social or emotional triggers for symptoms (possible); lack of evidence for other causes, including hyperthyroidism (anxiety can mimic other conditions and is therefore a diagnosis of exclusion)

> Panic attack: symptoms that peak within minutes; symptoms that can include palpitations, accelerated heart rate, shortness of breath, chest pain, dizziness, numbness or tingling, fear of losing control, fear of dying

Strategy for patient encounter

The likely scenario is a patient with localized numbness, likely carpal tunnel syndrome. The specified tasks could engage history, physical exam, investigations, or management.

History

Start by establishing the distribution of the symptoms, because this should point to a likely diagnosis: Where are you experiencing numbness? Ask about risk factors for diabetes (personal or family history), and workplace injury or repetitive tasks (relevant for carpal tunnel syndrome). Ask about a history of anxiety disorders and symptoms of panic attacks (recurrent surges of intense fear or discomfort that peak within minutes).

Physical exam
Perform a regional neurological exam of the affected area. Examine the skin for rashes (this is relevant for herpes zoster).

Investigations
For all patients, order a fasting glucose or glycated hemoglobin (HbA_{1c}) test to screen for diabetes. In possible carpal tunnel syndrome, nerve conduction studies may help in the diagnosis.

Management
Manage any underlying conditions. Consider referral to a plastic surgeon for patients with carpal tunnel syndrome.

REFERENCE

1 American Psychiatric Association. Diagnostic and statistical manual of mental disorders. 5th ed. Arlington, VA: American Psychiatric Association; 2013. 991 p.

96

Generalized pain disorders

MCC particular objective
Differentiate articular from nonarticular pain.

MCC differential diagnosis
with added evidence

FIBROMYALGIA OR CHRONIC FATIGUE SYNDROME
FIBROMYALGIA
This is a diagnosis of exclusion.

Signs and symptoms: female (more common); chronic, widespread pain for ≥ 3 months; pain that is bilateral, and above and below the waist; aching pain; fatigue; long sleep; restless legs syndrome; sleep apnea; impaired concentration, memory; dizziness; cramping (e.g., menstrual, abdominal); morning stiffness; numbness, tingling in the extremities; tender points; urinary symptoms (difficult or painful urination; irregular urination); sensitivity to noise, light, temperature

> Coexisting conditions (often): headaches, irritable bowel syndrome, interstitial cystitis

CHRONIC FATIGUE SYNDROME

Signs and symptoms: extreme fatigue unexplained by any underlying medical condition; symptoms that do not improve with rest; symptoms for ≥ 6 months

> Other symptoms: loss of memory or concentration; sore throat; enlarged lymph nodes (neck, armpits); muscle pain; pain that moves among joints without swelling or redness; headache of a new type, pattern, or severity; unrefreshing sleep; extreme exhaustion lasting > 24 hours after mental or physical exertion

POLYMYALGIA RHEUMATICA

Signs and symptoms: older than 50 (always); female (more common); northern European descent (higher incidence); history of giant cell temporal arteritis (many patients have this, but it may not be active at the same time as polymyalgia rheumatica); symmetrical symptoms (usual); shoulder pain (more common), hip pain, neck pain; stiffness (morning stiffness usually lasts ≥ 30 minutes, with inability to abduct shoulders past 90 degrees); pain that is worse with movement; synovitis and bursitis (many patients have distal musculoskeletal manifestations)

Investigations: elevated ESR (≥ 50 mm/h); elevated serum CRP

MENTAL HEALTH DISORDER (E.G., DEPRESSION, SOMATIC SYMPTOM DISORDER)

MAJOR DEPRESSIVE DISORDER[1(pp160–161)]

Signs and symptoms: symptoms that are present most of the time for ≥ 2 weeks; symptoms with significant impact on day-to-day life

> Key symptoms: depressed mood and/or loss of interest in usual activities

> Other symptoms: significant weight change; sleep disturbance; slowed or agitated mental processes; loss of concentration; recurrent thoughts of death or suicide

Risk factors: family history of mental health disorders (depression, anxiety, suicide); personal history of other mental health disorders; substance abuse; chronic illness (e.g., cancer, stroke, chronic pain)

SOMATIC SYMPTOM DISORDER[1(p311)]

Signs and symptoms: disproportionate and persistent thoughts about the seriousness of a health concern, and/or excessive and persistent anxiety about a health concern, and/or excessive time or energy devoted to a health concern; presence of symptoms for ≥ 6 months (the health concern involved may change); symptoms with significant impact on day-to-day life

Strategy for patient encounter

The likely scenario is a patient with generalized muscle pain. The specified tasks could engage history, physical exam, investigations, or management.

History

Causes of generalized pain can be difficult to separate.

Start with open-ended inquiry about the patient's symptoms: Please tell me about the pain you have been experiencing. What other symptoms do you have? Listen for evidence consistent with particular entities (e.g., the presence of morning stiffness in fibromyalgia and polymyalgia rheumatica; shoulder pain and pain that is worse with movement in polymyalgia rheumatica; enlarged lymph nodes in chronic fatigue syndrome; depressed mood combined with possible weight loss and/or suicidal thoughts in major depressive disorder). Ask specifically about morning stiffness and symptoms of depression, if the patient doesn't volunteer this information. Ask about a personal history of giant cell temporal arteritis (relevant for polymyalgia rheumatica), and a personal or family history of mental health disorders.

Physical exam

Perform a musculoskeletal exam looking for areas of tenderness. Palpate for tenderness over the temporal arteries.

Investigations

For all patients, order an erythrocyte sedimentation rate (ESR) or C-reactive protein (CRP) level. In suspected temporal arteritis, refer the patient to a surgeon for temporal artery biopsy.

Management

Polymyalgia rheumatica and temporal arteritis require immediate treatment with steroids. Patients with suicidal ideation (in major depressive disorder) may require hospitalization.

Pearls

The best way to treat fibromyalgia is through a multidisciplinary approach. A number of medications have been used with varying results, including antidepressants, nonsteroidal antiinflammatory drugs (NSAIDs), muscle relaxants, and antiepileptics. If medications are used at all, they should be combined with physical exercise and cognitive behavioural therapy.

REFERENCE

1 American Psychiatric Association. Diagnostic and statistical manual of mental disorders. 5th ed. Arlington, VA: American Psychiatric Association; 2013. 991 p.

97

Central or peripheral neuropathic pain

MCC particular objectives

None stated.

MCC differential diagnosis
with added evidence

METABOLIC CONDITION (E.G., DIABETIC NEUROPATHY)

DIABETIC NEUROPATHY

Signs and symptoms: symptoms in the legs and feet (most common); symptoms worse at night; numbness; tingling, burning sensations; sharp pains, cramps; hypersensitivity to touch; muscle weakness; loss of reflexes, especially in the ankles; loss of balance, coordination; foot ulcers, infections, deformities

> Diabetes: personal or family history of diabetes; history of diabetic complications and/or inadequate monitoring; polydipsia, polyuria, and/or weight loss

Investigations: neuromuscular signal conduction tests

NERVE ENTRAPMENT (E.G., CARPAL TUNNEL SYNDROME, LYMPHOMA, TRIGEMINAL NEURALGIA)

NERVE ENTRAPMENT OR COMPRESSION IN GENERAL

Signs and symptoms:

> Initial: numbness, pain, tingling; positive Tinel sign
>
> Subsequent: impaired function and muscle weakness; possible muscle atrophy

Investigations: nerve conduction studies

CARPAL TUNNEL SYNDROME

This is caused by compression or irritation of the median nerve within the carpal tunnel.

Signs and symptoms: numbness, tingling, weakness in the arm and hand

Risk factors: previous wrist injury or surgery; female; history of inflammatory conditions (e.g., rheumatoid arthritis); fluid retention from pregnancy (this resolves after delivery) or menopause; workplace factors such as working with vibrating tools, work that requires prolonged or repetitive flexing (e.g., assembly-line work), and working in cold temperatures

Investigations: X-ray (wrist, arm, or hand); EMG; nerve conduction study of the median nerve

LYMPHOMA

Enlarged lymph nodes may press on nerves, causing limb pain.

Signs and symptoms (non-Hodgkin lymphoma): constitutional symptoms (fatigue, fever, night sweats, weight loss), enlarged lymph nodes, chest pain, coughing, shortness of breath

> Hodgkin lymphoma (less common): constitutional symptoms (fatigue, fever, night sweats, weight loss); enlarged lymph nodes; itching or pain on drinking alcohol, or increased sensitivity to alcohol

Investigations: blasts or cancer cells on peripheral blood smear; excess blasts or cancer cells on bone marrow examination

TRIGEMINAL NEURALGIA

Compression of the trigeminal nerve near the brain stem may occur due to the effects on a nearby blood vessel because of trauma, stroke, or multiple sclerosis.

Signs and symptoms: severe, sudden, shock-like unilateral facial pain that last seconds to minutes with possible multiple episodes over hours; spontaneous pain or pain triggered by touch, air currents, eating, talking

INFECTION (E.G., POSTHERPETIC NEURALGIA)

POSTHERPETIC NEURALGIA

This involves pain > 4 months after the initial onset of rash from herpes zoster.

Signs and symptoms: advanced age (more common); involvement of thoracic (T4 to T6), cervical, trigeminal nerves; burning, sharp, stabbing pain that is constant or intermittent in areas of lost or impaired sensation; pain triggered by nonpainful stimuli (e.g., light touch); areas lacking sensation; deficits of thermal, tactile, pinprick, and vibration sensations with affected dermatomes

Severe: impaired sleep; decreased appetite; diminished libido

CENTRAL PAIN (E.G., PHANTOM LIMB PAIN, SPINAL CORD INJURY)

CENTRAL PAIN IN GENERAL

This is a delayed reaction that may come from amputation (phantom limb pain), spinal cord injury, trauma, tumours, stroke, and diseases such as multiple sclerosis and Parkinson disease.

Signs and symptoms: pain that is unrelenting, moderate to excruciating, localized or diffuse (localized in the case of phantom limb pain); burning sensations (common); pain with peculiar qualities (e.g., "skin coming off," "boring into bone marrow"); pain that is made worse by touch, movement, emotions, changes in temperature

Other: nausea, vomiting, hyperventilation, hypertonia

SYMPATHETIC PAIN (E.G., REFLEX SYMPATHETIC DYSTROPHY)

REFLEX SYMPATHETIC DYSTROPHY (COMPLEX REGIONAL PAIN SYNDROME)

Signs and symptoms: chronic unilateral pain in an arm or leg; history of trauma to the limb (many cases involve trauma; others may involve surgery, stroke, heart attack); pain out of proportion to the initial injury

Early symptoms in the affected limb: pain; swelling; redness; changes in skin temperature (from sweaty and hot to cold); cold, touch sensitivity

Later symptoms in the affected limb: changes in skin colour (pallor), texture (thin, shiny, tender), hair growth, and nail growth; muscle spasms

Investigations: sympathetic nervous system tests to detect disturbances; bone scan to detect possible bone changes; X-rays for later stage bone-mineral assessment

Strategy for patient encounter

The likely scenario is a patient with a history of herpes zoster who now has neuralgia. The specified tasks could engage history, physical exam, investigations, or management.

History

Use open-ended questions to take a thorough pain history: Where is the pain? What kind of pain is it (e.g., sharp, dull, throbbing)? How bad is the pain on a scale of 1 to 10? Where does the pain radiate? What makes the pain better? What makes it worse? What other symptoms do you have? The evidence should considerably narrow the differential diagnosis. Ask about psychosocial and functional impairment as a result of the pain.

Physical exam

Examine the affected area, paying particular attention to neuro-vascular examination.

Investigations

Consider a fasting glucose or glycated hemoglobin (HbA_{1c}) test in most patients to rule out diabetic neuropathy. Peripheral neuropathy (e.g., carpal tunnel syndrome) can be confirmed by nerve conduction studies, which can also indicate the urgency for surgery. Consider a chest X-ray to help rule out the presence of lymphoma. Patients with signs of vascular insufficiency should be referred for vascular studies.

Management

Treat any underlying conditions (e.g., diabetes, carpal tunnel syndrome). Discuss pharmacotherapy options. Counsel the patient regarding exercise and activity modification.

98

Palpitations

MCC particular objectives

Identify patients in need of urgent care.

Differentiate palpitations due to intrinsic heart disease from palpitations due to anxiety, exertion, or other systemic disease.

MCC differential diagnosis
with added evidence

SUPRAVENTRICULAR CONDITION

Sinus tachycardia

INCREASED DEMAND (E.G., PREGNANCY, ANEMIA)

PREGNANCY

Signs and symptoms: amenorrhea, especially during childbearing years (some experience spotting); sexual activity, especially without contraception or with inconsistent use of contraception; nausea, vomiting (common early sign); breast enlargement and tenderness; increased frequency of urination without pain or difficulty; fatigue

Investigations: blood or urine β-hCG

ANEMIA

Signs and symptoms: pallor, chest pain, palpitations, weakness, headache, dizziness, shortness of breath

Risk factors: intestinal disorders (Crohn disease, celiac disease), menstruation, pregnancy, chronic disease (e.g., cancer, kidney failure), family history of sickle cell disease

Investigations: CBC; visual examination of RBCs for unusual size, shape, colour

METABOLIC CONDITION (E.G., THYROTOXICOSIS, PHEOCHROMOCYTOMA)

THYROTOXICOSIS (INCLUDES HYPERTHYROIDISM)

A thyroid storm may lead to heart failure.

Signs and symptoms: tachycardia; palpitations; weight loss despite increased appetite; tremor; muscle weakness; sweating; fatigue; anxiety; poor concentration; heat intolerance; neck swelling; depression; eye irritation; eyelid swelling; warm moist skin; hair thinning; atrial fibrillation

Investigations: blood tests (findings: low thyrotropin, elevated free T_4 or T_3); ECG (findings: sinus tachycardia; increased QRS voltages; atrial fibrillation)

PHEOCHROMOCYTOMA

Signs and symptoms: tachycardia; pallor; headaches; shortness of breath; symptoms that occur in brief spells (up to 20 minutes) with no symptoms between (these spells may be mistaken for panic attacks); volatile or therapy-resistant hypertension

Investigations: plasma metanephrines or urinary fractionated metanephrines to measure catecholamines; abdominal and pelvic MRI or CT scan

ANXIETY[1(pp189–234)]

Examples of anxiety disorders listed in the *Diagnostic and Statistical Manual of Mental Disorders* (*DSM-5*) include generalized anxiety disorder, panic disorder, separation anxiety disorder, social anxiety disorder, and specific phobia. Anxiety disorders can provoke panic attacks (e.g., exposure to a phobic object). In the case of panic disorder, panic attacks occur spontaneously.

Signs and symptoms: history of anxiety disorder and/or symptoms consistent with a panic attack; history of social or emotional triggers for symptoms (possible); lack of evidence for other causes, including hyperthyroidism (anxiety can mimic other conditions and is therefore a diagnosis of exclusion)

> Panic attack: symptoms that peak within minutes; symptoms that can include palpitations, accelerated heart rate, shortness of breath, chest pain, dizziness, numbness or tingling, fear of losing control, fear of dying

DRUGS (E.G., COCAINE, CAFFEINE)

Atrial fibrillation or flutter

ATRIAL FIBRILLATION

Signs and symptoms: sustained irregular heart rhythm on pulse palpation or auscultation; shortness of breath; light-headedness or dizziness; focal neurological deficits; variable S_1 intensity and absence of S_4 on auscultation

Risk factors: hypertension, coronary heart disease, valvular heart disease, diabetes mellitus, sleep apnea

Investigations: ECG

> Findings: absence of P waves; irregular R-R intervals; narrow QRS complex (< 120 milliseconds) if no underlying bundle branch block

ATRIAL FLUTTER

Signs and symptoms: persistent or paroxysmal palpitations

> More severe: dizziness, chest pain, shortness of breath, anxiety

Investigations: AV conduction (findings: ventricular rate 140 to 150 beats per minute; AV conduction 2:1 or 4:1); 12-lead ECG (finding: flutter waves)

Supraventricular tachycardia (atrioventricular reentrant tachycardia), Wolff-Parkinson-White syndrome

SUPRAVENTRICULAR TACHYCARDIA

This is the most common arrhythmia in pediatrics.

Signs and symptoms: tachycardia (regular, fast cardiac rhythm of 150 to 270 beats per minute); episodes that last minutes to days; fatigue; light-headedness; chest pain; shortness of breath; anxiety; syncope

Investigations: ECG

> Findings: narrow QRS complex (< 120 milliseconds)

WOLFF-PARKINSON-WHITE SYNDROME

This is caused by congenital cardiac bypass tracts.

Signs and symptoms: young adult male (more common); tachycardia; palpitations; shortness of breath; syncope; fatigue; anxiety; chest pain, tightness; episodes that last seconds to hours, at rest or during exercise

Investigations: ECG (findings: short PR interval; delta waves; increased QRS interval)

Junctional tachycardia

This is a form of supraventricular tachycardia involving the atrioventricular node.

Causes include digitalis toxicity, theophylline, onset of acute coronary syndrome, and heart failure.

Signs and symptoms: tachycardia (either present or provoked by esophageal stimulation or invasive electrophysiological investigation); ventricular rate of 60 to 100 beats per minute; palpitations; fatigue, light-headedness; chest pain; shortness of breath; anxiety; polyuria; pounding sensation in the neck

> Automatic junctional tachycardia: irregular rhythm and heart rate; nonresponsiveness to vagal maneuvers (e.g., gagging, holding breath, coughing)

Investigations: ECG

> Findings: P wave that may be inverted in inferior leads (P wave can be before, during, or after QRS complex); narrow QRS complex (< 120 milliseconds)

Premature junctional complexes and premature atrial contractions

PREMATURE JUNCTIONAL COMPLEXES

Signs and symptoms: often asymptomatic, palpitations with hypotension (it may occur in healthy patients, or may be due to drug cardiotoxicity, electrolyte imbalance, mitral valve surgery, or cold water immersion)

Risk factors: stress; caffeine, nicotine, alcohol use

Investigations: ECG (findings: normal QRS complex, preceded by an abnormal P wave or no P wave)

PREMATURE ATRIAL CONTRACTIONS

Signs and symptoms: heart "skipping a beat"; occasionally strong heartbeat, fluttering sensation

Risk factors: stress, poor sleep, caffeine use, alcohol use

Investigations: ECG (findings: P wave with different morphology from preceding P waves; premature atrial complex followed by a noncompensatory pause)

VENTRICULAR CONDITION

Ventricular tachycardia

Sudden cardiac death or cardiac arrest is possible.

Causes include cardiomyopathy; structural or ischemic heart disease; heart failure; and oral macrolide antibiotics.

Signs and symptoms: palpitations, tachycardia, dizziness, syncope, fatigue, shortness of breath, angina, hypotension

Investigations: ECG (findings: ≥ 3 continuous beats of wide QRS with a pulse > 100 beats per minute)

Premature ventricular contractions (PVCs)

Signs and symptoms: feeling of heart "skipping a beat," or a strong beat, or chest suction; chest pain; light-headedness; fatigue; hyperventilation after exercise

Risk factors: alcohol, caffeine, cocaine, nicotine use; exercise; hypertension; hypercalcemia; anxiety; underlying heart disease

Investigations: ECG (**but** isolated PVCs may not be detected due to their infrequency); Holter monitor (this is a better detection method)

Ventricular fibrillation

This is associated with coronary artery disease.

Sudden cardiac death or arrest is a common initial presentation.

Signs and symptoms: underlying rhythm of cardiac arrest

Risk factors: ST-segment elevation and AV-conduction block during acute myocardial infarction

Investigations: ECG

Strategy for patient encounter

The likely scenario is a patient with heart palpitations. The likely tasks are history, physical exam, or investigations. The key is to identify individuals with palpitations due to intrinsic heart disease (as opposed to palpitations due to another systemic disease, or anxiety or exertion).

History

Start with open-ended inquiry about the patient's symptoms: Please tell me about the palpitations you've been experiencing. When do they happen? How long do they last? What accompanying symptoms have you noticed? Listen for symptoms consistent with intrinsic heart disease versus other causes (see the checklist). Ask specifically about symptoms of intrinsic heart disease if the patient doesn't volunteer them (chest pain; tachycardia or bradycardia; syncope). Ask about comorbid conditions, including anxiety, hyperthyroidism, and heart disease.

Physical exam

Obtain the patient's vital signs, and auscultate the heart and lungs. Note the rate and rhythm of the heart.

CHECKLIST

Symptoms of intrinsic heart disease versus other disorders

The following signs and symptoms are suggestive of intrinsic heart disease:

- chest pain
- tachycardia (higher than 100 beats per minute) or bradycardia (lower than 60 beats per minute)
- palpitations associated with syncope

The following symptoms are suggestive of anxiety, exertion, or systemic disease:

- current anxiety disorder or life stressors
- excessive intake of caffeine, alcohol, or nicotine
- hyperventilation, hand tingling, nervousness
- heat intolerance (hyperthyroidism)
- palpitations that can be stopped by deep breathing or changing body position

Investigations

Order an electrocardiogram (ECG) for all patients and be prepared to interpret the results (see the information this resource lists in the MCC differential diagnosis). If the ECG is not diagnostic, order a Holter monitor. Consider an echocardiogram to detect structural or functional abnormalities, and a thyrotropin (TSH) level to rule out thyroid disease. Measure serum electrolytes (potassium and magnesium).

REFERENCE

1 American Psychiatric Association. Diagnostic and statistical manual of mental disorders. 5th ed. Arlington, VA: American Psychiatric Association; 2013. 991 p.

99

Anxiety

MCC particular objectives
None stated.

MCC differential diagnosis
with added evidence
ANXIETY DISORDERS IN GENERAL
Signs and symptoms: symptoms with significant impact on day-to-day life (e.g., significant distress, significant impaired functioning); symptoms that last for weeks or months (as opposed to a few days)

GENERALIZED ANXIETY DISORDER[1(p222)]
Signs and symptoms: excessive anxiety across a number of contexts (e.g., work, school); anxiety that is difficult to control; presence of symptoms for most of the time for ≥ 6 months; **no** evidence of anxiety effects from drugs or medications (e.g., caffeine, alcohol, cannabis, phencyclidine, opioid, amphetamine, cocaine), or medical conditions (e.g., hyperthyroidism, Cushing syndrome)

Risk factors: female; family history of anxiety

POSTTRAUMATIC STRESS DISORDER[1(pp271–272)]
Signs and symptoms in adults: symptoms that begin after a traumatic event and last ≥ 1 month; intrusive symptoms (e.g., flashbacks, recurrent memories, recurrent dreams) about the event; negative changes to mood or perceptions (e.g., exaggerated negative beliefs about self, others, or the world; loss of interest in usual activities); marked changes in arousal or reactions (e.g., verbal or physical aggression with little provocation; self-destructive behaviour; hypervigilance)

> Traumatic events: exposure to death, threat of death, serious injury, or sexual violence through direct experience, witnessing, or repeated exposure (e.g., in the case of first responders), or learning of traumatic events involving close family or friends; **not** exposure via images (e.g., television, movies), unless this occurs through work

SEPARATION ANXIETY DISORDER[1(pp190–191)]
Signs and symptoms: excessive anxiety (e.g., distress, worry, nightmares) about separation from a particular person; physical symptoms provoked by anxiety (e.g., headaches, stomach aches)

Children and adolescents: presence of symptoms for
≥ 4 weeks

Adults: presence of symptoms for ≥ 6 months (usual)

PHOBIA[1(p197)]

SPECIFIC PHOBIA

Signs and symptoms: excessive anxiety about an object or situation
(e.g., insects, receiving an injection); presence of symptoms for
≥ 6 months

PANIC DISORDER[1(pp208–209)]

Signs and symptoms: recurrent unexpected panic attacks; anxiety
about future panic attacks; behaviours to avoid attacks for ≥ 1 month;
no evidence of anxiety effects from drugs or medications (e.g., caffeine,
alcohol, cannabis, phencyclidine, opioid, amphetamine, cocaine), or
medical conditions (e.g., hyperthyroidism, cardiopulmonary disorders)

Panic attack: symptoms that peak within minutes; symptoms
that can include palpitations, accelerated heart rate,
shortness of breath, chest pain, dizziness, numbness or
tingling, fear of losing control, fear of dying

ADJUSTMENT DISORDER[1(pp286–287)]

Signs and symptoms: excessive anxiety in response to an identifiable
stressor and within 3 months of the stressor; symptoms with significant
impact on day-to-day life; abatement of symptoms within 6 months of
cessation of stressor

Strategy for patient encounter

The likely scenario is a patient concerned about panic attacks.
The specified tasks could engage history, physical exam, investigations, or management.

History

Use open-ended inquiry to determine the patient's symptoms:
Please tell me about the symptoms you've been having. Listen for
evidence that:

- distinguishes true anxiety disorders from situational stress
  (see the checklist)
- is consistent with particular anxiety entities (e.g., persistent anxiety across many contexts with fatigue and
  muscle tension in generalized anxiety disorder)
- is consistent with hyperthyroidism (weight loss, tremor,
  weakness, diarrhea)

Ask about a personal or family history of mental illness. Ask about drug and medication use, including caffeine, alcohol, and recreational drugs (to rule these out as a source of the symptoms). Assess the patient for risk factors for self-harm: ask about substance addiction and abuse, and suicidal ideation. Ask about recent life stressors (e.g., job loss, divorce).

CHECKLIST
Distinguishing anxiety disorders from situational stress

Anxiety disorders have the following characteristics, compared to situational stress:

- They involve severe symptoms that significantly disrupt daily life.
- They can involve specific triggers (e.g., phobic objects in specific phobia).
- They have features of persistence: they occur in a variety of contexts and for longer periods of time.

Physical exam

Obtain the patient's vital signs, looking for tachycardia (relevant for hyperthyroidism) and hypertension (relevant for Cushing syndrome). Note any signs consistent with hyperthyroidism (enlarged thyroid, hyperpigmentation, hair loss, hyperactive reflexes) or Cushing syndrome (round red face, pronounced abdominal weight, hump on the upper back, thin arms and legs, high blood pressure, stretch marks, acne).

Investigations

Investigations are generally not needed in this context. In suspected hyperthyroidism, order a serum thyrotropin (TSH). In suspected Cushing syndrome, order a serum cortisol or dexamethasone suppression test.

Management

Ensure the immediate safety of the patient. A patient with specific and immediate plans for suicide requires admission to hospital for psychiatric assessment and monitoring. In patients not at immediate risk, consider referral to a psychiatrist. Treat any underlying or comorbid illness. Initiate treatment with pharmacological and/or psychological therapy, and ensure adequate follow-up.

REFERENCE

1 American Psychiatric Association. Diagnostic and statistical manual of mental disorders. 5th ed. Arlington, VA: American Psychiatric Association; 2013. 991 p.

100

Crying or fussing child

MCC particular objective
Identify pediatric emergencies.

MCC differential diagnosis
with added evidence

CRYING OR FUSSING IN GENERAL

Most crying or fussing expresses a need, and usually stops when the need is met, with fewer and shorter episodes after age 3 months.

Serious causes of crying (about 5% of cases) include cardiac, gastrointestinal, infectious, and traumatic conditions that are potentially life-threatening (heart failure, intussusception, volvulus, meningitis, and intracranial bleeding due to head trauma).

Red flags for pediatric emergencies include respiratory distress; bruising or abrasions; extreme irritability; fever; and inconsolability.

FUNCTIONAL CAUSES (E.G., HUNGER, IRRITABILITY)

COLIC
Signs and symptoms: excessive crying without any identifiable organic cause that occurs for ≥ 3 hours per day for ≥ 3 days per week for ≥ 3 weeks

TRAUMA
This may include obvious injury or occult injury secondary to abuse.

ILLNESS
Examples include common cold, otitis media, and other infections.

Strategy for patient encounter
This encounter will likely involve a parent discussing a child who has colic. The child will be absent on some pretext (e.g., a nurse is taking the child's vital signs and weight in another room). The specified tasks could engage history, physical exam, investigations, or management.

History

Use open-ended questions to determine the child's current symptoms, usual behaviours, and medical and immunization history.

- **Current symptoms:** How long has your child been fussing? How often does your child fuss like this? How well are you able to console your child? What other symptoms have you noticed? Listen for recurrent versus new-onset fussing (recurrent fussing suggests colic); and inconsolable fussing and fever (these are red flags).
- **Usual behaviours:** What is your child's usual sleep pattern? What is your child's usual feeding pattern? To what extent have these patterns changed recently? Listen for acute, marked changes in usual behaviours, which suggest acute illness.
- **Medical and immunization history:** What illnesses has your child had recently? What immunizations has your child had? Listen for recent infections and missed immunizations.

Physical exam

Examine the child for obvious immediate signs of an emergent condition. Because of the broad differential diagnosis for this clinical presentation, use a systems-check approach to avoid physical omissions (see the checklist).

(State that you will perform a physical exam. Because an actual pediatric patient is unlikely, the examiner may

---

CHECKLIST

Systems check for a crying or fussing child

The differential diagnosis for a crying or fussing child is broad, and includes both benign and life-threatening entities. A systematic approach is necessary to ensure that serious presentations are not missed.

- **Head and neck:** skull fracture; ocular or nasal foreign body; corneal abrasion; otitis media; oral thrush; tooth decay; stomatitis
- **Central nervous system:** meningitis, encephalitis
- **Cardiovascular system:** supraventricular tachycardia, myocarditis
- **Pulmonary system:** bronchiolitis, pneumonia, asthma
- **Gastrointestinal system:** appendicitis, gastroenteritis, pyloric stenosis, intussusception, volvulus, gastroesophageal reflux
- **Genitourinary system:** urinary tract infection, testicular torsion, incarcerated inguinal hernia
- **Musculoskeletal system:** fracture or dislocation, osteomyelitis, arthritis
- **Skin:** skin infection or abscess, insect bite, anal fissure
- **Sepsis**

interrupt, ask what you are looking for, and provide findings. State that you will thoroughly and systematically examine the child to rule out emergencies and identify organic illness.)

Investigations

Investigations will depend on the probable diagnosis determined through the history and physical exam. Imaging of the chest, heart, gastrointestinal tract, and head may be required.

Management

Management will depend on the specific entity diagnosed. If no organic disease is detected, counsel the parents to continue to observe the child at home, and bring the child back if new symptoms emerge or the child's condition changes.

101

Hypotonic infant

MCC particular objective

Recognize that hypotonic infants always require urgent attention.

MCC differential diagnosis
with added evidence

HYPOTONIC INFANT IN GENERAL

Signs and symptoms: reduced muscle tone and tension; "floppy infant" (infant seems like a rag doll when held); loosely extended elbows and knees while resting (normal position is flexed); poor head control; decreased spontaneous activity; decreased muscle resistance to stretch

NEUROLOGIC CONDITION (E.G., PERINATAL ASPHYXIA, SPINAL MUSCULAR ATROPHY, MYASTHENIA GRAVIS)

PERINATAL ASPHYXIA

This condition can result in hypoxic damage to most organs. Brain damage is of most concern.

Signs and symptoms: neurologic symptoms (low level of consciousness; seizures; stupor); symptoms of respiratory distress (cyanosis; low perfusion, responsiveness, muscle tone, reflexes, respiratory effort); generalized hypotonia; bradycardia; acidosis

Investigations: ultrasound of the head, MRI to detect brain injury, EEG to assess seizures

SPINAL MUSCULAR ATROPHY

Signs and symptoms: severe weakness that is symmetrical, progressive, more proximal than distal, in the arms more than the legs; poor head control; bilateral facial weakness; impaired tendon reflexes

> Other: hypotonia; severe joint contractures; respiratory failure; atrial septal defects; weak cry and cough; poor feeding

Investigations: genetic testing

MYASTHENIA GRAVIS

Signs and symptoms: ocular weakness (most common presentations: asymmetric drooping eyes; weakness in eye closure; double vision); painless, fluctuating, asymmetric muscle weakness (this may lead to respiratory failure); poor suck, head control; weak limbs

Investigations: serum anti-AChR antibody, single fibre electromyography

DISORDERS OF SKELETAL MUSCLE (E.G., MUSCULAR DYSTROPHY)

MUSCULAR DYSTROPHY

Signs and symptoms (myotonic dystrophy type 1): family history of muscular dystrophy; severe hypotonia and weakness; poor feeding; respiratory difficulties; positional malformations (e.g., club foot); delayed motor and intellectual development

Prenatal signs: reduced fetal movements or excess amniotic fluid

Investigations: genetic testing

GENETIC OR METABOLIC CONDITION (E.G., PRADER-WILLI SYNDROME, HYPOTHYROIDISM)

PRADER-WILLI SYNDROME

Signs and symptoms (adults and children in general): excess fat in the central body; small hands and feet; prominent nasal bridge; thin upper lip; downturned mouth; almond-shaped eyes; high narrow forehead; tapered fingers; soft, easily bruised skin; light skin and hair compared to family members; incomplete sexual development; frequent skin picking; delayed motor development

> Prenatal and neonate: reduced fetal movement; abnormal fetal position; excessive amniotic fluid; breech or cesarean birth; lethargy; hypotonia; poor sucking; hypogonadism

Children: delayed intellectual development; excessive sleeping; strabismus; scoliosis; cryptorchidism; speech delay; poor physical coordination; hyperphagia; excessive weight gain; sleep disorders; delayed puberty; short stature; obesity; extreme flexibility

Adults: infertility; hypogonadism; sparse pubic hair; obesity; hypotonia; learning and cognitive disabilities; diabetes (often)

Investigations: DNA-based methylation testing for Prader-Willi syndrome and Angelman syndrome

HYPOTHYROIDISM

Signs and symptoms in infants:

Early signs: jaundice; frequent choking; large, protruding tongue; puffy face

Later signs: constipation; poor muscle tone; sleepiness

Risk factors: family history of thyroid disease or autoimmune disease

SYSTEMIC ILLNESS (E.G., SEPSIS, DEHYDRATION)

SEPSIS

Definition: infection with systemic inflammatory response, dysfunction of ≥ 1 organ system

Infection usually occurs by vertical transmission. Examples include group B streptococci, *Escherichia coli*, *Staphylococcus aureus*, *Listeria monocytogenes*, *Streptococcus viridans*, *Haemophilus influenzae*, Cytomegalovirus, respiratory syncytial virus, human metapneumovirus, parainfluenza virus, human coronavirus, herpes simplex virus (HSV), HIV, *Candida albicans*, *Candida parapsilosis*, and *Aspergillus*.

Signs and symptoms: fever, tachycardia, tachypnea, poor muscle tone, poor feeding, vomiting, jaundice, abdominal distention, poor perfusion

Severe: oliguria; mental status changes; shortness of breath; extreme hypotension, unresponsive to fluid replacement (this indicates septic shock)

Risk factors: compromised immune system; wounds, burns; catheterization, intubation

Maternal factors: chorioamnionitis (intrauterine onset of infection); intrapartum maternal temperature ≥ 38° C; < 37 weeks gestation; membrane rupture > 18 hours before delivery

Investigations: CBC with differential (elevated neutrophils is a common finding); CRP; blood culture; cultures of other fluids (CSF, urine)

DEHYDRATION

Dehydration presenting with hypotension requires immediate aggressive isotonic fluid treatment.

Signs and symptoms: diminished skin turgor on skin pinch; decreased peripheral perfusion, delay in capillary refill; hypotension; increased pulse and respiratory rate; oliguria; irritability

Investigations: comparison of body weight change before and after rehydration; hypernatremia; elevated serum osmolality

Strategy for patient encounter

This encounter will likely involve a parent discussing an infant who is hypotonic. The infant will be absent on some pretext (e.g., a nurse is taking the infant's vital signs and weight in another room). The specified tasks could engage history, physical exam, investigations, or management.

History

Use open-ended questions to obtain a general history, obstetrical history, and perinatal history.

- **General history:** What symptoms does your baby have? For how long? How often does your baby have a wet diaper? What are your baby's stools like? What medical conditions run in the family? Listen for evidence of respiratory problems, neurologic symptoms, jaundice, constipation, fever, and dehydration; and a family history of genetic disorders.
- **Obstetrical history:** How many times have you been pregnant? How many times have you miscarried? What complications did you have during this pregnancy? What complications were there during the delivery? Listen for a history of repeated spontaneous abortions, and risk factors for infection (e.g., premature birth, intrapartum maternal fever, early membrane rupture in labour and delivery).
- **Perinatal history:** What was your baby's birth weight? What was your baby's Apgar score? How was your baby's health after the delivery?

Physical exam

Perform a thorough physical exam, including a neurological and musculoskeletal exam, and an assessment for dysmorphic features.

(State that you will perform a physical exam. Because an actual pediatric patient is unlikely, the examiner may interrupt, ask what you are looking for, and provide findings. State that you are looking for neurological and musculoskeletal abnormalities, and dysmorphic features.)

Investigations

Order tests for serum electrolytes, blood glucose, and arterial blood gases (ABG). Order a complete blood count (CBC), and tests for inflammatory markers to rule out sepsis. Order a CT scan or MRI of the brain and spine to detect structural abnormalities. Order a test for creatine kinase to look for muscle disorders. Perform a lumbar puncture and cerebrospinal fluid analysis to rule out neuroinfection. Nerve conduction and electromyogram studies, and muscle or nerve biopsy, may be necessary to diagnose specific disorders. Consider genetic studies if the diagnosis is not apparent or there is multisystem involvement.

Management

In addition to immediate supportive care, refer the patient to a neonatologist or pediatric neurologist. As these children will usually require long-term support, also ensure multidisciplinary follow-up.

Pearls

Neonates with severe neuromuscular symptoms (e.g., respiratory insufficiency, and lack of swallowing and tendon reflexes) have a very poor prognosis.

102

Pediatric respiratory distress

MCC particular objective
Consider respiratory rate in the context of the age of the child.

MCC differential diagnosis
with added evidence

UPPER AIRWAY PROBLEMS

Croup
This is due to swelling around the larynx, trachea, and bronchi in infants and children.

The common cause is viruses. Severe cases may be caused by bacteria.

Signs and symptoms: difficulty breathing; "barking" cough; stridor; hoarseness; fever; inflamed nasal mucous membranes; chest wall in-drawing; cyanotic nose and mouth

Foreign body aspiration
Signs and symptoms of airway obstruction (immediate intervention is required): no audible speech or cough, possibly with gagging or choking (this indicates complete upper airway obstruction; partial obstruction allows some phonation and breath sounds)

Laryngeal disorders
LARYNGEAL TUMOUR
Signs and symptoms: hoarseness, breathy voice, shortness of breath, difficulty swallowing, otalgia, hemoptysis
Investigations: biopsy

LARYNGOCELE
Signs and symptoms: hoarseness; airway obstruction; mass on the neck (if the laryngocele is external)
Investigations: CT scan (finding: smooth, ovoid, low-density mass)

Epiglottitis
This is a potentially life-threatening condition from inflammation or swelling of the epiglottis that blocks airflow to the lungs. The typical causes include infection or injury to the throat. The *Haemophilus influenzae* type B (Hib) vaccine has made it less common in Canada.

Signs and symptoms (these may develop within hours): fever; throat soreness or pain; difficulty breathing or stridor
Investigations: blood or throat culture to detect infection; CBC; X-ray of the neck or chest

Retropharyngeal abscess

This is a deep neck infection arising from an upper respiratory tract infection. It is rare. The mean age of incidence is 3 to 5 years.

The cause is often polymicrobial: group A streptococci, *Staphylococcus aureus*, methicillin-resistant *Staphylococcus aureus*, and/or respiratory anaerobes (*Fusobacteria, Prevotella, Veillonella*).

Signs and symptoms: moderate fever for several days; difficulty swallowing, pain on swallowing, or drooling; unwillingness to extend the neck; voice changes; stridor; tachypnea; neck swelling, mass, or lymphadenopathy

Investigations: increased WBCs; throat culture; blood culture (this is rarely positive); CT scan with contrast of the neck (this is the best imaging modality in this context) (findings: an area in the deep spaces of the neck with low attenuation, a surrounding enhanced ring, and possible central lucency)

Choanal atresia

This is a congenital obstruction (either partial or complete obstruction) of the nasal airway by tissue. It is the most common nasal abnormality in newborns and occurs twice as often in females.

Signs and symptoms: nasal obstruction on physical exam

Investigations: nasal endoscopy; CT scan to visualize abnormalities; sinus X-ray to detect structural deformities

LOWER AIRWAY, PULMONARY DISORDERS

Tracheitis, bronchiolitis

BACTERIAL TRACHEITIS

This is relatively rare and usually affects children younger than 6 years. It can result in severe respiratory distress, which requires immediate intubation.

Signs and symptoms: symptom onset during fall and winter (common); 3 days of viral upper respiratory tract infection (rhinorrhea, cough, fever) followed by respiratory distress, stridor, nonpainful cough, shortness of breath, fever, toxic appearance

Investigations: endoscopy (in severe respiratory distress); Gram stain of endoscopy exudates (findings: neutrophils and bacterial morphologies); X-ray of soft tissues in the lateral neck to detect severe airway obstruction (findings: narrowing of the subglottic trachea, tracheal edema, and sloughing of tracheal mucosa)

BRONCHIOLITIS

This often occurs in children younger than 2 years. It is a viral infection and is a common cause of illness.

Signs and symptoms: viral upper respiratory infection for the first few days (rhinorrhea, cough, fever) followed by lower respiratory tract infection (wheezing and/or crackles; increased respiratory rate; chest retractions, nasal flaring; tachypnea); symptoms that resolve in 5 days (usual); cough that resolves in 2 weeks (usual)

Investigations: none necessary

Pneumonia, atelectasis

PNEUMONIA

Signs and symptoms: fever, cough, and tachypnea that do not resolve

> Newborns: poor feeding; irritability, restlessness; tachypnea; hypoxemia
>
> Infants: cough, tachypnea, chest retractions, hypoxemia, fever, irritability, decreased feeding
>
> Adolescents: symptoms similar to younger children; possible constitutional symptoms (headache, pleuritic chest pain, vague abdominal pain)

Risk factors: lower socioeconomic status; crowded living conditions; secondhand smoke; recent viral upper respiratory tract infection; cardiopulmonary disorders; other medical conditions (congenital heart disease, bronchopulmonary dysplasia, cystic fibrosis, asthma, sickle cell disease, neuromuscular disorders)

Investigations: chest X-ray where there is clinical evidence for pneumonia

ATELECTASIS

This generally presents with few findings on physical exam, unless larger areas of the lung are atelectatic. It is sometimes incidentally found on ultrasound. Mucus plugging is the most common cause of atelectasis in children.

Signs and symptoms (when larger areas of the lung are atelectatic): localized decreased breath sounds; dullness with percussion; wheezing, rales on auscultation; **no** fever; grunting on expiration; neuromuscular weakness (atelectasis is common in these patients)

Investigations: X-ray to detect areas of pulmonary opacity, and assess mediastinal shift and extent of volume loss

Asthma, bronchospasm

Signs and symptoms (in general): recurrent wheezing; recurrent dry or productive cough; symptoms triggered by viral respiratory tract infection (often), allergens, exercise

> Asthma: shortness of breath; chest tightness, pain; disturbed sleep from symptoms

Risk factors (asthma): family history of asthma; secondhand smoke; exposure to air pollution; other allergic conditions (e.g., atopic dermatitis)

Investigations: pulmonary function testing; chest X-ray to detect specific inflation or structure abnormalities

Respiratory distress syndrome of the neonate

This is common in premature neonates due to deficiency of pulmonary surfactant.

Signs and symptoms: tachypnea; grunting; chest retractions; nasal flaring; cyanosis; apnea

Investigations: chest X-ray to detect ground-glass appearance, air bronchograms, low lung volume, absence of thymus

Tracheoesophageal fistula

This is a common, life-threatening congenital abnormality. It is diagnosed shortly after birth or in infancy.

Signs and symptoms: drooling; white frothy bubbles in the mouth and nose; choking; respiratory distress; inability to feed; abdominal distention; maternal polyhydramnios

Investigations: catheter insertion into stomach (this stops at 10–15 cm), with chest X-ray (this detects the catheter curled in the upper esophageal pouch); lateral chest X-ray to detect gas in the GI tract

PLEURAL DISORDER

Pleural effusion, empyema

Signs and symptoms (in general): chest pain, (sharp, stabbing pain that worsens on inspiration), especially if exudative effusion is present; pain that radiates to the shoulder (due to diaphragmatic irritation from pneumonic condition); fever; localized decreased breath sounds; tactile fremitus; dullness on percussion

Investigations: AP and lateral chest X-rays to distinguish pulmonary from cardiac etiologies for pleural fluid; pulmonary ultrasound to detect pleural effusion

Pneumothorax

SPONTANEOUS PNEUMOTHORAX

This occurs in the absence of any identified trauma.

Signs and symptoms: generally asymptomatic if the pneumothorax is small; adolescent male (more common); tall, thin body; family history of spontaneous pneumothorax; sudden-onset shortness of breath; chest pain (sharp, stabbing pain after a popping sensation); hyperresonance on percussion; decreased breath sounds in the affected lung; decreased chest excursion; **no** tactile fremitus

Investigations: ABG (in cases of respiratory distress)

SECONDARY PNEUMOTHORAX

Causes include use of inhaled drugs, undiagnosed asthma, foreign body aspiration, respiratory tract infection, and connective tissue disease.

Investigations: chest X-ray

   Findings for infants (large pneumothorax): hyperlucency

Findings for children (take X-rays in the upright position): pleural line; hyperlucency; attenuation of vascular and lung markings

NEUROLOGIC DISORDERS (E.G., DRUGS)

DRUGS

Examples include accidental or intentional drug overdose (especially from opiate and sedative medications).

Toxins (e.g., botulism) can also cause neurologic disorders with respiratory distress.

CARDIAC DISORDERS

Congestive heart failure (left-to-right shunt, left ventricular failure)

Signs and symptoms: excessive sweating, persistent tachypnea, tachycardia

Investigations: echocardiogram

Cardiac tamponade

Signs and symptoms: sharp chest pain, possibly worse on deep inhalation or coughing; difficulty breathing; palpitations; Beck triad (hypotension, high jugular venous pressure, muffled heart sounds)

Investigations: echocardiogram

Strategy for patient encounter

The likely scenario is an adolescent with asthma (the minimum age to play standardized patients is 16). The specified tasks could engage history, physical exam, investigations, or management.

Respiratory distress is possible in this clinical presentation. No matter what tasks the instructions for the encounter specify, start by checking the patient for respiratory distress.

The differential diagnosis for this clinical presentation is broad. A main objective is to differentiate cardiac causes from pulmonary, neuromuscular, and other causes.

Assessment for respiratory distress

Check the patient's airway, breathing, and circulation (mnemonic: **ABCs**). Check for tachypnea (see the tip on tachypnea). Provide emergency care to any patient with unstable vital signs.

If the child is not in distress, proceed to the history and physical exam.

History

Ask open-ended questions about the patient's symptoms: When did you start having difficulty breathing? What other symptoms have you noticed? Listen for evidence about onset (e.g., sudden onset is consistent with epiglottitis and pneumothorax; recurrent symptoms are consistent with asthma); suspected triggers for onset (e.g., trauma, upper respiratory infection, allergies); symptoms consistent with cardiac disorders (excessive sweating, tachycardia, chest pain, palpitations); and for symptoms consistent with particular disorders (e.g., barking cough in croup; fever in infectious entities; difficulty swallowing in laryngeal tumour and retropharyngeal abscess). Ask about a personal or family history of asthma.

> **TIP**
>
> **Pediatric tachypnea**
>
> The MCC specifies assessing a child's respiration rate in the context of the child's age. Many guidelines on pediatric respiration rates exist, with a variety of age breakdowns and ranges. In the context of the exam, if tachypnea is present, it will likely be pronounced, not borderline. For example:
>
> 0–3 years > 60 breaths/minute
>
> 4–10 years > 40 breaths/minute
>
> 11–18 years > 30 breaths/minute

Physical exam

Auscultate the lungs and heart. Examine the skin for cyanosis.

Investigations

Measure the patient's oxygen levels by pulse oximetry. Order a test for arterial blood gases (ABG) and a complete blood count (CBC).

Management

Provide supplemental oxygen. Consult pediatrics. Treat the underlying etiology identified.

103

Pelvic pain

MCC particular objectives

Identify patients with acute pain caused by life-threatening conditions.

Determine whether pregnancy is likely.

Stabilize hemodynamically unstable patients.

MCC differential diagnosis
with added evidence

PREGNANCY-RELATED CONDITION (E.G., ECTOPIC, MOLAR, ABRUPTION)

ECTOPIC PREGNANCY

Signs and symptoms: symptoms of pregnancy and/or positive pregnancy test; pelvic pain; vaginal bleeding; painful intercourse; shoulder pain; palpable tubal mass; pelvic tenderness and pain associated with 1 or both adnexa

> Severe symptom: syncope

Risk factors: previous ectopic pregnancy, pelvic inflammatory disease, pregnancy during intrauterine device (IUD) use

Investigations (pathognomonic): β-hCG above discriminatory zone (> 1500–2000 mIU/mL) **with** transvaginal ultrasound findings of a lack of intrauterine gestational sac, complex (mixed solid and cystic) masses in the adnexa, and free fluid in the cul-de-sac

MOLAR PREGNANCY (HYDATIDIFORM MOLE)

This is usually benign, but may progress to malignancy.

Signs and symptoms: symptoms similar to early pregnancy (missed menstrual periods; positive pregnancy test; vaginal bleeding; pelvic discomfort, pressure, or pain; hyperemesis gravidarum); uterus that is larger than expected for gestational age on pelvic exam or ultrasound

Risk factors: prior molar pregnancy or gestational trophoblastic disease; maternal age younger than 15 or older than 35; prior spontaneous abortion and infertility; vitamin A deficiency

Investigations: β-hCG (this is higher than for intrauterine or ectopic pregnancies of the same gestational age); ultrasound

> Ultrasound findings for complete moles may include **no** embryo or fetus; **no** amniotic fluid; central heterogeneous mass with numerous discrete anechoic spaces; and ovarian theca lutein cysts.

Ultrasound findings for partial moles may include a fetus (this may resemble a missed or incomplete abortion; if viable, it is often growth restricted); amniotic fluid, possibly with reduced volume; placenta with ≥ 1 abnormal findings (enlarged; cystic spaces in a "Swiss cheese" pattern; increased echogenicity of chorionic villi); increased transverse diameter of gestational sac; and **no** theca lutein cysts.

ABRUPTION (PLACENTAL)

Signs and symptoms: possibly asymptomatic; pregnancy > 20 weeks gestation; abrupt-onset vaginal bleeding; abdominal and/or back pain (mild to moderate); uterine contractions (high frequency, low amplitude); firm uterus that may be rigid and tender; maternal hypotension and nonreassuring fetal heart rate (clinically significant placental separation); disseminated intravascular coagulation

Risk factors: older maternal age, previous abruption, smoking, hypertension, asthma, family history of abruption

Investigations: ultrasound

> Classic finding: retroplacental hematoma (this is absent in many patients) with variable appearance (solid, complex; hypo-, hyper-, or isoechoic when compared to placenta)

GYNECOLOGIC CONDITION

Ovary (e.g., ruptured cyst, torsion)

RUPTURED CYST, TORSION

Signs and symptoms: pelvic pain; pain during intercourse; change in bowel habits; nausea, vomiting; fever; worsening or sudden onset of pain (this may indicate ovarian torsion); pelvic tenderness and pain associated with 1 or both adnexa

Investigations: enlarged ovary or ovaries on pelvic ultrasound or laparoscopy

Tube (e.g., pelvic inflammatory disease, endometriosis)

PELVIC INFLAMMATORY DISEASE

Signs and symptoms: lower abdominal and pelvic pain; pain during intercourse; fever; urinary symptoms; vaginal discharge; irregular menstruation; pelvic tenderness and pain associated with 1 or both adnexa

> History of gonorrhea, chlamydia, or risk factors for them (multiple partners, unprotected sex); intrauterine device (IUD); childbirth; gynecologic procedure

Investigations: cultures for gonorrhea and chlamydia; ultrasound (this has normal findings)

ENDOMETRIOSIS

Signs and symptoms: pelvic pain associated with menstruation (very common); excessive bleeding during menstruation; pain during intercourse; pain during urination or bowel movements; tenderness on pelvic exam; normal findings on abdominal exam (common)

Risk factors: family history of endometriosis; nulliparity; personal history of pelvic inflammatory disease

Investigations: ultrasound to detect ovarian cysts (common finding); laparoscopy with biopsy

Uterus (e.g., leiomyoma, endometriosis)

LEIOMYOMA

Signs and symptoms: commonly asymptomatic; premenopausal (usual); heavy or prolonged menstrual bleeding; pelvic, abdominal pressure; pain during intercourse; urinary symptoms (incontinence; frequent urination; difficulty emptying the bladder); constipation; pelvic mass or enlarged, irregular uterus on bimanual palpation

Risk factors: family history of leiomyoma; African descent

Investigations: ultrasound to detect mass ≥ 1 cm in diameter

ENDOMETRIOSIS—SEE ABOVE

OTHER (DYSMENORRHEA, OVULATION PAIN, DYSPAREUNIA)

DYSMENORRHEA (PRIMARY)

Primary dysmenorrhea (as opposed to secondary dysmenorrhea) occurs in women without disorders that could account for their symptoms (e.g., endometriosis, adenomyosis, uterine fibroids).

It occurs in 50% to 90% of reproductive-age women, and often improves with age and childbirth.

Signs and symptoms: recurrent pain during menstruation (midline, lower abdominal, suprapubic; mild to severe); **no** demonstrable disease; crampy, intermittently intense, and/or continuous dull ache with possible nausea, diarrhea, fatigue, headache; symptom onset 1 to 2 days before menstruation, diminishing over 12 to 72 hours; normal pelvic exam

Risk factors: younger than 30; body mass index (BMI) < 20 kg/m^2; smoking; menarche before age 12; longer menstrual cycles, durations of bleeding; irregular or heavy menstrual flow; family history of dysmenorrhea

OVULATION PAIN

Signs and symptoms: symptom onset 2 weeks before menstrual period; variable symptom duration (minutes to 48 hours); lower abdominal pain, just inside the hip bone, on the left or right side (the location depends on which ovary is active); uncomfortable pressure, twinges, sharp pains, or cramps

DYSPAREUNIA

Signs and symptoms: pain on penetration (sex, tampon insertion); new pain after previously pain-free intercourse

Risk factors: pelvic inflammatory disease, depression, anxiety, history of sexual abuse

SYSTEMIC CONDITION

Urologic (interstitial cystitis, renal colic)

INTERSTITIAL CYSTITIS

Signs and symptoms: increased frequency of urination; painful urination; pelvic pain and/or flank pain; fever; tenderness over the bladder

Investigations: urinalysis (positive for infection)

RENAL COLIC

Signs and symptoms: colicky flank pain; nausea, vomiting; fever; history of kidney stones (common); extreme tenderness at the costovertebral angle on abdominal examination; hematuria

Investigations (to detect stones): KUB X-ray; ureter ultrasound, abdominal CT scan

Musculoskeletal (fibromyalgia)

FIBROMYALGIA

This is a diagnosis of exclusion.

Signs and symptoms: female (more common); chronic, widespread pain for ≥ 3 months; pain that is bilateral, and above and below the waist; aching pain; fatigue; long sleep; restless legs syndrome; sleep apnea; impaired concentration, memory; dizziness; cramping (e.g., menstrual, abdominal); morning stiffness; numbness, tingling in the extremities; tender points; urinary symptoms (painful or difficult urination; irregular urination); sensitivity to noise, light, temperature

> Coexisting conditions (often): headaches, irritable bowel syndrome, interstitial cystitis

Gastrointestinal (irritable bowel syndrome, diverticulitis, inflammatory bowel disease, hernia)

IRRITABLE BOWEL SYNDROME[1]

Irritable bowel syndrome is commonly diagnosed by applying the Rome criteria.

Signs and symptoms (Rome criteria): ≥ 2 symptoms, present for ≥ 1 day/week for ≥ 3 months

> Symptoms: pain associated with defecation, pain associated with a change of stool frequency, pain associated with a change in stool consistency

DIVERTICULITIS

Signs and symptoms: constant left lower quadrant abdominal pain; abdominal tenderness; fever; nausea, vomiting; change in bowel habits (constipation and/or diarrhea)

Risk factors: advanced age; obesity; smoking; poor diet; lack of exercise

Investigations: CT scan

INFLAMMATORY BOWEL DISEASE

Signs and symptoms: younger than 30 (usually); family history of inflammatory bowel disease; fluctuating symptoms with periods of exacerbation and remission; diarrhea (possibly with nocturnal waking); blood in the stool; abdominal pain; weight loss; fever; fatigue; right lower quadrant and periumbilical pain; extraintestinal manifestations (e.g., uveitis, arthritis)

> Crohn disease: right lower quadrant mass, inflammation of the eyes, arthritis

Investigations: elevated CRP (this suggests active inflammation); fecal calprotectin; colonoscopy with biopsy (this is a standard diagnostic procedure); CT scan or MRI (findings: diagnostic structural changes associated with inflammatory bowel disease)

HERNIA (INGUINAL HERNIA)

Signs and symptoms: inguinal swelling that aches and enlarges with straining (usual); nausea, vomiting; constipation (this suggests an incarcerated hernia)

> Direct inguinal hernia: palpable bulge above the inguinal canal and **medial** to the internal inguinal ring
>
> Indirect inguinal hernia: palpable bulge above the inguinal canal and **lateral** to the internal inguinal ring

MENTAL HEALTH ISSUES

Depression, somatization

MAJOR DEPRESSIVE DISORDER[2(pp160–161)]

Signs and symptoms: symptoms that are present most of the time for ≥ 2 weeks; symptoms with significant impact on day-to-day life

> Key symptoms: depressed mood and/or loss of interest in usual activities
>
> Other symptoms: significant weight change; sleep disturbance; slowed or agitated mental processes; loss of concentration; recurrent thoughts of death or suicide

Risk factors: family history of mental health disorders (depression, anxiety, suicide); personal history of other mental health disorders; substance abuse; chronic illness (e.g., cancer, stroke, chronic pain)

SOMATIC SYMPTOM DISORDER[2(p311)]

Signs and symptoms: disproportionate and persistent thoughts about the seriousness of a health concern, and/or excessive and persistent anxiety about a health concern, and/or excessive time or energy devoted to a health concern; presence of symptoms for ≥ 6 months (the health concern involved may change); symptoms with significant impact on day-to-day life

Sexual, physical, and psychological abuse/domestic violence

People who suffer abuse often don't disclose it.

Pelvic pain in this context is most likely attributable to sexual abuse.

Signs and symptoms of sexual abuse: genital and pelvic bruising and injury; bruising and injury to other parts of the body

Strategy for patient encounter

The likely scenario is a female patient with acute pelvic pain (a female patient allows for a larger differential diagnosis, including obstetrical and gynecological causes). The likely tasks are history, physical exam, or investigations.

An actively bleeding patient is possible in this clinical presentation. No matter what tasks the instructions for the encounter specify, start by checking for active bleeding and follow up with an assessment of the patient's vital signs as indicated.

Active bleeding and vital signs

If the patient is actively bleeding, check the patient's airway, breathing, and hemodynamic status (mnemonic: **ABCs**). Provide emergency management, if indicated.

History

Use open-ended questions to take a menstrual and obstetric history, medical history, and pain history.

- **Menstrual and obstetric history:** What are your menstrual periods usually like? What changes have you noticed in your menstrual periods? When was your last period? How many times have you been pregnant? How many miscarriages have you had and at what stage of pregnancy? What complications have you had during previous pregnancies? Listen for evidence of painful menstruation, missed periods, previous miscarriage, and previous pregnancy complications (e.g., ectopic pregnancy). Ask about risk factors for pelvic inflammatory disease (history of sexually transmitted infections, use of an intrauterine device, multiple sexual partners, gynecological procedures).
- **Medical history:** What conditions have you been diagnosed with? Listen for entities listed in the MCC differential diagnosis. Ask about pelvic surgeries.

- **Pain and related symptoms:** What characterizes the pain you are experiencing? What other symptoms have you noticed? Listen for symptoms consistent with ectopic pregnancy (shoulder pain), ovarian cyst or ovarian torsion (abrupt-onset pain or worsening pain), endometriosis (pain with menstruation), dysmenorrhea or ovulation pain (regularly recurring pain), urologic conditions (flank pain), gastrointestinal conditions (pain focal to a lower quadrant or periumbilical pain), and symptoms relevant to particular entities such as vaginal discharge (pelvic inflammatory disease), vaginal bleeding (pregnancy-related condition), heavy or prolonged bleeding (leiomyoma), and changes in bowel habits (gastrointestinal conditions).

Ask if the patient could be pregnant.

Physical exam

If the patient is not actively bleeding, obtain the patient's vital signs, looking for fever (this suggests ruptured ovarian cyst, ovarian torsion, pelvic inflammatory disease, urologic infection, or renal colic) and hypotension (this suggests blood loss). Perform a pelvic and speculum exam.

(State you will perform a pelvic and speculum exam. Because these exams are not performed on standardized patients, the examiner will likely interrupt, ask what you are looking for, and provide findings. State that you are looking for masses, points of tenderness, injuries, and uterine abnormalities.)

Investigations

Order a pregnancy test for all female patients of childbearing age. Consider a pelvic ultrasound for most patients. Order other investigations if the history and physical exam point to a specific etiology (see the information this resource lists in the MCC differential diagnosis).

REFERENCE

1 Lacey B, Mearin F, Chang L, et al. Rome IV functional gastrointestinal disorders: disorders of gut-brain interaction. 4th ed. Vol. 2. Raleigh, NC: Rome Foundation; 2017. Chapter 11, Functional bowel disorders; 1393–1407.

2 American Psychiatric Association. Diagnostic and statistical manual of mental disorders. 5th ed. Arlington, VA: American Psychiatric Association; 2013. 991 p.

104

Periodic health encounter, preventive health advice

MCC particular objective

Determine the patient's risks for age- and sex-specific conditions.

MCC list of factors to consider

ALL AGES

Injury prevention (e.g., seatbelts, noise control, bike helmets)

Lifestyle modification (e.g., smoking cessation, physical activity, sun exposure)

Immunization

INFANTS AND CHILDREN

Nutrition, growth, and development

Behaviours

Other (e.g., hearing, amblyopia)

ADOLESCENTS

Sexual activity (e.g., contraception, sexually transmitted infections)

YOUNG ADULTS

Female reproductive health (e.g., Papanicolaou test, screening for sexually transmitted infections, folic acid)

MIDDLE-AGED ADULTS

Cardiovascular health risks (e.g., blood glucose, blood pressure, lipid profile)

Cancer screening (e.g., breast, colon, prostate, skin)

Osteoporosis

OLDER ADULTS

Fracture and fall prevention (e.g., osteoporosis screening)

Nutrition

Dementia screening

Strategy for patient encounter

The likely scenario is a middle-aged patient inquiring about routine screening. Also be prepared for the following scenarios, which the MCC specifies as possibilities for this clinical presentation: in-person visits, electronic or phone encounters, and consultations delegated by other health care team members. The specified tasks will likely include history and counselling on recommended screening maneuvers (see the checklist on screening guidelines).

History

Focus on the entities the MCC identifies for the patient's age group. In the case of a middle-aged person (the likely scenario), they are cardiovascular disorders, cancer, and osteoporosis.

Use open-ended questions to establish the patient's medical and family history: What health concerns do you currently have? What conditions have you been diagnosed with? Listen for a history of, or signs and symptoms consistent with, hypertension, heart disorders, dyslipidemia, diabetes, cancer, and osteoporosis. Ask whether any of these disorders run in the patient's family. Ask whether the patient smokes.

Counselling

Inform the patient that cardiovascular disorders, cancer, and osteoporosis are the priorities for screening in healthy middle-aged adults. Discuss with the patient any elements of the history that put them at higher risk of these entities.

CHECKLIST

Screening guidelines

As general preparation for this clinical presentation, familiarize yourself with the following resources, which you can find online.

- **Preventive Care Checklist Forms from the College of Family Physicians of Canada.** Recommendations for periodic health examinations are constantly evolving. The College of Family Physicians of Canada maintains up-to-date checklists.

- **Framingham risk score calculation.** The Canadian Cardiovascular Society has this under "calculators and forms," which is a section of "guideline resources."

- **FINDRISC calculator for type 2 diabetes.** The Canadian Task Force on Preventive Health Care has a version of this under "tools and resources."

- **Local screening guidelines for breast cancer, cervical cancer, and colorectal carcinoma.** You need to know your local guidelines, because these vary by region.

- **Osteoporosis Canada's clinical practice guidelines.** See especially the "quick reference guide."

In the scenario of a middle-aged adult inquiring about routine screening, the patient's concerns could revolve around the initiation of routine screening or the frequency of screening already in place.

In describing screening procedures for healthy adults, begin with procedures related to the entities where the patient's risk is higher.

SCREENING FOR CARDIOVASCULAR HEALTH

In middle-aged adults, this looks for:

- **Dyslipidemia:** Screening involves a lipid panel, which forms part of estimating the patient's risk of cardiovascular disease (e.g., with a Framingham risk score). Patients at low risk (Framingham risk score lower than 5%) should be rescreened every 3 to 5 years. Patients at intermediate and high risk (Framingham risk score higher than 5%) should be rescreened yearly.
- **Type 2 diabetes:** Screening first involves estimating the patient's risk of type 2 diabetes (e.g., with the FINDRISC calculator). Screening via blood tests (glycated hemoglobin or fasting blood glucose) is indicated for patients at high risk (every 3 to 5 years) and very high risk (yearly).
- **Hypertension:** This involves regular blood pressure monitoring (e.g., yearly in healthy adults).

SCREENING FOR CANCER

In middle-aged adults, this looks for:

- **Breast cancer:** Mammography is generally recommended every 2 to 3 years in asymptomatic women at low risk between the ages of 50 and 74.
- **Cervical cancer:** Papanicolaou testing is generally recommended every 3 years in asymptomatic women at low risk.
- **Colorectal cancer:** Screening via fecal immunochemical testing (FIT) is generally recommended every 1 to 2 years for asymptomatic patients at low risk between the ages of 50 and 74. Colonoscopy is generally recommended for patients at high risk (frequency varies by region) and always for symptomatic patients.

- **Prostate cancer:** The Canadian Task Force on Preventive Health Care **does not** recommend screening for prostate-specific antigen (PSA) in patients not previously diagnosed with prostate cancer, including patients with urinary symptoms (e.g., difficulty voiding) or benign prostatic hyperplasia.
- **Skin cancer:** The Canadian Cancer Society recommends a yearly visual exam in asymptomatic patients at low risk (e.g., no personal or family history of skin cancer).

SCREENING FOR OSTEOPOROSIS

In middle-aged adults, this starts with assessing risk factors for the disease (e.g., glucocorticoid use, smoking, family history). Osteoporosis Canada recommends bone mineral density (BMD) testing for adults at high risk, and for all adults older than 65 years.

Pearls

Screening for thyroid function, vitamin B_{12}, and vitamin D—though sometimes requested by patients—is not recommended for the general population. For vitamin D, use the "treat don't test" approach: counsel adults to take a supplement of 1000 IU/day.

105

Newborn assessment

MCC particular objectives

Identify significant abnormalities or risk factors.

Counsel parents on newborn care.

MCC differential diagnosis

None stated.

Strategy for patient encounter

The likely scenario is a mock newborn assessment in a recovery room following birth. The likely tasks are history, newborn assessment, or counselling.

History

Use open-ended questions to obtain a maternal history, perinatal history, and parental psychosocial history.

- **Maternal history:** How was your health during the pregnancy? What concerns or questions do you have about bonding with your baby? Ask about previous postpartum depression.
- **Perinatal history:** What method of feeding your baby do you plan to use? What concerns or questions do you have about your planned method?
- **Parental psychosocial history:** What are your living arrangements? What is your relationship situation? Ask about diagnosed psychiatric disorders in either parent. Ask about alcohol use and recreational-drug use in either parent.

Newborn assessment

Establish the baby's Apgar score. This is the first assessment done on a newborn, and is performed between 1 to 5 minutes after birth. Depending on the scenario, you may be performing this assessment, or the scenario may indicate that this assessment already been done (in which case, ask for the score). Babies with Apgar scores less than 3 require immediate resuscitation. The maximum score is 10 (see the checklist).

CHECKLIST

Apgar scoring for newborns

SIGN	FINDINGS THAT SCORE 0	FINDINGS THAT SCORE 1	FINDINGS THAT SCORE 2
Heart rate	Absent	< 100/minute	> 100/minute
Respiratory effort	Absent	Weak, irregular, or gasping	Crying
Muscle tone	Flaccid	Some flexion of extremities	Well-flexed/or active movements of extremities
Response to stimulation	No response	Grimace/weak cry	Good cry
Colour	Blue all over, or pale	Body pink, hands and feet blue	Pink all over

The initial physical exam for an infant includes assessing:

- birth weight: the average weight for term babies is about 3 kg (7 lbs)
- head circumference
- length
- temperature
- skin and eyes for jaundice
- presence of dysmorphic features
- pulse (normal is 120 to 160 beats per minute)
- respiratory rate (normal is 40 to 60 breaths per minute)
- head: check its appearance, shape, and presence of molding
- presence of bilateral red reflex
- presence and size of the fontanels
- clavicles: these may be broken during delivery
- mouth and palate: note the presence and strength of sucking reflex
- lungs sounds
- heart sounds
- femoral pulses: check for their presence and equality
- abdomen for masses and hernias
- genitalia and anus: in males, check the testicles for descent
- arms and legs for equal movement and development
- hips for dislocations
- primitive reflexes and tone
- spine for dysraphism (dimpling, hair)
- serum glucose: obtain a point-of-care glucose measurement
- bilirubin levels: use a point-of-care bilirubinometer or obtain a serum bilirubin

Counselling

Counsel the parents regarding feeding and infant nutrition, umbilical cord care, car seat use, prevention of sudden infant death syndrome (SIDS), and seeking medical attention for a fever in infants younger than 3 months.

Discuss newborn metabolic screening.

106

Preoperative medical evaluation

MCC particular objectives

Assess perioperative issues based on history and physical exam. Recommend strategies to minimize perioperative morbidity and mortality.

MCC assessment categories
with added evidence

OPTIMAL MANAGEMENT OF CHRONIC DISEASES (E.G., CORONARY ARTERY DISEASE, DIABETES MELLITUS)

CORONARY ARTERY DISEASE (CAD)

For risks associated with cardiac conditions, see *myocardial risk*, below.

Perioperative management of CAD: see the perioperative management checklist

Investigations: NT-proBNP level in at-risk patients, as identified on RCRI risk score (see the quick reference)

DIABETES MELLITUS

Patients with diabetes mellitus are at higher surgical risk if their diabetes is undetected, uncontrolled, and/or not properly monitored; and if they have comorbid conditions (e.g., cardiovascular disease, kidney damage, skin conditions, neuropathies).

> Signs and symptoms (undiagnosed diabetes mellitus): family history of diabetes; polydipsia, polyuria, and/or weight loss
>
> Perioperative management of diabetes: see the perioperative management checklist

Investigations: HbA_{1c} test (in clinically suspected, but undiagnosed, diabetes), glucose test, ECG (diabetic patients are at risk of silent myocardial ischemia due to diabetic neuropathy), tests for renal function

IDENTIFICATION OF PERIOPERATIVE RISKS

Cardiopulmonary risk

MYOCARDIAL RISK (E.G., ISCHEMIA, HEART FAILURE, ARRHYTHMIA)

Patients are at higher risk of cardiovascular complications if they have a history of cardiac events (myocardial infarction, congestive heart failure, valvular diseases, angina, arrhythmia, severe pulmonary hypertension); comorbid conditions (e.g., renal insufficiency, diabetes, chronic obstructive pulmonary disease, hypertension); reduced functional capacity (e.g., tolerance for < 4 metabolic equivalents of activity, such as walking ≤ 2 blocks without stopping); or abnormalities on physical exam (e.g., elevated venous pressure, pulmonary edema, third heart sound).

Other risk factors: dyslipidemia, smoking, current symptoms (e.g., chest pain, shortness of breath, claudication, syncope, presyncope)

Investigations: NT-proBNP level

PULMONARY RISK (E.G., CHRONIC OBSTRUCTIVE PULMONARY DISEASE, INFECTION)

CHRONIC OBSTRUCTIVE PULMONARY DISEASE (COPD)

Signs and symptoms: decreased breath sounds; wheezing; crackles; prolonged expiratory phase

Investigations: chest X-ray to detect COPD; FEV to establish risk in diagnosed COPD

High risk for postoperative complications: FEV1 < 40%

High risk for mortality in coronary bypass graft surgery: FEV1 < 60%

INFECTION

Risk factors for postoperative pulmonary infections include advanced age; planned thoracic or upper abdominal surgery; past or current lung disease; obesity; smoking; poorly controlled asthma; stroke; and chronic steroid use.

Anesthetic

SYSTEMIC RISK (E.G., MALIGNANT HYPERTHERMIA, SLEEP APNEA)

MALIGNANT HYPERTHERMIA (MH)

This is rare and hereditary, and can be fatal. In the context of surgical risk, it is triggered by volatile anesthetics (isoflurane, halothane, sevoflurane, desflurane). People with MH do not react on their first exposure to volatile anesthetics.

Risk factors: first degree relative with MH (50% risk); second degree relative with MH (25% risk); male (higher risk); muscle diseases (central core disease, minicore-multicore myopathy, nemaline myopathy); hypokalemic periodic paralysis; King-Denborough syndrome

Investigations: muscle biopsy for caffeine-halothane contracture test

OBSTRUCTIVE SLEEP APNEA

This can remain undiagnosed until a preoperative evaluation. Patients with this condition are at higher postoperative risk for sleep-disordered breathing, severe hypoxemia, hypercapnia, aspiration pneumonia, acute respiratory distress syndrome, and pulmonary embolism.

If also obese, they are additionally at risk of difficulties with endotracheal intubation and postoperative upper airway obstruction.

Signs and symptoms: excessive or loud snoring; disturbed sleep (e.g., not feeling rested in the morning); obesity (common); allergic rhinitis (sneezing, runny nose, eye irritation); morning headache; palpable masses in the oral cavity or neck

Investigations: sleep study (polysomnography); hypertrophic adenoid tissue on lateral neck X-ray

STOP-BANG questionnaire (patent self-evaluation questionnaire): **STOP-BANG** is a mnemonic for **s**noring, **t**ired, **o**bserved cessation of breathing during sleep by others, **p**ressure (hypertension), **B**MI > 35, **a**ge older than 50, **n**eck size (large), **g**ender (male).

INTUBATION AND AIRWAY (E.G., C-SPINE STABILITY)

C-SPINE STABILITY

Patients with C-spine instability risk spinal cord compression and/or the need for emergent airway protection during surgery.

Risk factors: C-spine trauma, rheumatoid arthritis, Down syndrome

Thromboembolic risk (prior deep vein thrombosis, thrombophilia)

Risk factors: older than 40; malignancy; immobilization; varicose veins; major vascular injury; cardiopulmonary disease (see *cardiopulmonary risk*, above); history of stroke, deep vein thrombosis, or thrombophilia; paralysis or spinal cord injury; hyperviscosity (due to malignancy or polycythemia vera); presence of current symptoms (leg pain, limb edema, calf tenderness)

Investigations: CBC, PT/INR, aPTT, platelets

Medication-related risk (e.g., prednisone, immunosuppressants)

PREDNISONE

Patients who regularly take prednisone or other steroids (e.g., to treat autoimmune and inflammatory diseases) are at higher postoperative risk of infection (e.g., pneumonia, peritonitis, urinary tract infections), delayed wound healing, hyperglycemia, hypertension, and neuropsychiatric conditions. They may require stress-dose steroids at the time of surgery to reduce the risk of adrenal suppression by exogenous steroid use.

IMMUNOSUPPRESSANTS

Patients taking immunosuppressants are at higher postoperative risk of sepsis, infections, and delayed wound healing.

ANTIREJECTION DRUGS

Investigations: renal function, liver function, metabolic assessment, CBC, acid-base fluid status, electrolytes, PT/INR, aPTT, platelets, plasma fibrinogen, 12-lead ECG, chest X-ray, echocardiogram, pulmonary function testing

CHEMOTHERAPY
Investigations: CBC, electrolytes, liver function, PT/INR, aPTT, platelets, plasma fibrinogen

ANTICOAGULANTS
Perioperative management of patients taking warfarin (see the perioperative management checklist) depends on an evaluation of the risk of thrombotic events versus the risk of bleeding events.

HIGH RISK OF THROMBOSIS
Risk factors: mitral valve or mechanical aortic valve (cage-ball or tilting-disk type); thromboembolism within last 3 months; history of thromboembolism on stopping warfarin; severe thrombophilia

INTERMEDIATE RISK OF THROMBOSIS
Risk factors: bileaflet-mechanical or bioprosthetic aortic valve; atrial fibrillation plus major risk factors for stroke (history of stroke, hypertension, diabetes, left ventricular condition, or older than 75)

LOW RISK OF THROMBOSIS
Patients have no major risk factors for stroke, and no thromboembolism for > 12 months.

Strategy for patient encounter
The likely scenario is a preoperative patient presenting for evaluation.

Preoperative evaluation involves a full history and physical exam with emphasis on conditions that may pose perioperative risks. Specified tasks could also engage perioperative management.

History
Use open-ended questions to gather evidence of potential risks.
- **Medical history:** What conditions have you been diagnosed with? Listen for a history of heart disease, diabetes, lung disease, renal problems, hypertension, dyslipidemia, and thrombotic risk factors (e.g., stroke, deep vein thrombosis, malignancy); and for risk factors associated with anesthetic (obstructive sleep apnea), intubation (rheumatoid arthritis, Down syndrome), and postoperative infection (e.g., asthma). Ask about a history of spinal trauma (this is relevant for intubation).

- **Current health status:** How has your health been lately? Listen for symptoms consistent with undiagnosed diabetes (polydipsia, weight loss, fatigue); undiagnosed obstructive sleep apnea (e.g., snoring, daytime fatigue, nighttime apnea observed by others); current thrombosis (leg pain, limb edema, calf tenderness); and current cardiopulmonary disorder (e.g., chest pain, shortness of breath, syncope).

- **History with anesthetics:** What is your experience with anesthetics? Ask about a family history of problems with anesthetics.

- **Current functional capacity:** How many blocks can you walk without stopping?

- **Medication history:** Obtain a full medication list, if possible, including over-the-counter medications. Otherwise, ask the patient what medications they take. (See the information about medication risks this resource lists in the MCC differential diagnosis.)

Determine the patient's risk for cardiovascular complications using the revised cardiac risk index (see the quick reference).

QUICK REFERENCE

Revised cardiac risk index (RCRI)

The RCRI scores patients' risk for postsurgical cardiovascular complications for noncardiac surgeries based on 6 variables. The website of the Canadian Cardiovascular Society includes the RCRI in its "guidelines library" (look under the menu item *guidelines*).

CHECKLIST

Mallampati score for assessing ease of intubation

Ask the patient to open their mouth and stick out their tongue as far as they can.

Scores are calculated (in increasing order of predicted intubation difficulty) as:

- **Mallampati 1:** Tonsillar pillars, soft palate and entire uvula are visible.

- **Mallampati 2:** Tonsillar pillars and soft palate are visible, but not the uvula.

- **Mallampati 3:** The soft palate is visible, but not the uvula.

- **Mallampati 4:** Only the hard palate is visible.

Reprinted by permission from Springer Nature: Canadian Anaesthetists' Society Journal, A clinical sign to predict difficult tracheal intubation: a prospective study, Mallampati SR, Gatt SP, Gugino LD, Desai SP, Waraksa B, Freiberger D, Liu PL, 1985.

Physical exam

Obtain the patient's vital signs. Examine the heart and lungs. Assess the predicted ease of intubation (see the checklist on Mallampati score).

Investigations

Routine surgeries on healthy patients do not necessarily require blood work or X-rays. In suspected undiagnosed diabetes, order a fasting glucose or glycated hemoglobin (HbA_{1c}) test. In patients with a higher risk of cardiovascular complications (patients 65 years or older, or with an RCRI score greater than 1, or age 45 to 64 with significant cardiovascular disease), order a test for N-terminal prohormone of brain natriuretic peptide (NT-proBNP). Target any other testing to the current status of preexisting conditions. Obtain a HbA_{1c} test for diabetic patients and a C-spine X-ray for rheumatoid arthritis patients.

Perioperative management

Communicate the risks of surgery to the patient and optimize care for existing conditions (see the checklist).

CHECKLIST

Perioperative management

CONDITION	MANAGEMENT
Cardiac condition	Counsel smoking cessation. Optimize therapy prior to surgery. This may include beta-blockers (do not start within 24 hours before surgery), statins, and surveillance.
Diabetes	Be alert to undiagnosed diabetes. Optimize glycemic control. This may include medication compliance or adjustments, and smoking cessation; and will include proper monitoring, appropriate diet, and adequate exercise.
Chronic obstructive pulmonary disease	Treat this aggressively. Treatment includes bronchodilators; smoking cessation; antibiotics and systemic steroids, as required, in suboptimal management despite therapy; and chest physical therapy.
Patients at risk of postoperative pulmonary infection	Counsel smoking cessation. Optimize asthma control, which may include medication adjustments or compliance, and avoiding triggers (e.g., environmental allergens, secondhand smoke).
Obstructive sleep apnea (OSA)	Be alert to undiagnosed OSA. Perioperative management involves nighttime continuous positive airway pressure with a ventilator.

Continued on next page

Continued from previous page

CONDITION	MANAGEMENT
Thrombosis	Provide prophylactic anticoagulants, especially in asymptomatic, high-risk patients scheduled for major or orthopedic surgery. Note that postoperative management for patients at risk of thrombosis includes early ambulation, graduated compression stockings, intermittent pneumatic compression devices, and resumption of oral anticoagulants.
Patients taking prednisone	Patients on high-dose steroids require supplemental perioperative doses of corticosteroids to reduce risk of adrenal crisis (hypotension, cardiovascular collapse). This should be given for 24 hours for moderate surgery, and for 48 to 72 hours for major surgery.
Patients taking antirejection drugs	Continue immunosuppressive therapy. Monitor blood levels of the immunosuppressive drug (e.g., tacrolimus or cyclosporine) daily.
Patients taking chemotherapy	Treat anemia and thrombocytopenia, as necessary. Optimize the patient's nutrition.
Patients taking anticoagulants	**High risk of thrombosis** Initiate bridging therapy (replace warfarin with injected short-acting anticoagulants 4 to 5 days before surgery; stop all anticoagulants 4 to 6 hours before surgery; resume warfarin immediately after surgery). Note that INR monitoring (aPTT) is required during bridging therapy if it uses intravenous (IV) unfractionated heparin. **Intermediate risk of thrombosis** Initiate bridging therapy on a case-by-case basis (e.g., initiate for surgeries or procedures with a high risk of bleeding events: neurologic, cardiac, major vascular, or major urologic surgery; joint replacement; lung resection; pacemaker or defibrillator insertion; intestinal anastomosis; kidney, prostate, or cervical cone biopsy; pericardiocentesis; colon polypectomy). **Low risk of thrombosis** Continue existing warfarin therapy.

107

Immunization

MCC particular objectives

Recommend an appropriate schedule of vaccinations.

Discuss the risks and benefits of vaccination.

MCC differential diagnosis

None stated.

Strategy for patient encounter

The likely scenario is parents discussing immunization for their child. The likely tasks are immunization history and counselling.

Immunization history

Obtain an immunization history: ask the parents (or patient) if they have an immunization record. If not, this information may be available from previous physicians or provincial public health services.

Determine whether the patient has a contraindication to immunization, including:

- allergies to vaccine components
- severe illness with or without fever
- immunodeficiency
- unstable neurological disease

The scenario may involve you giving an immunization (although this would not actually happen in the context of the exam). In this situation, be sure to obtain informed consent (see the checklist on informed consent).

CHECKLIST

Informed consent

- **Step 1:** Determine authority. If the patient is a minor, the person giving consent must be a parent or guardian.

- **Step 2:** Determine capacity. A person is capable of consenting if they understand the relevant information and appreciate the reasonably foreseeable consequences of actions based on that information.

- **Step 3:** Provide information. Describe the purpose of the intervention (in this case, immunization) and its risks and benefits.

- **Step 4:** Confirm understanding of the information.

- **Step 5:** Ask for, and answer, any questions.

- **Step 6:** Confirm consent.

- **Step 7:** Document consent or refusal.

Counselling

Counsel the parents (or patient) on possible reactions and how to manage them. Possible adverse reactions to a vaccine include local symptoms such as inflammation and tenderness at the site of injection. Systemic reactions include fever and rash (and crying in children). Allergic complications may include hives, stuffy or runny nose, and anaphylaxis. Local reactions should be managed by applying a cold compress to the injection site and by giving analgesic or antipruritic medication.

Parents who refuse vaccinations need to have their concerns heard. Listen respectfully to the concerns and address them. Correct any misconceptions that the parents may have. Give the message that vaccines are safe and effective, and that serious disease can occur to the child and others if they are not immunized.

Children are immunized on a schedule (see the immunization schedule checklist). Note that the schedule may vary from jurisdiction to jurisdiction.

CHECKLIST

TYPICAL IMMUNIZATION SCHEDULE FOR CHILDREN*

AGE	DTaP-IPV-Hib	DTaP-IPV	MMR	HepB	DTaP	VZ	Menin	Pneu	Infl**	RtV	HPV	MCV
2 mo	X						X	X		X		
4 mo	X						X	X		X		
6 mo	X						X	X	X			
1 y			X		X			X				
18 mo	X						X	X				
4–6 y		X	X			X						
Gr 5				X		X					X	
Gr 9					X							X

* This varies by jurisdiction: refer to local recommendations.

** Children 6 to 23 months should receive these yearly.

Abbreviations: DTaP: diphtheria, tetanus, acellular pertussis; DTaP-IPV: diphtheria, tetanus, acellular pertussis, polio; HepB: hepatitis B; Hib: hemophilus influenza B; HPV: human papillomavirus; Infl: influenza; MCV: meningococcal conjugate vaccine (groups A, C, W-135, and Y); Menin: meningococcal C conjugate; MMR: measles, mumps, rubella; Pneu: pneumococcal conjugate; RtV: rotavirus; VZ: varicella-zoster virus

For all healthy adults, the following vaccines are recommended:
- diphtheria and tetanus: every 10 years
- herpes zoster (shingles): 1 dose at 60+ years
- influenza: yearly
- pertussis (whooping cough): 1 dose as an adult
- pneumococcal: 1 dose at 65+ years

Depending on individual circumstances, the following may also be indicated:
- hepatitis A
- hepatitis B
- human papillomavirus (HPV): 1 dose at 26 years or younger
- measles, mumps, and rubella
- meningococcal (meningitis): 1 dose at 24 years or younger
- varicella-zoster virus (chicken pox): 1 dose
- travel vaccines

Pearls

Adverse drug reactions should be reported to the local health unit in your province or territory. The Government of Canada website has a form for this purpose: Adverse Events Following Immunization (AEFI).

108

Personality disorders

MCC particular objectives
Differentiate between a personality disorder and other mental illness.

Recognize the high prevalence of comorbidities.

Formulate a management plan.

MCC differential diagnosis
with added evidence
None stated. The following breakdown is offered as information.

GENERAL PERSONALITY DISORDER[1(pp646–647)]
Signs and symptoms: an enduring, inflexible pattern of behaviour that significantly deviates from cultural expectations, and has significant impact on day-to-day life; symptom onset no later than early adulthood; presence of symptoms across many contexts

> Key symptoms: deviations in perceptions, emotional response (e.g., range, intensity), interpersonal functioning, impulse control

PERSONALITY DISORDER TYPES[1(pp645–684)]
CLUSTER A PERSONALITY DISORDERS
General pattern: odd, eccentric behaviours

Paranoid personality disorder: distrust, suspiciousness

Schizoid personality disorder: detachment from social relationships; restricted emotional range

Schizotypal personality disorder: discomfort with close relationships; cognitive and perceptual distortions (e.g., about causal events or the meaning of events); eccentric behaviours

CLUSTER B PERSONALITY DISORDERS
General pattern: dramatic, emotional, and erratic behaviour; marked difficulty with impulse control and emotional regulation

Antisocial personality disorder: disregard for others, violating others' rights

Borderline personality disorder: instability in interpersonal relationships and self-image; impulsivity; suicidal behaviour

Histrionic personality disorder: excessive emotions, attention seeking

Narcissistic personality disorder: grandiosity, need for admiration, lack of empathy

CLUSTER C PERSONALITY DISORDERS

General pattern: anxiety, fearfulness

Avoidant personality disorder: social inhibition, feelings of inadequacy, hypersensitivity to criticism

Dependent personality disorder: submissive behaviour to satisfy an excessive need to be taken care of

Obsessive-compulsive personality disorder: preoccupation with orderliness, perfection, control

COEXISTING PSYCHIATRIC CONDITIONS (E.G., MOOD DISORDER)

MAJOR DEPRESSIVE DISORDER[1(pp160-161)]

Signs and symptoms: symptoms that are present most of the time for ≥ 2 weeks; symptoms with significant impact on day-to-day life

> Key symptoms: depressed mood and/or loss of interest in usual activities

> Other symptoms: significant weight change; sleep disturbance; slowed or agitated mental processes; loss of concentration; recurrent thoughts of death or suicide

Risk factors: family history of mental health disorders (depression, anxiety, suicide); personal history of other mental health disorders; substance abuse; chronic illness (e.g., cancer, stroke, chronic pain)

BIPOLAR DISORDER (TYPES I AND II)[1(pp123-134)]

Bipolar I disorder *always* involves at least 1 manic episode, and *may* involve hypomanic and/or major depressive episodes.

Bipolar II disorder *never* involves manic episodes, and *always* involves swings between hypomanic and major depressive episodes.

Family history of bipolar disorder is a risk factor for bipolar disorder.

MANIC EPISODE

Signs and symptoms: symptoms that are present most of the time for ≥ 1 week; symptoms with significant impact on day-to-day life, and that may pose a risk of harm to self and others

> Key symptoms: abnormally elevated (and/or irritable) mood, and goal-directed activity

> Other symptoms: increased self-importance, increased talking, racing thoughts, decreased need for sleep, risky pursuits (e.g., that could damage finances or relationships), psychosis (e.g., delusions, hallucinations)

HYPOMANIC EPISODE

Signs and symptoms: symptoms resembling a manic episode in presentation and duration, except:

> **No** significant impact on day-to-day life

> **No** risk of harm to self or others

> **No** psychosis (e.g., delusions, hallucinations)

MAJOR DEPRESSIVE EPISODE

Signs and symptoms: symptoms that are present most of the time for ≥ 2 weeks; symptoms with significant impact on day-to-day life

Key symptoms: depressed mood and/or loss of interest in usual activities

Other symptoms: significant weight change; sleep disturbance; slowed or agitated mental processes; loss of concentration; recurrent thoughts of death or suicide

Strategy for patient encounter

The likely scenario is a patient with a history of self-harm. The specified tasks could engage history, investigations, or management. Physical exam does not usually contribute useful information for diagnosing or managing personality disorders.

History

Start with open-ended questions about the patient's psychiatric history: What psychiatric conditions have you been diagnosed with? How long have you had problems with your mental health? What kinds of problems have you had? Listen for details that point to a diagnosis of personality disorder and/or a comorbid condition. In particular, note that personality disorders involve long-standing and enduring symptoms (inflexible behaviours); mood disorders involve episodic symptoms.

Perform a mental status exam (see the quick reference) to assess the patient's symptoms. Note symptoms unique to particular disorders (e.g., inappropriate

QUICK REFERENCE

Mental status exams (MSEs)

Many versions of MSEs exist. It's good general preparation for the exam to research MSEs, and choose or prepare a version for your own use (this is not the only clinical presentation where an MSE is appropriate). Your MSE could contain a series of ready-made descriptors that you check off, or it could be a framework for taking notes.

Note that MSEs use both observation and direct questioning to make assessments.

Generally, they assess:

- general appearance and behaviour
- mood
- speech: rate, tone, volume
- thought content: obsessions, preoccupations, hallucinations, delusions, suicidal ideation, homicidal ideation
- thought process: circumstantial, tangential, flight of ideas, loosening of associations
- orientation to time and place
- attention and concentration
- patient insight into their present condition

perceptions and emotional responses in personality disorders; loss of interest and fatigue in major depressive disorder; hallucinations in bipolar I disorder; alternating "up" and "down" moods in bipolar II disorder).

Ask about risk factors associated with personality disorders (e.g., suicidal ideation, substance abuse). Note the patient's insight into their condition, and their interest in changing their situation.

Investigations
Consider a urine drug screen in patients who may be abusing drugs.

Management
Initiate treatment for concurrent psychiatric illness. Consider referral to a psychiatrist or a clinical psychologist for cognitive behavioural therapy. Discuss a plan to treat any coexistent substance abuse.

Pearls
Personality disorders are not treatable by pharmacotherapy. Prescribe pharmacotherapy only in the context of coexisting psychiatric disorders.

Remember that pharmacotherapy involves the risk of abuse and overdose. In particular, prescriptions for sedative-hypnotics run the risk of diversion or abuse, and all psychotropic medications run the risk of overdose. These risks can be reduced by dispensing small quantities of medication (e.g., 1 week at a time) and arranging frequent follow-up with the patient.

REFERENCE

1 American Psychiatric Association. Diagnostic and statistical manual of mental disorders. 5th ed. Arlington, VA: American Psychiatric Association; 2013. 991 p.

109

Pleural effusion

MCC particular objective

Differentiate causes of pleural effusion based on pleural fluid analysis.

MCC differential diagnosis
with added evidence

TRANSUDATIVE (E.G., CONGESTIVE HEART FAILURE, NEPHROTIC SYNDROME, CIRRHOSIS)

TRANSUDATIVE PLEURAL EFFUSION IN GENERAL

This is caused by a combination of increased hydrostatic pressure and decreased plasma oncotic pressure.

Asymptomatic transudates require no treatment. Symptomatic transudates require thoracentesis, chest tube drainage, pleurodesis, pleurectomy, or a combination.

Signs and symptoms: **no** agreement with Light criteria (see *exudative*, below)

Risk factors: congestive heart failure; cirrhosis with ascites; hypoalbuminemia due to nephrotic syndrome

CONGESTIVE HEART FAILURE

Signs and symptoms: history of heart disease (or risk factors for heart disease: diabetes, hypertension, hyperlipidemia, and smoking) or hepatic vein thrombosis (Budd-Chiari syndrome); severe shortness of breath; elevated jugular venous pressure; edema in the abdomen and legs; pink phlegm; heart murmurs and extra cardiac sounds

Investigations: chest X-ray to detect pulmonary edema; NT-proBNP level; echocardiogram to distinguish forms of heart failure; cardiac stress testing, either with exercise or pharmacological agent

NEPHROTIC SYNDROME

Signs and symptoms: progressive lower extremity edema (ankles and feet); swelling around the eyes; weight gain (from water retention); foamy urine

Risk factors: conditions that damage the kidneys (e.g., diabetes, systemic lupus erythematosus, amyloidosis); use of nonsteroidal antiinflammatory drugs (NSAIDs), antibiotics; history of HIV, hepatitis B virus (HBV), hepatitis C virus (HCV), malaria

Investigations: urine (proteinuria, spot urine protein:creatinine ratio, lipuria); hyponatremia with low fractional sodium excretion; low serum albumin; high total cholesterol (hyperlipidemia); elevated BUN

CIRRHOSIS

Signs and symptoms: jaundice; easy bruising, bleeding; itching; ascites; spiderlike blood vessels on the skin; systemic symptoms (anorexia, weight loss, weakness, fatigue)

> History of chronic alcohol abuse; chronic viral HBV, HCV; hemochromatosis; nonalcoholic fatty liver disease
>
> HBV and HCV risk factors: autoimmune conditions, unprotected sex, intravenous drug abuse, blood transfusions, tattoos, body piercings, imprisonment, workplace exposure to body fluids

Investigations: liver function tests

EXUDATIVE

EXUDATIVE PLEURAL EFFUSION IN GENERAL

Signs and symptoms: symptoms that meet Light criteria

> Light criteria: ratio of pleural fluid protein to serum protein > 0.5; and/or ratio of pleural fluid lactate dehydrogenase (LDH) to serum LDH > 0.6; and/or pleural fluid LDH > 0.6 times the normal upper limit of a lab's serum LDH (labs define this differently)

Risk factors: pneumonia, malignancy, pulmonary embolism, viral infection, tuberculosis

Infectious/inflammatory causes (e.g., parapneumonic effusion, empyema, rheumatoid arthritis)

PARAPNEUMONIC EFFUSION

Signs and symptoms: cough; fever; pleuritic chest pain; shortness of breath and/or sputum production

UNCOMPLICATED PARAPNEUMONIC EFFUSION

Symptoms resolve with resolution of pneumonia.

Signs and symptoms: exudative, neutrophilic effusions (these result from inflammation associated with pneumonia); fluid that is sterile, and slightly cloudy or clear

COMPLICATED PARAPNEUMONIC EFFUSION

This requires drainage for resolution.

Signs and symptoms: fluid that is often sterile (false negative), but cloudy, with putrid odour

Investigations: increased neutrophils; pleural fluid acidosis; decreased glucose; increased LDH (> 1000 IU/L); anaerobic infection on Gram stain

EMPYEMA

Causes include complications of pneumonia, thoracotomy, abscesses (lung, liver, or subdiaphragmatic), and penetrating trauma with secondary infection.

Signs and symptoms: fever for several days (> 48 hours); malaise; frank pus in the pleural space (observed when drained by thoracentesis); pleural fluid that is thick, viscous, and opaque

> History of recent upper respiratory tract infection; bronchitis; pneumonia; recurrent aspiration (e.g., due to poor oral hygiene, alcoholism)

RHEUMATOID ARTHRITIS

Rheumatoid arthritis is among a group of systemic, inflammatory, autoimmune diseases that also includes systemic lupus erythematosus, scleroderma, temporal arteritis, and interstitial lung disease.

Signs and symptoms: fatigue, muscle weakness, fever, body aches, joint pain, skin rash

> Lung signs and symptoms: generally asymptomatic; small volume of pleural fluid, which is usually unilateral (left side) with high titres of rheumatoid factor and low glucose levels (< 25 mg/dL)

Neoplasm (e.g., primary, metastatic, mesothelioma)

Malignant pleural effusion is diagnosed with thoracentesis.

The pleura is more commonly involved in metastatic disease or advanced-stage tumours (lung, breast, lymphoma); mesothelioma; large primary tumours; and adenocarcinoma.

Malignant cells may be identified in cytologic examination of pleural fluid.

Signs and symptoms: shortness of breath, chest pain, malaise, dry cough

Pulmonary embolus

Signs and symptoms: sharp chest pain; shortness of breath; cough (possibly with blood); hypoxia; possible unilateral swelling of the lower limbs (this indicates deep vein thrombosis); elevated pulse and respiratory rate; arrhythmias; lung rales on auscultation; lower-lung dullness on percussion; motor or sensory deficits

Risk factors: heart failure; cancer; surgery; prolonged immobility (e.g., long plane trips); smoking; estrogen replacement therapy; oral contraceptives; current pregnancy; previous deep vein thrombosis, embolism, or stroke; family history of embolism

Investigations: elevated D-dimer level; area of reduced pulmonary perfusion on V/Q scan; CT angiography to detect blocked vessel

Gastrointestinal condition (e.g., ruptured esophagus, pancreatitis, chylothorax)

RUPTURED ESOPHAGUS (BOERHAAVE SYNDROME)

This is a life-threatening emergency (watch out for atypical presentations).

Signs and symptoms: male, middle-aged (common); recent severe vomiting or trauma; lower anterior chest or upper abdominal pain (other pain locations: the neck, back); subcutaneous emphysema; difficulty swallowing; shortness of breath; hematemesis; dark, tarry stools; history of dietary overindulgence, overconsumption of alcohol

> Mackler triad (classic presentation): chest pain, vomiting, subcutaneous emphysema

> Atypical presentation: shoulder pain, facial swelling, hoarseness, voice changes

Investigations: thoracentesis for pleural fluid (fluid has food fragments, pH < 6, elevated salivary amylase, leukocytosis); thoracic, cervical X-ray; contrast esophagram

PANCREATITIS

Pleural effusion is a complication in one-third of acute pancreatitis cases.

Signs and symptoms: constant upper abdominal pain that radiates to the back (sitting up and leaning forward may reduce the pain; pain occurs with coughing, vigorous movement, deep breathing); shortness of breath; nausea, vomiting; hypotension; fever; jaundice; abdominal tenderness

> History of gallstones or chronic alcoholism (usual); hyperlipidemia; hypercalcemia; change of medication

Investigations: serum amylase and lipase (levels are ≥ 3 times the upper limit of normal levels; elevated lipase indicates pancreatic damage); possible elevated calcium; possible elevated cholesterol; possible elevated ALT (this indicates associated liver inflammation); chest X-ray (this may show left-sided or bilateral pleural effusion; atelectasis); abdominal X-ray (this may show calcifications within pancreatic ducts; calcified gallstones; or localized ileus of a segment of small intestine); ultrasound

CHYLOTHORAX

Signs and symptoms: unilateral pleural effusion, right hemithorax involvement (often); decreased breath sounds; dullness to percussion

> Traumatic chylothorax: postoperative, cardiothoracic surgery (most common); pleural effusion on serial X-ray evaluations, or persistent drainage of pleural fluid from a preexisting chest tube

> Nontraumatic chylothorax: malignancy (e.g., lymphoma, chronic lymphocytic leukemia, metastatic cancer); gradual onset of symptoms; decreased exercise tolerance; shortness of breath; heavy feeling in the chest; fatigue; rarely fever or chest pain

Investigations: thoracentesis for pleural fluid (fluid is milky or opaque; triglyceride > 110 mg/dL confirms chylothorax; chylomicrons are present on electrophoresis, predominately lymphocytes); chest X-ray to detect the side of the chest with effusion; CT scan of the thorax and abdomen to identify site of thoracic duct rupture

Strategy for patient encounter

The likely scenario is a patient with shortness of breath and show-ing pleural effusion on X-ray. The specified tasks could engage history, physical exam, investigations, or management.

History

Start with open-ended questions to establish the patient's medi-cal history, relevant occupational exposures, and current health status: What conditions have you been diagnosed with? What do you do for a living? How has your health been lately? Listen for a history of conditions that cause edema states (e.g., heart failure); infectious disease, or symptoms consistent with infectious dis-ease (e.g., fever); neoplastic disease; and high-risk occupations for asbestos exposure (e.g., asbestos mining, construction, fire-fighting, industrial work).

When you identify an underlying condition, concentrate on the history of the condition and the seriousness of the symptoms the patient is experiencing. How long have you had this condi-tion? When did your current symptoms start? How have your symptoms changed?

Physical exam

Auscultate the heart and lungs, and percuss the lungs. Perform a focused exam based on the probable diagnosis identified from the history.

Investigations

Order a chest X-ray and be prepared to interpret the results. Identify indications for thoracentesis (for diagnosis or to relieve symptoms). Interpret the thoracentesis results (see the checklist) and use this to confirm the diagnosis.

Management

Specific management depends on the identified cause. Consider the need for referral to internal medicine or surgery.

CHECKLIST

Differentiating causes of pleural effusion based on pleural fluid analysis

CAUSES OF PLEURAL EFFUSION	PLEURAL FLUID ANALYSIS
Exudative	Cloudy; pH 7.3–7.45; positive Light criteria
Transudative	Clear; absolute total protein concentration < 3.0 g/dL; pH 7.4–7.55
Pulmonary embolus	Exudate
Rheumatoid arthritis	Exudate; low glucose level (< 25 mg/dL)
Ruptured esophagus	Exudate; amylase that exceeds upper limits of normal serum amylase; pleural fluid/serum amylase ratio > 1.0; low pH; ingested food fragments in fluid; low glucose concentration (< 60 mg/dL) or a pleural fluid/serum glucose ratio < 0.5
Pancreatitis	Exudate; amylase that exceeds upper limits of normal serum amylase; pleural fluid/serum amylase ratio > 1.0; > 10 000 nucleated cells/μL
Chylothorax	Exudate; milky to opaque; triglycerides > 110 mg/dL; chylomicrons; lymphocytosis
Parapneumonic effusion	Exudate; cloudy or clear; low glucose concentration (< 60 mg/dL) or a pleural fluid/serum glucose ratio < 0.5; > 50 000 nucleated cells/μL (neutrophilic)
Empyema	Exudate; fluid that has pus and putrid odour; thick, viscous, opaque; positive culture; LDH > 1000 IU/L; very low glucose concentration (sometimes undetectable) or a pleural fluid/serum glucose ratio < 0.5; > 50 000 nucleated cells/μL
Malignancy/neoplasm (primary, metastatic, mesothelioma)	Exudate; positive cytology; sometimes LDH > 1000 IU/L; low glucose concentration (30–50 mg/dL) or a pleural fluid/serum glucose ratio < 0.5; elevated levels of soluble mesothelin-related peptides or mesothelial cells in mesothelioma
Congestive heart failure	Transudate; serum-to-pleural-fluid albumin gradient > 1.2 g/dL; elevated blood NT-proBNP when Light criteria yield results in exudative range
Nephrotic syndrome	Transudate
Cirrhosis	Transudate; < 250 PMN cell count/mm^3; low protein (< 2.5 g/dL), albumin; pleural fluid/LDH ratio < 0.6; pleural fluid/serum bilirubin ratio < 0.6; pH > 7.4

Abbreviations: LDH: lactate dehydrogenase; NT-proBNP: N-terminal prohormone of brain natriuretic peptide; PMN: polymorphonuclear leukocyte

110

Poisoning

MCC particular objectives

Determine the nature of the toxicity and exposure.

Provide specific care based on this information.

MCC differential diagnosis
with added evidence

COMMON POISONS

Household or work items (e.g., cleaning substances, or other chemical products, cosmetics, plants)

A toxidrome is possible in this context (see the checklist on clinical signs of toxic syndromes).

Anticholinergics (e.g., antihistamines, tricyclics)

Signs and symptoms: possible anticholinergic toxidrome (see the checklist on clinical signs of toxic syndromes)

> Additional symptoms (mnemonic): "red as a beet, dry as a bone, hot as a hare, blind as a bat, mad as a hatter, full as a flask"

Sympathomimetic (e.g., cold remedies, amphetamines, cocaine)

Signs and symptoms: possible sympathetic toxidrome (see the checklist on clinical signs of toxic syndromes)

> Additional symptoms: hallucinations and/or psychosis; headache; sweating; increased motor activity; seizures; tremor

DEPRESSANTS (E.G., ALCOHOL, OPIATES, SEDATIVES, HYPNOTICS)

Signs and symptoms: possible sedative/hypnotic toxidrome (see the checklist on clinical signs of toxic syndromes)

> Additional symptoms: confusion, stupor, or coma; nystagmus; gait disturbance

Cholinergics (e.g., insecticides, nicotine)

Signs and symptoms: possible cholinergic toxidrome (see the checklist on clinical signs of toxic syndromes); muscarinic symptoms or nicotinic symptoms

> Muscarinic symptoms (most common) (mnemonic: **SLUDGE**): **s**alivation, **l**acrimation, **u**rination, **d**iarrhea, **g**astrointestinal pain, **e**mesis
>
> Nicotinic symptoms (less common): tremors; muscle weakness; fasciculations

SEROTONERGICS (E.G., SELECTIVE SEROTONIN REUPTAKE INHIBITORS)

Signs and symptoms (serotonin syndrome): agitation, restlessness, confusion, tachycardia, hypertension, dilated pupils, muscle symptoms (loss of control, twitching, rigidity), sweating, diarrhea, headache

> Severe: high fever, seizures, arrhythmia, coma

ANALGESICS (E.G., ACETYLSALICYLIC ACID, ACETAMINOPHEN)

SALICYLATE POISONING

Signs and symptoms: history of using skin products that contain salicylates, such as over-the-counter acne remedies; abdominal pain; tinnitus; nausea, vomiting (blood in the vomit); hyperthermia; mental status changes (agitation and seizures; or lethargy, central nervous system depression, and coma); mixed metabolic acidosis and respiratory acidosis

ACETAMINOPHEN POISONING

Signs and symptoms: nausea, vomiting; lethargy; pallor; liver enlargement and tenderness

CARDIOVASCULAR DRUGS (E.G., DIGOXIN, BETA-BLOCKERS, CALCIUM CHANNEL BLOCKERS)

DIGOXIN POISONING

Signs and symptoms: confusion, irregular pulse, fast heartbeat, nausea, vomiting, diarrhea

BETA-BLOCKER POISONING

Signs and symptoms: bradycardia; hypotension or shock; depressed level of consciousness; seizures

POISONING FROM CALCIUM CHANNEL BLOCKERS

Signs and symptoms: bradycardia, hypotension, cardiac arrest

OTHERS (E.G., HALLUCINOGENS)

Examples of hallucinogens include amphetamines, cannabinoids, and lysergic acid diethylamide (LSD).

Signs and symptoms: possible hallucinogenic toxidrome (see the checklist on clinical signs of toxic syndromes)

Additional symptoms: hallucinations, psychosis, sensory distortion

Strategy for patient encounter

The likely scenario is a patient with medication overdose. The specified tasks could engage history, physical exam, investigations, or management.

History

If the patient is conscious, ask for a history of ingestion, but consider that the patient may be impaired or not truthful. Always seek collateral information from accompanying caregivers on the ingested substance and dose, if possible.

Physical exam

Obtain the patient's vital signs and perform a physical examination with the goal of identifying a specific toxidrome (see the checklist).

CHECKLIST

Some clinical signs of toxic syndromes (toxidromes)[1]

TOXIDROME	HR	BP	RR	PUP	T
Anticholinergic	up	up	N	D	up
Cholinergic	down	up/down	up/N	C	N
Hallucinogenic	up/N	up/N	N	D/N	N
Sedative/hypnotic	N/down	N/down	N	N/C	down
Sympathetic	up	up	N/down	D	N

Abbreviations: HR, heart rate; BP, blood pressure; RR, respiration rate; PUP, pupils; T, temperature; D, dilated; C, constricted; N, normal.

Investigations

In the case of ingestion of acetaminophen or acetylsalicylic acid (ASA), order tests to determine the level of the ingested substance; or, if the ingested substance is unknown, assess toxic effects (arterial blood gases; anion and osmolar gaps). For un-known ingestions, consider a urine drug screen, but remember that some substances are commonly missed by this test (e.g., synthetic opioids).

Management

Measure and monitor the patient's vital signs and symptoms, in particular related to cardiac, respiratory, and neurological function. Airway and ventilation support may be needed in the most serious cases. Administer activated charcoal for decontamination or prevention of further absorption. Contact poison control. Administer specific antidotes if indicated (e.g., naloxone for opioid overdose, N-acetylcysteine for acetaminophen overdose). In patients with renal failure, or in severe poisoning without specific antidote, consider referral for dialysis. Consider referral for psychiatric assessment, if indicated.

REFERENCE

1 Baskin LB. Lab literacy for Canadian doctors. Edmonton, Canada: Brush Education Inc.; 2014. Chapter 9, Intoxication and toxidromes; 173–200 (Table 19, 178–179).

111

Hyperkalemia

MCC particular objective
Recognize the urgency of hyperkalemia associated with electro-cardiogram (ECG) abnormalities.

MCC differential diagnosis
with added evidence
HYPERKALEMIA IN GENERAL
Definition: serum potassium > 5.5 mmol/L

INCREASED INTAKE
The MCC notes that hyperkalemia is usually associated with low excretion.

REDISTRIBUTION
Decreased entry into cells (e.g., insulin deficiency, beta 2 blockade)
INSULIN DEFICIENCY: TYPE 1 DIABETES
Low insulin causes hyperglycemia, which moves fluid and potassium into blood circulation and leads to hyperkalemia. Low insulin can also result in diabetic ketoacidosis (DKA), which leads to *apparent* hyperkalemia. In DKA, a total body potassium deficit is present, which means that treatment with insulin can result in profound *hypokalemia* if potassium is not appropriately replaced.

Signs and symptoms: personal or family history of diabetes; history of diabetic complications and/or inadequate monitoring; polydipsia, polyuria, and/or weight loss

Investigations: fasting glucose or HbA_{1c} test; in suspected ketoacidosis: tests for blood glucose, electrolytes, blood pH, urine ketones

BETA 2 BLOCKADE
Nonselective beta-blockers decrease cellular potassium uptake, which leads to hyperkalemia. Beta-blockers also suppress catecholamine-stimulated renin release, decreasing aldosterone synthesis, which also leads to hyperkalemia.

Increased exit from cells (e.g., metabolic acidosis, rhabdomyolysis)
INCREASED POTASSIUM EXIT IN GENERAL
Conditions causing potassium exit from cells include volume

depletion, hyperchloremic metabolic acidosis, anion gap metabolic acidosis, respiratory acidosis, familial hyperkalemic periodic paralysis, rhabdomyolysis, hemolysis, tumour lysis syndrome, and trauma. Lab error (e.g., lysis during sample collection) is also possible.

METABOLIC ACIDOSIS

Signs and symptoms: chest pain, palpitations; headache; altered mental status; severe anxiety; decreased visual acuity; nausea, vomiting; abdominal pain; altered appetite and weight gain; muscle weakness; bone pain; joint pain; deep, rapid breathing

Investigations: ECG; electrolytes; glucose; renal function; CBC; urinalysis; arterial blood sampling (blood pH and anion gap) to detect renal tubular acidosis

RHABDOMYOLYSIS

Signs and symptoms: use of street drugs (especially cocaine, heroin, and amphetamines), statin medications, or anesthetics (i.e., during recent surgery); muscle weakness; recent severe trauma; fever and/or hypotension (possible: these are signs of malignant hyperthermia following anesthesia)

Investigations: elevated creatine kinase; elevated serum or urine myoglobin; elevated phosphate

REDUCED URINARY EXCRETION

Decreased glomerular filtration rate (e.g., acute or chronic kidney injury)

ACUTE OR CHRONIC KIDNEY INJURY

Kidney-related causes include acute renal failure or kidney injury; chronic kidney disease; diabetic nephropathy; systemic lupus erythematosus; and renal tubular acidosis type IV.

Signs and symptoms: often asymptomatic, muscle weakness, flaccid paralysis, paresthesia

Investigations: repeat test to rule out lab artifact (common occurrence); blood tests to assess kidney function and detect hyperglycemia (serum electrolytes, calcium, magnesium, BUN, creatinine, glucose); ECG to detect arrhythmia; spot urine potassium, creatinine; urine osmolality to calculate fractional excretion of potassium

Decreased secretion (e.g., aldosterone deficiency, drugs)

ALDOSTERONE DEFICIENCY

Chronic aldosterone-related hyperkalemia causes include mineralocorticoid (adrenal) deficiency (Addison disease, congenital adrenal hyperplasia, isolated hypoaldosteronism); hyporeninemic hypoaldosteronism (chronic kidney disease, diabetic nephropathy, lupus nephropathy, HIV nephropathy); and pseudohypoaldosteronism.

Investigations: low aldosterone, low cortisol, high renin, hyponatremia (adrenal insufficiency), low/normal renin, normal cortisol (hyporeninemic hypoaldosteronism)

DRUGS

Medications associated with hyperkalemia (renal tubular acidosis type IV) include ACE inhibitors; nonsteroidal antiinflammatory drugs (NSAIDs) (e.g., celecoxib, diclofenac, indomethacin); angiotensin II receptor blockers; potassium-sparing diuretics (e.g., spironolactone, eplerenone, triamterene); immunosuppressives (e.g., tacrolimus, cyclosporine); beta-blockers; digoxin; heparin; and antibiotics containing trimethoprim.

Strategy for patient encounter

The likely scenario is a patient with critically high potassium. The specified tasks could engage history, investigations, or management. Physical exam does not usually contribute useful information for diagnosing or managing hyperkalemia.

History

Ask open-ended questions to establish the patient's medical and medication history: What conditions have you been diagnosed with? What medications do you take? Listen for renal conditions, diabetes, aldosterone-related conditions (e.g., Addison disease), and cancer; and for beta-blockers, ACE inhibitors, nonsteroidal antiinflammatory drugs (NSAIDs), angiotensin II receptor blockers, diuretics, immunosuppressives, digoxin, heparin, and antibiotics. Ask about factors relevant to rhabdomyolysis (recent surgery, severe recent trauma, use of street drugs, use of statins).

Investigations

Order an electrocardiogram (ECG) to assess the physiologic severity of the hyperkalemia. Be prepared to interpret an ECG: the examiner may provide you with ECG results.

Order tests for serum creatinine and urine electrolytes to assess the cause.

Management

Address any underlying causes.

In severe hyperkalemia, or if ECG changes are present (tall peaked T waves with shorted QT interval; lengthened PR interval; wide QRS interval; absent P waves; sine-wave pattern), administer intravenous (IV) calcium to reduce cardiac toxicity.

Give IV glucose and insulin infusion to enhance potassium up-take by cells. Correct severe metabolic acidosis with IV sodium bicarbonate; if failure is present, consider nebulized ß-adrenergic agonist instead. Increase potassium excretion by administering loop diuretics or gastrointestinal cation-exchange medications (e.g., sodium polystyrene sulfonate). Provide emergency dialysis for severe hyperkalemia that is unresponsive to more conservative measures or in patients with complete renal failure.

112

Hypokalemia

MCC particular objective
Recognize the urgency of hypokalemia associated with muscle weakness and/or electrocardiogram (ECG) abnormalities.

MCC differential diagnosis
with added evidence
HYPOKALEMIA IN GENERAL
Definition: serum potassium < 3.5 mmol/L

DECREASED INTAKE (E.G., ANOREXIA NERVOSA)
ANOREXIA NERVOSA [1(pp338-339)]
Signs and symptoms: significantly low body weight; intense fear of gaining weight or persistent behaviour that interferes with gaining weight; excessive focus on body weight or shape in self-evaluation, or persistent lack of recognition of current low body weight

REDISTRIBUTION (E.G., ALKALEMIA, INSULIN, BETA 2-ADRENERGIC STIMULATING DRUGS)
Signs and symptoms (in general): often asymptomatic, muscle weakness, fatigue, anxiety, constipation, syncope, palpitations, respiratory distress, arrhythmias

> Alkalemia: arterial blood gas pH > 7.42 and arterial partial pressure of CO_2 < 38 mmHg

> Insulin: personal or family history of diabetes; history of diabetic complications and/or inadequate monitoring; signs

and symptoms of diabetes (polydipsia, polyuria, and/or weight loss)

Investigations: blood tests (electrolytes, magnesium, glucose, BUN, creatinine)

INCREASED LOSSES

Renal losses

Causes include medications (diuretics, mineralocorticoids, glucocorticoids, high-dose antibiotics) and chloride-responsive metabolic alkalosis.

Signs and symptoms: low blood pressure from hypovolemia

Investigations: 24-hour urine potassium excretion to differentiate renal loss (> 30 mmol) and extrarenal loss

Gastrointestinal losses (e.g., vomiting, diarrhea)

Strategy for patient encounter

The likely scenario is a patient with critically low potassium. The specified tasks could engage history, investigations, or management. Physical exam does not usually contribute useful information for diagnosing or managing hypokalemia. Take note, however, of obviously low body weight, which may indicate anorexia nervosa.

History

Start with open-ended questions to establish the patient's medical and medication history: What conditions have you been diagnosed with? What medications do you take? Listen for anorexia nervosa and diabetes; and for diuretics, insulin, beta 2-adrenergic stimulating drugs, mineralocorticoids, glucocorticoids, and antibiotics. Ask whether the patient has noticed any muscle weakness. Ask about vomiting and diarrhea.

Investigations

Order an ECG to identify life-threatening conduction abnormalities, and serum and urine electrolytes to distinguish the cause.

Management

Treat any underlying causes (vomiting, diarrhea, thiazide, and loop diuretics), and replace potassium. For potassium levels of 2.5–3.4 mmol/L, replace with oral potassium chloride (KCl).

Consider potassium-sparing diuretics in patients with normal renal function who are prone to significant hypokalemia.

For severe hypokalemia (< 2.5 mmol/L), apply a cardiac monitor and administer 40 mmol KCl in 1 L of normal saline with an infusion rate of 10 mmol/hour. Recheck the patient's serum potassium level after each 40 mmol of KCl. Also check the patient's magnesium ion (Mg^{2+}) level, because low magnesium may make it more difficult to control the potassium level. If the patient has low magnesium, initially give 4 mL of 50% magnesium sulfate ($MgSO_4$, 8 mmol).

REFERENCE

1 American Psychiatric Association. Diagnostic and statistical manual of mental disorders. 5th ed. Arlington, VA: American Psychiatric Association; 2013. 991 p.

113

Prenatal care

MCC particular objective

Use a shared decision-making model: enable patients to make informed decisions based on their needs.

MCC differential diagnosis

None stated.

Strategy for patient encounter

There are many possible scenarios for this patient encounter such as a patient with an unwanted pregnancy, a patient seeking breast-feeding advice, or a patient seeking counselling about a possible repeat cesarean section. The specified task will likely be counselling with an emphasis on shared decision making.

As basic preparation, inform yourself of standard local guidelines for prenatal testing, immunizations, and supplementation with folic acid.

Shared decision making

The MCC particular objective pertains to using a shared decision-making model. Shared decision making is an approach to person-centred care that is associated with improved health outcomes. It involves conferring agency to the patient by providing information and supporting them to make their own informed decisions.

The MCC identifies providing patients with generic information as common pitfall of the exam. To avoid this pitfall in the context of shared decision making, start by establishing the particulars of the patient's situation. Then ask for her concerns about the issue at hand. Use her response as the starting point for providing information. You need to provide a full range of information, but starting with information targeting the priorities of the patient shows you are listening.

The MCC may make the scenario clear in the notes it provides to introduce the case, but the notes may also just state that a pregnant patient is seeking advice. The best first step is open-ended inquiry about the patient's needs: Please tell me why you have come to see me today.

UNWANTED PREGNANCY

In this scenario, the patient has 3 options: parent the baby (despite not wanting it), opt for adoption, or opt for abortion. The stage of gestation may affect her choices, so begin those particulars: How do you know you are pregnant? When was the first day of your last period? Then ask

---

CHECKLIST

Breast milk versus formula

Breast milk suits infants' immature gastrointestinal tract, kidneys, immune system, and metabolic demands. It provides excellent nutrition and builds infants' immunity. Babies still need supplements of vitamin D.

Formula is a good substitute. Parents should use an iron-fortified brand and be consistent with 1 brand. Special formulas are available if needed (e.g., for protein hypersensitivity, lactose intolerance).

Note that cow's milk is not a good substitute for breast milk or formula in the first year due to high renal protein loading and poor iron absorption. From age 1 to 2 years, children should not drink reduced-fat milk (2% fat or lower): fat is required for neural development.

Maternal contraindications for breast-feeding

HIV/AIDS

Active or untreated tuberculosis

Regional herpes

Using alcohol/drugs

Chemotherapy or radiation therapy

the patient for her first concerns about being pregnant. She may describe her mental state or physical well-being, or her financial or social situation. Summarize her concerns, for example: "I think I hear you saying that you aren't ready to be pregnant." Ask for her response to your summary and listen for clarifications. Outline the option that best fits her concerns, including supports and resources available to navigate it. Then outline the other options. Ask for the patient's perspectives on the options, and offer support through referrals and follow-up appointments.

BREAST-FEEDING

In this scenario, the patient has 2 options: try to breast-feed or choose not to try (see the checklist on breast milk versus formula). Use open-ended inquiry to establish the patient's breast-feeding history: What are your experiences with breast-feeding? She may say she has no experience; or she may describe her reaction to seeing others breast-feed; or she may describe concerns from feeding children she already has. Ask what concerns she has about breast-feeding, if this is not clear. Summarize what she says and ask for clarifications. Describe the option that best fits her circumstances, and

CHECKLIST

VBAC advantages and risks

Most women (60% to 80%) can deliver vaginally after a C-section, even after 2 C-sections. The patient must deliver in a hospital with C-section capabilities. The procedure involves: admission as soon as labour starts; close monitoring of mother and baby; an attempt at vaginal delivery first; oxytocin for augmentation, if required (prostaglandins are not recommended); C-section, if required.

- **Advantages:** no surgical risks (e.g., infection, scarring); quicker recovery
- **Risks:** uterine rupture, which is higher if delivery for the current pregnancy takes place within 2 years of the last C-section, and which is sometimes solved with emergency hysterectomy
- **Contraindications:** prior inverted or classical C-section (due to risk of uterine rupture), previous uterine rupture, placenta previa

Repeat C-section advantages and risks

- **Advantages:** less risk of infection transmission to the baby (C-sections are often recommended in the context of maternal HIV, herpes); no risk of uterine rupture during labour
- **Risks (these increase with each repeated surgery):** uncontrolled postpartum bleeding, which is sometimes solved with hysterectomy; complications from internal scarring (e.g., adhesions that affect the bladder and bowel); placenta complications in future pregnancies (e.g., placenta accreta, placenta previa)

then describe the other option. Ask for the patient's perspectives on the options, and offer support through referrals and follow-up appointments.

VAGINAL BIRTH AFTER CESAREAN SECTION (VBAC)

In this scenario, the patient probably has 2 options, depending on the number and type of previous cesarean sections (C-sections): try for a vaginal birth or choose not to try. Use open-ended inquiry to obtain the patient's history with C-sections: How many C-sections have you had? What were the circumstances? What kind of C-sections have you had? When was your last C-section? How many vaginal deliveries have you had? Ask about the patient's delivery goals for her current pregnancy. Summarize what she says and ask for clarifications. Provide information on benefits and risks based on the options open to her (see the checklist on advantages and risks of VBAC versus repeat C-sections).

114

Intrapartum and postpartum care

MCC particular objective

Use a shared decision-making model: enable patients to make informed decisions based on their needs.

MCC differential diagnosis

None stated.

Strategy for patient encounter

The likely scenario is a pregnant woman with no previous prenatal care. It could address any topic in obstetrics. The MCC notes that intrapartum and postpartum care include labour and the 6 weeks after delivery. High-yield topics include the stages of labour and indications for labour induction (see the checklists).

CHECKLIST
Stages of labour

FIRST STAGE
This begins with the onset of contractions and ends when the cervix is dilated to 10 cm. It has 3 phases:

- **Early labour:** the period from the onset of contractions to 3 cm cervical dilation, characterized by contractions that are irregular and widely spaced
- **Active labour:** the period from 3 cm to 7 cm cervical dilation, characterized by contractions that are stronger and more regular
- **Transition:** the period from 7 cm to 10 cm cervical dilation

SECOND STAGE
This begins when the cervix is fully dilated and ends with delivery of the baby.

THIRD STAGE
This is delivery of the placenta.

CHECKLIST
Indications and contraindications for the induction of labour

INDICATIONS
Prolonged gestation (longer than 40 weeks)

Premature rupture of the membranes

Maternal health compromise (e.g., hypertension, preeclampsia, eclampsia)

Fetal growth restriction

Intrauterine fetal death

ABSOLUTE CONTRAINDICATIONS
Cephalopelvic disproportion

Placenta previa

Vasa previa

Cord prolapse

Transverse lie

Active primary genital herpes

Previous classical cesarean section

The specified tasks could engage history, physical exam, investigations, or management (with an emphasis on shared decision making).

History

In a woman presenting in labour without previous prenatal care, the goal of the history is to identify the stage of labour and risk factors for complications.

Ask open-ended questions about the onset of labour: When did your contractions start? How frequent are they? How regular are they? When did your water break?

Use open-ended questions to take an obstetrical history: How many children do you have? What complications have you had during previous pregnancies? What complications have you had during this pregnancy? Listen for a history of preterm labour, complicated labour (prolonged stage of labour, fever, or meconium-stained fluid), multiple gestation, and preeclampsia in previous pregnancies; and for vaginal bleeding or discharge during this pregnancy.

Establish key details of this pregnancy: whether it was planned, the estimated date of delivery, and the use of folate supplements prior to conception and during the pregnancy.

Ask about a history of diabetes, hypertension, blood-borne viruses (HIV, hepatitis B, hepatitis C), and other chronic diseases. Take a medication history.

Physical exam

Before you begin the physical exam, inform the patient of the need for the exam and for fetal monitoring. Make sure you obtain the patient's consent.

Obtain the patient's vital signs, looking for fever and hypertension. Perform a speculum exam, including swabs for group B streptococcus. Examine the abdomen and obtain a fundal height measurement.

(State that you will perform these examinations. Speculum exams are not performed on standardized patients, and a truly pregnant standardized patient is unlikely in any case. So, the examiner will likely interrupt, ask what you are looking for, and provide findings. State that you want to establish the degree of cervical dilation, take swabs for group B streptococcus, check for meconium-stained fluid, check for abnormal abdominal findings such as uterine tenderness, and measure fundal height to estimate gestational age.)

Investigations

Order an ultrasound of the fetus, looking for an enlarged liver, spleen, or heart, or ascites (these are possible signs of Rh antigen incompatibility). Test the mother's blood for the presence of anti-Rh antibodies. After the birth, test the umbilical cord blood for blood group, Rh factor, red blood cell count, antibodies, and bilirubin level.

Order a urinalysis, looking for proteinuria, and a urine culture and sensitivity, looking for infection. Order a fetal fibronectin and assess fetal well-being (ultrasound, fetal monitoring).

Shared decision making

The MCC lists using a shared decision-making model as the particular objective. Shared decision making is an approach to person-centred care that is associated with improved health outcomes. Shared decision making involves conferring agency to the patient by providing information and supporting them to make their own informed decisions.

Check if the patient has a birth plan. Review the plan, or create a plan with the patient. Discuss involving birth partners (e.g., the patient's spouse) and options for pain management.

115

Early pregnancy loss (spontaneous abortion)

MCC particular objectives

Provide supportive counselling to parents.

Investigate cases of recurrent miscarriage.

MCC differential diagnosis
with added evidence

SPONTANEOUS ABORTION IN GENERAL

This is defined as pregnancy loss before 20 weeks gestation, where the fetus or embryo is < 500 g.

Common causes include embryonic chromosomal abnormalities or teratogen exposure.

Signs and symptoms: uterine bleeding (from spotting to heavy bleeding); pelvic pain (severe or dull cramping); small-for-gestational-age uterus (this suggests spontaneous abortion)

> Asymptomatic patients: abnormalities incidentally discovered on Doppler or pelvic/transvaginal ultrasound (no fetal cardiac activity; abnormal gestational sac and yolk sac)

Risk factors: maternal age; reproductive factors; medication, drug, substance use; low folate level; high maternal body mass index (BMI); maternal fever; celiac disease; prior miscarriages

Investigations: decreasing serum β-hCG

GENETIC FACTORS (E.G., CHROMOSOMAL ABNORMALITIES)

CHROMOSOMAL ABNORMALITIES

Fetal chromosomal abnormalities in number or structure are the most common cause of spontaneous abortions and recurrent pregnancy loss.

> Aneuploidy: most common cause; increased risk with each spontaneous abortion
>
> Other causes: mosaicism, translocation, inversion, deletion, fragile sites; single-gene, X-linked, or polygenic disorders
>
> De novo genetic abnormalities: usually not inherited; possible increased risk associated with a first-degree relative with recurrent pregnancy loss of unknown etiology

REPRODUCTIVE TRACT ABNORMALITIES (E.G., UTERINE ANOMALIES)

UTERINE ABNORMALITIES

These can be congenital or acquired. They interfere with implantation and fetal growth, and are associated with recurrent miscarriages and preterm delivery.

Abnormalities include uterine septum, submucosal leiomyoma, and intrauterine adhesions.

> Women are often asymptomatic.
>
> Removal of the septum increases the live birth rate, even in women who were considered infertile before.

PROTHROMBOTIC FACTORS (E.G., THROMBOPHILIA)

THROMBOPHILIA

This results in recurrent miscarriages and uteroplacental circulation abnormalities.

Signs and symptoms: late or early fetal loss, stillbirths; intrauterine growth restriction (IUGR); placental disruption; preeclampsia

ENDOCRINOLOGIC FACTORS (E.G., POLYCYSTIC OVARY SYNDROME)

POLYCYSTIC OVARY SYNDROME

Signs and symptoms: symptom onset after puberty, with increased rate of hair growth and male-pattern hair growth; irregular menstruation; infertility; obesity; acne

Investigations: LH:FSH ratio (elevated: 2:1 or 3:1) (usual); elevated testosterone; ultrasound to detect ovarian cysts; normal prolactin levels; normal thyroid function

IMMUNOLOGIC FACTORS (E.G., ANTIPHOSPHOLIPID SYNDROME)

ANTIPHOSPHOLIPID SYNDROME

This is the only immune condition where spontaneous abortion (sometimes recurrent) is a diagnostic criterion (it also features elevated antiphospholipid antibodies).

Definition: ≥ 1 fetal deaths at ≥ 10 weeks gestation; ≥ 1 preterm deliveries at ≤ 34 weeks gestation due to preeclampsia; ≥ 3 consecutive spontaneous abortions at < 10 weeks gestation

Risk factors: autoimmune condition (e.g., systemic lupus erythematosus, Sjögren syndrome); syphilis; HIV/AIDS; hepatitis C virus (HCV); Lyme disease; use of hydralazine, quinidine, phenytoin, amoxicillin; family history of antiphospholipid syndrome

Strategy for patient encounter

The likely scenario is a patient with recurrent miscarriage. The likely tasks include history, investigations, or counselling. Physical exam does not usually contribute useful information for diagnosing the cause or managing the risk of miscarriage.

History

Use open-ended questions to obtain an obstetrical history: How old are you? How many times have you been pregnant? How easy has it been for you to become pregnant? How many miscarriages have you had, and at what stage of pregnancy? How many children do you have? What complications have you had during previous pregnancies? Listen for older maternal age; difficulty in becoming pregnant (this suggests reproductive tract abnormalities or endocrine conditions); intrauterine growth restriction (IUGR) in previous pregnancies (this suggests thrombophilia); preeclampsia in previous pregnancies (this suggests thrombophilia or immunologic factors); and late loss of pregnancy (this suggests immunologic factors).

Ask about medical history and medication history: What conditions have you been diagnosed with? What medications do you take? Listen for celiac disease, polycystic ovary syndrome, systemic lupus erythematosus, Sjögren syndrome, HIV/AIDS, hepatitis C virus (HCV), Lyme disease, and syphilis; and use of hydralazine, quinidine, phenytoin, and amoxicillin.

Ask about a family history of spontaneous abortions, heritable disorders, and antiphospholipid syndrome.

Investigations

Order an antiphospholipid antibody screen and karyotype, and a hysterosalpingogram. Depending on the history, consider other investigations (e.g., for polycystic ovary syndrome).

Counselling

Provide empathy and support for the parents' grief, and check risk factors for complicated grief (current or previous depression, anxiety, or other mental health disorders; and lack of social supports). Consider referral to a psychologist for parents at risk of complicated grief. Counsel the parents that it is safe to reattempt conception as soon as they are ready physically and psychologically. In spontaneous abortions with unknown etiology, reassure the parents that no evidence supports routine activities as the cause (e.g., stress, heavy lifting, sexual intercourse, bumping the abdomen). As appropriate, consider referral for specialized care (to an obstetrician-gynecologist and/or for medical genetics).

116

Preterm labour

MCC particular objective

Identify patients who need immediate transfer to a facility with neonatal intensive care.

MCC differential diagnosis
with added evidence

FETAL (E.G., MULTIPLE GESTATION, CONGENITAL ANOMALIES)

MULTIPLE GESTATION
This is found on ultrasound.

CONGENITAL ABNORMALITIES
These are often associated with a family history of congenital abnormalities, and are generally found on amniocentesis and/or imaging.

PLACENTAL (E.G., ABRUPTION, PLACENTAL INSUFFICIENCY)

ABRUPTION

This is most likely to occur in the last trimester of pregnancy.

Signs and symptoms: sudden vaginal bleeding (mild to life-threatening), abdominal pain, back pain; uterine tenderness and/or rigidity; rapid uterine contractions (high frequency and low amplitude, or similar to labour); suspicious fetal heart rate pattern

> Laboratory findings (during routine prenatal care): increased α-fetoprotein or β-hCG; decreased pregnancy-associated plasma protein A or unconjugated estriol

Risk factors: previous placental abruption; hypertension; smoking; abdominal trauma; substance abuse; premature rupture of the membranes; blood-clotting disorders; multiple gestation; maternal age older than 40

PLACENTAL INSUFFICIENCY

This is usually associated with asymmetry where the brain is spared, but weight and length are affected.

Signs and symptoms: late pregnancy (usual); oligohydramnios; late decelerations on fetal heart rate monitor

UTERINE (E.G., CERVICAL ANOMALIES)

CERVICAL ANOMALIES

Risk factors:

> Acquired (more common): cervical trauma from previous deliveries (e.g., forceps- or vacuum-assisted); previous rapid cervical dilation for gynecological procedures (e.g., uterine evacuation); treatment for cervical intraepithelial neoplasia

> Congenital: collagen disorders (e.g., Ehlers-Danlos syndrome); uterine anomalies; maternal diethylstilbestrol (DES) exposure

Investigations: ultrasound to measure the length of the cervix; uterine monitoring; swabs of vaginal secretions (not conclusive); maturity amniocentesis

MATERNAL (E.G., SUBSTANCE ABUSE, CHRONIC ILLNESS, INFECTION)

Signs and symptoms (in general): history of substance abuse, chronic illness (e.g., diabetes), or infection

INFECTION

BACTERIAL VAGINOSIS

Signs and symptoms: sometimes asymptomatic; vulvovaginal itching; unusual or foul smelling thin gray-white vaginal discharge; burning during urination

Investigations: Gram stain; wet mount microscopy of discharge; vaginal pH > 4.5

CHLAMYDIA TRACHOMATIS

Signs and symptoms: often asymptomatic; vaginal discharge; postcoital or intermenstrual bleeding; difficult or painful urination; pelvic and abdominal pain

Investigations: NAAT; vaginal swab culture; endocervical specimen in speculum exam

URINARY TRACT INFECTION

Signs and symptoms: frequent urination; painful urination; pelvic pain and/or flank pain; fever; tenderness over the bladder

Investigations: urinalysis, urine culture

CHORIOAMNIONITIS

Signs and symptoms: maternal fever; maternal and fetal tachycardia; uterine tenderness; foul-smelling amniotic fluid

Investigations: amniocentesis with confirmation of microbial growth; histology of placenta and umbilical cord

OTHER INFECTIONS

Examples include *Ureaplasma urealyticum*, *Mycoplasma genitalium*, vaginal *Escherichia coli*, and chronic hepatitis C virus (HCV).

IATROGENIC (INDICATED INDUCTION OF LABOUR—E.G., ECLAMPSIA, INTRAUTERINE GROWTH RESTRICTION, PREMATURE RUPTURE OF MEMBRANES)

ECLAMPSIA

Signs and symptoms: blood pressure > 160/110 mmHg; thrombocytopenia; compromised renal function; pulmonary edema; hemolytic anemia; seizures

INTRAUTERINE GROWTH RESTRICTION (AS INDICATION FOR INDUCED LABOUR)

This is defined as in-utero growth below the tenth percentile for a baby's gestational age.

Factors in decision to deliver: nonreassuring fetal assessment or complete absence of growth over 2 to 4 weeks

> American College of Obstetricians and Gynecologists recommendations: 38 to 39 weeks gestation for isolated fetal growth restriction; 34 to 37 weeks gestation for fetal growth restriction with additional adverse risk factors

> Royal College of Obstetricians and Gynecologists recommendations: by 32 weeks gestation for preterm fetus with absent umbilical artery or reversed end-diastolic velocities (earlier for viable fetus with umbilical vein pulsations or abnormal ductus venosus Doppler); by

37 weeks gestation for small-growth-for-age fetus detected
after 32 weeks

Investigations:

Ultrasound: umbilical artery Doppler; amniotic fluid index;
fetal biometry

Blood tests: infection screening; elevated β-hCG in first
and second trimester; low pregnancy-associated plasma
protein A; elevated vistafin

PREMATURE RUPTURE OF MEMBRANES

Signs and symptoms: rupture of the membranes > 1 hour before the
onset of labour; gush or slow leak of amniotic fluid

Risk factors: previous preterm birth; infection in the reproductive
system; vaginal bleeding during pregnancy; smoking

Investigations: lab tests to confirm amniotic fluid; ultrasound to confirm
levels of amniotic fluid

Strategy for patient encounter

The likely scenario is a woman in preterm labour. The specified tasks could engage history, physical exam, investigations, or
management.

History

Use open-ended questions to obtain an obstetrical history: How
old are you? How many times have you been pregnant? How many
miscarriages have you had, and at what stage of pregnancy? What
complications have you had during previous pregnancies? What
complications have you had during this pregnancy? Listen for evidence of multiple gestation, congenital abnormalities, abdominal
trauma, hypertension, diabetes, infection (e.g., fever, vaginal discharge, urinary symptoms), vaginal bleeding during pregnancy,
previous placental abruption, and previous forceps- or vacu-
um-assisted deliveries. Ask the patient whether they smoke.

Pay particular attention to identifying risk factors for preterm
labour: advanced maternal age, smoking, and prior preterm deliveries.

Physical exam

Obtain the patient's vital signs, looking for fever and hypertension. Perform a speculum exam, including swabs for group B
streptococcus. Examine the abdomen and obtain a fundal height
measurement.

(State that you will perform these examinations. Speculum exams are not performed on standardized patients, and a truly pregnant standardized patient is unlikely in any case. So, the examiner will likely interrupt, ask what you are looking for, and provide findings. State that you want to establish the degree of cervical dilation, take swabs for group B streptococcus, check for abnormal abdominal findings such as uterine tenderness, and measure fundal height to estimate gestational age.)

Investigations
Order a urinalysis, looking for proteinuria, and a urine culture and sensitivity, looking for infection. Order a fetal fibronectin and assess fetal well-being (with ultrasound or fetal monitoring).

Management
Refer the patient to an appropriate facility with a neonatal intensive care unit (NICU). Administer appropriate immediate interventions (antenatal steroids, group B streptococcus prophylaxis, tocolytics). Counsel the parents on the immediate and long-term health problems of premature infants.

117

Uterine prolapse, pelvic relaxation

MCC particular objectives
None stated.

MCC differential diagnosis
with added evidence
UTERINE PROLAPSE, PELVIC RELAXATION IN GENERAL
Signs and symptoms: feeling of heaviness or pressure in the area of the vagina; feeling that the uterus, bladder, or rectum is dropping out; problems with urination (urinary incontinence, urinary retention) or

with bowel movements; pelvic organs or small intestine that drop down and protrude into the vagina (or outside the body with severe symptoms); symptoms that occur when upright, straining, or coughing; symptoms that disappear when lying down or relaxing

>   Prolapsed rectum (rectocele): difficult bowel movements and constipation (women may be unable to empty their bowels completely)

>   Prolapsed small intestine (enterocele): generally asymptomatic; feeling of fullness, pressure, or pain in the pelvis or lower back

>   Prolapsed bladder (cystocele): coincident prolapsed urethra (urethrocele) (usual); stress incontinence (e.g., passage of urine during coughing, laughing); overflow incontinence (passage of urine when bladder becomes too full); urinary retention; problems with completely voiding the bladder; urinary tract infection; urge incontinence (an intense, irrepressible urge to urinate, resulting in passage of urine)

>   Prolapsed uterus: uterus that bulges into the upper part of the vagina, or into the opening of the vagina, or partly through the opening, or all the way through the opening (total uterine prolapse); often asymptomatic; pain in the lower back or over the tailbone (total uterine prolapse can cause pain during walking, difficulty with bowel movements; sores may develop on the protruding cervix and cause bleeding, discharge, and infection; possible uterine kink may hide urinary incontinence or make urinating painful)

Risk factors: multiple pregnancies and deliveries; obesity; advanced age

DAMAGE TO VAGINA AND PELVIC FLOOR SYSTEM: VAGINAL BIRTH, PRIOR PELVIC SURGERY, CHRONIC INCREASE IN INTRAABDOMINAL PRESSURE (E.G., CHRONIC COUGH)

Risk factors: multiple pregnancies and deliveries; prolonged labour; bearing down before full dilation; forceful delivery of the placenta

NEUROGENIC DYSFUNCTION OF PELVIC FLOOR

Signs and symptoms: personal or family history of neurologic disease or related conditions; abnormalities in speech or gross motor function; sensory abnormalities of the lumbosacral dermatomes on exam for light and sharp touch (performed with a small cotton swab and a sharp point)

Risk factors: spina bifida, diabetic neuropathy

CONNECTIVE TISSUE DISEASE

Signs and symptoms: personal or family history of connective tissue disease (e.g., Ehlers-Danlos syndrome, Sjögren syndrome)

GENETIC PREDISPOSITION

Signs and symptoms: family history of pelvic prolapse

Strategy for patient encounter

The likely scenario is a postmenopausal woman with uterine prolapse. The specified tasks could engage history, physical exam, or management. Lab investigations do not usually contribute useful information for diagnosing or managing uterine prolapse or pelvic relaxation.

History

Start with open-ended inquiry about the patient's concern: Please tell me about the problem you are experiencing. Listen for evidence consistent with uterine prolapse or pelvic relaxation (e.g., problems with urination, feeling that pelvic organs are dropping out). Take an obstetrical history: How many children do you have? What was the method of delivery for each child? What was the birth weight of each child? Ask about a history of spina bifida, diabetes, and connective tissue disease, and a family history of pelvic prolapse.

Physical exam

To make abnormalities more obvious on pelvic exam, ask the patient to stand with 1 foot on a stool, and to cough or bear down.

(State that you will perform this exam. Since pelvic exams are not performed on standardized patients, the examiner will likely interrupt, ask what you are looking for, and provide findings.)

Management

Discuss the benefits and limitations of treatment options (these include pelvic floor exercises, pessary, or surgery). Refer the patient to a gynecologist or, if appropriate, for surgery.

118

Proteinuria

MCC particular objective

Recognize the importance of proteinuria as a predictor of chronic kidney disease.

MCC differential diagnosis
with added evidence

ORTHOSTATIC PROTEINURIA

This is generally found incidentally on urinalysis for another condition (as a positive urine dipstick for protein).

Signs and symptoms: asymptomatic (generally); child or adolescent (it is uncommon in adults older than 30); elevated protein excretion while in upright position (daytime proteinuria), but normal in supine or recumbent position

Investigations:

> Protein to creatinine ratio in urine samples collected in recumbent and upright positions in the daytime and nighttime; elevated ratio in upright sample (> 20 mg protein/mg creatinine in children older than 2 years; > 0.5 mg protein/mg creatinine in infants 6 to 24 months); normal ratio in recumbent sample

> Urinary protein excretion rate in daytime and nighttime collections: normal rate in daytime collection (> 4 mg/m^2 per hour for children over an 8-hour period); normal rate in nighttime collection (< 4 mg/m^2 per hour)

TUBULOINTERSTITIAL PROTEINURIA (INTERSTITIAL NEPHRITIS)

INTERSTITIAL NEPHRITIS

Signs and symptoms: fever; rash; arthralgia; use of diuretics, antibiotics, analgesics

Investigations: urine eosinophils (this is suggestive); renal biopsy (definitive)

GLOMERULAR PROTEINURIA

Active urine sediment

PRIMARY (E.G., IgA NEPHROPATHY, MEMBRANOPROLIFERATIVE GLOMERULONEPHRITIS)

IgA NEPHROPATHY

Signs and symptoms: recurrent macroscopic hematuria (brown-coloured urine) or persistent microscopic hematuria (this is found incidentally on routine exam)

Risk factors: age 20 to 40 (peak incidence); male (more common); Caucasian, Asian, Indigenous descent (highest incidence); upper respiratory tract infection; cirrhosis; liver disease; celiac disease; HIV; family history of IgA nephropathy

Investigations: kidney biopsy with immunofluorescence or immunoperoxidase studies for IgA deposits

MEMBRANOPROLIFERATIVE GLOMERULONEPHRITIS

Signs and symptoms: asymptomatic (generally); nephrotic syndrome, or recurrent gross hematuria, or hypertension; proteinuria and hematuria on routine urinalysis; normal or elevated creatinine on blood work

> Nephrotic syndrome: progressive lower extremity edema (ankles and feet); swelling around the eyes; weight gain (from water retention); foamy urine

Risk factors: child, young adult (if idiopathic); Caucasian descent; history of hepatitis B virus (HBV), hepatitis C virus (HCV), cancer, autoimmune diseases

Investigations: renal biopsy; immunofluorescence microscopy; hypocomplementemia

SECONDARY (E.G., SYSTEMIC LUPUS ERYTHEMATOSUS, POSTINFECTION)

SYSTEMIC LUPUS ERYTHEMATOSUS

Signs and symptoms: personal or family history of systemic lupus erythematosus; malar rash; arthritis; cytopenias

Investigations: elevated ANA titre; elevated dsDNA level

POSTSTREPTOCOCCAL GLOMERULONEPHRITIS

Signs and symptoms: child 5 to 12 years, or adult older than 60 (increased risk); asymptomatic (often); gross hematuria (brown or cloudy urine); proteinuria; edema; hypertension; acute kidney injury; recent skin or throat infection due to nephritogenic strains of group A ß-hemolytic streptococcus

Investigations: elevated serum creatinine; positive throat or skin culture for recent infection; decreased total complement activity in the first 2 weeks of disease (C3, CH50); elevated antibody titres for extracellular streptococcal products (positive for ASO, AHase, ASKase, anti-NAD, anti-DNase B)

Nonactive urine sediment

PRIMARY (E.G., MINIMAL CHANGE, FOCAL SEGMENTAL GLOMERULOSCLEROSIS)

MINIMAL CHANGE DISEASE

This is a major cause of nephrotic syndrome in children (mostly younger than 6) and adults (the average age of onset is 40).

Signs and symptoms: facial edema that is preceded by an upper respiratory tract infection, allergic reaction to a bee sting, use of nonsteroidal antiinflammatory drugs (NSAIDs), or cancer; malaise; fatigue; weight gain; hypovolemia; hypertension (often in adults, less commonly in children), thromboembolism, or infection; wet retina; dependent and subungual edema; muscle wasting; thinning of the skin; growth failure in children if prolonged proteinuria

Investigations: profound proteinuria (> 40 mg/h/m^2 in children; > 3.5 g/24 h/1.73 m^2 in adults); random albumin to creatinine ratio > 5; slightly elevated plasma creatinine

FOCAL SEGMENTAL GLOMERULOSCLEROSIS

Signs and symptoms: asymptomatic proteinuria (usual)

> If symptomatic: nephrotic syndrome (progressive lower extremity edema; swelling around the eyes; weight gain from water retention; foamy urine)
>
> Severe symptoms: severe hypertension; massive proteinuria; poor response to corticosteroids

Investigations: histology

SECONDARY (E.G., DIABETES, AMYLOID)

DIABETES MELLITUS

Signs and symptoms: personal or family history of diabetes; history of diabetic complications and/or inadequate monitoring; polydipsia, polyuria, and/or weight loss

> In the context of proteinuria: heavy proteinuria (protein excretion > 3.5 g in a 24-hour urine collection) with or without nephrotic syndrome

AMYLOIDOSIS

Signs and symptoms: male, older than 50 (higher incidence); asymptomatic until advanced; enlarged tongue (this causes swallowing difficulty, shortness of breath); skin symptoms (thickening; easy bruising; purpura around the eyes); numbness, tingling, pain in the extremities; diarrhea or constipation; feeling full quickly on eating, with weight loss; variable additional symptoms depending on the organ or system affected

> Renal amyloidosis: nephrotic syndrome, heavy proteinuria
>
> Cardiac amyloidosis: shortness of breath; cardiac arrhythmia; diastolic and systolic heart failure symptoms (edema of the ankles and feet; fatigue; weakness; nausea)

Liver amyloidosis: enlarged liver; elevated serum alanine aminotransferase (ALT); elevated alkaline phosphatase (ALP)

Gastrointestinal amyloidosis: decreased appetite; diarrhea; nausea; abdominal pain; weight loss

Investigations: detection of monoclonal paraprotein in serum or urine (primary amyloidosis)

Strategy for patient encounter

The likely scenario is a diabetic patient with proteinuria. The specified tasks could engage history, physical exam, investigations, or management.

In this clinical presentation, the diagnosis of proteinuria has already been made—a diagnosis based largely on lab tests and subsequent ancillary testing. The key to this patient encounter is to focus on the patient's risk of chronic kidney disease.

History

Ask about a personal or family history of kidney problems, and conditions associated with kidney problems (diabetes, hypertension).

Physical exam

Obtain the patient's vital signs, looking for hypertension. Except for this, physical exam will not likely contribute useful information.

Investigations

For all patients, obtain a qualitative measure of the proteinuria (albumin:creatinine ratio, random or 24-hour collection). If the diagnosis is still in doubt, order tests for underlying causes (blood glucose for diabetes; serum protein electrophoresis for amyloidosis and multiple myeloma).

Management

The goals of management are to treat any underlying causes (hypertension and diabetes). Consider treatment with an ACE inhibitor.

119

Pruritus

MCC particular objectives

Differentiate excoriations due to scratching from skin lesions.

Identify skin lesions, if present.

If no skin lesions are present, identify the underlying cause of pruritus.

MCC differential diagnosis
with added evidence

SKIN LESIONS

Primary skin disease

BLISTERS (E.G., DERMATITIS HERPETIFORMIS)
DERMATITIS HERPETIFORMIS

Signs and symptoms: rash (bumps, blisters) that is extremely itchy and bilaterally symmetrical; located on the elbows, knees, back, buttocks (common); sensitivity to gluten

Investigations: skin biopsy; tTG antibodies (to rule out celiac disease)

RASH (E.G., PSORIASIS, LICHEN PLANUS)
PSORIASIS (GUTTATE PSORIASIS)

Note that chronic plaque psoriasis is another form of psoriasis, but it is usually not itchy.

Signs and symptoms: numerous, small pink papules and plaques 2–15 mm in diameter with fine overlying scale; an upper respiratory tract infection 2 to 3 weeks before the appearance of symptoms; located on the trunk and proximal extremities, or on the scalp, hands, feet, nails

LICHEN PLANUS

This is a common, chronic inflammatory condition of the skin (common locations: inner wrists, forearms, lower legs, lower back) and/or mucous membranes (locations: mouth, vagina).

Signs and symptoms (skin): acute lesions that are planar, purple, polygonal, pruritic, papules (mnemonic 5 Ps); lesion diameter of 2–4 mm; Wickham striae on lesions (lacy white lines, particularly visible on mucous membranes) (often)

Investigations: biopsy

Parasitosis (e.g., scabies, pediculosis)

SCABIES

Signs and symptoms: thin, grayish, reddish-brownish threadlike elevated lines in the superficial epidermis, 2–15 mm long (from female mites burrowing under the skin)

> Location in adults: sides of fingers and webbed spaces between fingers; inside surfaces of the wrists, elbows; armpits; belt line; feet; scrotum; areolae (women); **not** the head
>
> Location in children: the palms, soles, head
>
> Location in the elderly: the back (appearing as excoriations)

PEDICULOSIS

Finding nits and lice confirms the diagnosis.

Signs and symptoms: itchy skin with excoriations

> Head lice: on the scalp; persistent pyoderma around the neck or ears
>
> Body lice: on the shoulders, buttocks, abdomen; small red spiky spots; excoriations on the trunk and neck; urticaria; superficial bacterial infection
>
> Pubic lice: on the lower abdomen, proximal thighs, buttocks

Allergy (e.g., eczema, allergic dermatitis, urticaria)

ECZEMA (ATOPIC DERMATITIS)

Signs and symptoms: chronic symptoms that flare and subside; onset before 5 years (usual); scaly, itchy rash; family or personal history of asthma, allergies

> Location (most common): hands; feet; ankles; wrists; neck; upper chest; eyelids; inside the elbows and knees; face, scalp (infants)

ALLERGIC DERMATITIS

This is a type of contact dermatitis. Examples of allergens include nickel (e.g., jewellery), hair dye, topical antibiotics, and perfumes.

Signs and symptoms: red, sore, or inflamed skin; severely itchy; history of direct contact of symptomatic skin with a substance (no reaction occurs on first exposure; reaction occurs 24 to 48 hours after subsequent exposures, but may occur after months of exposure); personal or family history of allergies or specific allergic reactions

Investigations: patch testing to detect allergens

URTICARIA (HIVES)

Common causes include infections (viral, bacterial, parasitic), allergic reactions (medications, insect bites, latex, foods), and contact with radio-contrast agents.

Signs and symptoms: rash that is itchy, painless; lesions that are circumscribed, raised (round, oval, or with wavy margins; < 1 cm to several cm in diameter); plaques with central pallor; located anywhere on the body

Duration: < 6 weeks (acute); > 6 weeks, recurrent (chronic)

Investigations: allergy tests for specifically suspected allergens (otherwise, lab tests are not helpful)

Arthropod bites

Signs and symptoms: red, sore bump at the site of a bite; mild pain and itching; swelling, burning, numbness, or tingling

Risk for complications: personal or family history of allergies; type of arthropod

Factitious dermatitis

Signs and symptoms: red bumps, blisters, or dry, cracked lesions; located on the face, lower extremities, hands, forearms, torso (common)

History: low health-related quality of life; perception of skin condition; possible psychosocial stressor; substance abuse; psychiatric disorder (e.g., somatic symptom disorder)

Investigations: skin biopsy to rule out underlying pathologies

NO SKIN LESIONS

Dry skin

Signs and symptoms: older age; frequent washing or bathing

Drugs or food

MEDICATIONS AND DRUGS

Causes include opiates, with intrathecal or epidural administration, and anticancer agents (EGF inhibitors, tyrosine kinase inhibitors, BRAF inhibitors, MEK inhibitors).

Recreational drugs: opioids, cocaine, amphetamines

Signs and symptoms: itch without skin manifestations (skin lesions from scratching and rubbing are present: lichenified plaques, excoriations, prurigo nodules)

FOOD (ALLERGY)

Signs and symptoms: personal or family history of allergies

Obstructive biliary disease

Causes of blocked bile ducts include cysts or tumours; inflammation or scarring within the bile ducts; and gallstones.

Signs and symptoms: history of liver disease, gallstones; itching that affects the whole body; normal-looking skin, except for excoriations; abdominal pain; nausea; pale stools; dark urine; jaundice; fever

Investigations: increased bilirubin and liver enzymes (these can indicate biliary distress); imaging to detect blocked bile ducts

Uremia or kidney injury

UREMIC PRURITUS

Pruritus is common in patients with end-stage renal disease.

Signs and symptoms: itching whose duration ranges from a few minutes per day to continuous; xerosis

> Worse: at night (leading to sleep disruption); in hot temperatures; when sweating excessively; during stress

> Better: in cool temperatures; with physical activity

> Location: first, the back; then, the arms, head, abdomen (common)

Investigations: blood tests (GFR, blood urea nitrogen, creatinine, potassium, phosphate, calcium, sodium); 24-hour urine collection; nuclear medicine radioisotope (iothalamate) clearance (this is the best test, but it is expensive), or modification of diet in renal disease (MDRD), or Cockcroft-Gault formula

Hematological (anemia, leukemia)

ANEMIA

Signs and symptoms: itch with dry or rough skin (no skin lesions); fatigue; weakness; headache; irritability; exercise intolerance

LEUKEMIA

Signs and symptoms: fever; chills; persistent fatigue and weakness; frequent or severe infections; weight loss; pallor; swollen lymph nodes; enlarged liver or spleen; easy bleeding and bruising; recurrent nosebleeds; petechiae; excessive sweating; bone pain or tenderness

Investigations: CBC; peripheral blood smear; flow cytometry; bone marrow aspiration and biopsy

Carcinoma or carcinoid syndrome

Carcinoid tumour most commonly occurs in the gastrointestinal tract or lungs and is generally discovered incidentally.

Carcinoid syndrome results from secretions into the blood by advanced tumours.

Signs and symptoms (carcinoid syndrome): skin flushing on the face and upper chest; facial lesions; diarrhea; breathing difficulty; rapid heart rate

Investigations: blood and urine tests to detect specific molecules such as serotonin and 5-HIAA respectively; CT scan or MRI of chest or abdomen

Endocrine disorder (diabetes, thyroid disease)

DIABETES

Pruritus occurs in diabetic patients with associated disorders; otherwise, itching does not occur at a higher rate in diabetic patients.

Examples of causes include dermatophyte infections; xerosis; pruritus in the lower extremities, scalp, or trunk due to diabetic neuropathy; anogenital pruritus due to *Candida* infections; and pruritus vulvae due to poorly controlled diabetes.

THYROID DISEASE

HYPERTHYROIDISM

Signs and symptoms: changes in menstrual patterns, enlarged thyroid, tachycardia, palpitations, diarrhea, muscle weakness, tremor, hyperactive reflexes, weight loss, sweating

> Skin: itching; warm skin; sweating; onycholysis and softening of the nails; hyperpigmentation; hair loss

Investigations: decreased thyrotropin (TSH)

HYPOTHYROIDISM

Signs and symptoms: cold intolerance, decreased reflexes, weight gain, impaired cognition

> Skin: dry, itchy, pale skin; decreased sweating; skin discolouration (yellowish tinge or hyperpigmentation); coarse hair; brittle nails; hair loss; nonpitting edema

Investigations: elevated thyrotropin (TSH)

PSYCHIATRIC OR EMOTIONAL DISORDERS

In psychogenic excoriation, patients excessively pick and scratch normal skin.

Signs and symptoms: personal or family history of mental health disorders; recent psychological stress (e.g., death of a friend or family member; divorce; job loss); scattered, linear, crusted skin lesions on the extremities or anywhere the patient can reach to scratch

Strategy for patient encounter

The likely scenario is a patient with generalized pruritus. The likely tasks are history, physical exam, or investigations.

History

Use open-ended questions to obtain a history of the pruritus, a general medical history, and an occupational history: When did the itching start? What other symptoms have you noticed? What conditions have you been diagnosed with? What do you do for a living? Listen for acute versus slow or recurrent onset (acute onset suggests acute stress or an exposure as a cause); evidence about the presence and location of skin lesions (this information focuses the differential diagnosis considerably); celiac disease, liver disease, kidney disease, anemia, leukemia, cancer, diabetes, thyroid disease, and psychiatric disorders; and occupations with relevant exposure risks (e.g., day care worker and lice).

Ask about medications and over-the-counter drugs.

Physical exam

The main purpose of the physical exam is to determine the character and distribution of any skin lesions, and to differentiate pruritus associated with skin lesions from that without skin lesions. Since rashes are difficult to reliably show on simulated patients, expect pruritus without skin lesions.

Investigations

If the patient has no skin lesions, order investigations to diagnose systemic disorders (see the information this resource lists for the entities without skin lesions in the MCC differential diagnosis).

120

Psychosis

MCC particular objective

In acute psychosis, differentiate a primary psychotic disorder from delirium, psychosis due to a medical condition, and substance-induced psychosis.

MCC differential diagnosis
with added evidence

PSYCHOTIC DISORDERS (E.G., SCHIZOPHRENIA, SCHIZOAFFECTIVE DISORDER)

SCHIZOPHRENIA[1(p99)]

Schizophrenia is the most common primary disorder associated with psychosis.

Signs and symptoms: presence of active symptoms for ≥ 1 month, and continuous presence of symptoms (active, and prodromal and/or residual) for ≥ 6 months

> Key symptoms: delusions, hallucinations, and/or disorganized speech

> Other symptoms: disorganized or catatonic behaviour; negative symptoms (e.g., reduced emotional response)

SCHIZOAFFECTIVE DISORDER[1(p105)]

Signs and symptoms: manic or major depressive episode that occurs at the same time as delusions, hallucinations, and/or disorganized speech; presence of delusions or hallucinations for ≥ 2 weeks over the total duration of the illness, during times when a manic or major depressive episode is not present

MANIC EPISODE[1(pp123–134)]

Signs and symptoms: symptoms that are present most of the time for ≥ 1 week; symptoms with significant impact on day-to-day life, and that may pose a risk of harm to self and others

> Key symptoms: abnormally elevated (and/or irritable) mood, and goal-directed activity

> Other symptoms: increased self-importance, increased talking, racing thoughts, decreased need for sleep, risky pursuits (e.g., that could damage finances or relationships), psychosis (e.g., delusions, hallucinations)

MAJOR DEPRESSIVE EPISODE[1(pp123–134)]

Signs and symptoms: symptoms that are present most of the time for ≥ 2 weeks; symptoms with significant impact on day-to-day life

> Key symptoms: depressed mood and/or loss of interest in usual activities

> Other symptoms: significant weight change; sleep disturbance; slowed or agitated mental processes; loss of concentration; recurrent thoughts of death or suicide

PSYCHOTIC DISORDER DUE TO A MEDICAL CONDITION (E.G., SEIZURE DISORDERS, CENTRAL NERVOUS SYSTEM TUMOURS)

SEIZURE DISORDERS

Signs and symptoms: history of seizures; behavioural or other abnormalities; history of complications during gestation (e.g., toxin exposure such as alcohol) and/or delivery; neurologic abnormalities; growth abnormalities; dysmorphic features; hypothyroidism; exposure to lead

CENTRAL NERVOUS SYSTEM TUMOUR

Signs and symptoms: headache that gets worse over time (common symptom: 50% of cases); vision impairment; balance problems; personality or behaviour changes; seizures; drowsiness

Risk factors: exposure to radiation (e.g., to treat leukemia in childhood); family history (rare); neurofibromatosis type 1 or type 2; tuberous sclerosis; Von Hippel-Lindau disease; Li-Fraumeni syndrome; immune system disorders

SUBSTANCE-INDUCED PSYCHOTIC DISORDER (E.G., CORTICOSTEROIDS, COCAINE)

CORTICOSTEROIDS

These are used to treat inflammatory diseases (e.g., rheumatologic diseases).

Psychiatric symptoms occur in 1 out of every 2 to 3 patients. They typically develop 3 to 4 days after beginning therapy. Symptoms with features of hypomania, mania, and psychosis are the most common.

ABUSE OF COCAINE OR AMPHETAMINE

Signs and symptoms: persecutory delusions (typical); visual, auditory, tactile hallucinations; physical evidence of drug abuse such as nasal septum perforation (from long-term cocaine use), track marks on the arms

ALCOHOL WITHDRAWAL

This is the most common cause of substance-induced psychosis.

Symptoms: agitation; irritability; confusion; delirium; fatigue; restlessness; body tremors; sensitivity to light, sound, or touch; seizures; hallucinations

Strategy for patient encounter

The likely scenario is a patient with psychotic ideation. The likely tasks are history, risk assessment, or management.

History

The first task of the history is to differentiate primary psychotic disorder from delirium and other causes of psychotic disorder (medical conditions, substances). Obtain collateral information (e.g., from an accompanying caregiver), if possible. Start with open-ended questions about the patient's medical history and medication history: What conditions have you been diagnosed with? What medications do you take? Listen for a history of psychotic disorders, seizure disorder, and inflammatory diseases; use of corticosteroids; and evidence consistent with delirium (e.g., sudden-onset changes in level of consciousness following recent surgery or substance withdrawal). Ask about symptoms of central nervous system tumour (headaches; vision impairment; balance problems; personality or behaviour changes; seizures;

drowsiness). Ask about use of cocaine, amphetamines, and alcohol.

Risk assessment

Perform a mental status exam to assess the patient's capacity, and to identify risk factors for self-harm or harming others (see the quick reference).

Management

Ensure the immediate safety of the patient and others.

A patient with specific and immediate plans for suicide or homicide requires admission to hospital for psychiatric assessment and monitoring. If a patient at risk of committing suicide or homicide refuses admission, consider involuntary admission. The regulations for involuntary admission vary by jurisdiction, but generally require a written order by 2 physicians.

If the patient is not at immediate risk, refer the patient to psychiatry. Provide antipsychotic pharmacotherapy for the patient's acute symptoms and for maintenance therapy. Treat any underlying comorbidity. Ensure the patient has monitoring and regular follow-up to assess their capacity and possible need for a substitute decision maker. Involve the patient's family members, or friends, as appropriate, and consider referring the patient, and family and friends, for counselling about psychosis and support.

QUICK REFERENCE
Mental status exams (MSEs)

The MCC recommends an MSE in this case.

Many versions of mental status exams exist. It's good general preparation for the exam to research MSEs, and choose or prepare a version for your own use (this is not the only clinical presentation that calls for an MSE). Your MSE could contain a series of ready-made descriptors that you check off, or it could be a framework for taking notes.

Note that MSEs use both observation and direct questioning to make assessments.

Generally, they assess:
- general appearance and behaviour
- mood
- speech: rate, tone, volume
- thought content: obsessions, preoccupations, hallucinations, delusions, suicidal ideation, homicidal ideation
- thought process: circumstantial, tangential, flight of ideas, loosening of associations
- orientation to time and place
- attention and concentration
- patient insight into their present condition

REFERENCE

1 American Psychiatric Association. Diagnostic and statistical manual of mental disorders. 5th ed. Arlington, VA: American Psychiatric Association; 2013. 991 p.

121

Acute kidney injury (anuria or oliguria)

MCC particular objective
Recognize when urgent intervention is required.

MCC differential diagnosis
with added evidence

ACUTE KIDNEY INJURY IN GENERAL
Definition: rising serum creatinine over a short period of time

Investigations: increase in serum creatinine by ≥ 26 μmol within 48 hours, or ≥ 1.5 times baseline; or urine volume < 0.5 mL/kg/hour for 6 hours

PRERENAL CAUSE

PRERENAL CAUSE IN GENERAL
Signs and symptoms: thirst; reduced fluid intake; blood or fluid loss (from vomiting, diarrhea, bleeding, severe burns)

Renal hypoperfusion (e.g., hepatorenal syndrome, ACE inhibitor with bilateral renal artery stenosis)

RENAL HYPOPERFUSION IN GENERAL
Predisposing conditions for localized renal hypoperfusion include renal artery obstruction due to expanding abdominal aortic aneurysm; hypercalcemia; renal artery stenosis or occlusion; and use of medications including nonsteroidal antiinflammatory drugs (NSAIDs), COX-2 inhibitors, angiotensin II receptor blockers, norepinephrine, radio-contrast agents, amphotericin B, and calcineurin inhibitors. **ACE inhibitors are contraindicated for patients with bilateral renal artery stenosis.**

HEPATORENAL SYNDROME
Signs and symptoms: renal dysfunction (progressive or rapid) in the context of cirrhosis with ascites; arterial hypotension; circulatory dysfunction; signs of liver disease (jaundice, edema, ascites); history of bacterial peritonitis, cirrhosis, hepatitis, alcohol use

Investigations: BUN:creatinine ratio > 20:1; blood tests (electrolytes, WBCs, CRP, culture); urine tests (proteinuria, microhematuria, sodium, osmolality, culture)

Systemic hypoperfusion (e.g., shock, hypovolemia)

CIRCULATORY SHOCK

Signs and symptoms: persistent hypotension; tachycardia; acute ischemia; heart failure; chest trauma; cold cyanotic extremities; poor organ perfusion; history of heart failure, coronary artery disease, infarction, angina

Investigations: blood tests (cardiac troponin; ABG; lactate)

HYPOVOLEMIA

Signs and symptoms: weakness; lethargy; change in thirst or drinking pattern; dry mucous membranes; sunken eyes; slow capillary refill; hypotension; resting tachycardia; orthostatic changes

> History of acute or chronic illness (gastrointestinal illness, cirrhosis, nephrotic syndrome, heart failure, prolonged fever, difficulty swallowing, blood loss); use of diuretics, laxatives, antidiuretic hormone (ADH) antagonists, lithium, narcotics, alcohol; medical procedures including surgery, nasogastric suction, enemas, tube feeding

Investigations: ECG; chest X-ray; BUN:creatinine ratio > 20:1; decreased urinary sodium (unless on diuretics); blood tests (electrolytes, osmolality, glucose, calcium); nonactive urine sediment

RENAL CAUSE

RENAL CAUSE IN GENERAL

Signs and symptoms: fatigue; weight loss; fever; muscle and joint pain; cough with blood

Tubulointerstitial condition (e.g., acute tubular necrosis, interstitial nephritis)

ACUTE TUBULAR NECROSIS

Causes include ischemic injury (e.g., prolonged kidney hypoperfusion) and toxic injury (e.g., from calcineurin inhibitors, radio-contrast agents, or antibiotics such as aminoglycoside and amphotericin B).

Investigations: BUN:creatinine ratio 10:1–20:1; signs of tubular necrosis (urinary sediment with muddy brown casts, renal tubular epithelial cells, granular casts); urine osmolality < 350–400 mmol/kg; urine sodium > 40 mmol/L; blood electrolytes

ACUTE INTERSTITIAL NEPHRITIS

Signs and symptoms: fever; rash; arthralgia; use of diuretics, antibiotics, analgesics (usual); history of autoimmune disorders

Investigations: urine eosinophils (their presence is suggestive); urinalysis (normal findings for RBCs, proteinuria, and red cell casts); blood tests (normal creatinine; normal complement level); renal biopsy (definitive)

Glomerular condition (e.g., glomerulonephritis, thrombotic thrombocytopenic purpura, or hemolytic uremic syndrome)

INFECTION-RELATED GLOMERULONEPHRITIS AND MEMBRANOPROLIFERATIVE GLOMERULONEPHRITIS

The common cause for infections is *Streptococcus* in the upper respiratory tract or skin. Contributing factors include alpha-interferon treatment, hepatitis B virus (HBV), hepatitis C virus (HCV), HIV, and hematologic abnormalities.

Signs and symptoms: hypertension; edema, oliguria, or anuria (infection related); frothy urine; gross hematuria

THROMBOTIC THROMBOCYTOPENIC PURPURA

Signs and symptoms: neurologic symptoms (headache, seizures, coma, sensory-motor deficits, transient ischemic attacks); skin symptoms (purpura, jaundice, pallor); use of associated medications (quinine, ticlopidine, mitomycin C, cyclosporine A); microangiopathic hemolytic anemia; thrombocytopenia; decreased ADAMTS13 activity

HEMOLYTIC UREMIC SYNDROME

This commonly follows infection from Shiga toxin–producing *Escherichia coli.*

Signs and symptoms: gastrointestinal symptoms (abdominal pain, bloody diarrhea); anemia (fatigue, weakness, pallor); neurologic symptoms (irritability, confusion, seizures); peripheral edema (this is a sign of renal failure); thrombocytopenia

Investigations: blood tests (BUN, creatinine, electrolytes, peripheral smear); urinalysis (to detect proteinuria and RBCs); elevated PT/INR

POSTRENAL CAUSE OR OBSTRUCTION (E.G., PROSTATIC HYPERTROPHY, CERVICAL CANCER, CALCULI)

POSTRENAL CAUSE OR OBSTRUCTION IN GENERAL

Predisposing conditions for ureteral or urethral obstruction include nephrolithiasis; benign prostatic hyperplasia or hypertrophy; and prostate or cervical cancer.

Signs and symptoms: palpable bladder, enlarged prostate (prostatic hypertrophy), pelvic mass (cervical cancer), history of kidney stones

Investigations: renal ultrasound to detect obstruction; noncontrast CT scan to see calculi; PSA or Pap test for prostate or cervical conditions

Strategy for patient encounter

The likely scenario is a patient with new-onset renal failure. The specified tasks could engage history, physical exam, investigations, or management.

History

Begin the history with questions that target prerenal, renal, and postrenal causes. This will help structure the interview and narrow the possible diagnosis.

- **Prerenal causes:** Ask about increased thirst, and recent sources of fluid loss (e.g., vomiting, diarrhea, bleeding, severe burns). Ask about a history of bilateral renal artery stenosis.
- **Renal causes:** Ask about a pattern of fatigue, weight loss, and fever.
- **Postrenal causes:** Ask about a history of kidney stones, prostate trouble, and cervical cancer.

Next, use open-ended inquiry to establish the patient's related symptoms and medical history: What other symptoms do you have? What conditions have you been diagnosed with? Listen for evidence consistent with the likely cause (e.g., cyanosis and heart disease, or jaundice and liver disease, in prerenal causes; rash and autoimmune disorders, or hematuria and *Streptococcus* infection, or neurologic symptoms and *Escherichia coli*, in renal causes).

Finally, take a medication history. Listen for medications relevant to the likely cause (e.g., ACE inhibitors in the context of bilateral renal artery stenosis in prerenal causes; calcineurin inhibitors and antibiotics in renal causes).

Physical exam

Obtain the patient's vital signs, looking for shock and hypovolemia. Examine the abdomen looking for masses and a palpable bladder.

Investigations

Order a urinalysis and urine sediment analysis, and tests for serum creatinine, urine electrolytes, and serum electrolytes. Order a renal ultrasound and CT scan to assess for renal or bladder obstruction.

Management

Assess the need for urgent intervention, which could include dialysis, fluid resuscitation, or urinary catheterization. Institute dialysis in patients with a glomerular filtration rate (GFR) < 15 mL/minute, and with 1 or more of the following: symptoms or signs of uremia (progressive fatigue; anorexia; nausea, vomiting; muscle atrophy; tremors; mental function changes; shallow breathing; metabolic acidosis); inability to control hydration status or blood pressure; and inability to maintain nutritional status. Refer the patient to a nephrologist.

122

Chronic kidney injury

MCC particular objectives
None stated.

MCC differential diagnosis
with added evidence

PRERENAL CAUSES (E.G., BLOOD PRESSURE)

HYPERTENSION
Signs and symptoms: systolic blood pressure $\geq$ 140 mmHg and/or diastolic blood pressure $\geq$ 90 mmHg

> History of renal conditions, diabetes, adrenal or thyroid conditions, vascular conditions, catecholamine excess, obstructive sleep apnea, family history of hypertension

Risk factors: lack of exercise; high-sodium diet; obesity

RENAL CAUSE

Glomerular condition (e.g., IgA nephropathy, diabetic nephropathy)

GLOMERULAR CONDITION IN GENERAL
Signs and symptoms: hematuria (gross or microscopic, often following a urinary tract infection); proteinuria; dysmorphic red blood cells (RBCs) in urine

IGA NEPHROPATHY
Signs and symptoms: often asymptomatic; low-grade fever; loin pain; hypertension; edema
Investigations: renal biopsy

DIABETIC NEPHROPATHY

Signs and symptoms: usually asymptomatic; hypertension; edema

Investigations: elevated albumin to creatinine ratio in urine (i.e., albuminuria)

Tubulointerstitial condition (e.g., drug toxicity)

DRUG TOXICITY

ANALGESIC NEPHROPATHY

There is conflicting evidence on the risk of chronic kidney disease from analgesic use (nonsteroidal antiinflammatory drugs, aspirin, lithium).

Signs and symptoms: headache; anemia (fatigue, pallor, dizziness, shortness of breath, tachycardia); hypertension; pyuria; proteinuria; possible renal papillary necrosis and chronic interstitial nephritis (on CT scan) due to capillary sclerosis

DECREASED GLOMERULAR FILTRATION RATE

Chemotherapy can cause kidney disease. Examples of chemotherapeutic drugs include cisplatin, ifosfamide, methoxyamine, pemetrexed, and bisphosphonates.

Signs and symptoms: features of uremia (progressive fatigue; anorexia; nausea, vomiting; muscle atrophy; tremors; mental function changes; shallow breathing; metabolic acidosis)

Investigations: GFR < 60 mL/min; BUN; creatinine; elevated cystatin C; proteinuria; albuminuria; urine sediment abnormalities

OTHER

Kidney injury (acute or chronic) can be caused by use of ACE inhibitors, angiotensin receptor blockers, diuretics, and nonsteroidal antiinflammatory drugs (NSAIDs) in combination (the first 3 drugs are often used in combination to treat hypertension and heart failure); antimicrobials including aminoglycosides, sulfa-based antibiotics, vancomycin, ciprofloxacin; and herbal supplements.

Ischemic condition

RENAL ARTERY STENOSIS

The common cause is atherosclerosis.

Signs and symptoms: usually asymptomatic; sudden-onset hypertension; bruits from arteries in the kidneys on auscultation

Risk factors: older than 55; hypertension; hyperlipidemia; diabetes; obesity; family history of heart disease; smoking; lack of exercise

Investigations: blood tests (GFR, BUN, electrolytes); urinalysis (protein, blood, pH); renal ultrasound with Doppler

Congenital condition (e.g., dysplasia, polycystic kidney disease)

MULTICYSTIC DYSPLASTIC KIDNEY

This is usually detected on prenatal ultrasound.

Signs and symptoms: palpable mass in abdomen

AUTOSOMAL DOMINANT POLYCYSTIC KIDNEY DISEASE

This is the most common inherited cause of kidney disease.

It may not be detected in patients younger than 30.

Signs and symptoms: family history of polycystic kidney disease; hypertension with pain (abdomen, flank, lower back); hematuria; urinary tract infections (UTIs)

Investigations: renal ultrasound; genetic testing; serum creatinine and GFR to assess disease; urine tests (hematuria, micro or gross; culture to detect UTI or cyst infection)

AUTOSOMAL RECESSIVE POLYCYSTIC KIDNEY DISEASE

This is usually detected on prenatal ultrasound.

Signs and symptoms: enlarged kidney (neonates, infants); bilateral flank or abdominal masses; tachypnea; grunting, respiratory distress; impaired renal function

POSTRENAL CAUSE (E.G., OBSTRUCTIVE UROPATHY)

OBSTRUCTIVE UROPATHY

Signs and symptoms: flank pain; fever; nausea, vomiting; weight gain; edema; frequent urge to urinate; difficulty voiding or abnormal urine stream; reduced urine volume; hematuria

Investigations: ultrasound or CT scan of the pelvis, abdomen; intravenous pyelogram; voiding cystourethrogram; renal nuclear scan

Strategy for patient encounter

The likely scenario is a diabetic patient with long-standing elevated creatinine. The specified tasks could engage history, physical exam, investigations, or management.

The differential diagnosis for this clinical presentation is large and complex. Keep in mind that the most common conditions associated with chronic kidney injury are diabetes and hypertension.

History

Use open-ended questions to establish the patient's medical history and symptoms: What conditions have you been diagnosed with? What medications do you take? How has your health been lately? Listen for a history of diabetes, hypertension, kidney disease, or heart disease; drugs such as chemotherapeutic drugs, analgesics, ACE inhibitors, and antimicrobials; urinary problems (e.g., urinary tract infections, hematuria); and symptoms of uremia (e.g., progressive fatigue; tremors; mental function changes). Ask about a family history of kidney problems.

Physical exam

Obtain the patient's vital signs, looking for hypertension and fever (fever suggests IgA nephropathy or obstructive uropathy). Examine the abdomen for masses.

Investigations

Order blood work for creatinine, electrolytes, and glucose. Order a urinalysis and a serum protein electrophoresis. Some causes will require a kidney biopsy for diagnosis.

Management

Manage immediately life-threatening metabolic abnormalities (fluids, electrolytes, acidosis). Institute immediate measures to prevent further loss of renal function (blood pressure control, steroids for autoimmune disorders). Refer the patient to a nephrologist.

Institute dialysis in patients with a glomerular filtration rate (GFR) < 15 mL/minute, and with 1 or more of the following: symptoms or signs of uremia; inability to control hydration status or blood pressure; and inability to maintain nutritional status.

123

Scrotal mass

MCC particular objective

Differentiate malignant testicular tumours from other types of scrotal masses.

MCC differential diagnosis
with added evidence

CYSTIC MASS (E.G., HYDROCELE)

HYDROCELE

Causes include injury or infection (filariasis from *Wuchereria bancrofti* infection) of the scrotum. (In infants, the cause is an unsealed opening between the abdomen and the scrotum, which resolves by age 1 year.)

Signs and symptoms: painless (often) swelling of the scrotum; scrotal pain or discomfort; heavy or full feeling of the scrotum; swelling and irritation of the skin around the scrotum

Investigations: light test to detect solid masses in the sac; or ultrasound to detect fluid collection surrounding the testis, which are avascular on Doppler

SOLID MASS

Benign (e.g., hematoma)

HEMATOMA

This is common after a vasectomy or other trauma. It usually resolves on its own within 4 to 8 weeks.

Signs and symptoms: asymptomatic (small hematoma); scrotal swelling, bruising, pain (large hematoma)

Investigations: lack of colour on Doppler flow ultrasound, isoechoic/hyperechoic region in the affected testicle

Malignant (e.g., seminoma)

SEMINOMA

This is a testicular germ cell tumour that is treatable and curable if discovered in early stages.

It is the most common malignancy in males age 15 to 35.

Signs and symptoms: Caucasian descent (more common); painless testicular mass (noticeable from days to months)

Investigations: abnormal semen findings (possible subfertility); scrotal ultrasound (homogenous intratesticular mass; lower echogenicity than normal testicle; well-defined, oval, without invasion; usually confined to tunica albuginea); AFP level (if elevated, it is not seminoma)

Inflammatory or infectious (e.g., orchitis, scrotal abscess)

ORCHITIS

The common cause is mumps (more common in children).

Signs and symptoms: acute symptoms that resolve in 3 to 10 days (usual); enlarged, firm, tender testis; enlarged epididymis; red scrotal skin; prostatitis; fever; chills; nausea; headache; fatigue; myalgias

SCROTAL ABSCESS

For superficial abscesses, common causes include infected hair follicles, infections of scrotal lacerations, and minor scrotal surgeries (confined to scrotal wall).

For intrascrotal abscesses, common causes include bacterial epididymitis and tuberculous infection in the epididymis.

Signs and symptoms (superficial, intrascrotal): penile discharge; frequent urination and urge to urinate; difficult or painful urination; red, swollen, tender scrotum

Strategy for patient encounter

The likely scenario is a young man with a scrotal mass. The specified tasks could engage history, physical exam, investigations, or management.

The differential diagnosis for scrotal masses is fairly small. Pay particular attention to the instructions for the patient encounter: these may provide details that point to a likely diagnosis. See also the clinical presentation on scrotal pain for other diagnostic possibilities.

History

Start with open-ended questions: When did you find the mass? How did you find the mass? What have you noticed about the mass? Listen for details consistent with malignancy (slow onset, no pain, no fever). Ask about recent scrotal trauma or surgery. Ask about risk factors for infection (prolonged travel in the tropics, which is relevant for lymphatic filariasis; lapsed immunizations, which is relevant for mumps; exposure to tuberculosis).

Physical exam

Obtain the patient's vital signs, looking for fever. Examine the scrotum and look for enlargement of the inguinal lymph nodes.

(State that you will perform a scrotal exam. Since this is not done on standardized patients, the examiner will likely interrupt, ask what you are looking for, and provide findings. State that you are looking for masses, tenderness, swelling, and redness.)

Investigations

For all patients, order a scrotal ultrasound (with Doppler to assess blood flow) and/or a CT scan.

Management

Consider referral to a urologist.

Pearls

Varicoceles are usually unilateral (sometimes bilateral) and, if unilateral, are almost always on the left side. Unilateral right-side varicoceles are rare and may indicate a retroperitoneal mass.

124

Scrotal pain

MCC particular objective

Sudden-onset pain requires emergent investigation for testicular torsion.

MCC differential diagnosis
with added evidence

TESTICULAR TORSION

This is common in boys age 12 to 16 years (but it can occur at any age, including neonates).

Testicular torsion requires emergency surgery to save the testicle and preserve future fertility. Surgery within 6 hours of pain onset has a high success rate (up to 100%); surgery after 12 hours has a ≤ 50% success rate.

Signs and symptoms: sudden severe pain with swelling in the scrotum; a testicle that is higher than normal or at an abnormal angle; swollen, tender, firm, erythematous testicle; nausea, vomiting

Investigations: scrotal ultrasound

INFLAMMATION (E.G., ACUTE EPIDIDYMITIS, ORCHITIS, TRAUMA)

ACUTE EPIDIDYMITIS

This is the most common cause of scrotal pain in adults.

It is most commonly due to sexually transmitted infection (chlamydia, gonorrhea) in men younger than 35.

Signs and symptoms: symptoms that last < 6 weeks (acute condition); testicular swelling, pain, tenderness, firmness

ORCHITIS

The common cause is mumps (more common in children).

Signs and symptoms: acute symptoms that resolve in 3 to 10 days (usual); enlarged, firm, tender testis; enlarged epididymis; red scrotal skin; prostatitis; fever; chills; nausea; headache; fatigue; myalgia

TRAUMA

Examples of trauma include scrotal avulsion; blunt and penetrating trauma; and injury to scrotal contents. Causes include animal attacks, car accidents, self-mutilation, assaults, and machinery-related accidents.

Signs and symptoms: age 10 to 13 years (most common group); acute scrotal pain, swelling, bruising, associated skin loss; injured right testicle (more common than left)

Investigations: ultrasound to detect intratesticular and extratesticular hematomas (consider testicular torsion in cases of minor injuries with nonperfusion of testis on ultrasound and extensive scrotal pain, swelling, and bruising)

INCARCERATED HERNIA

Signs and symptoms: palpable mass or swelling in the abdomen, groin, or upper thigh; rapid-onset acute pain at the site of the mass or swelling; nausea, vomiting; constipation; history of abdominal surgery (this is common in ventral hernias)

Risk factor (ventral hernia): obesity

Investigations: ultrasound or CT scan

HEMORRHAGE INTO TESTICULAR TUMOUR

Testicular tumours can hemorrhage to produce swelling and pain. The tumours themselves are often painless lumps or swellings on either testicle.

Some men have acute pain secondary to bleeding into the testis from extravasation of tumour vessels.

Strategy for patient encounter

The age of the patient will help point to a diagnosis. If the patient is a young boy (the likely scenario), the setting for this encounter will probably be an emergency room, where the patient has temporarily left the room with a caregiver on some pretext (e.g., to use the toilet), leaving a parent to give you a history. The likely tasks include history, physical exam, or emergency management.

History

In all patients, start with open-ended questions about the onset of the pain and other symptoms: When did the pain start? How quickly did the pain develop? What other symptoms have you noticed? Listen for sudden versus gradual onset (sudden onset suggests testicular torsion or incarcerated hernia), symptoms consistent with mumps (enlarged, tender unilateral or bilateral salivary glands), masses or lumps (this suggests tumour or hernia), and constipation (this suggests hernia). Ask whether the patient's immunizations are up to date (lapsed immunizations are a risk factor for mumps) and about a history of abdominal surgery (this a risk factor for ventral hernia).

If the patient is an adult, ask about risk factors for sexually transmitted infections (unprotected sex, multiple sexual partners).

Physical exam

Obtain the patient's vital signs, looking for fever. Examine the scrotum for abnormalities (e.g., masses, swelling, redness, tenderness, abnormal position of the testes). Examine the abdomen for masses and tenderness.

(State that you will perform a physical exam. Since children cannot play standardized patients, and since scrotal exams are not done on standardized patients in any case, the examiner will likely interrupt, ask what you are looking for, and provide findings.)

Emergency management

In suspected testicular torsion, order an emergent ultrasound of the testes.

Testicular torsion is a medical emergency that requires immediate surgical assessment.

125

Seizures or epilepsy

MCC particular objectives

Differentiate a seizure from other transient nonseizure conditions (e.g., syncope, pseudoseizure).

Consider seizure in the context of episodic neurological symptoms (e.g., inattention, psychosis).

Outline a plan for the emergent treatment of a patient presenting with a seizure.

MCC differential diagnosis
with added evidence

PRIMARY NEUROLOGICAL DISORDERS (E.G., IDIOPATHIC EPILEPSY, HEAD TRAUMA, ENCEPHALITIS)

IDIOPATHIC EPILEPSY

This presents with generalized seizures or partial (focal) seizures. Cognition is normal. In children, it often resolves on its own at a later age.

Risk factors: family history of epilepsy

IDIOPATHIC GENERALIZED EPILEPSY

Signs and symptoms:

Childhood absence epilepsy: age 4 to 10 years; absence seizures (brief losses of awareness with staring, eye blinking, lip smacking); episodes of loss of consciousness without loss of body tone that are brief (4 to 20 seconds) and frequent (up to 10 times a day) (hyperventilation provokes episodes); electroencephalograph (EEG) showing generalized spike wave activity at 2.5–5 Hz

Juvenile absence epilepsy: onset at age 10 to 12 years; absence seizures; generalized tonic-clonic seizures (possible; these are not seen in childhood absence epilepsy)

Juvenile myoclonic epilepsy (this disorder does not completely resolve in adulthood, so it requires lifelong therapy): myoclonic jerks, generalized tonic-clonic seizures, and absence seizures (absence seizures begin several years before the onset of other seizure types); seizures that are provoked by sleep deprivation or waking; EEG showing spike wave at 4–6 Hz

IDIOPATHIC FOCAL EPILEPSY

Signs and symptoms:

Benign epilepsy of childhood with centrotemporal spikes: onset at age 3 to 13 years (peak incidence age 7 to 9 years); seizures with facial numbness or twitching, guttural vocalizations, hypersalivation, drooling, dysphasia, speech arrest (**no** loss of consciousness); nighttime seizures or on waking; EEG showing centrotemporal sharp waves

Panayiotopoulos syndrome: onset before age 5 years; seizures with vomiting, sudden loss of muscle tone, unresponsiveness, pale skin, incontinence, coughing, hypersalivation; nighttime seizures (duration > 5 minutes); interictal EEG showing occipital spikes and epileptiform activity from other or multiple areas

Benign occipital epilepsy of childhood: onset at age 8 to 9 years; seizures with blindness, visual hallucinations, hemiclonic activity, automatisms, migraines, versive movements; daytime seizures (duration < 5 minutes); interictal EEG showing epileptiform activity that is mostly occipital and long bursts of spike-wave activity on closing the eyes

SEIZURES OR EPILEPSY DUE TO HEAD TRAUMA

Head trauma includes bullet wounds, severe sports-related injuries, and other severe physical trauma to the head.

Early posttraumatic seizures (these develop within days of trauma) are usually focal.

Late posttraumatic seizures (these develop within weeks of trauma) are associated with a high risk of later epilepsy (posttraumatic epilepsy).

Prompt treatment of active seizures (with intravenous phenytoin and sodium valproate) is needed to prevent further damage.

Investigations: MRI

SEIZURES OR EPILEPSY DUE TO ENCEPHALITIS

Seizures are common in encephalitis.

Viral infection is the most common cause: herpes simplex virus, type 1 and type 2 (HSV-1, HSV-2); Epstein-Barr virus (EBV); varicella-zoster virus; Enterovirus (e.g., Coxsackievirus); and insect-borne viruses (e.g., West Nile disease, Lyme disease).

Signs and symptoms: altered mental status (e.g., decreased level of consciousness, lethargy, personality change, behaviour change), fever, headache, nausea, vomiting

Infants and neonates: poor feeding, irritability, lethargy

Children and adolescents: irritability; movement disorder; ataxia; stupor; coma; hemiparesis; cranial nerve defect; status epilepticus (severe)

Adults: motor or sensory deficits; speech or movement impairment; flaccid paralysis

Investigations: blood tests (CBC, differential, platelets; electrolytes; glucose; BUN; creatinine; aminotransferases; coagulation); MRI to detect brain edema, inflammation of the cerebral cortex, gray-white matter junction, thalamus, basal ganglia; CSF tests (perform lumbar puncture after results of MRI; order CSF protein, glucose, cell count, differential, Gram stain, bacterial culture); EEG (usually abnormal) to differentiate from nonconvulsive seizure activity

SYSTEMIC DISORDER (E.G., HYPOGLYCEMIA, ELECTROLYTE DISORDERS)

HYPOGLYCEMIA

Hypoglycemic seizures are common in diabetic patients who take excessive insulin or oral hypoglycemics.

Signs and symptoms: palpitations, pallor, sweating, nightmares, fatigue, hunger

Severe: confusion, disorientation, blurred vision, seizures, coma

ELECTROLYTE DISORDERS

Status epilepticus in older adults is associated with electrolyte imbalance.

Signs and symptoms:

Hyponatremia (this is a medical emergency): serum sodium < 135 mmol/L (severe: < 115 mmol/L); in adults, generalized seizures; in children, acute symptomatic nonfebrile seizures; nonspecific findings on EEG

Hypocalcemia: plasma calcium < 2.12 mmol/L; mental status changes and generalized tonic-clonic or focal motor seizures, with or without muscular tetany (acute hypocalcemia); positive Chvostek sign; Trousseau sign; EEG showing background rhythm with evolution from alpha to theta, diffuse increase in slow wave activity in theta and delta range

Hypomagnesemia: plasma magnesium < 1.6 mmol/L (severe: < 0.8 mmol/L); generalized tonic-clonic seizures (severe hypomagnesemia); neuromuscular irritability; cardiac arrhythmia; higher risk of hypomagnesemia in HIV-positive patients

Hypophosphatemia (symptoms usually arise only in cases of chronic and severe phosphate depletion: < 0.32 mmol/L): paresthesias; generalized seizures; impaired muscle contractility; history of chronic alcoholism, refeeding syndrome, Fanconi syndrome

OTHER (E.G., FEBRILE SEIZURE, WITHDRAWAL)

FEBRILE SEIZURE

Signs and symptoms: young child (age 3 months to 6 years; peak incidence age 12 to 18 months); fever > 38°C; symptoms of cold, influenza, ear infection (febrile seizure is usually the first sign of illness); **no** intracranial infection, central nervous system (CNS) inflammation, acute systemic metabolic abnormality; **no** previous afebrile seizures

Simple febrile seizure (most common): generalized tonic-clonic phase (loss of consciousness, followed by both arms and legs shaking uncontrollably); generalized convulsions lasting ≤ 15 minutes; quick return to baseline after convulsions (**no** confusion, agitation, drowsiness); **no** recurrence within 24 hours

Complex febrile seizure: younger child with abnormal development; focal convulsions (1 limb or 1 side of the body shakes); convulsions lasting > 15 minutes

Risk factors for recurrence: first febrile seizure at younger than 18 months; family history of febrile seizure; high fever; viral infection

WITHDRAWAL SEIZURES (ALCOHOL)

Signs and symptoms: chronic alcoholism (onset at age 40 to 50); tonic-clonic seizures; single seizure or a brief period of multiple seizures that occur 12 to 48 hours after the last alcoholic drink

Strategy for patient encounter

This encounter will likely involve parents discussing a child, who has had a febrile seizure. The child will be absent on some pretext (e.g., a nurse is taking the child's height and weight in another room). The specified tasks could engage history, physical exam, investigations, or management.

History

A main goal of the history is to differentiate a true seizure from nonseizure conditions.

Start with open-ended inquiry seeking information relevant to true seizures (which is the likely scenario): Please tell me about your child's seizure. How was your child before it happened? How was your child after it happened? What conditions does your child have? Listen for seizure symptoms consistent with epilepsy and febrile seizure (see the information this resource lists in the MCC differential diagnosis), triggers (fever, infection, head trauma), and coexisting medical conditions (diabetes).

Ask about a family history of epilepsy. If the child is diabetic, ask about insulin routines, looking for possible noncompliance with medication.

Physical exam

Obtain the child's vital signs looking for fever. Perform a neurological examination looking for focal neurologic signs.

(State that you will perform these exams. Since an actual pediatric patient is unlikely, the examiner may interrupt, ask what you are looking for, and provide findings.)

Investigations

If the diagnosis is in doubt, order tests for serum glucose and electrolytes to rule out underlying medical conditions; a CT scan or MRI of the head to rule out intracranial pathology; and an electroencephalograph (EEG) to investigate the seizure type.

Management

In febrile seizure, provide the parents with information and reassurance. In suspected primary neurological disorder, refer the child to a neurologist. Manage any coexisting medical conditions.

Pearls

Patients taking antiseizure medications often experience weight gain and develop high lipids. These are complications that require monitoring.

126

Abnormal pubertal development

MCC particular objectives

Distinguish normal variants of pubertal development from serious underlying disorders.

Provide supportive counselling on the psychosocial aspects of puberty.

MCC differential diagnosis
with added evidence

DELAYED PUBERTY

DELAYED PUBERTY IN GENERAL

Signs and symptoms:

> Girls: no breast development by age 13; no menstruation for ≥ 5 years after first appearance of breast tissue

> Boys: no testicle development by age 14; incomplete development of male organs 5 years after first signs of testicle development

Variant of normal constitutional delay of puberty

This describes the absence of pubertal development before age 14, with evidence of sexual maturation by age 18.

It is more common in males.

It may generate anxiety in adolescents and their families, and contribute to psychosocial difficulties for some children.

Signs and symptoms: family history of delayed sexual development; stature that is small for age, but with normal growth rate

> **No** evidence of growth hormone deficiency; hypothyroidism; systemic conditions interfering with puberty; hypogonadism

Investigations: blood tests to exclude other possible causes

Primary gonadal disorders

CONGENITAL: CHROMOSOMAL (E.G., TURNER AND KLINEFELTER SYNDROMES), CONGENITAL MALFORMATIONS

TURNER SYNDROME

This is the most common chromosomal abnormality in women (45,X).

Signs and symptoms: ovarian insufficiency (no or minor breast development; primary or secondary amenorrhea); short stature with webbed neck and widely spaced nipples; cubitus valgus; Madelung deformity of the forearm and wrist; normal intelligence (usual)

> Neonates (possible signs and symptoms): lymphedema of the hands and feet; nail dysplasia; high-arched palate; short fourth metacarpals and/or metatarsals
>
> As girls age: hearing loss, hypothyroidism, liver dysfunction
>
> Adult women: mildly elevated liver enzymes

Investigations: elevated FSH; presence of anti-Müllerian hormone; karyotyping

KLINEFELTER SYNDROME

This is the most common congenital abnormality causing hypogonadism in men (most common karyotype: 47,XXY).

Signs and symptoms: small, firm testes or cryptorchidism; small penis; gynecomastia; infertility; decreased virilization; long legs due to long bone abnormality; difficulty with social interactions; learning disabilities; impaired attention without impulsivity

Investigations: low sperm count; elevated FSH and LH; low serum testosterone; karyotyping

CONGENITAL MALFORMATIONS

These result from genetic or environmental factors (half of all cases have an unknown cause). They are either structural or functional. Structural abnormalities are likely identifiable at birth; functional abnormalities can take months or years to identify.

ACQUIRED GONADAL DISORDERS (E.G., GONADAL INFECTION, TRAUMA, NEOPLASM)

Signs and symptoms:

> Gonadal infection: history of infection (e.g., mumps orchitis)
>
> Ovarian neoplasm: abdominal pain, palpable mass
>
> Testicular neoplasm: painless scrotal mass

Secondary gonadal disorders

FUNCTIONAL (E.G., CHRONIC ILLNESS, MALNUTRITION)

CHRONIC ILLNESS

DIABETES

Signs and symptoms: personal or family history of diabetes; history of diabetic complications and/or inadequate monitoring; polydipsia, polyuria, and/or weight loss

Investigations: fasting glucose or HbA_{1c} test

CYSTIC FIBROSIS

Signs and symptoms: family history of cystic fibrosis; recurrent pneumonia; shortness of breath; productive cough; failure to thrive; fever; wheezing on lung auscultation

Investigations: positive sweat chloride test

KIDNEY DISEASE

Signs and symptoms: history of kidney disease, chronic renal failure, and/or current renal dialysis; bilateral lower limb swelling; shortness of breath; paroxysmal nocturnal dyspnea; orthopnea

Risk factors: diabetes, diabetic complications, and/or inadequate monitoring; hypertension; smoking

MALNUTRITION: ANOREXIA NERVOSA[1(pp338-339)]

This causes secondary amenorrhea.

Signs and symptoms: significantly low body weight; intense fear of gaining weight or persistent behaviour that interferes with gaining weight; excessive focus on body weight or shape in self-evaluation, or persistent lack of recognition of current low body weight

HYPOTHALAMIC DYSFUNCTION (E.G., HYPERPROLACTINEMIA)

HYPERPROLACTINEMIA

The most common cause is prolactinoma (which usually presents in adulthood).

Signs and symptoms:

> Girls: delayed puberty, amenorrhea, galactorrhea
>
> Boys: delayed puberty, gynecomastia, galactorrhea, impaired vision, headaches

PITUITARY DYSFUNCTION (E.G., CENTRAL NERVOUS SYSTEM TUMOUR)

CENTRAL NERVOUS SYSTEM (CNS) TUMOUR

Signs and symptoms: headache that gets worse over time (this is a common symptom: 50% of cases); vision impairment; balance problems; personality or behaviour changes; seizures; drowsiness

> Pituitary adenomas or cysts can press on gonadotrophs, causing disrupted function, decreased prolactin (reduced galactorrhea), and decreased gonadotropins (e.g., LH, FSH).

Risk factors: exposure to radiation (e.g., to treat leukemia in childhood); family history (rare); neurofibromatosis type 1 or type 2; tuberous sclerosis; Von Hippel-Lindau disease; Li-Fraumeni syndrome; immune system disorders

PRECOCIOUS PUBERTY

PRECOCIOUS PUBERTY IN GENERAL

Signs and symptoms:

> Girls, before age 6–7 years: breast development, menarche
>
> Boys, before age 9 years: enlarged testicles and penis; facial hair (usually upper lip); voice change
>
> Both sexes: pubic and underarm hair; rapid growth; acne; adult body odour

Central precocious puberty (gonadotropin dependent)

Central precocious puberty is related to the hypothalamus or pituitary gland.

IDIOPATHIC

CENTRAL NERVOUS SYSTEM (E.G., NEOPLASMS, HYDROCEPHALUS)

CNS NEOPLASM

Signs and symptoms: headache, vision impairment

Hamartoma is the most common type of CNS neoplasm to cause precocious puberty in very young children and infants. It is usually benign, often found incidentally. Pubertal development stops on removal. Signs and symptoms include gelastic seizures; other types of seizures; convulsions; intellectual developmental delay; and behavioural disorders.

Risk factors: exposure to radiation (e.g., to treat leukemia in childhood); family history (rare); neurofibromatosis type 1 or type 2; tuberous sclerosis; Von Hippel-Lindau disease; Li-Fraumeni syndrome; immune system disorders

Investigations: brain MRI

HYDROCEPHALUS

Excess fluid accumulation, and pressure from dilated third ventricle on the hypothalamus, results in accelerated or precocious puberty.

Signs and symptoms: early morning headaches in children with possible nausea and vomiting; changes in behaviour (e.g., irritability, unruliness, loss of interest); changes in vital signs (bradycardia, hypertension, altered respiratory rate); dilated or prominent scalp veins; double vision; papilledema; impaired upward gaze; spasticity in the legs, extremities

As hydrocephalus progresses: lethargy and drowsiness

Peripheral precocious puberty (gonadotropin independent)

PERIPHERAL PRECOCIOUS PUBERTY IN GENERAL

This is abnormal development of secondary sex characteristics not related to the hypothalamus or pituitary gland.

Investigations: high serum androgen or estrogen levels

AUTONOMOUS GONADAL FUNCTION (E.G., OVARIAN CYSTS, LEYDIG CELL TUMOURS OF OVARIES OR TESTES)

OVARIAN CYSTS

Large functioning follicular ovarian cysts are the most common cause of peripheral precocity in girls. They appear and regress spontaneously. They can cause ovarian torsion.

Signs and symptoms: early breast development; vaginal bleeding once cysts regress

Investigations: pelvic ultrasound

LEYDIG CELL TUMOURS OF OVARIES OR TESTES (ARRHENOBLASTOMA)

In girls, these produce androgens. They are usually benign (90%). Signs and symptoms include virilization precocity.

In boys, they produce asymmetric testicular enlargement. They are usually benign (90%). Signs and symptoms include feminization (if estrogen-secreting) or pubertal precocity (if androgen-secreting).

Investigations: pelvic ultrasound; histology (in boys, sample the larger testicle, if present, regardless of the presence of a mass)

ADRENAL PATHOLOGY (E.G., TUMOURS, CONGENITAL ADRENAL HYPERPLASIA)

ADRENAL TUMOURS

In girls, granulosa cell tumours cause gender-conforming precocity (unlike Leydig cell tumours which cause virilization precocity—see above).

In boys, hCG-secreting germ cell tumours increase testosterone production, which causes increased testicular size.

Investigations: pelvic and adrenal ultrasound

CONGENITAL ADRENAL HYPERPLASIA (CAH)

CAH is an enzyme defect in adrenal steroid biosynthesis. The most common cause is deficiency in 21-hydroxylase. Most patients are identified as neonates or infants.

In neonate boys (1 to 4 weeks), severe 21-hydroxylase deficiency can cause salt wasting (signs and symptoms include difficulty feeding, failure to thrive, vomiting, dehydration, volume depletion, hyponatremia, hyperkalemia, and shock).

Signs and symptoms: premature pubic hair growth

> Infant girls: virilization; ambiguous genitals
>
> Infant boys: undervirilization; normal genitals
>
> Later in childhood (in cases of mild 21-hydroxylase deficiency): accelerated growth and skeletal maturation; enlarged genitalia

Risk factors: Ashkenazi Jewish descent, Eastern European descent

Investigations for CAH due to 21-hydroxylase: high serum concentration of 17-hydroxyprogesterone (> 30 nmol/L); elevated adrenal androgens (DHEA-S); genetic testing

EXOGENOUS SEX HORMONE EXPOSURE

Examples include the use by parents or caregivers of estrogen-containing products (e.g., to treat menopause: creams, ointments, sprays with estrogen) and androgen creams (e.g., to treat low testosterone levels). Other sources include food contaminated with hormones and foods high in phytoestrogens (soy, lavender oil, tea tree oil).

Strategy for patient encounter

This encounter will likely involve parents discussing a child with delayed puberty. The child will be absent on some pretext (e.g., someone has taken the child to use the toilet). The specified tasks could engage history, physical exam, investigations, or management.

History

There is a wide range of possible entities for this patient encounter.

Start with open-ended inquiry, which will quickly establish whether the issue is delayed or precocious puberty: What are your concerns about your child's development? Make sure, based on the age of the child and the symptoms, that delayed or precocious puberty is really at issue (see the definitions this resource lists in the MCC differential diagnosis).

In apparent delayed puberty, ask for details about what the parent has noticed. Listen for signs consistent with Turner syndrome (in girls; short stature, webbed neck, widely spaced nipples); Klinefelter syndrome (in boys; small genitals or cryptorchidism); and prolactinoma (galactorrhea). Ask about headache, seizures, abnormal movement, or changes in personality (these suggest central nervous system tumour). Ask about a history of mumps, kidney disease, anorexia nervosa, exposure to radiation, and use of steroids (for example, to treat skin conditions). Ask about a family history of diabetes and cystic fibrosis.

In apparent precocious puberty, ask how the child's health has generally been. Listen for symptoms consistent with central nervous system (CNS) neoplasm (headaches, vision problems) and hydrocephalus (headaches, nausea, behaviour changes, spasticity). Ask about possible exposure to hormone-containing products from adult caregivers (e.g., to treat menopause or low testosterone).

Ask about the age at which the patient's parents and siblings went through puberty.

Physical exam

Perform a physical exam to determine the child's stage of pubertal development, and to look for specific physical signs of entities you suspect from the history (e.g., cryptorchidism in Klinefelter syndrome, palpable masses in gonadal neoplasm).

CHECKLIST

Tanner staging for normal puberty

	GIRLS	BOYS
Stage 1	Prepubertal Growth in height: 5–6 cm/year Breast growth: papillar elevation only Pubic hair (villus hair only)	Prepubertal Growth in height: 5–6 cm/year Testicular length: < 2.5 cm No penis growth No pubic hair
Stage 2	Typical age: 8–13 years Growth in height: 7–8 cm/year Breast growth: areolae enlargement, palpable breast buds Age 9–13: pubic hair growth near labia	Typical age: 10–14 years Growth in height: 5–6 cm/year Testicular length: 2.5–3.2 cm Increase in penis length and width Minimal pubic hair at base of penis
Stage 3	Typical age: 9–14 years Growth in height (peak): 8 cm/year Breast growth: further enlargement of breasts and areolae, elevation of breast contour Increase in pubic hair volume, coarseness, and pigmentation, with spread over mons pubis Development of axillary hair and acne Menarche	Typical age: 11–16 years Growth in height: 7–8 cm/year Testicular length: 3.6 cm Increase in penis length and width Increase in pubic hair volume, coarseness, and pigmentation, with spread over the pubis Changes in voice Increase in muscle mass
Stage 4	Typical age: 10–15 years Growth in height: 7 cm/year Breast growth: areola that forms a mound on breast Adult-like pubic hair, but no spread to junction of medial thigh with perineum Menarche	Typical age: 12–16 years Growth in height (peak): 10 cm/year Testicular length: 4.1–4.5 cm Adult-like pubic hair, but no spread to junction of medial thigh with perineum Around age 14: presence of axillary hair, acne, and voice changes
Stage 5	Typical age: 16 years No further growth in height Adult breast contour with recessed areola Adult distribution of pubic hair, which spreads to medial thigh (no spread to linea alba)	Typical age: 15–17 years No further growth in height after 17 years Testicular length: > 4.5 cm Mature penis size Adult distribution of pubic hair, which spreads to medial thigh (no spread to linea alba) Facial hair, mature male physique, no gynecomastia

Reproduced from Archives of Disease in Childhood, Marshall WA, Tanner JM, Vol. 44, pp 291–303, 1969, and Vol. 45, pp 13–23, 1970, with permission from BMJ Publishing Group Ltd.

(State that you will perform a physical exam. Because an actual pediatric patient is unlikely, the examiner may interrupt, ask what you are looking for, and provide findings. State that you are looking for evidence of the child's Tanner stage. Be prepared to describe Tanner staging in full—see the checklist. You should also state signs of entities you suspect from the history.)

Investigations

In suspected neoplasm, order CNS or pelvic imaging. In suspected genetic abnormality, order karyotyping.

Order other specific tests if indicated by the results of the history and physical exam (see the information this resource lists in the MCC differential diagnosis).

Management

Specialist referral to a pediatrician or endocrinologist will usually be indicated.

REFERENCE

1 American Psychiatric Association. Diagnostic and statistical manual of mental disorders. 5th ed. Arlington, VA: American Psychiatric Association; 2013. 991 p.

127

Sexually concerned patient

MCC particular objective

Demonstrate acceptance of, and appropriate care for, patients of all gender identities.

MCC differential diagnosis
with added evidence

SEXUAL DYSFUNCTION

SEXUAL DYSFUNCTION IN GENERAL

Signs and symptoms: in men, erectile dysfunction (recurring inability to get and maintain an erection; reduced sexual desire); in women, recurring reduced sexual desire or response, anorgasmia, and/or pain with intercourse

Psychological or emotional condition (e.g., depression, abuse)

MAJOR DEPRESSIVE DISORDER[1(pp160–161)]

Signs and symptoms: symptoms that are present most of the time for ≥ 2 weeks; symptoms with significant impact on day-to-day life

> Key symptoms: depressed mood and/or loss of interest in usual activities

> Other symptoms: significant weight change; sleep disturbance; slowed or agitated mental processes; loss of concentration; recurrent thoughts of death or suicide

Risk factors: family history of mental health disorders (depression, anxiety, suicide); personal history of other mental health disorders; substance abuse; chronic illness (e.g., cancer, stroke, chronic pain)

INTIMATE PARTNER ABUSE

Signs and symptoms: disclosed abuse (physical; psychological or emotional; sexual; economic; social isolation); bruising, scars, healed fractures; recurrent symptoms or injuries; resistance by the partner to having the patient interviewed alone (usual)

> Note: victims do not always disclose abuse.

Risk factors: pregnancy; threat to leave; partner's history of violence or substance abuse

Hormonal condition (e.g., menopause)

MENOPAUSE

Menopause has occurred when 12 months have passed since a woman's last menstrual period. This can occur naturally (usually around age 50); or because of surgical removal of the ovaries, or chemotherapy or radiation therapy.

Signs and symptoms: dry, inelastic vaginal tissue, which leads to difficult or painful intercourse; hot flashes; irritability; weight gain

Neurologic dysfunction (e.g., spinal cord injury)

In addition to spinal cord injury, common causes include brain injury, stroke, and multiple sclerosis.

Vascular insufficiency (e.g., diabetes mellitus)

DIABETES

Signs and symptoms: personal or family history of diabetes; history of diabetic complications and/or inadequate monitoring; polydipsia, polyuria, and/or weight loss

Investigations: fasting glucose or HbA_{1c} test

Drug side effects (e.g., beta-blockers)

Trauma (e.g., episiotomy)

PARAPHILIAS (E.G., PEDOPHILIA)

PEDOPHILIC DISORDER[1(p697)]

Signs and symptoms: age 16 or older; symptoms that are present ≥ 6 months; recurrent fantasies or urges about sexual activity with children (at least 5 years younger than the individual); symptoms with significant impact on day-to-day life, including acting on the urges or fantasies

GENDER IDENTITY DISORDERS

GENDER DYSPHORIA IN ADOLESCENTS AND ADULTS[1(pp452–453)]

Signs and symptoms: incongruence between the expressed gender and the assigned gender of an individual (e.g., rejection of the sex characteristics of the assigned gender; desire for the sex characteristics of the expressed gender; desire to be treated as a member of the expressed gender); symptoms that are present ≥ 6 months; symptoms with significant impact on day-to-day life

SPECIAL POPULATIONS

People with disabilities

Possible issues include personal and social acceptance of the sexuality of people with disabilities; depression, anxiety due to lack of acceptance; appropriate contraception (e.g., women with reduced mobility have higher risk of thrombosis from oral contraceptives);

genetic concerns, if the disability is congenital; and adaptive practices (e.g., use of sex aids).

Lesbian, gay, bisexual, transgender people
Possible issues include personal and social acceptance of sexual identity; depression, anxiety due to lack of acceptance; violence and bullying due to sexual identity; risks associated with sexual orientation (e.g., men who have sex with men have a higher risk of sexually transmitted diseases: HIV, hepatitis, human papillomavirus, herpes simplex, gonorrhea, chlamydia, syphilis).

Children and adolescents
Possible issues include sexual identity, consent, sexual abuse, bullying, contraception, and safe sex.

Elderly people
Possible issues include sexual dysfunction from declining general health, depression; erectile dysfunction; urogenital atrophy causing difficult or painful intercourse (women); and institutionalization, resulting in a lack of privacy with partners.

SEXUAL ADDICTION
The *Diagnostic and Statistical Manual of Mental Disorders (DSM-5)* does not include sexual addiction as a disorder because of lack of peer-reviewed evidence, but notes that some clinicians talk about it as a behavioural disorder like gambling.

Strategy for patient encounter
The likely scenario is a patient with gender identity questions. The specified tasks could engage history, physical exam, investigations, or management.

The MCC identifies setting the patient at ease as a key aspect of this clinical presentation (see the tip).

History
Start with open-ended inquiry, which will quickly establish

TIP

Setting patients at ease
It's good general preparation for the exam to plan steps to help patients who are embarrassed or reluctant to discuss their concerns. Any standardized patient in any encounter may test your skill to elicit information.

Some general strategies include:

- maintaining eye contact
- remaining calm and respectful
- expressing support for the patient's decision to seek your help
- expressing confidence in your ability to provide help
- assuring the patient that you will listen and provide care without judging the patient

the nature of the patient's problem: Please tell me about the problem you've been having.

Where appropriate (for example, if the patient expresses concerns about sexual orientation or identity), establish the patient's sexual development (socially and physically), sexual orientation, and comfort with their orientation. For example, ask: How long have you had these concerns? What brought the concerns to the surface? What has been your experience with your physical sexual maturation? What has been your experience with sexual relationships? How have your experiences affected your relationships with family and friends? How do you regard your sexual orientation?

In male erectile dysfunction, concentrate on identifying treatable causes (e.g., diabetes, hypertension).

Physical exam
In male erectile dysfunction, remember to obtain the patient's vital signs (looking for hypertension).

Investigations
Where relevant, screen for diabetes.

Management
Manage treatable causes. Counsel and educate the patient. Consider psychological support and referral.

REFERENCE

1 American Psychiatric Association. Diagnostic and statistical manual of mental disorders. 5th ed. Arlington, VA: American Psychiatric Association; 2013. 991 p.

128

Urticaria, angioedema

MCC particular objective

Determine if the condition is acute and/or life-threatening, and requires immediate treatment.

MCC differential diagnosis
with added evidence

URTICARIA, ANGIOEDEMA IN GENERAL

Signs and symptoms: symptoms that can be chronic with frequent, unpredictable recurrence

> Urticaria (this affects the upper dermis): hives (red or white welts), usually on the face, trunk, arms, legs; itching

> Angioedema (this affects the dermis, subcutaneous tissue, mucosa, submucosa): swelling with pain or burning that can affect the eyes, cheeks, lips, hands, feet, genitals, inside the throat

IDIOPATHIC

ASSOCIATED WITH IDENTIFIABLE CAUSES

Allergic reaction (e.g., drugs, insects, food)

DRUGS

Anaphylaxis is possible and requires emergent intervention.

Common reactions:

> Antibiotics (e.g., penicillins, cephalosporins): IgE-mediated (acute) urticaria that occurs within minutes to 2 hours of exposure (**but** vancomycin allergy causes diffuse erythema or flushing with urticaria: the reaction is due to direct mast cell activation; it is not IgE-mediated)

> Muscle relaxants (e.g., atracurium, vecuronium, succinylcholine, curare): symptoms associated with direct mast cell activation (IgE-mediated anaphylaxis is also possible)

INSECTS

Anaphylaxis is possible and requires emergent intervention.

Common reactions:

> Urticarial lesions: bees, wasps, hornets, fire ants

> Papular urticarial lesions on the lower extremities (resolve over weeks): bedbugs, fleas, mites

FOOD

Anaphylaxis is possible and requires emergent intervention.

Common reactions:

> IgE-mediated reactions in children (on ingestion): milk, eggs, peanuts, tree nuts, soy, wheat
>
> IgE-mediated reactions in adults (on ingestion): shellfish, fish, tree nuts, peanuts
>
> Direct mast cell activated reactions in young children (on contact or ingestion): tomatoes, strawberries
>
> Direct physical contact with food allergens (e.g., kitchen or food-processing workers): urticaria; IgE-mediated allergic reactions

Direct mast cell release (e.g., opiates, radio-contrast agents)

OPIATES

Examples include dextromethorphan in cough syrup, morphine, and codeine.

Common reaction: acute urticaria with flushing, sweating, asthma, hypotension, sneezing

RADIO-CONTRAST AGENTS

Examples include benzoic acid molecules: ionic monomers, ionic dimer, nonionic monomer, nonionic dimer.

Common reaction: urticaria with angioedema, flushing, bronchospasm, wheezing, laryngeal edema, stridor that occurs within 5 minutes to 1 hour on intravenous (IV) injection of radio-contrast agent

Complement-mediated condition (e.g., serum sickness, infection)

SERUM SICKNESS

This is a less common cause of urticaria. It involves reaction to exogenous proteins, medications, or infectious agents. Examples include antiseizure medications, antibiotics (cefaclor, penicillin, amoxicillin, trimethoprim-sulfamethoxazole), and vaccines (rabies; diphtheria; botulinum; spider or snake venom).

Signs and symptoms: symptoms that present 1 to 3 weeks after exposure (symptoms resolve within a few weeks of exposure cessation); urticarial rash; fever; malaise; polyarthralgia; pruritic rash (not on mucous membranes)

INFECTION

BACTERIAL AND VIRAL INFECTIONS

Causes include urinary tract infections, upper respiratory tract infections, gastrointestinal infections, and pharyngitis.

Signs and symptoms: acute urticaria (especially in children); history of recent illness with fever, sore throat, cough, rhinorrhea, headache, diarrhea, vomiting

PARASITIC INFECTION

Causes include ascariasis, strongyloidiasis, schistosomiasis, and trichinosis.

Signs and symptoms: acute urticaria with eosinophilia; history of ingesting contaminated raw or undercooked fish; travel to endemic areas

> *Anisakis simplex*: urticaria, angioedema, abdominal pain, and/or anaphylaxis 2 to 24 hours after ingestion

Investigations: stool examination to detect ova and parasites

Physical (e.g., dermatographism, cold)

DERMATOGRAPHISM

This is the most common type of physical urticaria.

Signs and symptoms: rapid-onset (within several minutes) urticaria following physical irritation of the skin (e.g., pressure, scratching, rubbing); welts whose orientation follows the pattern of irritation (e.g., scratching produces linear welts)

COLD

This is a chronic condition that affects young adults and that resolves in 5 to 6 years. Patients with cold urticaria risk anaphylaxis and drowning if they swim in cold water.

Signs and symptoms: urticaria with or without angioedema that forms after cold exposure (e.g., contact with cold air, objects, liquids)

Strategy for patient encounter

The likely scenario is a patient with recurrent urticaria. The specified tasks could engage history, physical exam, investigations, or management.

Anaphylaxis is possible in this clinical presentation. No matter what tasks the instructions for the encounter specify, start by checking the patient's airway and hemodynamic status.

Airway and hemodynamic status

Check the patient's vital signs, including blood pressure (looking for hypotension) and pulse (looking for tachycardia).

Check for key symptoms (e.g., itchiness, swelling, shortness of breath).

Note that a patient presenting with allergic symptoms can develop anaphylaxis minutes or hours after the triggering event. Stay alert to changes in the condition of any patient who presents with urticaria or angioedema.

Provide emergency care to any patient with unstable vital signs.

History

Ask open-ended questions about symptom onset, duration, and triggers: When did you start having symptoms? When you have symptoms, how long do they last? What triggers the symptoms, or what triggers do you suspect? Listen for evidence of chronic versus acute symptoms, and association of symptoms with systemic disease (serum sickness, infection).

Physical exam

Examine the skin for rashes and urticaria.

Investigations

In an unstable patient, attach a pulse oximeter and blood pressure cuff. After the patient is stable, consider serum IgG tests for specific antigens if the offending agent is unknown.

Management

In patients undergoing anaphylaxis, provide supportive therapy and administer epinephrine, antihistamines, or steroids. Obtain intravenous (IV) access, and ensure the patient is in a monitored setting.

Discuss avoidance of triggers and appropriate medication (e.g., antihistamines, steroids). Consider prescribing injectable epinephrine (EpiPen), and counsel the patient about its use.

129

Sleep-wake disorders

MCC particular objectives
None stated.

MCC differential diagnosis
with added evidence

EXTERNAL FACTORS (E.G., SLEEP DISRUPTION DUE TO POOR SLEEP ENVIRONMENT)

POOR SLEEP ENVIRONMENT
Poor sleep environments may have too much light, too much noise, uncomfortable temperatures (too hot or cold), or cosleepers with sleep disorders (e.g., snoring).

INTRINSIC SLEEP DISORDERS (E.G., CIRCADIAN RHYTHM DISORDERS, INSOMNIA, SLEEP-DISORDERED BREATHING)

CIRCADIAN RHYTHM SLEEP-WAKE DISORDERS
Signs and symptoms: symptoms that last > 3 months; chronic or recurrent pattern of insomnia and/or excessive sleepiness; associated daytime distress or impairment

> Delayed sleep-wake disorder: adolescents and young adults (high incidence); late bedtime (2 am or later) and late wake time (e.g., 3 pm); undisturbed sleep once initiated; with early rising (e.g., for school or work), daytime sleepiness and impaired performance

> Advanced sleep-wake disorder: older person (high incidence); early bedtime (6 pm to 9 pm) and early wake time (1 am to 5 am); insomnia; sleepiness in the late afternoon to early evening

> Irregular sleep-wake disorder: children with developmental disorders (common); adults with Alzheimer, Parkinson, or Huntington disease (common); no clearly defined circadian rhythm of sleeping and waking

> Non-24 hour sleep-wake rhythm disorder: blind patients (common); reduced sleep time; poor sleep quality at night; sleepiness during the daytime

INSOMNIA

Signs and symptoms: impaired daytime function (difficulty with paying attention, concentration, memory); daytime sleepiness; difficulty falling asleep; difficulty staying asleep; earlier than desired wake time

> Short-term insomnia: symptoms that last < 3 months; symptoms related to stressors such as pain, grief, medications, illness, altered sleep environment; resolution of symptoms on cessation of stressor or patient adaptation to stressor

> Chronic insomnia: symptoms that last > 3 months and occur ≥ 3 times/week; symptoms related to depression, chronic stress, chronic pain, chronic illness, some medications; in children and young adults, sleep latency or wake periods of > 20 minutes; in adults: sleep latency or wake periods of > 30 minutes

> Other insomnia: symptoms of insomnia without meeting the criteria for short-term or chronic insomnia

Risk factors: female (more common); older age; mental health disorder or medical condition; high stress

SLEEP-DISORDERED BREATHING

A common cause is obstructive sleep apnea.

Signs and symptoms: abnormal respiration (apneas or hypopneas); disrupted sleep with snoring, restlessness, resuscitative snorts; difficulty breathing during sleep (during sleep, breathing stops for ≥ 10 seconds despite inspiration efforts); excessive daytime sleepiness, fatigue, poor concentration; nocturnal hypoxemia; morning headache; poorly controlled hypertension

Risk factors (these increase with age): obesity; male; craniofacial and upper airway abnormalities

Investigations: formal sleep test

COMORBID CONDITIONS (E.G., PSYCHIATRIC DISORDERS, NEUROLOGIC DISORDERS, SUBSTANCE ABUSE, DYSPNEA)

Psychiatric disorders often present with sleep disruption (e.g., depression, anxiety).

Neurologic disorders (e.g., Alzheimer disease, Parkinson disease, disorders with chronic pain) can present with insomnia associated with physical limitations, reduced social participation, and fatigue.

Substance abuse can cause sleep disruption: insomnia in alcohol abuse; reduction in sleep latency in cannabis use; difficulty falling asleep in cannabis withdrawal; increased sleep latency in cocaine use; and poor sleep efficiency and reduced sleep time in opioid use.

Dyspnea is a sign and symptom of comorbid insomnia.

Strategy for patient encounter

The likely scenario is a shift worker with disturbed sleep. The specified tasks could engage history, physical exam, investigations, or management.

History

Start with open-ended inquiry about the patient's sleep-wake disorder: Please tell me about the problems you've been having with sleep. Listen for evidence of external factors (shift work, sleep environment), intrinsic factors (pain, illness, emotional stress, dysfunctional circadian rhythms, obstructive sleep apnea), and comorbid conditions (psychiatric conditions, neurological conditions, substance abuse). Note that patients may be reluctant to disclose substance abuse, so ask about this directly if the patient does not volunteer the information.

Ask if the patient has a sleep log or diary with them. If so, ask to review it. If not, obtain a sleep history: What time do you usually go to bed? What time do you usually wake up? How well do you usually sleep? What do you usually do before you go to bed?

Obtain collateral information on the patient's sleep routine from a family member, if possible.

Physical exam

Obtain the patient's vital signs including blood pressure, height, and weight. Calculate the patient's body mass index (BMI).

Investigations

Consider ordering a sleep study (polysomnograph), if the diagnosis is in doubt.

> **TIP**
>
> **Tailoring information to individual patients**
>
> Try to avoid the common exam error of providing patients with generic information.
>
> Instead, provide strategies that target the patient's specific situation.
>
> In the case of a shift worker with disordered sleep, first establish what kind of shift work is at issue (e.g., continuous night shifts, rotating shifts).
>
> For continuous night shifts, workers should try to maintain as constant a sleep schedule as possible, even on their days off.
>
> For rotating shifts, workers should try for a regular rotation that allows them to establish a routine to adjust their sleep schedule. Strategic napping (e.g., short naps before starting a shift) and breaks for walks (to avoid extended sitting) can help with on-the-job sleepiness.
>
> Sleep hygiene is also important. This includes avoiding caffeine and alcohol before sleeping, and maintaining a cool, dark, quiet sleep environment.

Management

Screen the patient for safety concerns (e.g., excessive work-time somnolence).

Counsel the patient on managing their sleep disorder. Treat comorbidities (e.g., substance abuse, obesity).

130

Hypernatremia

MCC particular objective

Recognize that most cases of hypernatremia occur in the frail elderly from water depletion.

MCC differential diagnosis
with added evidence

WATER DEPLETION (DEHYDRATION)
DEHYDRATION IN GENERAL

Symptoms: postural dizziness; headache; malaise; muscle weakness; lethargy or somnolence; change in activity or mental status; restlessness; irritability; agitation; reduced urine output; acute weight loss; constipation

> Severe: seizures, coma

> Signs on physical examination: dry mucous membranes; sunken-appearing eyes; slow capillary refill; hypotension; resting tachycardia; orthostatic changes; flat neck veins in supine position; oliguria; reduced or abnormal skin turgor; recent change of consciousness; increased postural pulse, decreased postural blood pressure

Risk factors: elderly, acute illness, chronic conditions, no intact thirst mechanism, dementia, reduced kidney function, high percentage fat, low muscle mass, dehydrating medication (e.g., diuretics, laxatives, antidiuretic hormone antagonists, lithium, alcohol, narcotics), reduced fluid intake

Investigations:

> Blood tests: electrolytes including sodium (> 145 mmol/L), potassium, chloride, bicarbonate; BUN; creatinine; osmolality; glucose; calcium

Urine tests: spot sodium concentration; specific gravity; osmolality

Decreased intake of water (e.g., impaired thirst)

IMPAIRED THIRST

Patients in long-term care may have a combination of factors, including altered thirst, decreased cognitive function (e.g., delirium, depression, sedation, dementia), and higher fluid losses.

Increased loss

RENAL LOSS (E.G., OSMOTIC DIURESIS)

OSMOTIC DIURESIS

The most common cause is hyperglycemia due to diabetes.

Signs and symptoms: personal or family history of diabetes; history of diabetic complications and/or inadequate monitoring; polydipsia, polyuria, and/or weight loss

Investigations: fasting glucose or HbA_{1c} test

GASTROINTESTINAL LOSS (E.G., DIARRHEA)

INCREASED INSENSIBLE LOSS (E.G., PROLONGED EXERCISE)

SODIUM GAIN (E.G., HYPERTONIC FLUID REPLACEMENT)

HYPERTONIC FLUID REPLACEMENT

Examples include hypertonic dialysis and administration of hypertonic saline.

Strategy for patient encounter

The likely scenario is a patient with hypernatremia found on blood work. The likely tasks include interpreting lab tests, history, physical exam, further investigations, or management.

Interpreting lab tests

The diagnosis of hypernatremia necessarily starts with a lab test. Expect this patient encounter to rely heavily on lab test interpretation. As a first step, ask to see the results of any blood work that has already been done. (The patient or the examiner may give you this information.)

History

Ask open-ended questions to elicit evidence of common triggers and risk factors for hypernatremia: How has your health been generally? What chronic conditions do you have? What medications do you take? Listen for recent illness, diabetes, use of dehydrating medications, and diarrhea.

Ask whether the patient feels thirsty (hypernatremia with lack of thirst suggests impaired thirst mechanism). Ask about recent prolonged exercise and hypertonic fluid replacement.

In elderly patients, listen for habitation in a long-term care facility (where they may rely on others to get water) and medications that impair cognition.

Physical exam
Obtain the patient's vital signs. Assess the patient for volume status. Pay attention to neurological symptoms (these suggest an impaired thirst mechanism, or may be secondary to the hypernatremia itself) and the patient's mental status (dehydration can lead to mental status changes).

Further investigations
Estimate the level of water deficit. Order a blood glucose test and brain imaging (to detect conditions that impair the thirst mechanism, such as lesions on the hypothalamus).

Management
Management depends on the specific entity identified. Consider referral to an endocrinologist or nephrologist.

Pearls
Overly rapid correction of hypernatremia carries the risk of convulsions and cerebral edema. The rate of correction should not exceed 1 mmol/L per hour. Over a 24-hour period, the rate of correction should not exceed 10–12 mmol/L.

131

Hyponatremia

MCC particular objective

Recognize that severe hyponatremia can be life-threatening.

MCC differential diagnosis
with added evidence

HYPONATREMIA IN GENERAL

Signs and symptoms: anorexia, nausea, malaise (early); decreased reaction times, slow cognition, ataxia (moderate to chronic); headache, muscle cramps, irritability, drowsiness, confusion, weakness (worse than moderate); coma, respiratory arrest (severe)

HYPONATREMIA WITH NORMAL SERUM OSMOLALITY (E.G., HYPERLIPIDEMIA)

HYPERTRIGLYCERIDEMIA

Signs and symptoms: usually asymptomatic; recurrent pancreatitis

Skin: eruptive xanthomas (yellow papules on the back, chest, proximal extremities); palmar xanthomas (yellow creases on the palms); tuberous xanthomas (red/orange shiny nodules on finger extensors); tendinous xanthomas (Achilles tendon); xanthelasma (yellow plaques on the eyelids)

Contributing medications: atypical antipsychotics; beta-blockers; estrogens; immunosuppressives; isotretinoin; protease inhibitors; thiazide-type diuretics; tamoxifen; clomiphene; herbal or botanical supplements

Risk factors: diabetes; history of coronary heart disease or noncoronary atherosclerosis (e.g., abdominal aortic aneurysm); family history of cardiovascular disease; smoking; hypertension; obesity

Investigations: fasting serum triglycerides (< 1.7 mmol/L is normal; 2.3–5.6 mmol/L is high; > 5.6 mmol/L is very high)

HYPERCHOLESTEROLEMIA

Signs and symptoms: usually asymptomatic

Risk factors: diet high in processed foods and fat; obesity; large waist circumference; lack of exercise; smoking; diabetes

Contributing medications: progestins, anabolic steroids, corticosteroids, protease inhibitors

Investigations: total cholesterol (< 5.2 mmol/L is normal; > 6.2 mmol/L is high); LDL-C (< 2.59 mmol/L is optimal; > 4.90 mmol/L is very high)

HYPONATREMIA WITH HIGH SERUM OSMOLALITY (E.G., HYPERGLYCEMIA)

HYPERGLYCEMIA

Serum sodium decreases by 2.4 mmol/L for each increase of 5.6 mmol/L serum glucose. Sodium correction in hyperglycemia is:

$$Na = Measured\ Sodium + 0.016 \times (Glucose - 100)$$

Risk factors: personal or family history of diabetes; history of diabetic complications and/or inadequate monitoring

Investigations: serum and urine osmolality; serum glucose and lipids

HYPONATREMIA WITH LOW SERUM OSMOLALITY

Low total body water volume, elevated antidiuretic hormone (ADH) level (e.g., gastrointestinal loss, diuretic use)

Signs and symptoms: history of diarrhea or diuretic use

Normal total body water volume (e.g., syndrome of inappropriate ADH secretion, hypothyroidism, adrenal insufficiency)

SYNDROME OF INAPPROPRIATE ADH SECRETION (SIADH)

Signs and symptoms: general symptoms of hyponatremia (see above)

Investigations: hyponatremia; hypoosmolality; urine osmolality > 100 mmol/kg; urine sodium concentration > 40 mmol/L; normal serum potassium concentration; no acid-base disturbance; low serum uric acid concentration (often)

HYPOTHYROIDISM

Signs and symptoms: history of hypothyroidism or symptoms of hypothyroidism (cold intolerance, decreased reflexes, dry skin, weight gain, impaired cognition)

Investigations: elevated thyrotropin (TSH)

ADRENAL INSUFFICIENCY

Signs and symptoms: symptoms that develop slowly (often over several months); hyperpigmentation; fatigue; weight loss; dizziness; muscle and/or joint pain; salt craving

Investigations: serum sodium, potassium, cortisol, ACTH; ACTH stimulation test (this involves artificial stimulation of the adrenal gland) to determine adrenal gland function; CT scan of the adrenal gland

High total body water volume, elevated ADH level (e.g., congestive heart failure, nephrotic syndrome, cirrhosis)

CONGESTIVE HEART FAILURE

Signs and symptoms: history of heart disease (or risk factors for heart disease: diabetes, hypertension, hyperlipidemia, and smoking) or hepatic vein thrombosis (Budd-Chiari syndrome); severe shortness of breath; elevated jugular venous pressure; edema in the abdomen and legs; pink phlegm; heart murmurs and extra cardiac sounds

Investigations: chest X-ray to detect pulmonary edema; NT-proBNP level; echocardiogram to distinguish forms of heart failure; cardiac stress testing, either with exercise or pharmacological agent

NEPHROTIC SYNDROME

Signs and symptoms: progressive bilateral lower extremity edema (ankles and feet); swelling around the eyes; weight gain (from water retention); foamy urine

Risk factors: conditions that damage the kidneys (e.g., diabetes, systemic lupus erythematosus, amyloidosis); use of nonsteroidal antiinflammatory drugs (NSAIDs), antibiotics; history of HIV, hepatitis B virus (HBV) infection, hepatitis C virus (HCV) infection, malaria

Investigations: urine (proteinuria; spot urine protein:creatinine ratio; lipuria); hyponatremia with low fractional sodium excretion; low serum albumin; high total cholesterol (hyperlipidemia); elevated BUN

CIRRHOSIS

Signs and symptoms: jaundice; easy bruising, bleeding; itching; ascites; spiderlike blood vessels on the skin; systemic symptoms (anorexia, weight loss, weakness, fatigue)

>History of chronic alcohol abuse; chronic viral HBV or HCV infection; hemochromatosis; nonalcoholic fatty liver disease

>HBV and HCV risk factors: autoimmune conditions, unprotected sex, intravenous drug abuse, blood transfusions, workplace exposure to body fluids, tattoos, body piercings, imprisonment

Investigations: liver function tests

Strategy for patient encounter

The likely scenario is a patient with hyponatremia found on blood work. The likely tasks are interpreting lab tests, history, physical exam, further investigations, or management.

Interpreting lab tests

The diagnosis of hyponatremia necessarily starts with a lab test. Expect this patient encounter to rely heavily on lab test interpretation. The instructions for this encounter may give you lab test results. If not, as a first step, ask to see the results of any blood work that has already been done. (The patient or the examiner may give you this information.)

History

Use open-ended inquiry about the patient's medical history: What conditions have you been diagnosed with? Listen for conditions listed in the MCC differential diagnosis.

Physical exam

Obtain the patient's vital signs. Assess the patient for volume status. Pay attention to the patient's mental status because severe hyponatremia may lead to confusion.

Further investigations

For all patients, order tests for plasma and urine osmolality, and urine electrolytes. Order additional specific tests as outlined by this resource in the MCC differential diagnosis.

Management

Management will depend on the specific entity identified. Consider referral to an endocrinologist or nephrologist.

Pearls

Overly rapid correction of hyponatremia can lead to central pontine myelinolysis. Risk factors for central pontine myelinolysis include alcoholism, liver disease, malnutrition, and a baseline serum sodium of < 120 mmol/L. Do not correct by more than 6–8 mmol/L over 24 hours.

132

Sore throat and/or rhinorrhea

MCC particular objectives
None stated.

MCC differential diagnosis
with added evidence

INFECTION (E.G., VIRAL, BACTERIAL, CANDIDAL)

VIRAL INFECTION

Examples include the common cold, influenza, and mononucleosis.

Signs and symptoms: sore throat; rhinorrhea; sneezing; cough; fatigue; myalgia; symptoms that last < 2 weeks (average: 1 week), followed by continued coughing and fatigue

> Influenza: fever, chills, headache, myalgias

> Mononucleosis (classic triad): fever, sore throat, lymphadenopathy (usually posterior cervical)

Investigations (mononucleosis): CBC to detect lymphocytosis (> 50%); peripheral blood smear to detect atypical lymphocytes; heterophile antibody test (e.g., Monospot); EBV-specific serology testing (definitive)

BACTERIAL INFECTION

Examples include group A streptococci and bacterial rhinosinusitis.

Signs and symptoms: sudden-onset sore throat; fever; rhinorrhea; symptoms that last > 10 days or that continue to become worse after 1 week

Investigations: rapid antigen test to detect group A streptococci

CANDIDA (YEAST) INFECTION

This is common in healthy infants; immunocompromised patients; patients using antibiotics or inhaled glucocorticoids, or undergoing chemotherapy or radiation.

Signs and symptoms: sore throat; white plaques on the tongue, buccal mucosa, oropharynx, or palate

ALLERGIC CONDITION (E.G., CHRONIC ALLERGIC RHINOSINUSITIS)

CHRONIC ALLERGIC RHINOSINUSITIS

Patients may develop hypersensitivity to allergens over time (sensitivity to low levels of allergens). They often do not seek medical attention until symptoms are severe.

Signs and symptoms: sudden attacks of sneezing; clear rhinorrhea; nasal itching; post nasal drip; cough; irritability; fatigue; **no** fever; **no** myalgia

> Perennial allergies (more common) are caused by indoor allergens: dust mites, mold spores, animal dander, and insects.
>
> Seasonal allergies are caused by outdoor allergens: pollens from trees, grasses, and weeds.

OTHER (E.G., TRAUMA, NEOPLASM, FOREIGN BODY)

TRAUMA

Trauma can cause cerebrospinal-fluid rhinorrhea, which is due to nasal or skull fractures.

Signs and symptoms: clear nasal discharge (unilateral or bilateral) without mucosal inflammation

NEOPLASM

Signs and symptoms: chronic sinus congestion; recurrent nasal obstruction; nasal discharge; nosebleeds; unilateral symptoms (**unlike** rhinitis, chronic sinusitis, or nasal polyps, which have similar presentations)

FOREIGN BODY

Patients are often young children and those with intellectual disabilities. Foreign bodies can be lodged high in the nasal cavities or paranasal sinuses.

Signs and symptoms: unilateral symptoms (acute or chronic); history of foreign nasal body insertion; sometimes bloody or foul-smelling discharge

Strategy for patient encounter

The likely scenario is a patient with recurrent sore throat. The specified tasks could engage history, physical exam, investigations, or management.

History

Start with open-ended questions, such as: When did the sore throat start? What other symptoms have you noticed? How often do you get sore throats? Listen for recurrent sore throat and rhinorrhea (this suggests chronic allergy); symptoms of infection (fever, myalgia, sudden onset); and unilateral versus bilateral rhinorrhea.

Remember to ask about possible relationships to environmental exposure: Do you get more sore throats depending on the season?

Physical exam

Obtain the patient's vital signs (looking for fever). Visually inspect the nose and oropharynx (inflammation suggests infection; plaques suggest yeast infection). Examine the neck for cervical lymphadenopathy (this suggests mononucleosis). Listen to the lungs (congestion suggests infection).

Investigations

Based on the history and physical exam, determine the need for a swab for group A streptococci (for rapid antigen test), a heterophile antibody test (e.g., Monospot), and tests for nonallergy causes of rhinorrhea.

Management

Bacterial and fungal infections require treatment, but most viral infections do not. First-line treatment for allergic rhinitis is intranasal steroids or antihistamines.

133

Abnormal stature

MCC particular objectives

Determine whether the growth pattern is pathologic or normal.
Determine whether the child has dysmorphic features.

MCC differential diagnosis
with added evidence

TALL STATURE

Genetic (e.g., Marfan syndrome)
MARFAN SYNDROME
This is a connective tissue disorder.
Signs and symptoms: tall stature; long arms, legs, fingers (disproportionate); high arched palate, crowded teeth; heart murmurs; severe myopia; curved spine; flat feet
Risk factors: family history of Marfan syndrome

Investigations: bone X-rays to determine maturity and growth potential; echocardiogram to detect cardiac abnormalities

Endocrine disorder (e.g., excess growth hormone)

EXCESS GROWTH HORMONE

The common cause is pituitary tumour (usually benign).

Signs and symptoms: large body stature; delayed puberty; large hands and feet with widening distal phalanges; large forehead, jaw, tongue, nose, lips; underbite; wide teeth spacing

Pituitary tumour (other signs and symptoms): headache, vision impairment

Investigations: IGF-1; growth hormone suppression test; bone X-rays to determine maturity and growth potential; imaging to detect pituitary tumour, if suspected

SHORT STATURE

SHORT STATURE IN GENERAL

Definition: ≥ 2 standard deviations below the mean height for children of the same sex and chronological age in a given population (below the 2.3rd percentile)

Genetic cause (e.g., Down syndrome)

DOWN SYNDROME

Signs and symptoms: characteristic dysmorphic features (small head, flattened facial features, protruding tongue, upward slanting eyes, small hands and feet, short fingers, single crease on the palms of the hands)

> Other: ligamentous laxity

Risk factors: older maternal age, siblings with Down syndrome

Investigations: genetic testing (karyotyping will also detect other genetic causes such as Turner syndrome), X-rays of target areas to assess development

Systemic disorder (e.g., chronic disease and treatment complications)

Almost any serious systemic disease can cause growth failure. Typical causes include undernourishment from Crohn disease, celiac disease, cystic fibrosis, and cancer; increased energy expenditure from cancer and cardiac disease; cytokine production from rheumatologic disease; and irregular hormone regulation from renal disease.

Therapies (radiation, chemotherapy, stimulants, glucocorticoids) can have transient or permanent effects on growth.

Investigations: tests for nutritional status and hormones; X-rays for bone assessment

Environmental cause

MALNUTRITION

This includes insufficient nutrition (inadequate food supply; self-imposed restriction; underlying systemic disease that interferes with food intake or absorption, or increases energy needs) and vitamin deficiency.

Signs and symptoms: low weight for height

Investigations: blood and urine tests to determine nutritional status, hormones, and drug use; X-rays (wrist or hand) to detect bone age

TOXINS OR DRUGS

Examples of toxins include lead poisoning (common sources for children are dust in older buildings and lead-based paint), and alcohol and tobacco exposure in utero, which can cause intrauterine growth restriction.

Examples of drugs include glucocorticoids and chemotherapy.

Intrauterine growth restriction (IUGR)

This is in-utero growth below the tenth percentile for a baby's gestational age. After delivery, growth and development depend on the severity and cause of IUGR.

Causes include:

> Placental problems: placental insufficiency; placental malformation; abruptio placentae; placental ischemia or infarction
>
> Maternal problems: medical conditions (hypertension, diabetes mellitus, renal disease, autoimmune diseases); medications (anticonvulsants, anticoagulants, heparin, antineoplastics, cyclophosphamide); malnutrition; smoking; use of alcohol or illicit drugs; low prepregnancy weight; low socioeconomic status; younger than 16 or older than 35; use of assisted reproductive technology; current pregnancy complications (e.g., preeclampsia, threatened miscarriage with heavy bleeding)
>
> Fetal problems: genetic syndrome; intrauterine infection (toxoplasmosis, Cytomegalovirus, rubella, varicella-zoster virus, malaria, syphilis, herpes simplex virus, HIV)

Investigations: ultrasound to measure fluid around the baby, and the baby's growth, movements, and blood flow

Strategy for patient encounter

This encounter will likely involve parents discussing concerns about the stature of their child. The child will be absent on some pretext (e.g., someone has taken the child to use the toilet). The specified tasks could engage history, physical exam (including plotting of growth curve), investigations, or management.

History

Start with a family history: Does anyone in your family have abnormal stature? Does your family have a history of genetic disorders?

Obtain a birth history. Ask about the gestational age of the child at birth and a history of intrauterine growth restriction (IUGR).

Check for underlying conditions such as chronic illnesses and environmental factors (e.g., toxin exposure, malnutrition).

Physical exam

Perform a physical exam looking for dysmorphic features and other physical abnormalities. Measure the child's height, weight, and head circumference, and plot these on a growth chart. Interpret your findings with consideration to the height of family members.

(State that you will perform a physical exam. Because an actual pediatric patient is unlikely, the examiner may interrupt, ask what you are looking for, and provide findings.)

Investigations

Order an X-ray of the left wrist for bone age and a karyotype to identify chromosomal abnormalities. Consider other tests for specific abnormalities (see the information this resource lists in the MCC differential diagnosis).

Management

In suspected abnormal stature, refer the patient to a pediatrician or medical geneticist for diagnosis and further management.

134

Strabismus and/or amblyopia

MCC particular objective

Determine the type of strabismus and the necessary urgency of treatment to prevent severe amblyopia.

MCC differential diagnosis
with added evidence

STRABISMUS AND AMBLYOPIA IN GENERAL

Risk factors: premature birth; low birth weight; family history of strabismus or amblyopia; developmental disability (e.g., Down syndrome, cerebral palsy); head injury

Investigations: cover test; light reflex test

ESOTROPIA (CONVERGENT, INTERNAL, CROSS-EYE): CONGENITAL AND ACQUIRED

CONGENITAL

Signs and symptoms: present at birth; variable angle of deviation (the angle can exceed 50%)

ACQUIRED

Signs and symptoms: onset at age 2 to 5 years (usual); relatively small angle of deviation

TRANSIENT (E.G., PRESENT AT YOUNGER THAN 4 MONTHS OF AGE)

Signs and symptoms: strabismus that resolves in early infancy (age 4 months)

> If no resolution by 4 months, test for strabismus (early treatment can prevent permanent disorder).

> Consider pseudostrabismus: some babies have broad epicanthal folds in 1 or both eyes at the inner corner of the eyelids. These reduce the sclera visible toward the nose and make the baby appear cross-eyed.

IDIOPATHIC (ESOTROPIA AND EXOTROPIA)

NEUROGENIC STRABISMUS (E.G., CRANIAL NERVE PARESIS)

CRANIAL NERVE PARESIS

Impairment of cranial nerves III, IV, and VI can cause the eyes to turn away from the respective muscle. Causes in children include trauma (e.g., birth trauma; head or neck injury); neoplasm; infection (e.g., abscess, varicella-zoster virus, meningitis, Cytomegalovirus); vascular disorder (e.g., diabetes); intracranial disorders (e.g., aneurysm); and neurologic disorder (e.g., pseudotumour cerebri).

Signs and symptoms: strabismus, double vision, drooping eyelid(s), papilledema, history of possible cause (see above)

Investigations: neuroimaging

MYOGENIC STRABISMUS (E.G., MECHANICAL RESTRICTION; NEUROMUSCULAR JUNCTION DEFECT; MUSCLE DISEASE OR INFLAMMATION)

MECHANICAL RESTRICTION

Causes include congenital muscle fibrosis, muscle fibrosis from thyroid disorders (this usually affects adults), and blowout fracture.

Signs and symptoms: compensatory head turning

NEUROMUSCULAR JUNCTION DEFECT

MYASTHENIA GRAVIS

Signs and symptoms: ocular weakness (usually just this) with drooping eyelid(s), blurred vision, or double vision; oropharyngeal weakness (difficulty speaking; hoarseness; chewing and swallowing difficulty); limb weakness with difficulty climbing stairs, working with elevated arms; fluctuating weakness that is asymmetrical and worse with sustained exercise

Investigations: single fibre electromyography; serum anti-AChR antibody

MUSCLE DISEASE OR INFLAMMATION

INHERITED MUSCLE DISEASE

Signs and symptoms: family history of muscle disease (e.g., oculopharyngeal muscular dystrophy, congenital myopathy)

> Oculopharyngeal muscular dystrophy: onset at age 40 to 60; drooping eyelid(s); difficulty swallowing; ocular dysfunction including strabismus

> Congenital myopathy: onset during infancy (sometimes); strabismus; drooping eyelid(s); hypotonia; facial weakness; weak sucking and crying; respiratory distress; dysmorphic features

ORBITAL MYOSITIS

Signs and symptoms: sudden onset of symptoms; periocular pain; swollen, red eyelids; restricted eye movement; strabismus

Investigations: CT scan or MRI to detect inflammation of the extraocular muscles

SENSORY STRABISMUS (LOSS OF VISION DUE TO ORGANIC OCULAR ANOMALIES CAUSING STRABISMUS)

Signs and symptoms: unilateral cataract (this is the most common cause; the cataract can be congenital or due to trauma)

Adolescents or adults: exotropia (usual)

Children (relatively uncommon): onset age 0 to 5 years; esotropia (usual)

AMBLYOPIA WITHOUT STRABISMUS

The usual cause is untreated impaired vision in 1 eye in early life, which leads to the brain's reduced reliance on the impaired eye for vision, and altered nerve pathways between the retina and the brain.

Strategy for patient encounter

This patient encounter will likely involve parents discussing a child with strabismus. The child will be absent on some pretext (e.g., someone has taken the child to use the toilet). The likely tasks are history, physical exam, or referral.

History

Ask when the strabismus was identified and by whom. Ask about risk factors for strabismus: premature birth; low birth weight; family history of strabismus or amblyopia; developmental disability (e.g., Down syndrome, cerebral palsy); and head injury.

Physical exam

Differentiate pseudostrabismus (e.g., lid configuration) from true strabismus by performing a cover test and a light reflex test.

- **Cover test:** Cover 1 eye and wait 1 to 2 seconds. While this eye remains covered, observe the uncovered eye for any shift in fixation.
- **Light reflex test:** Shine a light in the patient's eyes and observe where the light reflects off the corneas. In normal ocular alignment, the light reflects symmetrically from both corneas. Within each cornea, the reflection is slightly off-centre (toward the nose).

(State that you will perform these tests. Because an actual pediatric patient is unlikely, the examiner may interrupt, ask what the tests and examinations involve, and provide findings.)

In an older child, or in an adult, also test the patient's visual acuity and perform a cranial-nerve examination.

Referral
Refer patients with strabismus to an ophthalmologist for immediate management.

135

Substance-related or addictive condition

MCC particular objectives
Identify the issue.

Identify potential consequences.

Provide immediate and continuing support and intervention.

MCC differential diagnosis
with added evidence

ADDICTION IN GENERAL
Signs and symptoms: need to use a substance, or engage in a behaviour, every day; increasing need for the substance or behaviour; maintaining the substance use or behaviour despite negative consequences (e.g., financial trouble; jeopardized relationships); taking risks because of the substance use or behaviour (e.g., driving under the influence; unprotected sex; bankruptcy); unsuccessful attempts to quit; experiencing withdrawal symptoms on attempts to quit

SUBSTANCE USE

Stimulants
Examples of stimulants include cocaine, amphetamines, and methamphetamine.

Signs and symptoms: increased alertness, energy; restlessness; aggression; irritability; paranoia; rapid speech; insomnia; anorexia or weight loss; hypertension; pupillary dilation; feeling of excess confidence and exhilaration; depression as the effects of the drug wear off

> Withdrawal: dysphoria; excessive sleep; hunger; severe psychomotor retardation; **no** effect on vital functions

Depressants

Examples of depressants include sedative hypnotics (e.g., barbiturates, benzodiazepines).

Patients with chronic pain are at a higher risk of overdose.

Signs and symptoms: drowsiness; dizziness; ataxia; euphoria or an exaggerated feeling of well-being; slurred speech; lack of coordination; impaired concentration and memory; nystagmus; low blood pressure; slowed breathing; depression

> Withdrawal (symptoms start 2 to 10 days after abrupt discontinuation): psychomotor and autonomic dysfunction; other symptoms that resemble alcohol withdrawal (see below)

Other substances

OPIOIDS

Signs and symptoms: low respiratory rate; pinpoint pupils; feeling of euphoria; drowsiness; psychomotor retardation; slurred speech; impaired memory, concentration, judgement; skin abrasions from scratching (track marks or pock marks if the opioid is injected); possible avoidance of physical exam, lab tests, treatment referrals

> Withdrawal: rhinorrhea, sneezing, yawning, tears, abdominal and leg cramping, goose bumps, nausea, vomiting, diarrhea, dilated pupils

ALCOHOL

Signs and symptoms: tremor in the hands or tongue; unexplained trauma; signs of malnutrition (delayed wound healing, frequent severe infections, wasting, cachexia); cirrhosis; liver disease; oral cancer; gynecomastia in men

> Mild withdrawal (symptoms start within 24 hours of last alcoholic drink): tremulousness, insomnia, anxiety, hyperreflexia, sweating, gastrointestinal upset, mild autonomic hyperactivity

> Moderate withdrawal (symptoms start within 24 to 48 hours of last drink): tremors, insomnia, intense anxiety, excessive adrenergic symptoms

> Severe withdrawal (symptoms start > 48 hours after last drink): disorientation, agitation, hallucinations, tremulousness, tachycardia, tachypnea, hyperthermia, sweating

NICOTINE

Signs and symptoms: smoking > 20 cigarettes/day or smoking the first cigarette within 30 minutes of waking up; giving up activities (e.g., visiting nonsmoking family or friends) because of smoking

> Withdrawal: increased appetite; anxiety; irritability; impaired concentration; depressed mood; insomnia; constipation or diarrhea

Risk factors for relapse: other smokers in the household; other substance use or alcohol use; depression or other psychiatric disorder; high levels of stress

CANNABIS

Signs and symptoms: heightened sense of visual, auditory, and taste perception; hypertension and tachycardia; red eyes; dry mouth; decreased coordination and reaction time; impaired memory and concentration; increased appetite; paranoia

> Withdrawal: mood changes (depressed mood, irritability, anxiety); changes in sleep patterns; changes in appetite; nausea; stomach pain

PROCESS (BEHAVIOURAL) ADDICTIONS (E.G., GAMBLING)

GAMBLING DISORDER[1(p585)]

Signs and symptoms: symptoms that are present for ≥ 1 year; symptoms that can include gambling with increasing amounts of money, unsuccessful attempts to quit gambling, continuing to gamble despite negative consequences (e.g., jeopardized relationships, work), reliance on others for money because of gambling, irritability (or edginess) on attempts to quit

ADVERSE CHILDHOOD OR TRAUMATIC EXPERIENCES

These include abuse (physical, sexual, emotional); neglect (physical, emotional); exposure to domestic violence; and family dysfunction due to divorce (or separation), substance abuse, mental illness, or imprisonment.

EPIGENETIC CHANGES

Drug-specific epigenetic changes occur mainly in the nucleus accumbens of the brain.

Substances that cause epigenetic changes include cocaine (with chronic use and addiction); opioids and methadone; and alcohol (with acute and chronic use).

COMORBID ILLNESS (E.G., MENTAL ILLNESS, CHRONIC DISEASE STATES, TRAUMA)

Patients may abuse substances to manage the symptoms of comorbid illnesses.

Patients with chronic disease and/or chronic pain can require opioids to manage their symptoms, and are at risk of opioid addiction. They may also use illicit drugs and alcohol to manage associated depression and anxiety.

PSYCHOSOCIAL STRESSORS (E.G., UNEMPLOYMENT, SOCIAL ISOLATION)

Strategy for patient encounter

The likely scenario is a patient seeking to refill an opioid prescription. The likely tasks include history, risk assessment, physical exam, investigations, or management.

History

Obtain a medical history: What conditions have you been diagnosed with? What chronic illnesses do you have? What medications do you take? Do you have a history of addictions or substance abuse? Identify the possible need for collateral information (e.g., from an accompanying caregiver) if the patient is unable to answer or if you suspect the answers may not be accurate.

Obtain a family and social history. Ask where the patient lives and with whom; who is in their family; whether the family has a history of abuse (e.g., physical, sexual) or a history of substance abuse; whether the patient is in a relationship; whether the patient has children, and if so, where the children are; whether the patient works; and whether the patient has been in trouble with the law or has been to prison.

Risk assessment

The CAGE questionnaire is a brief, commonly used screening tool for alcohol addiction. You can adapt it for drug addiction. (**CAGE** is a mnemonic for cut down, annoyed, guilty, eye-opener).

- Have you ever felt the need to cut down on your drinking?
- Have people annoyed you by criticizing your drinking?
- Have you ever felt guilty about drinking?

- Have you ever felt you needed a drink first thing in the morning (eye-opener)?

See the quick reference on screening tools for other options, including screening tools for gambling addiction.

In suspected addiction, assess the risk of harm to the patient. Ask about financial problems; problems with relationships; problems with work or school performance; risk-taking behaviours such as impaired driving and unprotected sex while impaired; and withdrawal symptoms on trying to quit using a substance.

Physical exam
Obtain the patient's vital signs to look for evidence of drug or alcohol withdrawal (tachycardia, hyperthermia).

Investigations
Consider the need to screen for liver disease (in suspected alcohol abuse), and HIV and hepatitis (in suspected intravenous drug use).

Management
In suspected addiction, provide a referral for the patient (and, as appropriate, the patient's family) to addiction treatment or counselling. Refer the patient for other supportive services (mental health, community, medical), as needed. Provide specific treatment for substance withdrawal, if needed (see the checklist for treating withdrawal syndromes).

Administer antidotes in the event of acute intoxication (e.g., naloxone for opioids, flumazenil for benzodiazepines).

QUICK REFERENCE
Online addiction-screening tools
These free online tools are available to clinicians to screen for addictive behaviours.

- **American Psychiatric Association DSM-5 Level 1 Cross-Cutting Symptom Measure for Adults.** This questionnaire can help identify substance abuse and comorbid mental illness.

- **American Psychiatric Association DSM-5 Level 2 Substance Use Questionnaire for Adults.** This questionnaire helps identify particular substances of abuse and the degree of abuse.

- **Brief Biosocial Gambling Screen.** This is a 3-question tool developed by researchers at Cambridge Health Alliance.

- **Problem Gambling Severity Index.** This questionnaire is from the Canadian Consortium for Gambling Research.

CHECKLIST

Treatment for withdrawal syndromes

SYNDROME	TREATMENT
Alcohol withdrawal syndrome	Treat with sedative-hypnotic drugs (benzodiazepines, barbiturates, propofol). Moderate-to-severe withdrawal requires inpatient treatment with admission to intensive care (ICU). Mild withdrawal can be treated on an outpatient basis.
Sedative-hypnotic withdrawal syndrome	Treat with long-acting benzodiazepine or phenobarbital. Provide a maintenance dose for a few days followed by decreasing doses over 2 to 3 weeks.
Opioid withdrawal syndrome	Treat with a long-acting opioid agonist (20–35 mg/d methadone or 4–16 mg/d buprenorphine, followed by tapering over days to weeks). A dose of 0.1-0.2 mg every 4 to 8 hours decreases the severity of symptoms. Long-acting benzodiazepines can be added to control insomnia and muscle cramps.
Stimulant withdrawal syndrome	There are no specific medications to treat this syndrome. Observe the patient.

REFERENCE

1 American Psychiatric Association. Diagnostic and statistical manual of mental disorders. 5th ed. Arlington, VA: American Psychiatric Association; 2013. 991 p.

136

Substance withdrawal

MCC particular objective
Identify the need for immediate and continuing support and intervention.

MCC differential diagnosis
with added evidence

CHEMICAL DEPENDENCY (E.G., ALCOHOL, ILLICIT DRUGS, TOBACCO, PRESCRIPTION DRUGS)

ALCOHOL
Signs and symptoms (withdrawal):

Mild withdrawal (symptoms start within 24 hours of last alcoholic drink): tremulousness, insomnia, anxiety, hyperreflexia, sweating, gastrointestinal upset, mild autonomic hyperactivity

Moderate withdrawal (symptoms start within 24 to 48 hours of last drink): tremors, insomnia, intense anxiety, excessive adrenergic symptoms

Severe withdrawal (symptoms start > 48 hours after last drink): disorientation, agitation, hallucinations, tremulousness, tachycardia, tachypnea, hyperthermia, sweating

ILLICIT DRUGS

COCAINE, METHAMPHETAMINE
Signs and symptoms (withdrawal): dysphoria; excessive sleep; hunger; severe psychomotor retardation; **no** effect on vital functions

CANNABIS
Signs and symptoms (withdrawal): irritability, anxiety, insomnia, bad dreams, weight loss, depressed mood, at least 1 physical symptom (abdominal pain; tremors or shakiness; sweating; fever; chills; headache)

TOBACCO
Signs and symptoms (withdrawal): increased appetite; anxiety; irritability; impaired concentration; depressed mood; insomnia; constipation or diarrhea

Risk factors for relapse: other smokers in the household; alcohol use or other substance use; depression or other psychiatric disorder; high levels of stress

PRESCRIPTION DRUGS (AND HEROIN)

OPIOIDS

Signs and symptoms (withdrawal): rhinorrhea, sneezing, yawning, tears, abdominal and leg cramping, goose bumps, nausea, vomiting, diarrhea, dilated pupils

> Heroin: peak symptoms at 36 to 72 hours; symptom duration 7 to 10 days

> Methadone: peak symptoms at 72 to 96 hours; symptom duration 2 weeks

Strategy for patient encounter

The likely scenario is a patient with opioid withdrawal. The specified tasks could engage history, physical exam, investigations, or management.

History

Start with open-ended questions about the patient's substance use: What are you using? How often and for how long? When was the last time you used? In the case of drugs, determine whether the drugs are street or prescription drugs. Identify the possible need for collateral information (e.g., from an accompanying caregiver) if the patient is unable to answer or if you suspect the answers may not be accurate.

Obtain a family and social history. Ask where the patient lives and with whom; who is in their family; whether the family has a history of abuse (e.g., physical, sexual) or a history of substance abuse; whether the patient is in a relationship; whether the patient has children, and if so, where the children are; whether the patient works; and whether the patient has been in trouble with the law or has been to prison.

QUICK REFERENCE

Mini–mental status exams (MMSEs)

A mini–mental status exam is a common way to assess for cognitive impairment.

Several versions of MMSEs exist. It's good general preparation for the exam to research MMSEs, and choose or prepare a version for your own use (this isn't the only clinical presentation where an MMSE may be appropriate).

MMSEs generally assess:

- orientation to time and place
- recall (e.g., remembering a short list of words)
- calculation (e.g., spelling a word backwards)
- language comprehension (e.g., naming objects; following a written command, a verbal command, and a complex instruction; repeating back a spoken phrase)

Physical exam

Assess the patient's mental status. You could use a mini–mental status exam (see the quick reference), if appropriate (available time may determine your decision, because a typical MMSE takes 5 to 10 minutes). Otherwise, ask the patient for their full name and date of birth. Ask them to state where they are and how they got here.

Obtain the patient's vital signs, and assess balance and gait. Look for tremulousness, agitation, and disorientation.

Investigations

Consider a urine drug screen to confirm which classes of drugs are being used.

Management

Identify the type of withdrawal syndrome based on patient history and symptoms (see the evidence this resource lists in the MCC differential diagnosis). Assess the need for emergency supportive measures (airway, fluid resuscitation, pain management). Ensure a safe environment (hospital, recovery centre). Provide specific treatment based on the withdrawal syndrome (see the checklist). If appropriate, initiate a referral to an addiction program, and to family counselling and mental health services.

CHECKLIST

Treatment for withdrawal syndromes

SYNDROME	TREATMENT
Alcohol withdrawal syndrome	Treat with sedative-hypnotic drugs (benzodiazepines, barbiturates, propofol). Moderate-to-severe withdrawal requires inpatient treatment with admission to intensive care (ICU). Mild withdrawal can be treated on an outpatient basis.
Sedative-hypnotic withdrawal syndrome	Treat with long-acting benzodiazepine or phenobarbital. Provide a maintenance dose for a few days followed by decreasing doses over 2 to 3 weeks.
Opioid withdrawal syndrome	Treat with a long-acting opioid agonist (20–35 mg/d methadone or 4–16 mg/d buprenorphine, followed by tapering over days to weeks). A dose of 0.1-0.2 mg every 4 to 8 hours decreases the severity of symptoms. Long-acting benzodiazepines can be added to control insomnia and muscle cramps.
Stimulant withdrawal syndrome	There are no specific medications to treat this syndrome. Observe the patient.

137

Sudden infant death syndrome (SIDS)

MCC particular objectives

Evaluate fully the possible risk factors and/or causes.

Counsel the family.

MCC breakdown of SIDS risk and protective factors

SIDS IN GENERAL

The MCC notes SIDS appears to arise from the following factors:
1) an underlying genetic or anatomic predisposition, 2) a trigger
(e.g., maternal smoking; airflow obstruction), and 3) the coincidence of
the first 2 factors with a vulnerable stage of development.

It notes that risk factors and protective factors are known.

RISK FACTORS FOR SIDS

Maternal factors

Young maternal age (younger than 20)

Maternal smoking during pregnancy

Maternal alcohol and drug abuse during pregnancy

Late or no prenatal care

Infant factors

Preterm birth or low birth weight

Prone sleeping position

Sleeping on a soft surface, or with bedding accessories (e.g., blankets, pillows)

Sibling of a SIDS victim

Environmental factors

Exposure to secondhand smoke

Bed sharing

Overheating

Swaddling

Protective factors

Room sharing

Pacifier use
Breastfeeding
Fan use
Immunizations

Strategy for patient encounter

The likely scenario is parents who have had a previous SIDS death and are worried about future pregnancies. The likely tasks are history or counselling.

History

The goal here is to get a detailed history of the SIDS event.

Start with open-ended inquiry about the event: Please tell me about the circumstances of your baby's death. Listen for details that point to identified risk factors. Use follow-up questions as necessary: What position did your baby sleep in? What was your baby's bed like? How warm was your baby's room? Ask about secondhand smoke, bed sharing, and swaddling (wrapping baby up).

Take an obstetrical history, looking for maternal risk factors, premature birth, and/or low birth weight.

Ask about a family history of genetic disorders.

Review the autopsy report, if available.

Counselling

Counsel the parents on the risk of recurrence of SIDS. The risk of a SIDS death in the general population is about 1:8500. However, the risk of subsequent SIDS deaths in the same family is considerably higher due to common genetic or environmental factors (as high as 1:100). Note any risk factors present for the previous death from SIDS. Discuss identified protective factors.

Assess the parents' need for short- and long-term bereavement support, and refer them to a psychologist as necessary.

138

Brief resolved unexplained event (BRUE)

MCC particular objectives

Evaluate risk factors and possible causes.

In idiopathic BRUE, use risk categorization to determine the need for further investigations.

MCC differential diagnosis
with added evidence

BRUE IN GENERAL (FORMERLY KNOWN AS APPARENT LIFE-THREATENING EVENT, OR ALTE)

The American Pediatric Society (APS) defines BRUEs as nonspecific, resolved events in infants aged 1 year or younger that last < 1 minute, and typically last 20 to 30 seconds. The MCC notes that BRUEs are idiopathic in most infants, and may involve cyanosis, breathing abnormalities (decreased, absent, irregular breathing), and hyper- or hypotonia.

Risk factors (APS guidelines):

Lower risk: first BRUE; older than 60 days; full term (if premature, gestational age at birth ≥ 32 weeks and current postconceptional age ≥ 45 weeks); event duration < 1 minute; **no** cardiopulmonary resuscitation necessary; **no** abnormal findings from history or physical exam

Higher risk: younger than 2 months; premature (gestational age at birth < 32 weeks and current postconceptional age < 45 weeks); > 1 BRUE

MISINTERPRETATION OF NORMAL INFANT PHYSIOLOGY

The MCC gives the following examples: transient choking because of rapid feeding, or because of coughing during feeding, and periodic pauses in breathing of 5 to 15 seconds.

INFECTIOUS DISEASE (E.G., RESPIRATORY INFECTION, SEPSIS, MENINGITIS, ENCEPHALITIS)

INFECTIOUS DISEASE IN GENERAL

Signs and symptoms: fever, persistent respiratory symptoms

RESPIRATORY SYNCYTIAL VIRUS

This is the most common cause of respiratory infection in infants.

Signs and symptoms:

> Initial: apnea (common in infants younger than 6 months), upper respiratory symptoms (e.g., cough, nasal congestion), fever (common in infants older than 6 months and in children)

> Subsequent (these develop over a few days): shortness of breath; cough; wheezing and/or crackles on chest auscultation

Investigations (it is generally diagnosed clinically): rapid antigen test of nasal washing or swab; RT-PCR; viral culture

SEPSIS

Definition: infection with systemic inflammatory response, dysfunction of ≥ 1 organ system

In neonates, infection usually occurs by vertical transmission. Examples include group B streptococci, *Escherichia coli*, *Staphylococcus aureus*, *Listeria monocytogenes*, *Streptococcus viridans*, *Haemophilus influenzae*, Cytomegalovirus, respiratory syncytial virus, human metapneumovirus, parainfluenza virus, human coronavirus, herpes simplex virus (HSV), HIV, *Candida albicans*, *Candida parapsilosis*, and *Aspergillus*.

Signs and symptoms: fever, tachycardia, tachypnea, poor muscle tone, poor feeding, vomiting, jaundice, abdominal distention, poor perfusion

> Severe: oliguria; mental status changes; shortness of breath; extreme hypotension unresponsive to fluid replacement (this indicates septic shock)

Risk factors: compromised immune system; wounds, burns; catheterization, intubation

> Maternal factors: chorioamnionitis (intrauterine onset of infection); intrapartum maternal temperature ≥ 38° C; < 37 weeks gestation; membrane rupture > 18 hours before delivery

Investigations: CBC with differential (elevated neutrophils is a common finding); CRP; blood culture; cultures of other fluids (CSF, urine)

ENCEPHALITIS

Viral infection is the most common cause: herpes simplex virus, type 1 and type 2 (HSV-1, HSV-2); Epstein-Barr virus (EBV); varicella-zoster virus; Enterovirus (e.g., Coxsackievirus); and insect-borne viruses (e.g., West Nile disease, Lyme disease).

Signs and symptoms: seizures, altered mental status (e.g., decreased level of consciousness, lethargy, personality change, behaviour change), fever, headache, nausea, vomiting

> Infants and neonates: poor feeding, irritability, lethargy

Investigations: blood tests (CBC, differential, platelets, electrolytes, glucose, BUN, creatinine, aminotransferases, coagulation); MRI (to detect brain edema; inflammation of the cerebral cortex, gray-white matter junction, thalamus, basal ganglia); CSF tests (perform lumbar puncture after results of MRI; order CSF protein, glucose, cell count, differential, Gram stain, bacterial culture); EEG (usually abnormal) to differentiate from nonconvulsive seizure activity

CARDIOPULMONARY ABNORMALITIES (CENTRAL OR OBSTRUCTIVE SLEEP APNEA, ARRHYTHMIA)

CENTRAL OR OBSTRUCTIVE SLEEP APNEA

Obstructive sleep apnea involves a mechanical blockage from soft tissues in the throat. It is a common cause of airway obstruction in infants and children, and is underdiagnosed. Central sleep apnea involves episodes of absent respiration without mechanical obstruction.

Signs and symptoms: recurring pauses in breathing of ≥ 20 seconds; possible cyanosis, hypotonia, bradycardia, and/or pallor

> Central sleep apnea: absence of chest wall motion; premature birth (more common)

> Obstructive sleep apnea: enlarged tonsils, adenoids; obesity; craniofacial abnormalities (e.g., micrognathia); mucopolysaccharidoses; conditions that affect muscle tone (e.g., Down syndrome, cerebral palsy, muscular dystrophy)

ARRHYTHMIA

Signs and symptoms: family history of sudden, unexplained death (parent, sibling); irritability; pallor; disinterest in feeding; bradycardia, tachycardia, or arrhythmia

Investigations: ECG

NEUROLOGIC DISEASE (E.G., EPILEPSY)

EPILEPSY

Epilepsy is difficult to diagnose in infants.

Signs and symptoms: episodes of jerking movements with possible changes in expression, breathing, and/or heart rate; recurring episodes with the same symptoms and duration; episodes that occur during awake hours and during sleep; episodes that do not resolve with caregivers' attempts to resolve; episodes that interrupt other activities (e.g., feeding)

CHILD ABUSE (E.G., INTENTIONAL SUFFOCATION, NONACCIDENTAL HEAD INJURY)

CHILD ABUSE (INFANTS) IN GENERAL

The suspicion of child abuse rises with repeated BRUEs with no medical cause, and with evidence of other injuries (e.g., burns, bruises, fractures).

Signs and symptoms (in caregivers): inconsistency in descriptions of the circumstances surrounding the BRUE; inappropriate expectations about infant behaviour

Risk factors: history of substance abuse by the parents or caregiver; unstable living situation of the parents or caregiver

ABUSIVE HEAD TRAUMA

Signs and symptoms: extreme irritability or sleepiness; disrupted breathing; disinterest in feeding; vomiting, seizures; loss of consciousness

METABOLIC DISEASE (E.G., INBORN ERROR OF METABOLISM)

INBORN ERROR OF METABOLISM

Signs and symptoms: failure to thrive; family history of metabolic disease (e.g., glycogen storage disease, Gaucher disease, Niemann-Pick disease)

OTHER (E.G., TOXIC INGESTION, POISONING)

POISONING

The common cause is over-the-counter cold medication.

Other causes recorded in cases of BRUE include acetaminophen, amphetamine, benzodiazepines, cocaine, codeine, meperidine, methadone, phenobarbital, and phenothiazine.

Investigations: urine toxicology screen

Strategy for patient encounter

This encounter will likely involve parents discussing an infant who has a history of BRUE. The infant will be absent on some pretext (e.g., a nurse is taking the infant's vital signs and weight in another room). The specified tasks could engage history, physical exam, investigations, or management.

History

Use open-ended questions to obtain a detailed history.

- **History of the event:** What were your child's symptoms during the episode? How long did it last? How often has this happened? Listen for symptoms consistent with particular entities (e.g., breathing pauses in apnea; jerky movements in epilepsy); episodes lasting longer than 1 minute; and recurrent episodes. Ask whether the infant required cardiopulmonary resuscitation.

- **Infant history:** How was your child's health before the episode? How was it after the episode? What medications does your child take? What conditions has your child been diagnosed with? Listen for symptoms of infection (e.g., fever, cough); persistent symptoms that suggest enduring disorders (e.g., persistent irritability, persistent disinterest in feeding); use of cold medications and acetaminophen; and Down syndrome and cerebral palsy (these can contribute to sleep apnea).
- **Maternal and obstetrical history (relevant for neonatal patients):** What was your child's gestational age at birth? What complications were there during the delivery? Listen for premature delivery and risk factors for vertical transmission of infection (e.g., intrapartum maternal fever, early membrane rupture in labour and delivery). In premature delivery, ask about risk factors for BRUE: birth at less than 32 weeks gestation and/or current postconception age less than 45 weeks.
- **Family history:** What conditions run in your family? Listen for heart abnormalities (e.g., long QT syndromes) and muscular dystrophy. Ask about a history of sudden death in first-degree relatives.
- **Parental psychosocial history:** What are your living arrangements? What is your relationship situation? Ask about diagnosed psychiatric disorders in either parent. Ask about alcohol use and recreational-drug use in either parent.

Physical exam

Obtain the infant's vital signs, looking for fever and arrhythmia. Examine the skin for unexplained bruising, and look for a torn labial or lingual frenulum (these are signs of possible child abuse). Auscultate the lungs for wheezing and respiratory symptoms. Auscultate the heart for abnormal sounds, rate, and rhythm.

(State that you will examine the infant. Because an actual pediatric patient is unlikely, the examiner may interrupt, ask what you are looking for, and provide findings.)

Investigations

Order respiratory viral and pertussis testing in all patients.

In patients at higher risk of BRUE (see the checklist), order an overnight polysomnograph; a complete blood count (CBC); urinalysis and urine culture; chest X-ray; cerebrospinal fluid (CSF) analysis and culture; and a workup for inborn errors of metabolism (tests for serum lactic acid, serum bicarbonate, electrolytes, calcium, ammonia, venous or arterial blood gases, blood glucose, urine organic acids, plasma amino acids, and plasma acylcarnitines).

CHECKLIST

Risk factors for BRUE

The American Pediatric Society identifies the following risk factors for BRUE:

- **Lower risk:** first BRUE; older than 60 days; full term (if premature, gestational age at birth 32 or more weeks and current postconceptional age 45 or more weeks); event duration less than 1 minute; **no** cardiopulmonary resuscitation necessary; **no** abnormal findings from history or physical exam

- **Higher risk:** younger than 2 months; premature (gestational age at birth less than 32 weeks and current postconceptional age less than 45 weeks); more than 1 BRUE

Management

Consider a period of brief observation with continuous pulse oximetry for infants with lower-risk BRUE. Admit higher-risk patients for cardiorespiratory monitoring. Refer the parents for cardiopulmonary resuscitation (CPR) training.

139

Suicidal behaviour

MCC particular objectives

Determine the degree of risk.

Institute appropriate management.

MCC differential diagnosis
with added evidence

PSYCHIATRIC DISORDER (E.G., DEPRESSION, SCHIZOPHRENIA)

MAJOR DEPRESSIVE DISORDER[1(pp160-161)]

Signs and symptoms: symptoms that are present most of the time for ≥ 2 weeks; symptoms with significant impact on day-to-day life

Key symptoms: depressed mood and/or loss of interest in usual activities

Other symptoms: significant weight change; sleep disturbance; slowed or agitated mental processes; loss of concentration; recurrent thoughts of death or suicide

Risk factors: family history of mental health disorders (depression, anxiety, suicide); personal history of other mental health disorders; substance abuse; chronic illness (e.g., cancer, stroke, chronic pain)

SCHIZOPHRENIA[1(p99)]

Schizophrenia is the most common primary disorder associated with psychosis.

Signs and symptoms: presence of active symptoms for ≥ 1 month, and continuous presence of symptoms (active, and prodromal and/or residual) for ≥ 6 months

Key symptoms: delusions, hallucinations, and/or disorganized speech

Other symptoms: disorganized or catatonic behaviour; negative symptoms (e.g., reduced emotional response)

PSYCHOSOCIAL STRESSORS (E.G., DIVORCE, ADVERSE CHILDHOOD EXPERIENCE)

Examples of psychosocial stressors include recent divorce, job loss, financial ruin, death of a friend or family member, and serious medical diagnoses.

Adverse childhood experiences include abuse (physical, sexual, emotional); neglect (physical, emotional); exposure to domestic violence; and family dysfunction due to divorce (or separation), substance abuse, mental illness, or imprisonment.

SUBSTANCE USE

Signs and symptoms: family or personal history of substance abuse; physical signs of substance abuse (track marks on the arms; nasal septum perforation, which indicates long-term cocaine use); tachycardia; tremor and/or sweating

OTHER (E.G., SERIOUS CHRONIC DISEASE)

Examples of serious chronic disease include heart disease, multiple sclerosis, Parkinson disease, and chronic pain.

Strategy for patient encounter

The likely scenario is a depressed patient with suicidal ideation. The likely tasks include risk assessment, physical exam, or management.

Risk assessment

Assess the patient for imminent risk of suicide (see the checklist). Ask if they have specific suicidal plans and intent, and if they have the means to carry out their suicide plan. Ask about previous psychiatric history and previous suicide attempts. Ask about recent life stresses and life events.

CHECKLIST

Indicators of suicide risk

Patients are at risk of suicide if they have suicidal thoughts, a plan, and intent.

The following additional factors put them at high risk of suicide:

- a history of suicide attempts
- access to firearms
- a psychiatric disorder or disorders (e.g., depression, bipolar disorder, schizophrenia, alcohol or substance abuse, personality disorder, anxiety disorder)
- current substance abuse
- male
- lack of social support (e.g., they live alone)
- for children and adolescents: exposure to abuse, violence, victimization, or bulling; family history of suicides; member of a minority in sexual orientation

Physical exam

Assess the patient for obvious signs of intoxication and/or drug impairment.

Management

A patient with specific and immediate plans for suicide requires admission to hospital for psychiatric assessment and monitoring.

If a patient at risk of suicide refuses admission, consider involuntary admission. The regulations for involuntary admission vary by jurisdiction, but generally require a written order by 2 physicians.

If the patient is not at immediate risk, initiate management of the underlying problems—for example, treat depression with a selective serotonin reuptake inhibitor (SSRI), or refer the patient for counselling about psychosocial stressors. Involve family members as appropriate. Ensure the patient has monitoring and regular follow-up (especially if the patient's life, work, or social situation changes) and a psychiatric referral.

REFERENCE

1 American Psychiatric Association. Diagnostic and statistical manual of mental disorders. 5th ed. Arlington, VA: American Psychiatric Association; 2013. 991 p.

140

Syncope and presyncope

MCC particular objectives

Differentiate syncope from seizure.

Identify patients with syncope due to serious underlying disease.

MCC differential diagnosis
with added evidence

CARDIOVASCULAR CONDITION

Cardiac arrhythmia

Signs and symptoms: light-headedness or fainting; shortness of breath; tachycardia or bradycardia; hypotension

Investigations: ECG

Reduced cardiac output (e.g., aortic stenosis, myocardial infarction)

AORTIC STENOSIS

Signs and symptoms: chest pain; feeling faint, fainting with exertion; shortness of breath, especially on exertion; fatigue, especially during and after exertion; palpitations

Risk factors: bicuspid aortic valve; older age; history of rheumatic fever

Investigations: echocardiogram; chest X-ray; coronary angiography; CT scan; MRI; ECG to measure electrical impulses from the heart muscle; exercise testing

MYOCARDIAL INFARCTION

Presyncope signs and symptoms: symptom onset over hours to weeks; fatigue; palpitations; sleep disturbance; chest discomfort

> Other symptoms: shortness of breath; nausea, vomiting; weakness; sweating; chest pain or pressure usually in substernal region radiating to the neck, jaw, left shoulder, left arm; pain on exertion (often)

Syncope signs and symptoms: sudden collapse (the patient is unresponsive to touch and sound; is not breathing or has abnormal breathing such as gasping); hypertension or hypotension; bradycardia or tachycardia (possible: vital signs are often unremarkable)

Investigations: ECG to identify type of infarction (STEMI, NSTEMI); cardiac troponin (preferred diagnostic biomarker)

Reflex or underfilling (e.g., vasovagal, orthostatic)

VASOVAGAL SYNCOPE

This is the most common type of syncope, and is common in young and healthy patients with or without cardiac or neurologic disease, and in athletes.

Signs and symptoms: triggered by emotional or orthostatic distress (fear; pain; prolonged standing; seeing or using needles) (diagnostic)

> Older patients: triggered by cough, urination, defecation, swallowing (possible)

ORTHOSTATIC HYPOTENSION

This is the most common cause of syncope among the elderly. It may be idiopathic or a sequela of Parkinson disease.

Signs and symptoms: light-headedness or dizziness on standing after sitting or lying down

> Blood pressure signs: normal blood pressure when upright; on standing after lying down for 5 minutes, ≥ 20 mmHg fall in systolic pressure and ≥ 10 mmHg fall in diastolic pressure within 2 to 5 minutes (diagnostic)

CEREBROVASCULAR CAUSES (E.G., CAROTID ARTERY DISEASE, TRANSIENT ISCHEMIC ATTACK)

CAROTID ARTERY DISEASE

Signs and symptoms: dizziness; loss of balance; blurred vision or loss of vision; confusion; loss of memory or sensation; speech or language problems; weakness in the face or limbs; bruits in carotid arteries in the neck on auscultation

Investigations: serum lipids and glucose levels; ultrasound of the carotid arteries to observe the quality of blood flow; angiography to examine blood vessels in the neck and brain

TRANSIENT ISCHEMIC ATTACK (TIA)

TIAs ("ministrokes") cause no permanent damage, but 1 in 3 patients have a stroke within a year.

Signs and symptoms: symptoms that resolve within a few minutes (usual); weakness, numbness, paralysis (unilateral); slurred speech; difficulty understanding others; loss of vision in 1 or both eyes, double vision; dizziness; loss of balance and/or coordination

> Embolic TIA: symptoms that last hours, or are infrequent, or that present differently (depending on the migration of the emboli)

Risk factors: family or personal history of TIA or stroke; older than 55; anemia or sickle cell disease; hypertension; high cholesterol; cardiovascular disease; diabetes; obesity; smoking; excessive alcohol intake

OTHER

Metabolic disorder (e.g., hypoglycemia)

HYPOGLYCEMIA

Metabolic disorders rarely cause syncope. Hypoglycemia is the most common metabolic cause and is usually due to diabetes treatment.

Signs and symptoms: palpitations, pallor, nightmares, fatigue, hunger

> Severe: confusion, disorientation, blurred vision, seizures, coma

Investigations: low plasma glucose level (symptoms typically develop at concentrations ≤ 3.0 mmol/L)

Drugs (e.g., antihypertensive medications)

Psychiatric disorder (e.g., panic disorders)

PANIC ATTACKS[1(pp189-234)]

Panic attacks can arise from anxiety disorders, such as generalized anxiety disorder, panic disorder, separation anxiety disorder, social anxiety disorder, and specific phobia. In panic disorder, panic attacks occur spontaneously. In other anxiety disorders, panic attacks can have specific triggers (e.g., phobic objects in specific phobia).

Signs and symptoms: history of anxiety disorder and/or symptoms consistent with a panic attack; history of social or emotional triggers for symptoms (possible); lack of evidence for other causes, including hyperthyroidism (anxiety can mimic other conditions and is therefore a diagnosis of exclusion)

> Panic attack: symptoms that peak within minutes; symptoms that can include palpitations, accelerated heart rate, shortness of breath, chest pain, dizziness, numbness or tingling, fear of losing control, fear of dying

Strategy for patient encounter

The likely scenario is a patient who has had a vasovagal episode. The specified tasks could engage history, physical exam, investigations, or management.

The differential diagnosis for this clinical presentation is challenging and includes a common, benign entity (vasovagal syncope) as well as a number of life-threatening entities. Often, extensive investigations are needed to determine a cause. In addition, the MCC objectives emphasize differentiating syncope and seizure (see the checklist).

History

Start with open-ended questions focused on the circumstances surrounding the attack: What were you doing? What happened? Listen for evidence consistent with particular entities (e.g., shortness of breath in cardiac arrhythmia; chest pain in aortic stenosis; triggers such as fear or prolonged standing in vasovagal syncope, or standing after sitting in orthostatic syncope; vision disturbances and slurred speech in cerebrovascular causes).

Use open-ended questions to establish the patient's medical and medication history: What conditions do you have? What medications do you take? Listen for hypertension, diabetes, heart disease, Parkinson disease, and epilepsy; and for antihypertensives, antidepressants, and antiarrhythmics.

Ask about previous similar episodes and a family history of sudden death.

CHECKLIST

Differentiating syncope and seizure

SYNCOPE
This is an abrupt, transient, complete loss of consciousness that results in postural tone loss. It is followed by spontaneous recovery.

Loss of consciousness has rapid onset and short duration.

It occurs when the patient is in an upright position and resolves when the patient is supine. Tilt-table testing, which changes the patient's position from supine to upright, is useful in diagnosing syncope.

SEIZURE
Epileptic tonic-clonic seizures can induce syncope. This is characterized by a longer duration of unconsciousness than other types of syncope.

Urinary incontinence and tongue biting during an episode suggest seizure rather than syncope.

Electroencephalography confirms seizures.

Physical exam

Obtain the patient's vital signs, including supine and standing blood pressure (looking for orthostatic hypotension). Auscultate the heart and lungs. Auscultate the carotid arteries listening for bruits. Perform a neurological exam looking for focal neurological deficits. Palpate the abdomen looking for an abdominal aortic aneurism.

Investigations

For all patients, order an electrocardiogram (ECG) to look for cardiac rhythm disturbances, a complete blood count (CBC) to look for anemia, and a serum glucose test to look for diabetes. In a suspected arrhythmic cause, order a 24-hour (Holter) ECG monitor. For patients with a history of heart disease or an abnormal ECG, order an echocardiogram to look for valvular disease. For patients with unexplained syncope, order tilt-table testing to look for bradycardia or hypotension suggestive of reflex-mediated syncope. In patients with a probable cerebrovascular cause (with disturbance in vision, focal neurologic signs, carotid bruit), order an electroencephalogram (EEG), carotid Doppler, and CT scan or MRI of the brain.

Management

Specific management will depend on the probable cause identified from history, physical exam, and investigations. Patients with an unknown cause should be referred to an internist for further investigations.

Pearls

In elderly patients, consider the possibility of abdominal aortic aneurism as a cause of unexplained syncope.

REFERENCE

1 American Psychiatric Association. Diagnostic and statistical manual of mental disorders. 5th ed. Arlington, VA: American Psychiatric Association; 2013. 991 p.

141

Fever and hyperthermia

MCC particular objective
Rule out life-threatening conditions, such as meningococcal meningitis.

MCC differential diagnosis
with added evidence

INFECTIOUS CAUSES

Bacteria (e.g., group A streptococcus, *Escherichia coli*)
GROUP A STREPTOCOCCUS

When this infection occurs with fever, it is typically centred in the throat ("strep throat").

Signs and symptoms: sudden-onset fever and sore throat; enlarged lymph nodes in the neck; swollen tonsils, possibly with white spots or pus; red spots at the top of the mouth

Investigations: rapid antigen test, throat culture

ESCHERICHIA COLI

Signs and symptoms: abdominal cramping, diarrhea, nausea, vomiting, fever

Investigations: stool analysis

MENINGOCOCCAL MENINGITIS

Signs and symptoms: fever, headache, Kernig sign (flexing the patient's hip 90 degrees, then extending the knee, causes pain), Brudzinski neck sign (flexing the patient's neck causes flexion of hips and knees)

> Neonates: poor feeding, lethargy, irritability, apnea, listlessness, apathy, hypothermia, seizures, jaundice, bulging fontanelle, pallor, shock, hypotonia, hypoglycemia

> Infants and children: nuchal rigidity, opisthotonos, convulsions, photophobia, alterations of the sensorium, irritability, lethargy, anorexia, nausea, vomiting, coma

Investigations: positive culture in CSF; meningeal inflammation (increased pleocytosis, low glucose in CSF); CSF absolute neutrophil count $\geq$ 1000/μL; CSF protein level $\geq$ 80 mg/dL; peripheral blood absolute neutrophil count $\geq$ 10 000/μL; CT scan, MRI

URINARY TRACT INFECTION

Signs and symptoms: frequent urination; painful urination; pelvic pain and/or flank pain; fever; tenderness over the bladder

Investigations: urinalysis, urine culture

Viruses (e.g., influenza, measles)

INFLUENZA

Signs and symptoms: fever, muscle aches, fatigue, chills, sweats, dry cough

Investigations: throat or nose swab for antigens

MEASLES

Signs and symptoms: fever, dry cough, sore throat, runny nose, inflamed eyes (conjunctivitis), light sensitivity, rash (large flat blotches), Koplik spots (these are pathognomonic: tiny white spots with blue-white centres inside the cheek lining that are present before the rash appears)

> Progression from exposure: asymptomatic during incubation (10–14 days); followed by mild fever, nonspecific symptoms (2–3 days); followed by acute illness and rash, beginning with the face (4 days)

Risk factors: unvaccinated for measles; international travel; vitamin A deficiency

Investigations: blood or saliva IgM test

Parasites (e.g., malaria)

MALARIA

Signs and symptoms: travel to an endemic area (equatorial tropical and subtropical regions, including sub-Saharan Africa, Asia, Central America, South America); recurrent symptoms that begin a few weeks after a bite from an infected mosquito (but some types remain dormant for up to a year); shaking chills, high fever, sweating (common); headache; vomiting; diarrhea

Investigations: blood smears to detect malaria parasites

Fungi (e.g., Cryptococcus)

CRYPTOCOCCOSIS

Signs and symptoms: history of immune-system compromise (e.g., HIV/ AIDS, lymphoma, use of steroids, splenectomy), fever, pulmonary symptoms (cough, shortness of breath, chest pain)

> Later symptoms (cryptococcal meningitis): headache, neck pain, cognitive changes

Investigations: chest X-ray, cryptococcal antigen testing (blood, CSF, sputum)

INFLAMMATORY AND MALIGNANT CONDITIONS (E.G., SYSTEMIC LUPUS ERYTHEMATOSUS, LYMPHOMA)

SYSTEMIC LUPUS ERYTHEMATOSUS

Signs and symptoms: personal or family history of systemic lupus erythematosus; malar rash; arthritis; cytopenias

Investigations: elevated ANA titre; elevated dsDNA level

LYMPHOMA

Signs and symptoms: constitutional symptoms (weight loss, fever, night sweats), enlarged lymph nodes

Investigations: blasts or cancer cells on peripheral blood smear; excess blasts or cancer cells on bone marrow examination

DRUGS (E.G., BLEOMYCIN, INTERFERON)

BLEOMYCIN, INTERFERON

Fever is a common short-term side effect of these cancer therapies.

INCREASED HEAT LOAD (E.G., HEAT STROKE)

This is a multisystem illness characterized by central nervous system (CNS) dysfunction (encephalopathy), and additional organ and/or tissue damage, and high body temperature.

Examples of causes include heat exposure and extreme exertion.

Signs and symptoms:

Two criteria: core temp > 40°C; CNS dysfunction

CNS dysfunction: disorientation; headache; irritability; irrational behaviour; emotional instability; confusion; altered consciousness; collapse (usually from hypertrophic cardiomyopathy in younger athletes) or coma; seizure

Other signs and symptoms: tachycardia, hypotension, hyperventilation, dehydration, dry mouth, thirst, muscle cramps, loss of muscle function, ataxia

Investigations: chest X-ray (to detect pulmonary edema); ECG (to detect dysrhythmia; conduction disturbance; nonspecific ST-T wave changes; heat-related myocardial ischemia and/or infarction); CBC; serum electrolytes; BUN; creatinine; hepatic transaminases; PT; PTT; ABG; toxicologic screening (to detect medication effects)

DIMINISHED HEAT DISSIPATION (E.G., MEDICATIONS, ILLICIT DRUGS)

Drugs and medications that cause hyperthermia include psychotropic medications such as selective serotonin reuptake inhibitors (SSRIs), monoamine oxidase inhibitors (MAOIs), and tricyclic antidepressants; stimulants such as amphetamines, cocaine, phencyclidine (PCP), lysergic acid diethylamide (LSD), and 3,4 methylenedioxymethamphetamine (MDMA); common anesthetic agents (e.g., halothane) or paralytic agents (e.g., succinylcholine); anticholinergics (muscarinic antagonists); and drugs that decouple oxidative phosphorylation (e.g., 2,4-dinitrophenol, used as a weight-loss drug).

FACTITIOUS FEVER

Patients generally have complex medical histories, health care experience or knowledge, and an underlying psychiatric disorder (e.g., somatic symptom disorder).

Strategy for patient encounter

The likely scenario is a patient with elevated temperature. The specified tasks could engage history, physical exam, investigations, or management.

History

Start with open-ended questions: When did your symptoms start? What other symptoms do you have? What medications do you take? What drugs do you use? What conditions have you been diagnosed with? Listen for sudden-onset symptoms following exertion, heat exposure, or drug use; infectious symptoms (e.g., cough, dysuria, diarrhea, rash); constitutional symptoms (these suggest malignancy: weight loss, night sweats); a history of using relevant medications and street drugs (see the information this resource lists in the MCC differential diagnosis); and evidence of immune compromise (e.g., HIV/AIDS, splenectomy, corticosteroid use). Ask about a family history of cancer or systemic lupus erythematosus. Ask about travel to malaria-endemic areas. Ask about relevant immunizations (e.g., measles).

Physical exam

Obtain the patient's vital signs. Perform a full physical exam, looking in particular for sources of infection.

Investigations

Order imaging (chest X-ray, and pelvic ultrasound or CT scan), urinalysis, blood cultures, and lumbar puncture for cerebrospinal fluid (CSF) analysis and culture. Order tests for C-reactive protein (CRP), lactate dehydrogenase (LDH), creatine kinase (CK), thyrotropin (TSH), electrolytes, liver function, antinuclear antibodies (ANA), rheumatoid factor, Epstein-Barr virus (EBV), Cytomegalovirus (CMV), HIV, and tuberculosis (purified protein derivative skin test). In children, consider tests for common pediatric infections (see the checklist).

Common infections in infants and children

NEONATES YOUNGER THAN 3 DAYS	NEONATES OLDER THAN 3 DAYS	INFANTS UP TO 3 MONTHS OF AGE	CHILDREN AGED 3 MONTHS TO 6 YEARS
Group B streptococci	Coagulase-negative staphylococci	Respiratory syncytial virus	Viruses
Escherichia coli	Pseudomonas	Influenza A	Pneumococcus
Staphylococcus aureus	Enterobacter	Enterobacter	Haemophilus influenzae type b
Klebsiella	Citrobacter	Group B streptococci	Neisseria meningitidis
Enterococcus	Serratia	Listeria monocytogenes	Salmonella
Streptococcus	Klebsiella	Salmonella enteritidis	
Listeria monocytogenes	Salmonella	Escherichia coli	
Fungi	Haemophilus influenzae	Neisseria meningitidis	
Herpes simplex virus		Pneumococcus	
		Haemophilus influenzae type b	
		Staphylococcus aureus	

Management

Unstable patients (septic shock) require resuscitation and admission to an intensive care unit (ICU). Administer acetaminophen or ibuprofen for symptom management, and consider evaporative cooling. Treat any treatable underlying cause (e.g., administer antibiotics or antifungals). Adjust antimicrobial therapy based on culture and sensitivity. In cases of infection, consider referring the patient to an infectious disease specialist. In cases of malignancy, refer the patient to surgery or oncology.

142

Fever in the immune-compromised host or recurrent fever

MCC particular objectives

Determine whether a patient with recurrent fever is immuno-compromised and the likely nature of the immune defect.

Perform appropriate investigations to diagnose the source of infection.

Manage, based on the type and severity of the immunosuppression.

MCC differential diagnosis
with added evidence

HOST DEFENSE DEFECTS

Cellular (e.g., HIV, steroids)

HIV

The most common cause of fever in HIV patients is bacterial infection, especially *Streptococcus pneumoniae* and *Staphylococcus aureus*.

> Other causes: viral illnesses; focal or systemic bacterial infections; occult bacteremia; HIV-associated opportunistic infections; malignancy; acute retroviral syndrome (in adolescents)

Investigations: WBCs; blood culture; urinalysis and urine culture; chest and sinus X-rays; lumbar puncture (CSF: cell counts; protein and glucose concentrations; bacterial, mycobacterial, fungal, viral studies; cryptococcal and other fungal antigen tests; cytology)

> Prolonged fever (> 8 days) with no apparent diagnosis requires more extensive testing.

STEROIDS

The degree of immunocompromise depends on dose.

Signs and symptoms: fever; chills; sore throat; cough; frequent urination; increased thirst; pain (muscles, back, ribs, arms, legs, hips, shoulders, stomach, throat); swollen feet or lower legs; redness; sores

Investigations: neutrophilic leukocytosis; decreased IgG levels with high doses or chronic use (possible)

Humoral (e.g., congenital)

CONGENITAL HUMORAL DEFECTS

Signs and symptoms: recurrent upper and lower respiratory tract infections including otitis media (common in children, less common in adults), sinusitis, pneumonia

> Other infections: gastrointestinal infections (e.g., giardiasis), bacterial meningitis, viral encephalitis, severe hepatitis B (HBV)

Investigations: IgG, IgA, IgM tests to detect antibody deficiencies; T cells and B cells to detect deficiencies

Neutropenia (e.g., medication induced)

NEUTROPENIA IN GENERAL

Agranulocytosis is an acute and severe leukopenia, most commonly of neutrophils, causing neutropenia in circulation.

> Neutropenia: absolute neutrophil count < 1500/μL

Signs and symptoms: female (twice as common as males); age 50 or older (50% of cases)

MEDICATION-INDUCED

The most common medications include methimazole, sulfasalazine, and trimethoprim-sulfamethoxazole.

> Other: bone marrow suppressors (e.g. methotrexate, cyclophosphamide, colchicine, azathioprine, ganciclovir); calcium dobesilate (Doxium); psychotropic drugs and anticonvulsants (clozapine, olanzapine); deferiprone; thioamides; ticlopidine; rituximab; quinine; cocaine; heroin

Signs and symptoms: onset 3 to 6 days after taking drug; oral ulcerations with or without fever; possible sepsis

Investigations: CBC; white cell differential; peripheral smear; low absolute neutrophil count (neutrophil count recovers after drug cessation); negative for anemia, thrombocytopenia; bone marrow aspiration and biopsy (hypocellular with low granulocytic precursors)

Strategy for patient encounter

The likely scenario is an HIV patient with recurrent fever. The specified tasks could engage history, physical exam, investigations, or management.

History

Start with open-ended questions about the timing and duration of the fever: When did the fever start? How often do you get a fever? How high is the fever?

Ask open-ended questions to establish associated symptoms and past medical history: What conditions do you have? How has your health been generally? What medications do you take? Listen for a history of immunosuppression (HIV, malignancy, immunosuppressant medications), chronic illnesses, and recurrent infections.

If the patient is HIV positive, ask if they have a recent CD4 count. Ask about retroviral therapy: Have you been able to take your therapy consistently?

Physical exam

Obtain the patient's vital signs looking for a current fever and hypotension (this is a possible sign of septic shock). Perform a physical exam looking for signs of focal infection and inflammation.

Investigations

Order a complete blood count (CBC). Is there neutropenia? Fever in an immunosuppressed patient may be difficult to localize and often requires cultures to find the source (blood culture; urinalysis and urine culture; chest X-ray; lumbar puncture).

Management

Start immediate empirical antibiotic treatment for all febrile neutropenic patients (modify treatment, as appropriate, based on culture results). Hospitalize all unstable patients, and patients with abnormal liver or renal function. Other patients can generally be treated as outpatients, unless their fever began in hospital. Prescribe oral ciprofloxacin, and amoxicillin and clavulanic acid, as first-line empiric treatment. In patients with a history of fungal infection or significant mucosal damage, add empiric antifungal treatment with oral posaconazole, fluconazole, or itraconazole. In patients who are seropositive for herpes simplex virus (HSV) with stem cell transplants, or in those who had an HSV reactivation with previous chemotherapy, add oral acyclovir or valacyclovir. Continue treatment until the absolute neutrophil count is > 500–1000/mm^3, or until cultures identify a specific etiology.

Consult an infectious disease specialist.

143

Hypothermia

MCC particular objective
Recognize the severity of hypothermia and provide urgent therapy.

MCC differential diagnosis
This is listed for information: the cause of hypothermia will not likely be the focus of the scenario (emergency management will).

DECREASED HEAT PRODUCTION (E.G., HYPOTHYROIDISM)

INCREASED HEAT LOSS (E.G., EXPOSURE)

IMPAIRED THERMOREGULATION (E.G., NEUROLOGIC DISORDER, METABOLIC DISORDER, ALCOHOL)

Strategy for patient encounter
The likely scenario is a patient in the emergency room with hypothermia from environmental exposure. Patient simulations using "dummies" are quite advanced and could be used for this clinical presentation. The likely task is emergency management.

Emergency management
Perform a history and physical exam at the same time.

HISTORY
The patient will likely be unconscious, so obtain a brief history from accompanying caregivers: What happened?

PHYSICAL EXAM
Obtain the patient's vital signs, including core body temperature. Obtain intravenous (IV) access. Provide supplemental oxygen and attach a cardiac monitor.

Determine the degree of hypothermia using the following criteria (this will guide subsequent treatment):

- **Mild hypothermia (stage I):** 32°C to 35°C; vigorous shivering, cold white skin
- **Moderate hypothermia (stage II):** 28°C to < 32°C; mental status changes (amnesia, confusion, apathy); slurred speech; hyporeflexia; loss of fine motor coordination; reduced shivering
- **Severe hypothermia (stages III and IV):** 24°C to < 28°C (stage III), < 24°C (stage IV); no shivering; cold edematous skin; areflexia; oliguria; fixed, dilated pupils; hypotension; pulmonary edema; bradycardia

TIP

Working with nurses to provide emergency care

The MCC identifies unclear directions to nurses as a common exam error.

To avoid this error, work out some standard directions for nurses in emergency scenarios. Emergency scenarios are likely to involve nurses, and likely to involve similar procedures to stabilize the patient. For example, if 1 nurse is present:

- Ask the nurse to take the patient's vital signs and obtain intravenous access.
- You start ventilation and attach the cardiac monitor.

If 2 nurses are present:

- Ask for the first name of each nurse present.
- Ask a specific nurse by name to start ventilation and attach the cardiac monitor.
- Ask a specific nurse by name to take the patient's vital signs and obtain intravenous access.

INVESTIGATIONS

There are generally no investigations indicated for acute management situations.

TREATMENT

Treatment depends on the severity of the hypothermia.

- **Mild hypothermia (stage I):** Provide passive external rewarming; get the patient actively moving; provide high-carbohydrate liquids and foods.
- **Moderate hypothermia (stage II):** Provide full-body insulation, active rewarming.
- **Severe hypothermia (stage III):** In addition to stage II steps, provide airway management; use a defibrillator (single shocks) for ventricular fibrillation or tachycardia;

consider invasive warming (e.g., extracorporeal membrane oxygenation or cardiopulmonary bypass).

- **Severe hypothermia (stage IV):** In addition to stage III steps, provide cardiopulmonary resuscitation (CPR); defibrillation; 1 mg epinephrine (up to 3 doses); invasive rewarming.

PEARLS

Remember the rule of thumb that a patient is not dead until they are warm and dead. This means that in arrested patients rewarming is necessary before stopping resuscitation, especially in a child.

144

Tinnitus

MCC particular objective

Understand the distress caused by this usually benign condition.

MCC differential diagnosis
with added evidence

AUDITORY

TINNITUS FROM AUDITORY CAUSES IN GENERAL

This is commonly a sign of hearing loss or cochlear injury.

Signs and symptoms: intermittent or continuous ringing or other sounds (buzzing, clicking) without an external source; variable apparent location of sounds (1 or both ears; within or around the head; distant)

External or middle ear (e.g., otitis, wax)

OTITIS MEDIA

Signs and symptoms: ear pain; fever; hearing loss with possible discharge from the ear

> Otoscopy exam: tympanic membrane that is erythematous (typically) or opaque, white, yellow, or green (this indicates pus behind the tympanic membrane); loss of bony landmarks

Risk factors: upper respiratory tract infection; allergic rhinitis; chronic rhinosinusitis; crowded living conditions; contact with infected persons; exposure to secondhand smoke; family history of otitis media

> Children: attending a day care; bottle feeding or pacifier use; age 6 to 24 months

WAX

Signs and symptoms: hearing loss; pain; tinnitus; vertigo; feeling of fullness; history of recent mechanical cleaning of ears (e.g., Q-Tip use); cerumen impaction on otoscopy exam

Cochlear-vestibular end organ (e.g., medications, otosclerosis, environmental exposure)

MEDICATIONS

Common ototoxic medications include antibiotics (some: e.g., gentamicin), ACE inhibitors, antimalarial drugs, bismuth, calcium channel blockers, cisplatin, COX-2 inhibitors, local anesthetics, tricyclic antidepressants, valproic acid, and aspirin (in large amounts: tinnitus stops when aspirin intake stops).

OTOSCLEROSIS

Signs (on imaging): missing ossicular bones (part or all); intratympanic muscle changes; facial nerve aberrant course

ENVIRONMENTAL EXPOSURE

Noise exposure can lead to temporary tinnitus, but long-term exposure can lead to permanent tinnitus.

Common exposures include workplace saws, drills, and machines, and portable music devices.

Cochlear nerve (e.g., acoustic neuroma)

ACOUSTIC NEUROMA

Signs and symptoms: ear or mastoid pain; facial weakness; dizziness or vertigo

Brainstem or cortex (e.g., ischemia, infection)

Signs and symptoms (in general): history of stroke, trauma, multiple sclerosis, encephalitis

Strategy for patient encounter

The likely scenario is a patient with chronic tinnitus. The specified tasks could engage history, physical exam, investigations, or management.

History

Start with open-ended questions to establish the patient's symptoms, and medical and medication history: When did the tinnitus start? How frequent is it? What other symptoms have you noticed? What conditions do you have? What medications do you take? Listen for a history of trauma, stroke, multiple sclerosis, or encephalitis; constant versus intermittent symptoms; hearing loss; fever, pain, vertigo; and ototoxic medications. Ask about occupational noise exposure.

The MCC's objective for this clinical presentation is recognition of the distress tinnitus can cause. Be sure to pursue this: How is the ringing in your ears affecting your daily life? How are you doing emotionally?

Physical exam

Perform an otoscopy, looking for infection and impacted wax. Examine the head and neck looking for mastoid pain (this suggests infection), and muscle weakness (this suggests acoustic neuroma or stroke).

Investigations

Order an audiogram to assess for hearing loss. If there are associated neurological symptoms, order a CT scan of the head.

Management

Management will depend on the cause of symptoms.

If impacted earwax is present, removal can decrease symptoms.

If an ototoxic medication is being taken, it should be discontinued or substituted.

For cases caused by hearing loss or without known cause, the use of noise suppression may help. Options include white noise machines, hearing aids, and masking devices.

Counselling and the use of tricyclic antidepressants (e.g. amitriptyline, nortriptyline) or anxiolytics may be useful in some patients.

145

Trauma

MCC particular objectives

None stated.

MCC differential diagnosis

This is listed for information: the cause of injury will not likely be the focus of the scenario (emergency management will).

BLUNT TRAUMA (E.G., BLAST INJURIES, DECELERATION INJURIES)

PENETRATING TRAUMA (E.G., STABBING, SHOOTING)

Strategy for patient encounter

The likely scenario is an unstable trauma patient in the emergency room. The likely task is emergency management.

Emergency management

This patient encounter will likely test your management of an unstable patient. Patient simulations using "dummies" are quite advanced and could be used for this clinical presentation. Follow the Advanced Trauma Life Support (ATLS) guidelines, including primary and secondary surveys to ensure all external evidence of injury is assessed.

TIP

Working with nurses during primary surveys

This scenario is likely to involve nurses. The MCC identifies unclear directions to nurses as a common exam error.

To avoid this error, work out some standard directions for nurses during primary surveys. For example, if 1 nurse is present:

- Ask the nurse to perform the airway and cervical spine tasks (protect the spine, provide oxygen, and assess the airway) and then the expose tasks (assess temperature, undress, cover).
- You perform the tasks for breathing, circulation and hemorrhage control, and disability.

If 2 nurses are present:

- Ask for the first name of each nurse present.
- Ask a specific nurse by name to perform the airway and cervical spine tasks.
- Ask a specific nurse by name to perform the expose tasks.

PRIMARY SURVEY

Perform a primary survey first, consisting of these steps (mnemonic **ABCDE**):

- **Airway and cervical spine:** Protect the C-spine (immobilize the patient with a collar), provide oxygen, assess the airway.
- **Breathing:** Inspect the chest for abnormality; assess pulse oximetry and arterial blood gases (ABG).
- **Circulation and hemorrhage control:** Assess shock; assess tissue perfusion; control bleeding from the chest and abdomen; monitor blood pressure.
- **Disability:** Perform a brief neurological exam; assess the patient's level of consciousness with the Glasgow

CHECKLIST

Glasgow coma scale

ASSESSMENT FOCUS	FINDING	SCORE
Eyes	Do not open to any stimulus	1
	Open in response to pain	2
	Open in response to speech	3
	Open spontaneously	4
Limbs	Do not respond to any stimulus	1
	Extend in response to pain	2
	Flex abnormally in response to pain	3
	Withdraw in response to pain	4
	Exhibit localized pain (patient can point to area)	5
	Respond to commands	6
Speech	Patient does not speak	1
	Makes incomprehensible sounds	2
	Uses inappropriate words	3
	Makes confused conversation	4
	Communicates well	5

Interpretation

Score < 9 severely reduced consciousness; score 9–12 moderately reduced consciousness; score 13–14 mildly reduced consciousness; score 15 normal consciousness

Reprinted from The Lancet, Vol. 2, Teasdale G and Jennett B, Assessment of coma and impaired consciousness: a practical scale, pages 81–84, 1974, with permission from Elsevier.

coma scale (see the checklist); check the pupils; monitor blood sugar.
- **Expose:** Assess temperature, undress, cover.

SECONDARY SURVEY

When you have completed the primary survey, immediately start on a secondary survey, which includes:
- **History:** Ask about the mechanism of the injury to determine the likely severity of the injury and the possibility of other associated injuries. Listen carefully and seek clarification through follow-up questions. If the patient is unable to give a history, seek information from an accompanying caregiver.
- **Complete regional physical exam:** The purpose of this exam is to identify all injuries.

INVESTIGATIONS

Based on the findings of the primary and secondary surveys, identify investigations that are useful to managing the injury (e.g., imaging, electrocardiogram). Remember that investigations should be deferred in unstable patients. Order a complete blood count (CBC), and type and screen in case the patient needs a blood transfusion.

NEXT STEPS

Start intravenous (IV) access with normal saline or Ringer's lactate, and give supplemental oxygen. Activate the trauma protocol specific to the institution. In the absence of a trauma protocol, obtain an emergent consultation with general surgery or trauma surgery.

Reassess the patient's response to resuscitation.

146

Abdominal injuries

MCC particular objectives

None stated.

MCC differential diagnosis

This is listed for information: the cause of injury will not likely be the focus of the scenario (emergency management will).

BLUNT TRAUMA (E.G., BLAST INJURIES, DECELERATION INJURIES)

PENETRATING TRAUMA (E.G., STABBING, SHOOTING)

Strategy for patient encounter

The likely scenario is a patient in the emergency room with abdominal trauma. The likely task is emergency management.

Emergency management

AIRWAY AND HEMODYNAMIC STATUS

Check the patient's airway, breathing, and circulation (mnemonic: **ABCs**). Begin resuscitation, as required. For serious injuries, provide an emergency referral to a trauma team, or activate the local trauma protocol.

HISTORY

Perform a history and physical exam at the same time. If the patient is unable to give a history, seek information from an accompanying caregiver.

Ask about the mechanism of the injury to determine the likely severity of the injury and the possibility of other associated injuries: How did the injury happen? Listen carefully and seek clarification through follow-up questions. Ask about preexisting medical conditions, previous surgeries, and medications and allergies.

PHYSICAL EXAM

Remember that abdominal injuries commonly occur in association with other serious injuries, including thoracic and spinal injuries. Hypovolemia and/or shock are common signs of abdominal injury. Look for tachycardia; hypotension; tachypnea; sweating; cold, pale, or bluish skin; altered level of consciousness; and swelling of the abdomen due to excess blood. Palpate the spine for tenderness; listen to the heart and lungs; and check the lower limbs for sensation and motor function.

INVESTIGATIONS

Order a complete blood count (CBC), looking for anemia due to intraabdominal blood loss. Note, however, that in acute situations hemoglobin may be normal even with significant blood loss. Order a blood type and screen in case the patient needs a blood transfusion. In suspected intraabdominal blood loss, perform a peritoneal lavage. Order a urinalysis looking for hematuria, which may indicate injury to the bladder, kidneys, or ureter. Order an ultrasound or CT scan without contrast of the abdomen to investigate the extent of the injury and identify associated occult injuries.

PEARLS

Blunt trauma typically involves a larger area of impact on the abdomen, and so has a greater risk of multisystem injury. This is especially true in events such as impact with an object, fall from a height, or a motor vehicle accident.

TIP

Working with nurses to provide emergency care

The MCC identifies unclear directions to nurses as a common exam error.

To avoid this error, work out some standard directions for nurses in emergency scenarios. Emergency scenarios are likely to involve nurses, and likely to involve similar procedures to stabilize the patient. For example, if 1 nurse is present:

- Ask the nurse to take the patient's vital signs and obtain intravenous access.
- You start ventilation.

If 2 nurses are present:

- Ask for the first name of each nurse present.
- Ask a specific nurse by name to start ventilation.
- Ask a specific nurse by name to take the patient's vital signs and obtain intravenous access.

147

Bone or joint injury

MCC particular objectives

None stated.

MCC differential diagnosis
with added evidence

HIGH ENERGY TRAUMA

Common causes include motor vehicle accidents, industrial accidents (e.g., explosions), and falls from heights. These injuries usually occur with other emergent injuries.

NONACCIDENTAL INJURY (E.G., DOMESTIC VIOLENCE, CHILD ABUSE)

ADULT OR INTIMATE PARTNER ABUSE

Signs and symptoms: disclosed abuse (victims do not always disclose abuse); bruising, scars, healed fractures; recurrent symptoms or injuries; resistance by the partner to having the patient interviewed alone (usual)

Risk factors: pregnancy; threat to leave; partner's history of violence or substance abuse

CHILD ABUSE

Signs and symptoms: disclosed abuse (victims do not always disclose abuse); resistance by the parent or caregiver to having the patient interviewed alone (usual); inconsistency between an injury and the explanation for the injury and/or the developmental stage of the child; other injuries (e.g., facial contusions; marks on the neck or limbs; burn marks; ligature marks on the wrists and ankles; bite marks; lash marks)

Risk factors: history of substance abuse by the parents or caregiver; unstable living situation of the parents or caregiver; dysfunctional domestic dynamics

FALLS

Examples include slipping, tripping, or loss of balance.

Causes include vertigo, gait disturbances (e.g., due to Parkinson disease), syncope, cognitive impairment, substance abuse, medications (e.g., antipsychotics, narcotics, antihypertensives), environmental factors (e.g., loose rugs), decreased vision, and urinary urgency (e.g., due to urinary tract infection).

PATHOLOGIC CONDITIONS PREDISPOSING TO INJURY (E.G., OSTEOPOROSIS, LIGAMENTOUS LAXITY)

PATHOLOGIC CONDITIONS IN GENERAL

These are fractures that occur with minimal force in bone weakened by a disorder.

In addition to the disorders listed here (which come from the MCC's objectives for the exam), malignancy is a possible cause. Bone lesions can result from primary malignancy (e.g., multiple myeloma), or metastatic malignancy (e.g., breast, prostate, lung).

OSTEOPOROSIS

Common sites of fracture are the hip, wrist, and spine.

Signs and symptoms: back pain, loss of height, stooped posture

Risk factors: postmenopausal patients; Caucasian or Asian descent; family history of osteoporosis; history of hyperthyroidism, eating disorders, bariatric surgery, bowel-removing surgery, celiac disease, inflammatory bowel disease, kidney disease, liver disease, cancer, lupus, multiple myeloma, rheumatoid arthritis; use of steroids or medications for seizures, gastric reflux, cancer, transplant rejection; diet low in calcium

Investigations: bone density scan

LIGAMENTOUS LAXITY

Signs and symptoms: hypermobile joints (joints bend beyond the normal range of motion); family history of ligamentous laxity; chronic joint pain; frequent injuries such as sprains, dislocations

Strategy for patient encounter

The likely scenario is a patient with a fracture from a minor fall. The specified tasks could engage history, physical exam, investigations, or management.

History

Use open-ended inquiry to establish the mechanism of the injury: How did the injury happen? Listen carefully and seek clarification through follow-up questions.

Screen for a history of recurrent falls. Identify symptoms and signs that suggest abuse (e.g., recurrent injuries in an adult and/ or resistance by the patient's intimate partner to having the patient interviewed alone).

Physical exam

Examine the injured area, paying particular attention to neurological and vascular status.

Perform a targeted examination to exclude other life-threatening injuries, paying particular attention to spinal injuries.

Investigations
Order an X-ray or CT scan of the injured area.

Management
Fractures require reduction and immobilization in a cast. Refer the patient to orthopedic surgery for injuries that cannot be reduced or require internal fixation.

Pearls
Remember that unexplained fractures in children may signal abuse.

148

Chest injuries

MCC particular objective
Patients often present in shock or with respiratory distress, so pay particular attention to prompt resuscitation.

MCC differential diagnosis
This is listed for information: the cause of injury will not likely be the focus of the scenario (emergency management will).

BLUNT TRAUMA (E.G., BLAST INJURIES, DECELERATION INJURIES)

PENETRATING TRAUMA (E.G., STABBING, SHOOTING)

Strategy for patient encounter
The likely scenario is a patient in the emergency room with chest trauma. The likely task is emergency management.

Emergency management

Patient simulations using "dummies" are quite advanced and could be used for this clinical presentation.

AIRWAY AND HEMODYNAMIC STATUS

Check the patient's airway, breathing, and circulation (mnemonic: **ABCs**). Begin resuscitation, as required. For serious injuries, provide an emergency referral to a trauma team, or activate the local trauma protocol.

HISTORY

Perform a history and physical exam at the same time. If the patient is unable to give a history, seek information from an accompanying caregiver.

Ask about the mechanism of the injury to determine the likely severity of the injury and the possibility of other associated injuries: How did the injury happen? Listen carefully and seek clarification through follow-up questions. Ask about preexisting medical conditions, previous surgeries, medications, and allergies.

PHYSICAL EXAM

Examine the chest (front and back). Palpate the spine for tenderness. Listen to the heart and lungs. Keep the most common life-threatening chest injuries in mind: aortic rupture, pericardial tamponade, tension pneumothorax, and massive hemothorax.

> **TIP**
>
> **Working with nurses to provide emergency care**
>
> The MCC identifies unclear directions to nurses as a common exam error.
>
> To avoid this error, work out some standard directions for nurses in emergency scenarios. Emergency scenarios are likely to involve nurses, and likely to involve similar procedures to stabilize the patient. For example, if 1 nurse is present:
>
> - Ask the nurse to take the patient's vital signs and obtain intravenous access.
> - You start ventilation.
>
> If 2 nurses are present:
>
> - Ask for the first name of each nurse present.
> - Ask a specific nurse by name to start ventilation.
> - Ask a specific nurse by name to take the patient's vital signs and obtain intravenous access.

INVESTIGATIONS

Order a chest X-ray and/or CT scan. Order electrocardiography (defer this if the patient is unstable).

149

Drowning (near drowning)

MCC particular objectives

None stated.

MCC differential diagnosis

This is listed for information: the cause of the near drowning will not likely be the focus of the scenario (emergency management will).

INABILITY TO SWIM (E.G., OVERESTIMATION OF CAPABILITY)

RISK-TAKING BEHAVIOUR/BOAT ACCIDENTS

ALCOHOL AND SUBSTANCE ABUSE (> 50% OF ADULT DROWNING DEATHS)

INADEQUATE ADULT SUPERVISION

CONCOMITANT CLINICAL DIFFICULTIES

Trauma

Seizure

Cerebrovascular accident

Cardiac event

Strategy for patient encounter

The likely scenario is a patient in the emergency room who has experienced near drowning. Patient simulations using "dummies" are quite advanced and could be used for this patient encounter. The likely task is emergency management.

Note that history taking will not be helpful in this clinical presentation, other than to establish that you are treating a victim of near drowning (this is likely to be stated in the case scenario).

Emergency management

AIRWAY AND HEMODYNAMIC STATUS

Check the patient's airway, breathing, and circulation (mnemonic:

ABCs). Initiate cardiopulmonary resuscitation (CPR) if needed. Be sure to demonstrate appropriate airway management: positive-pressure bag and mask, and endotracheal intubation.

PHYSICAL EXAM

Monitor the patient's core body temperature. Identify any coexisting trauma (including spinal cord injury) and implement appropriate precautions.

INVESTIGATIONS

Order investigations for suspected complications, as clinically indicated: arterial blood gases (ABG), chest X-ray, complete blood count (CBC),

---

TIP
Working with nurses to provide emergency care

The MCC identifies unclear directions to nurses as a common exam error.

To avoid this error, work out some standard directions for nurses in emergency scenarios. Emergency scenarios are likely to involve nurses, and likely to involve similar procedures to stabilize the patient. For example, if 1 nurse is present:

- Ask the nurse to take the patient's vital signs and obtain intravenous access.
- You start ventilation.

If 2 nurses are present:

- Ask for the first name of each nurse present.
- Ask a specific nurse by name to start ventilation.
- Ask a specific nurse by name to take the patient's vital signs and obtain intravenous access.

---

electrolytes, electrocardiography (this is recommended), prothrombin time/international normalized ratio (PT/INR), partial thromboplastin time (PTT), urinalysis, drug screen, and urine myoglobin.

MANAGEMENT

Initiate additional supportive therapy: oxygen, intravenous fluid therapy, and correction of hypothermia. (CPR must continue until the patient's body temperature is 32–35°C.)

Recognize possible complications: cerebral edema; anoxic or ischemic encephalopathy; cardiovascular collapse; cardiac dysrhythmia; acute respiratory distress syndrome; and coexisting trauma.

PEARLS

The primary focus of treatment is to recover adequate ventilation, oxygenation, and perfusion: hypoxia is the most common cause of death by drowning.

150

Facial injuries

MCC particular objectives

Assess and control vital functions.

Give management priority to life-threatening injuries.

MCC differential diagnosis

This is listed for information: the cause of injury will not likely be the focus of the scenario (emergency management will).

TRAUMA (E.G., BLUNT, PENETRATING, CRUSH INJURIES)

BURNS

Strategy for patient encounter

The likely scenario is a patient with facial trauma. The likely task is emergency management.

Emergency management

AIRWAY AND HEMODYNAMIC STATUS
Check the patient's airway, breathing, and circulation (mnemonic: **ABC**s).

- **Airway:** This may be blocked by blood, broken teeth, posterior retraction of the tongue, edema from neck damage, or foreign objects.

TIP

Working with nurses to provide emergency care

The MCC identifies unclear directions to nurses as a common exam error.

To avoid this error, work out some standard directions for nurses in emergency scenarios. Emergency scenarios are likely to involve nurses, and likely to involve similar procedures to stabilize the patient. For example, if 1 nurse is present:

- Ask the nurse to take the patient's vital signs and obtain intravenous access.
- You start ventilation.

If 2 nurses are present:

- Ask for the first name of each nurse present.
- Ask a specific nurse by name to start ventilation.
- Ask a specific nurse by name to take the patient's vital signs and obtain intravenous access.

- **Breathing:** Facial injury can be associated with brain injury, which can compromise breathing.
- **Circulation:** The patient may be actively bleeding through the nose or ears, and possibly into the brain.

For serious injuries, provide an emergency referral to a trauma team, or activate the local trauma protocol.

HISTORY

Perform a history and physical exam at the same time. If the patient is unable to give a history, seek information from an accompanying caregiver.

Ask about the mechanism of the injury to determine the likely severity of the injury and the possibility of other associated

CHECKLIST

Glasgow coma scale

ASSESSMENT FOCUS	FINDING	SCORE	
Eyes	Do not open to any stimulus	1	
	Open in response to pain	2	
	Open in response to speech	3	
	Open spontaneously	4	
Limbs	Do not respond to any stimulus	1	
	Extend in response to pain	2	
	Flex abnormally in response to pain	3	
	Withdraw in response to pain	4	
	Exhibit localized pain (patient can point to area)	5	
	Respond to commands	6	
Speech	Patient does not speak	1	
	Makes incomprehensible sounds	2	
	Uses inappropriate words	3	
	Makes confused conversation	4	
	Communicates well	5	

Interpretation

Score < **9** severely reduced consciousness; **score 9–12** moderately reduced consciousness; **score 13–14** mildly reduced consciousness; **score 15** normal consciousness

Reprinted from The Lancet, Vol. 2, Teasdale G and Jennett B, Assessment of coma and impaired consciousness: a practical scale, pages 81–84, 1974, with permission from Elsevier.

injuries: How did the injury happen? Listen carefully and seek clarification through follow-up questions. Ask about preexisting medical conditions, previous surgeries, medications, and allergies.

PHYSICAL EXAM

Expose the face and head to assess all injuries.

Check for neurological dysfunction (this may occur if the force causing the facial injury also fractured the skull or damaged the brain). Assess the patient's level of consciousness with the Glasgow coma scale (see the checklist). Assess the patient's cognitive, sensory, and motor status, and pupillary response.

INVESTIGATIONS

Depending on the nature of the injury, obtain facial X-rays and/ or a CT scan of the head.

NEXT STEPS

For facial fractures or significant cosmetic injuries, refer the patient for cosmetic surgery. In the case of open trauma, once the patient is stable, consider tetanus immunization.

151

Hand and/or wrist injuries

MCC particular objectives

None stated.

MCC differential diagnosis
with added evidence

DAMAGE TO TENDONS (E.G., LACERATION, TENDONITIS)

TENDON LACERATION

Signs and symptoms: pain, swelling, bruising, deformity in the area of the tendon; inability to fully extend joints; obvious laceration of soft tissue

Investigations: ultrasound, CT scan, MRI

TENDONITIS

This is inflammation of the tendons.

Signs and symptoms: pain with palpation or tendon loading; crepitus (this is a "crackling" or "creaking" tendon on movement); observable tendon thickening for superficial tendons; inflammation in the affected area (swollen, hot, red); palpable fluid or lump in the tendon lining

Investigations: ultrasound, MRI for tendon appearance; X-ray to detect calcium deposits around tendon

DAMAGE TO NERVES (E.G., CARPAL TUNNEL SYNDROME)

CARPAL TUNNEL SYNDROME

This is caused by compression or irritation of the median nerve within the carpal tunnel.

Signs and symptoms: numbness, tingling, weakness in the arm and hand

Risk factors: previous wrist injury or surgery; female; history of inflammatory conditions (e.g., rheumatoid arthritis); fluid retention from pregnancy (this resolves after delivery) or menopause; workplace factors such as working with vibrating tools, work that requires prolonged or repetitive flexing (e.g., assembly-line work), and working in cold temperatures

Investigations: X-ray (wrist, arm, or hand); EMG; nerve conduction study of the median nerve

DAMAGE TO BONES AND/OR JOINTS (E.G., FRACTURE, DISLOCATION)

Signs and symptoms (in general): pain and swelling on dorsum of the wrist or proximal hand; dorsal tenderness over the wrist bone; limited range of wrist motion due to pain

Investigations: imaging to describe fractures including precise location, geometry (e.g., transverse, oblique, spiral, longitudinal), and comminution

> X-ray: poor sensitivity for wrist fractures
>
> CT scan: identification of fracture or dislocation, assessing joint surfaces (highly accurate)
>
> MRI: acute and chronic bony and soft tissue injuries, occult fractures, early vascular problems
>
> Arthrography: ligament tears

Strategy for patient encounter

The likely scenario is a patient with tendonitis. The specified tasks could engage history, physical exam, investigations, or management.

History

In cases of trauma, determine the mechanism and timing of the injury. For other presentations, ask about the characteristics of the patient's symptoms. Use open-ended inquiry: Please tell me about your symptoms. When did your symptoms start? Listen for evidence of constant versus sudden-onset symptoms (sudden-onset symptoms suggest fracture); alleviating or aggravating factors (e.g., pain with tendon loading in tendinitis; pain with movement in fracture or dislocation); and symptoms consistent with particular entities (e.g., tingling and numbness in nerve injuries).

Obtain an occupational and recreational history, looking for risk factors for repetitive strain injury (e.g., sports, typing, assembly-line work).

Physical exam

Perform a neurovascular assessment of the affected area. Note its colour and temperature, and the presence of swelling. Palpate the areas of common tendonitis (medial and lateral epicondyles). Assess 2-point discrimination, light touch, and motor function in the affected area. Examine the unaffected hand or wrist, and compare findings with the affected hand or wrist.

Investigations

For fractures and dislocations, order an X-ray of the affected area. For suspected carpal tunnel syndrome, order electromyography (EMG) and conduction velocity studies to confirm the diagnosis.

Management

In all cases, it is important to recognize the potential for long-term impact on function.

Tendonitis is treated with pain management, antiinflammatory medication, icing, splinting, and referral to physiotherapy.

For carpal tunnel syndrome, refer the patient to a plastic surgeon.

Fractures require reduction and immobilization in a cast. Dislocations require only reduction.

In all cases, counsel the patient regarding return to work and recreational activities.

152

Head trauma, brain death, transplant donations

MCC particular objectives

Determine an appropriate management plan, and select appropriate imaging and ongoing surveillance.

When brain death has occurred, activate appropriate organ-donation protocol.

MCC differential diagnosis
with added evidence

This is listed for information: diagnosis will not likely be the focus of the scenario.

HEAD TRAUMA IN GENERAL

Head trauma may result in closed or open head injury, depending on penetration and the status of the scalp. Some brain injuries are not clinically evident and require imaging.

Signs and symptoms:

> Severe injury or complications: altered consciousness; seizures; cerebrospinal fluid buildup; infection; blood vessel damage; nerve damage (this primarily presents as sensory problems); intellectual, emotional, or behavioural problems; communication problems

> Indications for imaging: patients with more than transiently impaired consciousness; Glasgow coma score < 15; focal neurologic findings; persistent vomiting; seizures; a history of loss of consciousness; clinically suspected fractures

SKULL FRACTURE, PENETRATING INJURY

HEMORRHAGE, HEMATOMA (SUBDURAL, EPIDURAL, SUBARACHNOID, SHAKEN BABY SYNDROME)

CEREBRAL CONTUSION

EDEMA (MIDLINE SHIFT)

Strategy for patient encounter

This patient encounter will likely involve the assessment and diagnosis of brain death following head trauma, and the discussion of organ donation with the family of the injured individual.

Note that the scenario may include imaging or other studies already done to diagnose the extent and nature of the head injury, but further investigations are not likely needed.

Physical exam

Three findings are needed to diagnose brain death: coma, absence of brainstem reflexes, and apnea.

Discussion of organ donation

In discussing the case with the family, first offer condolences and determine the extent of their understanding of the medical condition of their relative.

Determine if the patient is an organ donor. The family may know the answer to this. If not, they may have the patient's wallet, which might have a driver's license (which often lists organ donor status) or an organ donor card.

If the patient is not a donor, counsel the family about the possibility of organ donation. If the family consents to donation, determine which organs they are consenting to.

If the patient is an organ donor or the family consents to donation, contact the organ transplant team.

> **TIP**
>
> **Truth telling**
>
> This case engages the need for truth telling. Truth telling involves communicating difficult information clearly.
>
> - Ask about friends, family, or spiritual mentors who could provide support. Help the family make a plan to contact these people, or to use community support services or hospital spiritual care services.
>
> - Use direct, clear language. Make eye contact. Avoid technical terms and jargon.
>
> - Check for understanding. Answer any questions.
>
> - Revisit the family's plan for seeking support.

153

Nerve injury

MCC particular objectives

Identify the peripheral nerve involved.

Identify the level and type of involvement.

MCC differential diagnosis

This is listed for information: the cause of the injury will not be the focus of the scenario.

COMPRESSION, STRETCH

CONTUSION

LACERATION

Strategy for patient encounter

The likely scenario is a patient with peripheral nerve injury. The specified tasks could engage history, physical exam, investigations, or management.

History

Ask about the nature and timing of the injury: What happened and when? Ask whether the patient has had loss of sensation and/or loss of motor function.

Physical exam

Perform a neurological exam of the affected area to determine which nerve is involved. This should include both sensory assessment (2-point discrimination, light nerve tap, pinching, icing, brushing) and motor assessment (strength of muscle movement; reflexes; walking and balance for lower extremity nerve injuries; muscle tone; abnormal or involuntary movements). Examine the same area on the unaffected side and compare findings.

Investigations

Consider electromyography (EMG) and a nerve conduction

velocity study to help classify and isolate affected nerves in cases of chronic injury (e.g., carpal tunnel syndrome).

Management

Management will depend on the severity of the injury.

Closed injuries with partial sensory loss and no motor loss do not require surgery. Consider managing these with analgesics, anticonvulsants, and corticosteroids.

Clean, open nerve cuts require referral to plastic surgery for microneural surgical repair within 7 days of injury. Note that the nature of the injury may delay needed surgery (e.g., crush nerve injuries). Nerve injuries may also show insufficient healing with time: these injuries usually require nerve grafts.

Prescribe physical therapy and/or orthotic devices as required.

Pearls

Remember to inquire if the injury was related to employment. Workers injured on the job can make a workers' compensation claim.

154

Skin wounds

MCC particular objectives

Before closing a wound, look for damage to underlying structures (tendon, nerve, blood vessel), foreign bodies, and signs of infection.

Consider tetanus immunization (in the case of lacerations).

MCC differential diagnosis

This is listed for information: the cause of the injury will not be the focus of the scenario.

LACERATIONS

PUNCTURE WOUNDS (E.G., BITES, NEEDLE STICKS)

CRUSH INJURIES

OTHER (E.G., AVULSIONS, ABRASIONS)

Strategy for patient encounter

The likely scenario is a health care worker with a needle-stick injury (closure of a wound could be simulated, but is unlikely as a scenario for a clinical skills exam). The specified tasks could engage history, physical exam, investigations, or management.

History

Needle-stick injuries involve sharp objects that have been in contact with blood, tissue, or other body fluids from another individual.

Use open-ended questions to establish the circumstances of the injury: When did the injury happen? What happened? Listen for evidence of injury from hollow-bore needles (these carry a higher risk of disease transmission than solid needles, such as suture needles). Ask whether the patient's immunizations are up to date (especially tetanus), and whether they have been immunized against hepatitis B virus (HBV). Ask about the patient's current HBV, hepatitis C virus (HCV), and HIV status. Ask whether the HBV, HCV, and HIV status of the other individual is known.

Physical exam

Examine the site of the injury for signs of skin infection.

Investigations

Order HBV, HCV, and HIV serology.

Management

Treat any skin infection.

If the wound is open and the patient is not up to date with tetanus prophylaxis, administer a tetanus vaccine.

Report needle-stick injuries to the hospital's or institution's occupational health officer, and follow the institution's protocol for antiviral prophylaxis until the HBV, HCV, and HIV status of the other individual is known.

155

Spinal trauma

MCC particular objective

Pay particular attention to the initial immobilization of the patient, and to maintaining airway and ventilation.

MCC differential diagnosis
with added evidence

TRAUMATIC (FRACTURE/DISLOCATION OF VERTEBRAL COLUMN, PENETRATING INJURY)

SPINAL TRAUMA IN GENERAL

Signs and symptoms: spinal pain; head injury (this increases the possibility of spinal trauma); confusion or coma; weakness and/or loss of sensation

> High cervical cord injury: impaired breathing
>
> Thoracic level injury: leg symptoms
>
> Lumbar sacral injury: symptoms that affect 1 or both legs, and bowel and bladder control
>
> Emergency signs and symptoms: extreme pain or pressure in the area of the injury; weakness or paralysis in any part of the body; numbness, tingling, loss of sensation in limbs and extremities; urinary or bowel incontinence; impaired balance, difficulty walking; difficulty breathing

ACUTE DISK RUPTURE

Signs and symptoms: pain; numbness or tingling; weakness (the location of symptoms depends on the location of the disk rupture)

> Lower back disk rupture: leg symptoms
>
> Neck disk rupture: shoulder or arm symptoms

Strategy for patient encounter

The likely scenario is a patient in the emergency room with spinal trauma. Patient simulations using "dummies" are quite advanced and could be used for this clinical presentation. The specified tasks could engage history, physical exam, investigations, or management. The likely objective (and key task) is the initial stabilization of the patient.

Patient stabilization

Address the patient's airway, breathing and circulation (mnemonic: **ABCs**). Ensure that the patient is properly immobilized with a cervical collar and spinal board.

After immobilization, obtain intravenous (IV) access. Catheterize the bladder. (Catheterization is not done on standardized patients, so state that you will perform this procedure. The examiner will likely interrupt and acknowledge the procedure as complete.)

History

Start with open-ended questions to obtain a history of the injury either from the patient or caregivers with the patient: How were you injured? When were you injured? What symptoms did you notice immediately following the injury? What symptoms do you have now? Listen for evidence of loss of motor function or sensation. Take a medical and medication history. Ask about allergies. Ask about the patient's history of surgery.

Physical exam

Consider the possibility of other injuries (pelvic fracture, intraabdominal injury). Patients with spinal injuries may not have symptoms typical of these other injuries.

To the extent possible, examine the heart and lungs. Perform a screening neurological exam to determine motor function and sensation in the limbs and abdomen. Perform a screening exam of the major cranial nerves.

TIP

Working with nurses to provide emergency care

The MCC identifies unclear directions to nurses as a common exam error.

To avoid this error, work out some standard directions for nurses in emergency scenarios. Emergency scenarios are likely to involve nurses, and likely to involve similar procedures to stabilize the patient. For example, if 1 nurse is present:

- Ask the nurse to take the patient's vital signs and obtain intravenous access.
- You start ventilation.

If 2 nurses are present:

- Ask for the first name of each nurse present.
- Ask a specific nurse by name to start ventilation.
- Ask a specific nurse by name to take the patient's vital signs and obtain intravenous access.

Investigations

Imaging is generally deferred until the patient is stable and immobilized.

Management

Obtain an urgent neurosurgical consultation.

156

Urinary tract injuries

MCC particular objective

Consider trauma to the bladder or posterior urethra in patients with pelvic fracture.

MCC differential diagnosis
with added evidence

URINARY TRACT INJURY IN GENERAL

The common cause is blunt, rather than penetrating, trauma.

Signs and symptoms: pain in the pelvis and lower abdomen with urination; abdominal or bladder distention or bloating; hematuria; difficulty with urination

KIDNEY INJURY

This is associated with posterior rib or spine fractures, and abdominal injuries.

Signs and symptoms: bruising, pain, tenderness in the abdomen or flank; gross or microscopic hematuria; shock; fever

BLADDER AND/OR URETHRA INJURY

Distal urethra (e.g., straddle injuries from bicycle riding, monkey bars)

Note that straddle injuries can cause urethral stricture, which may appear years after injury.

Proximal urethra (e.g., pelvic fracture, abdominal injuries)

PELVIC FRACTURE AND ABDOMINAL INJURIES IN GENERAL

Common causes include car accidents and falls from heights.

> These injuries usually occur with other emergent injuries.

> Car accidents usually lead to posterior urethral injuries in the case of pelvic fracture.

> Abdominal injuries that cause urinary tract injury also usually cause bladder injury.

> Men have a higher risk of urethral injury than women.

Signs and symptoms: penile and vaginal bleeding; hemodynamic instability; shock (hypotension, tachycardia, pallor, sweating, decreased alertness, drowsiness, coma)

Investigations: bedside ultrasound; if the patient is hemodynamically unstable, diagnostic peritoneal aspiration and X-ray

Strategy for patient encounter

This clinical presentation is generally associated with blunt trauma. The scenario will likely involve a motor vehicle accident, which means other injuries may be present. The likely task is emergency management.

Emergency management

AIRWAY AND HEMODYNAMIC STATUS

Check the patient's airway, breathing, and circulation (mnemonic: **ABCs**). Begin resuscitation, as required. For serious injuries, provide an emergency referral to a trauma team, or activate the local trauma protocol.

HISTORY

Perform a history and physical exam at the same time. If the patient is unable to give a history, seek information from an accompanying caregiver.

TIP

Working with nurses to provide emergency care

The MCC identifies unclear directions to nurses as a common exam error.

To avoid this error, work out some standard directions for nurses in emergency scenarios. Emergency scenarios are likely to involve nurses, and likely to involve similar procedures to stabilize the patient. For example, if 1 nurse is present:

- Ask the nurse to take the patient's vital signs and obtain intravenous access.
- You start ventilation.

If 2 nurses are present:

- Ask for the first name of each nurse present.
- Ask a specific nurse by name to start ventilation.
- Ask a specific nurse by name to take the patient's vital signs and obtain intravenous access.

Obtain a history of the injury. How were you injured and when? Ask about blood in the urine and difficulty voiding.

PHYSICAL EXAM

Remember that urethral injury may occur with multiple other injuries sustained in an accident. Examine the abdomen looking for pain.

Examine the urethral meatus looking for blood and evidence of trauma. In males, perform a digital rectal exam to examine the prostate for injury. Examine the perineum looking for swelling.

(State that you will perform these exams. Since these exams are not performed on standardized patients, the examiner will likely interrupt, ask what you are looking for, and provide findings.)

INVESTIGATIONS

Order a retrograde urethrogram (for urethral injury), cystogram (for bladder injury), and/or CT scan (for fractures and/or renal injury).

157

Vascular injury

MCC particular objective

Act quickly to ensure revascularization.

MCC differential diagnosis
with added evidence

PENETRATING TRAUMA (E.G., LACERATION)

BLUNT TRAUMA (E.G., CONTUSION, SPASM, COMPRESSION)

The following are examples of acute vascular injuries.

ACUTE LIMB ISCHEMIA

Signs and symptoms: variable depending on the location of vessel occlusion and presence of prior occlusive vascular disease

Occlusive vascular disease: symptoms that develop over hours to days; new or worsening claudication; sudden paralysis of the affected limb

No vascular disease (mnemonic **6 Ps**): **p**aresthesia, **p**ain, **p**allor, **p**ulselessness, **p**oikilothermia, **p**aralysis

Risk factors: cardiovascular disorders (e.g., atrial fibrillation, recent myocardial infarction, aortic atherosclerosis); vascular disorders (e.g., larger vessel aneurysmal disease, arterial trauma, deep vein thrombosis, prior lower extremity revascularization)

COMPARTMENT SYNDROME

Signs and symptoms:

Initial: burning or deep aching pain when stretched (locations include the upper and lower extremities, abdomen, buttocks); decreased peripheral sensation

Subsequent: lack of distal pulse; hypoesthesia; paresis of the injured compartment; ischemic necrosis of the affected compartment if untreated

Investigations: CK concentration ≥ 1000–5000 U/mL; myoglobinuria

RETROPERITONEAL HEMORRHAGE

Signs and symptoms: flank bruising; flank or lower back discomfort; femoral nerve palsy; urinary symptoms (if the bladder is compressed)

Late sign: flank ecchymosis

Investigations: falling hematocrit; abdominal CT scan to detect vascular injury and differentiate from tumour and abscess

Strategy for patient encounter

The likely scenario is a patient with compartment syndrome. The specified tasks could engage history, physical exam, investigations, or management. Note that all acute presentations of vascular injury involve emergency consultation with a vascular surgeon.

History

Start with open-ended questions about the onset of symptoms: When did they start? How did they start? Listen for sudden versus gradual onset, and indications of trauma, burns, or recent extreme exercise.

Ask whether the patient smokes, and about a history of diabetes, cardiovascular disease, peripheral vascular disease, and stroke.

Physical exam

Examine the affected limb looking at temperature, colour, and the presence of pulses. Examine pulses with a Doppler probe.

Investigations

Use Doppler ultrasound to confirm lack of pulses in an ischemic limb, if needed (history and physical exam generally make the diagnosis).

In compartment syndrome, pressure can be assessed with an intramuscular pressure monitor. Measurement of serum creatine kinase (CK) may be useful in diagnosing compartment syndrome.

Management

In a fracture or dislocation resulting in limb ischemia, prompt reduction of the fracture may restore blood flow. However, emergency referral to a surgeon (vascular, plastic, or general, depending on the location of the blockage) is generally needed. In retroperitoneal hemorrhage (considered an unlikely scenario for this clinical presentation), a high index of suspicion is needed following trauma to the abdomen.

158

Dysuria, urinary frequency and urgency, and/or pyuria

MCC particular objectives
None stated.

MCC differential diagnosis
with added evidence

URINARY TRACT INFECTION (E.G., CYSTITIS, PROSTATITIS, PYELONEPHRITIS)
Signs and symptoms (in general): frequent urination; painful urination; pelvic pain and/or flank pain; fever; tenderness over the bladder; history of prostatism

Investigations: urinalysis, urine culture

SEXUALLY TRANSMITTED INFECTION
Signs and symptoms: lower abdominal and pelvic pain; pain during intercourse; fever; urinary symptoms (often); vaginal or urethral discharge (anal discharge in anal sex); irregular menstruation

Risk factors: unprotected sex, multiple sexual partners

Investigations: cultures to detect gonorrhea and/or chlamydia

NONINFECTIOUS URINARY TRACT INFLAMMATION (E.G., TRAUMA, INTERSTITIAL CYSTITIS, BLADDER CARCINOMA, BLADDER STONES, URETHRAL STRICTURE)

NONINFECTIOUS URINARY TRACT INFLAMMATION IN GENERAL
Signs and symptoms: weak urine stream, dribbling; painful urination; increased urinary frequency or urgency; inability to empty bladder; nocturia; pelvic pain; abdominal pain; abdominal distention

TRAUMA
Examples of trauma include blunt trauma, penetrating wounds, pelvic fracture, straddle injury, and surgery.

INTERSTITIAL CYSTITIS (PAINFUL BLADDER SYNDROME)
Signs and symptoms: chronic symptoms (≥ 6 weeks), often relapsing and remitting; bladder or pelvic discomfort or pressure, spreading to the lower abdomen and back; tenderness at affected areas; symptoms

triggered by coffee, tea, alcohol, carbonated drinks, tomatoes, bananas, citrus (possible); history of urinary tract infections, autoimmune disorders, irritable bowel syndrome

Investigations: urinalysis; urine cytology; pelvic and/or abdominal imaging

BLADDER CARCINOMA

Signs and symptoms: gross or microscopic hematuria; painless

> Advanced or metastatic cancer: pain in the flank, abdomen, pelvis, bone

Investigations: cystoscopy with transurethral resection and biopsy; upper urinary tract imaging

BLADDER STONES

Signs and symptoms: often asymptomatic; recurrent severe pain in the lower abdomen and back; nausea, vomiting; chills; fever; hematuria; cloudy or dark urine

Investigations: urinalysis; ultrasonography; X-ray; cytoscopy

URETHRAL STRICTURE

This is a narrowing of the urethra due to injury, instrumentation, or infection.

Signs of injury: blood along the perineum or at the urethral meatus; high-riding prostate gland

> Extreme traumas: shock (pallor, tachycardia)

Investigations: urethrogram (X-ray); cytoscopy

VULVOVAGINITIS

VULVOVAGINAL CANDIDIASIS (MOST COMMON)

Signs and symptoms: thick, white, clumpy ("curd-like") vaginal discharge; vulvar pruritus, burning, soreness; thrush patches loosely adherent to the vulva; erythema and edema of the vestibule, labia majora, labia minora

Risk factors: diabetes; pregnancy; estrogen therapy; recent antibiotic use; contraceptive devices; immunosuppression

Investigations: normal vaginal pH (4–4.5); wet-mount test of discharge with potassium hydroxide preparation to detect yeast

ATROPHIC VAGINITIS

Signs and symptoms: postmenopausal patients (most common); vaginal pain, soreness; painful vaginal discharge; painful intercourse; vaginal bleeding, spotting

Investigations: wet mount to detect WBCs and decrease in *Lactobacillus*

VULVAR VESTIBULITIS

Signs and symptoms: vaginal pain, soreness, burning; vulvar burning; symptoms that are aggravated by stress, exercise, tight clothing, intercourse, tampon insertion; irritating vaginal discharge; erythema around the vestibular glands

CONTACT DERMATITIS

Signs and symptoms: use of scented panty liners, pads, soaps, lotions, detergents, bubble baths; use of douches, spermicides, certain topical drugs (e.g., povidone-iodine); vaginal or vulvar pruritus, pain, burning; red, edematous skin; erosions; ulcers; necrosis

Strategy for patient encounter

The likely scenario is a patient with a urinary tract infection (UTI). The specified tasks could engage history, physical exam, investigations, or management.

The key objective is to differentiate infectious causes, such as UTI and sexually transmitted infection (STI), from noninfectious causes.

History

Start with open-ended questions about the urinary symptoms: When did they start? What did you notice when they started? Listen for information about the onset of symptoms (sudden onset is usual in infectious causes); fever or flank pain (these suggest UTI); and genital rash or other lesions (these suggest STI).

Establish whether the patient is sexually active and whether the symptoms appeared following sex (this suggests UTI or STI).

In men, ask about the symptoms of prostatism: nocturia and frequent voiding.

Physical exam

Palpate over the bladder looking for tenderness. Examine the urethral meatus looking for redness and other lesions (note that this exam is not necessary in straightforward UTIs). In males, perform a prostate exam looking for enlargement and tenderness.

(State that you will perform exams of the urethral meatus and prostate. Since these exams are not performed on standardized patients, the examiner will likely interrupt, ask what you are looking for, and provide findings.)

Investigations

Order a urinalysis and urine culture. In possible STI, perform a vaginal or urethral swab for chlamydia and gonorrhea. In recurrent UTI, order an ultrasound to determine the presence of a predisposing condition (e.g., urine stasis; presence of a stone or foreign body).

Management
Management will depend on the specific diagnosis. In recurrent UTIs related to sexual activity, antibiotic prophylaxis may be indicated.

Pearls
UTI is the most common cause of dysuria, but it needs to be differentiated from other, potentially more serious, causes (including STI, which can lead to infertility).

159

Polyuria and/or polydipsia

MCC particular objectives
None stated.

MCC differential diagnosis
with added evidence

WATER DIURESIS

Excessive intake (primary polydipsia)
Risk factors: middle-aged, female; use of phenothiazine (psychiatric patients); sarcoidosis; hypothalamic lesions

Investigations: low plasma sodium concentration (the lower limit of normal is 134–135 mmol/L) with low urine osmolality (urine osmolality is less than serum osmolality)

Excessive loss (diabetes insipidus)
DIABETES INSIPIDUS (DI) IN GENERAL
Signs and symptoms: excessive urine excretion or loss (3–30 L/day)

Investigations: high-normal plasma sodium concentration (> 142 mmol/L); low urine specific gravity; low urine osmolality

CENTRAL DI

This is caused by deficient secretion of antidiuretic hormone (ADH) due to hypothalamic-pituitary disorders. Most cases are idiopathic. Other common causes include trauma, pituitary surgery, and hypoxic or ischemic encephalopathy.

Signs and symptoms: sudden-onset symptoms (usual in adult patients); polyuria; nocturia; polydipsia; neurologic symptoms (with underlying neurological disease); decreased bone mineral density at the lumbar spine and femoral neck

> Moderate to severe hypernatremia occurs in patients with hypodipsia because of central nervous system lesions (plasma sodium concentration > 160 mmol/L); in infants and young children who cannot freely access water; and in postoperative patients with unrecognized DI.

NEPHROGENIC DI

This is caused by renal resistance to antidiuretic hormone (ADH) (patients have normal ADH excretion). It is common in elderly people, those with underlying renal disease, and those with a long-term history of lithium use. In children, it is mostly caused by inherited defects: X-linked hereditary nephrogenic DI is due to mutations in the *AVPR2* gene encoding the ADH receptor V2; autosomal recessive and dominant nephrogenic DI is due to mutations in the aquaporin-2 gene.

Signs and symptoms: gradual onset (usual)

OSMOTIC DIURESIS

Sugar: diabetes mellitus

Signs and symptoms in addition to polydipsia, polyuria: personal or family history of diabetes; history of diabetic complications and/or inadequate monitoring; weight loss, or obesity, or current pregnancy (gestational diabetes); blurred vision; thirst; fatigue; hunger

Investigations: fasting glucose or HbA_{1c} test

Urea: chronic renal disease

This is also known as chronic kidney disease (CKD). It is often not reversible. It is more common in the elderly, and is associated with increased risk of cardiovascular disease, end-stage renal disease, infection, cancer, and mortality.

Definition: kidney damage (urinary albumin excretion of $\geq$ 30 mg/day) or decreased glomerular filtration rate (GFR) (< 60 mL/min/1.73 m^2 for at least 3 months)

Five stages of CKD:

> Stage 1: normal or increased GFR (> 90 mL/min/1.73 m^2)
>
> Stage 2: mild reduction in GFR (60–89 mL/min/1.73 m^2)
>
> Stage 3a, 3b: moderate reduction in GFR (3a: 45–59 mL/min/1.73 m^2; 3b: 30–44 mL/min/1.73 m^2)
>
> Stage 4: severe reduction in GFR (12–29 mL/min/1.73 m^2)
>
> Stage 5 (renal failure): GFR < 15 mL/min/1.73 m^2

Signs and symptoms:

Stages 1–3: asymptomatic

Stages 4–5: fluid and electrolyte imbalance (volume overload, hyperkalemia, metabolic acidosis, hyperphosphatemia); hormonal or systemic dysfunction (anorexia, nausea, vomiting, fatigue, hypertension, anemia, malnutrition, hyperlipidemia, bone disease); pericarditis; pleuritis; central nervous system (CNS) abnormalities (loss of concentration, confusion, lethargy, seizures); depression; pruritus

Salts: organic anions

Signs and symptoms: acute onset; polyuria; volume expansion due to large volumes of intravenous saline or to the release of bilateral urinary tract obstruction

Investigations: urine osmolality > 300 mmol/kg; increased total solute excretion (normal water diuresis is 600–900 mmol/day)

Strategy for patient encounter

The likely scenario is a patient with polyuria. The specified tasks could engage history, physical exam, investigations (including interpreting lab results), or management.

History

Start with open-ended questions about the symptoms: When did the polyuria or polydipsia start? What other symptoms have you noticed? Listen for evidence consistent with particular entities (e.g., sudden-onset symptoms, nocturia, and neurologic symptoms in central diabetes mellitus; weight loss in diabetes mellitus).

Ask open-ended questions to establish the patient's medical and medication history: What conditions do you have? What conditions run in your family? What medications do you take? Listen for a history of diabetes or sarcoidosis, and use of phenothiazine or lithium.

Physical exam

Obtain the patient's vital signs and look for peripheral edema (this suggests chronic kidney disease). If the symptoms suggest intracranial pathology, perform a neurological exam.

Investigations

Order glucose or glycated hemoglobin (HbA_{1c}) tests to check for diabetes. Order a urinalysis to look for proteinuria. Order tests for serum electrolytes, serum osmolality, urine electrolytes, urine specific gravity, and urine osmolality. (For interpretations of these tests, see the information this resource lists in the MCC differential diagnosis.)

Management

Patients with diabetes should be prescribed glucose-lowering medications. Patients with chronic kidney disease require referral to a nephrologist. Patients with diabetes insipidus require referral to an endocrinologist.

Pearls

It is important to distinguish true polyuria from frequent urination. The latter may be due to infection or urinary obstruction.

160

Urinary tract obstruction

MCC particular objectives

None stated.

MCC differential diagnosis
with added evidence

URINARY TRACT OBSTRUCTION IN GENERAL

Signs and symptoms: pain (e.g., costovertebral tenderness or abdominal tenderness from bladder distention); change in urine output; hypertension; hematuria

Investigations: elevated serum creatinine; ultrasound

INFECTION AND INFLAMMATION (E.G., CYSTITIS, PROSTATITIS)

CYSTITIS

Signs and symptoms: frequent urination; painful urination; pelvic pain and/or flank pain; fever; tenderness over the bladder

Investigations: urinalysis, urine culture

PROSTATITIS

PROSTATITIS IN GENERAL

This condition affects men of all ages.

Risk factors: young and middle-aged men; previous prostatitis; previous bladder infections or urinary tract infections (UTIs); pelvic trauma (e.g., from biking or horseback riding); previous use of urinary catheter; HIV/AIDS; previous prostate biopsies

CHRONIC PROSTATITIS

This is the most common form of prostatitis.

Signs and symptoms: urinary, genital, and/or pelvic pain for ≥ 3 months of the past 6 months; pain in the perineum, lower abdomen, testicles, penis, or with ejaculation; difficulty with urination

Investigations: negative urine culture

CHRONIC BACTERIAL PROSTATITIS

This is due to chronic or recurrent UTIs that enter the prostate.

Signs and symptoms: UTI symptoms (frequent and urgent urination; difficult or painful urination; perineal discomfort; low grade fever); pain in the perineum, lower abdomen, testicles, penis, or with ejaculation; blood in the semen (sometimes)

Investigations: urine culture (if positive, it is usually *E. coli*)

ACUTE BACTERIAL PROSTATITIS

This is the least common form of bacterial prostatitis.

Signs and symptoms: fever; chills; muscle pain; malaise; urinary frequency and urgency; nocturia; pelvic and genital pain; difficult or painful urination; cloudy urine; tender prostate that is warm, firm, edematous on prostate exam

Investigations: CBC for peripheral leukocytosis; urinalysis and culture for pyuria, bacteriuria (*E. coli*); elevated CRP; elevated ESR

STRUCTURAL CONDITION (E.G., STONES, TUMOUR, BENIGN PROSTATIC HYPERTROPHY)

STONES

Stones can occur in adults of all ages.

Signs and symptoms: severe flank pain; severe renal or ureteral colic pain (associated with obstruction due to ureteral stone); nausea, vomiting; difficult or painful urination; urinary urgency; gross hematuria

Investigations: CT scan

TUMOUR

Tumours can cause external compression that leads to intrarenal and urethral obstruction, and renal failure, in cancer patients.

Signs and symptoms: older adult (more common); pain if mass is present

BENIGN PROSTATIC HYPERTROPHY

A flow rate < 15 mL/second suggests obstruction.

Signs and symptoms: older male; urinary frequency, urgency, hesitancy, intermittency; nocturia; dribbling, incomplete bladder emptying; bladder distention (sometimes); nontender, enlarged prostate with rubbery consistency and lack of median furrow on digital rectal exam, urodynamic studies

Investigations: transrectal ultrasound of the prostate

MEDICAL CONDITIONS (E.G., DIABETES MELLITUS, MULTIPLE SCLEROSIS)

DIABETES

Signs and symptoms: personal or family history of diabetes; history of diabetic complications and/or inadequate monitoring; polydipsia, polyuria, and/or weight loss

Investigations: fasting glucose or HbA_{1c} test

MULTIPLE SCLEROSIS

Signs and symptoms: variable depending on lesion location

> Spinal cord: sensory or motor dysfunction; Lhermitte sign (paresthesias radiating down the extremities or trunk with neck flexion); bowel, bladder or erectile dysfunction
>
> Brainstem: double vision; swallowing, speech difficulties; vertigo; pseudobulbar palsy
>
> Cerebrum: cognitive impairment; depression; upper motor neuron signs; unilateral motor or sensory deficits
>
> Cerebellum: problems with balance and coordination; vertigo
>
> Other symptoms: tonic spasms; fatigue; pain; exercise intolerance; temperature sensitivity; painful unilateral loss of visual acuity

Risk factors: younger than 50, female

Investigations: brain and spinal cord MRI, including advanced MRI techniques, with established occurrence of multiple episodes; CSF fluid analysis

DRUGS (E.G., ANTICHOLINERGICS, OPIOIDS)

Strategy for patient encounter

The likely scenario is a male patient with nocturia. The specified tasks could engage history, physical exam, investigations, or management.

History

Start with open-ended questions about the urinary symptoms: When did the symptoms start? What is it like when you urinate? What other symptoms have you noticed with urination? Listen for evidence consistent with obstruction: frequent urination or frequent urge to urinate; nighttime urination; blood in the urine; and pain with urination. If the patient indicates frequent urination, ask if the quantity voided is large or small (it is large and frequent in diabetes).

Ask open-ended questions to establish the patient's medical and medication history: What conditions do you have? How has your health been generally? What medications do you take? Listen for a history of, or symptoms consistent with, diabetes (polydipsia, weight loss, fatigue), multiple sclerosis (e.g., sensory or motor dysfunction; Lhermitte sign; bowel or erectile dysfunction; fatigue); or infection (fever; pelvic, bladder, or genital pain). Listen for use of anticholinergics or opioids.

Physical exam

Examine the abdomen looking for masses, tenderness, and a palpable bladder. In females, perform a pelvic exam looking for an enlarged uterus or other masses. In males, perform a rectal exam looking for an enlarged prostate.

(State that you will perform a pelvic or rectal exam. Since these exams are not performed on standardized patients, the examiner will likely interrupt, ask what you are looking for, and provide findings.)

Investigations

For all patients, order a urinalysis looking for infection or blood. Order a creatinine test to assess renal function. If a diagnosis is not obvious from the history, physical exam, and the above investigations, order imaging of the bladder, kidneys, and pelvis (ultrasound, CT scan, or MRI) to look for sources of obstruction. In males with an enlarged prostate, consider ordering a test for prostate-specific antigen (PSA).

Management

Management will depend on the specific diagnosis, but in all cases be aware of the risk of impaired renal function and consequent uremia. Patients with impaired renal function require urgent referral to a urologist.

161

Vaginal bleeding: excessive, irregular, abnormal

MCC particular objectives

None stated.

MCC differential diagnosis
with added evidence

PREMENARCHAL CONDITION (E.G., TRAUMA, SEXUAL ABUSE)

TRAUMA

Most vaginal trauma in girls is unintentional and due to blunt, nonpenetrating minor vaginal injuries that commonly occur in car accidents, falls in the bathroom at home, and accidents from bicycles, the playground, or swimming pool.

Penetrating injuries that lacerate the vaginal wall can cause life-threatening hemorrhage. Causes of these injuries include: high pressure water jets from water slides or fountains; water- or jet-skiing accidents; and intercourse.

CHILD SEXUAL ABUSE

Signs and symptoms: disclosed abuse (victims do not always disclose abuse); resistance by the parent or caregiver to having the child interviewed alone (usual); coexisting signs of physical or emotional abuse (bruising, scars, healed fractures; developmental delay and/or behavioural problems)

Risk factors: history of substance abuse by the parents or caregiver; unstable living situation of the parents or caregiver; dysfunctional domestic dynamics

PREMENOPAUSAL CONDITION

Ovulatory condition

INTERMENSTRUAL CONDITION (E.G., ORAL CONTRACEPTIVES, BENIGN GROWTHS)

ORAL CONTRACEPTIVES

Symptoms differ by type of oral contraceptive:

> Progestin-only: irregular uterine bleeding or amenorrhea
>
> Estrogen-progestin: unscheduled bleeding, especially in the first 3 months of use

BENIGN GROWTHS

Examples include leiomyoma, adenomyosis, and cervical polyps.

LEIOMYOMA

This is the most common pelvic tumour in women (usually in reproductive-age women).

Signs and symptoms: commonly asymptomatic; premenopausal (usual); heavy or prolonged menstrual bleeding; pelvic, abdominal pressure; pain on intercourse; urinary symptoms (incontinence; frequent urination; difficulty emptying the bladder); constipation; pelvic mass or enlarged, irregular uterus on bimanual palpation

Risk factors: family history of leiomyoma; African descent

Investigations: ultrasound to detect mass ≥ 1 cm in diameter

ADENOMYOSIS

This is often diagnosed by microscopic examination of the uterus at the time of hysterectomy.

Signs and symptoms: asymptomatic (often: a third of cases); parity (more common than nulliparity); heavy and prolonged menstrual bleeding; dysmenorrhea; enlarged uterus; pelvic pain

Investigations: ultrasound and MRI (T2) (this is increasingly used for clinical decision making)

CERVICAL POLYPS

Signs and symptoms: older than 40 (common); if symptomatic, bleeding and excessive discharge

Investigations: histology (cervical polyps rarely become malignant, but this should be confirmed)

MENORRHAGIA

Signs and symptoms: change from a woman's normal menstrual cycle that interferes with her quality of life; pain during menstruation; containment problems; anemia (fatigue, pallor, dizziness, shortness of breath, tachycardia)

Investigations: CBC with platelets; tests for coagulation disorders (rare); thyrotropin (TSH) to detect thyroid disorders; transvaginal or transabdominal ultrasound; endometrial biopsy to detect cancer

NEOPLASMS OR COAGULATION DISORDERS

NEOPLASMS—SEE BELOW

COAGULATION DISORDERS

Signs and symptoms: use of anticoagulants; easy bruising or bleeding

OTHER (E.G., ENDOMETRITIS, HYPOTHYROIDISM)

ENDOMETRITIS

Signs and symptoms: pelvic pain associated with menstruation (very common); excessive bleeding during menstruation; pain during intercourse; pain during urination or bowel movement

Risk factors: family history of endometriosis; nulliparity; personal history of pelvic inflammatory disease; tenderness on pelvic exam; normal findings on abdominal exam (common)

Investigations: ultrasound to detect ovarian cysts (common finding); laparoscopy with biopsy

HYPOTHYROIDISM

Signs and symptoms: history of hypothyroidism or symptoms of hypothyroidism (cold intolerance, decreased reflexes, dry skin, weight gain, impaired cognition)

Investigations: elevated thyrotropin (TSH)

Anovulatory condition

AGE-RELATED ENDOCRINE OR METABOLIC CONDITION (E.G., THYROID)

HYPOTHYROIDISM—SEE ABOVE

HYPERTHYROIDISM

Signs and symptoms: changes in menstrual patterns; history of hyperthyroidism or symptoms of hyperthyroidism (weight loss, tremor, weakness, diarrhea)

Investigations: decreased thyrotropin (TSH)

NEOPLASM (E.G., PROLACTINOMA, OVARIAN TUMOUR)

PROLACTINOMA

This is a benign tumour.

Signs and symptoms of microprolactinoma:

> General: galactorrhea; clinical signs of estrogen deficiency (vaginal dryness, painful intercourse, decreased bone density in the lower spine and forearm)

> Reproductive-age women: menstrual disturbance (oligomenorrhea, amenorrhea, irregularity) and/or infertility

> Younger women: delayed menarche

> Prepubertal females: hyperprolactinemia

Signs and symptoms of macroprolactinoma: headaches when stretching, vision problems (bitemporal hemianopsia)

Investigations: elevated serum prolactin (> 20 ng/mL); MRI of the head to detect mass in the sella turcica

OVARIAN TUMOUR

Signs and symptoms: child, adolescent, or postmenopausal female (usual); asymptomatic in early stage (usual); abdominal bloating, discomfort, distention (ascites); ovarian or pelvic mass; urinary urgency, frequency; abnormal vaginal bleeding; fatigue; gastrointestinal symptoms (nausea, heart burn, diarrhea, constipation, early satiety); shortness of breath

Investigations: transvaginal and abdominal ultrasound; CA 125 blood test; pelvic or abdominal CT scan; analysis of ascitic fluid; biopsy

OTHER (E.G., POLYCYSTIC OVARY SYNDROME; WEIGHT LOSS, EXERCISE, OR STRESS; STRUCTURAL DISEASE)

POLYCYSTIC OVARY SYNDROME

Signs and symptoms: symptom onset after puberty, with increased rate of hair growth and male-pattern hair growth; irregular menstruation; infertility; obesity; acne

Investigations: LH:FSH ratio (elevated: 2:1 or 3:1) (usual); elevated testosterone; ultrasound to detect ovarian cysts; normal prolactin levels; normal thyroid function

WEIGHT LOSS, EXERCISE, OR STRESS

Signs and symptoms: history of recent weight loss, prolonged exercise, or personal stress (e.g., death of a friend or family member, divorce, job loss)

STRUCTURAL DISEASE

ENDOMETRIAL POLYPS

Signs and symptoms: intermenstrual bleeding in premenopausal women, usually light; incidence increases with age

Pregnancy-related condition

FIRST TRIMESTER BLEEDING

SPONTANEOUS ABORTION

Signs and symptoms: uterine bleeding, from spotting to heavy bleeding; pelvic pain (severe or dull cramping); uterus that is small for gestational age of the fetus

Risk factors: maternal age; family history of genetic disorders; medication, drug, or substance use; low folate level; high maternal body mass index (BMI); maternal fever, celiac disease, previous miscarriages

Investigations: decrease in β-hCG by at least 21%

ECTOPIC PREGNANCY

Signs and symptoms: symptoms of pregnancy and/or positive pregnancy test; pelvic pain; vaginal bleeding; painful intercourse; shoulder pain; palpable tubal mass; pelvic tenderness and pain associated with 1 or both adnexa

Severe symptom: syncope

Risk factors: previous ectopic pregnancy, pelvic inflammatory disease, pregnancy during intrauterine device (IUD) use

Investigations (pathognomonic): β-hCG above discriminatory zone (> 1500–2000 mIU/mL) **with** transvaginal ultrasound findings of a lack of intrauterine gestational sac, complex (mixed solid and cystic) masses in the adnexa, and free fluid in the cul-de-sac

IMPLANTATION

Signs and symptoms: spotting or minimal bleeding 10 to 14 days after fertilization

PATHOLOGY OF THE CERVIX, VAGINA, OR UTERUS—SEE NEOPLASM, STRUCTURAL DISEASE, GENITAL TRACT DISEASE

SECOND AND THIRD TRIMESTER BLEEDING

This is not as common as first trimester bleeding.

PLACENTA PREVIA

Signs and symptoms: bleeding before or after 20 weeks gestation (any time in the second half of the pregnancy); uterine contractions without abdominal pain, but with vaginal bleeding

Investigations: ultrasound

ABRUPTIO PLACENTAE

Signs and symptoms: symptom onset before 20 weeks gestation; bleeding, cramping, placental separation

Investigations note: ultrasound not helpful

POSTMENOPAUSAL DISORDER: STRUCTURAL, SYSTEMIC

Genital tract disease (excluding trauma)

ENDOMETRIAL POLYPS—SEE ABOVE

VAGINAL ATROPHY

Signs and symptoms: light bleeding or spotting; vaginal epithelium that is pale, dry, shiny, smooth; patchy erythema, petechiae, bleeding, discharge (if there is inflammation)

ENDOMETRIAL HYPERPLASIA OR CARCINOMA

Signs and symptoms: spotting or heavier bleeding

Endometrial hyperplasia: uterus not enlarged on exam

Endometrial carcinoma: pelvic mass, possibly enlarged uterus on exam

Investigations: biopsy

Neoplastic systemic disease

LEUKEMIA

Signs and symptoms: fever; chills; persistent fatigue and weakness; frequent or severe infections; weight loss; pallor; swollen lymph nodes; enlarged liver or spleen; easy bleeding and bruising; recurrent nosebleeds; petechiae; excessive sweating; bone pain or tenderness

Investigations: CBC; peripheral blood smear; flow cytometry; bone marrow aspiration and biopsy

LYMPHOMA

Signs and symptoms (non-Hodgkin): constitutional symptoms (fatigue, fever, night sweats, weight loss), enlarged lymph nodes, chest pain, coughing, shortness of breath

> Hodgkin lymphoma (less common): constitutional symptoms (fatigue, fever, night sweats, weight loss); enlarged lymph nodes; itching or pain on drinking alcohol, or increased sensitivity to alcohol

Investigations: blasts or cancer cells on peripheral blood smear; excess blasts or cancer cells on bone marrow examination

METASTATIC CANCER

Signs and symptoms: history of cancer; constitutional symptoms (weight loss, fever, night sweats)

Investigations: blood tests (CBC with differential; platelet count; ESR); CT scan; tissue biopsy or fine needle aspiration biopsy for histology/cytology and immunophenotyping

Drugs (e.g., hormone replacement therapy, anticoagulants)

Strategy for patient encounter

The likely scenario is a premenopausal woman with irregular vaginal bleeding. The specified tasks could engage history, physical exam, investigations, or management.

An actively bleeding patient is possible in this clinical presentation. No matter what tasks the instructions for the encounter specify, start by checking the patient's airway and hemodynamic status.

Airway and hemodynamic status

Check the patient's airway, breathing, and circulation (mnemonic: ABCs). Look in particular for hypotension and tachycardia. In unstable patients, establish large bore intravenous (IV) access and provide fluid resuscitation.

History

The differential diagnosis is extensive for this clinical presentation. Ask open-ended questions and listen for information that will help narrow the possibilities: What is the bleeding like? When did it start? When does it occur? What are your periods usually like? What medical conditions do you have? What medications do you take?

In a woman of childbearing age, ask whether she could be pregnant.

Physical exam

Perform a pelvic exam, unless contraindicated (e.g., placenta previa), looking for enlarged or tender uterus and adnexa.

(State that you will perform a pelvic exam. Since this exam is not performed on standardized patients, the examiner will likely interrupt, ask what you are looking for, and provide findings.)

Investigations

Order a pregnancy test and complete blood count (CBC). In suspected thyroid disease, order a thyrotropin (TSH) level. Order other specific tests as listed by this resource in the MCC differential diagnosis.

Management

Management will depend on the specific diagnosis. In pregnant patients, order an urgent ultrasound. Other causes may require ultrasound or other pelvic imaging, and referral to an obstetrician-gynecologist.

162

Vaginal discharge, vulvar pruritus

MCC particular objective

Distinguish sexually transmitted infections (STIs) from other causes.

MCC differential diagnosis
with added evidence

PHYSIOLOGIC DISCHARGE AND CERVICAL MUCOUS PRODUCTION

This discharge is caused by pregnancy, puerperium, lactation, premenstrual changes, ovulation, sexual excitement, oral contraceptives, and emotional stress.

GENITAL TRACT INFECTIONS (BACTERIAL VAGINOSIS, YEAST, SEXUALLY TRANSMITTED INFECTION)

BACTERIAL VAGINOSIS

Signs and symptoms: often asymptomatic; foul vaginal odour; mild to moderate increase in vaginal discharge (homogenous, thin, gray, white, green); vulvar pruritus

Risk factors: unprotected sex with multiple partners or new partners; frequent douching; natural lack of *Lactobacillus*; recent antibiotic use

Investigations: vaginal pH $\geq$ 4.5; saline smear to detect clue cells

YEAST: VULVOVAGINAL CANDIDIASIS

Signs and symptoms: thick, white, clumpy ("curd-like") vaginal discharge; vulvar pruritus, burning, soreness; thrush patches loosely adherent to the vulva; erythema and edema of the vestibule, labia majora, labia minora

Risk factors: diabetes; pregnancy; estrogen therapy; recent antibiotic use; contraceptive devices; immunosuppression

Investigations: normal vaginal pH (4–4.5); wet-mount test of discharge with potassium hydroxide preparation to detect yeast

SEXUALLY TRANSMITTED INFECTION (STI)

STIs include chlamydia and gonorrhea (very common), syphilis, human papillomavirus (HPV), HIV, hepatitis B virus (HBV), hepatitis C virus (HCV), and trichomonas.

Signs and symptoms (symptoms vary with the specific STI):

often asymptomatic; vaginal or urethral discharge; ulcerative or nonulcerative genital disease; pelvic pain

Risk factors: unprotected sex with multiple or new partners; sex-trade work or sexual contact with sex workers; age 15 to 24; prior STIs

GENITAL TRACT INFLAMMATIONS (E.G., IRRITANTS)

IRRITANTS

Signs and symptoms: vulvar pruritus; erythema

Risk factors: use of scented panty liners, pads, soaps, lotions, detergents, bubble baths; use of douches, spermicides, certain topical drugs (e.g., povidone-iodine)

Strategy for patient encounter

The likely scenario is a young woman with vaginal itching and discharge. The specified tasks could engage history, physical exam, investigations, or management.

History

Start with open-ended questions about the symptoms: When did they start? What have you noticed? Listen for evidence consis- tent with particular entities (e.g., foul odour and thin grey, white, or green discharge in bacterial infection; clumpy discharge with itching in yeast infections; pelvic pain and/or genital ulcers in STIs). Ask about factors that make the symptoms better or worse, such as possible irritants.

Establish the likely phase of the patient's menstrual cycle, and whether the patient is pregnant: When was your last period? Are you pregnant? Are you sexually active?

Check risk factors for STIs: unprotected sex with multiple partners or new partners; working in the sex trade; sexual contact with sex workers; age 15 to 24; and prior STIs.

Physical exam

Examine the abdomen for tenderness. Perform a bimanual pelvic exam and a speculum exam for adnexal or uterine tenderness; skin or mucosal abnormalities; and discharge.

(State that you will perform these exams. Since these exams are not performed on standardized patients, the examiner will likely interrupt, ask what you are looking for, and provide find- ings.)

Investigations

Test for yeast and bacterial vaginosis. If the patient has risk factors for STIs, swab for gonorrhea and chlamydia, and consider testing for HIV, hepatitis B virus (HBV), and hepatitis C virus (HCV).

Management

Positive gonorrhea and chlamydia tests require specific antibiotic treatment and reporting to public health authorities. Treat yeast infections with oral or intravaginal antifungals. Treat bacterial vaginosis with intravaginal antibiotics. In the case of chemical irritants, the treatment is to avoid the causative agent.

Pearls

In practice, the diagnosis of bacterial vaginosis, yeast infection, and trichomonas is usually done together with swabs, rather than with pH and wet mount or potassium hydroxide (KOH) smears.

163

Child abuse

MCC particular objectives

Be aware of presentations that may indicate child abuse.

In suspected abuse, manage with particular attention to safety and prevention.

In disclosed abuse, construct a prevention plan.

MCC differential diagnosis
with added evidence

CHILD ABUSE IN GENERAL

Signs and symptoms: disclosed abuse (victims do not always disclose abuse); resistance by the parent or caregiver to having the patient interviewed alone (usual)

> **No** evidence of medical conditions that could mimic abuse (e.g., malabsorption; developmental delay due to

complications during gestation or delivery; genetic or metabolic disorders)

Risk factors: history of substance abuse by the parents or caregiver; unstable living situation of the parents or caregiver

PHYSICAL ABUSE

This is purposeful action with the intent to physically harm a child. It includes hitting and beating; using an object to hit; kicking; burning; holding under water; tying up; and severely shaking a baby.

Signs and symptoms: inconsistency between an injury and the explanation for the injury and/or the developmental stage of the child; facial contusions; marks on the neck or limbs; burn marks; ligature marks on the wrists and ankles; bite marks; lash marks; bruises or broken bones unexplainable by usual activities; unexplained loss of consciousness in an infant

SEXUAL ABUSE

This is an action done with a child for the sexual arousal and gratification of an adult or significantly older child (greater than a 4-year age difference, chronologically or in mental or physical development).

Signs and symptoms: behaviour and knowledge that is inappropriate for the child's age; pregnancy or sexually transmitted infection (STI); blood in the child's underwear; trouble walking or sitting, or complaints of genital pain; sexual abuse of other children by the victim

PSYCHOLOGICAL ABUSE

This is injuring a child's self-esteem or emotional well-being. It includes verbal and emotional assault (continually belittling, berating, threatening, intimidating, isolating, or rejecting a child); not providing a child with a safe environment; and withholding or omitting positive contributions to a child's emotional well-being.

Signs and symptoms: problems in school; eating disorders leading to weight loss or poor weight gain; emotional issues (anxiety, low self-esteem); depression; extreme behaviour (acting out to seek attention); trouble sleeping

NEGLECT

Neglect involves failure to provide all or some basic physical, emotional, educational, and medical needs. Examples include rejecting a child and not giving love; not feeding a child; not dressing a child in proper clothing; not giving needed medical or dental care; and abandonment by leaving a child at home alone for a long time.

Signs and symptoms: not attending school regularly; poor hygiene, dental care; malnutrition; reports by the child suggesting lack of physical and/or emotional care at home

EXPOSURE TO DOMESTIC VIOLENCE
This involves witnessing an abusive situation within a family, such as violence between parents.

Signs and symptoms: excessive anxiety or crying; fearfulness; difficulty sleeping; depression; social withdrawal; difficulty in school; running away from home; violent tendencies and/or unhealthy tolerance for abuse

Strategy for patient encounter
The likely scenario is a family member seeking advice about a child whom a relative may be abusing. The likely tasks include history, fulfilling a duty to report, and a developing a prevention plan.

History
Ask whether the child has disclosed abuse to the relative you are interviewing. If this has not happened (victims of abuse often do not disclose abuse), ask why the relative suspects abuse.

Duty to report
Abuse of a minor, or danger of abuse, must be reported to the appropriate authorities. Depending on your region, this may be social services, a child protection agency, or the police. Know what is required in your region.

Prevention plan
Outline a safety plan that the relative could help the child prepare, including safe places where the child can go (e.g., safe friends and relatives); leaving the room if they are witnessing abuse; how to call 911; and knowing their full name and address.

Advise the relative about counselling and mental health services that are available for the child, the family, and caregivers.

Encourage the relative to get the child to a doctor for evaluation.

164

Elder abuse

MCC particular objectives

Given a state of distress or unexplained findings in an elderly patient, inquire about potential elder abuse.

Identify the immediate level of risk.

MCC differential diagnosis
with added evidence

ELDER ABUSE

Signs and symptoms: disclosed abuse (physical, sexual, psychological, economic, financial or material, neglect); resistance by a caregiver to having the patient interviewed alone (usual); fear of the patient towards a caregiver; isolation; depression; unexplained changes in financial situation; bruising, scars, healed fractures; poor hygiene; sudden weight loss, malnutrition

> Note: victims do not always disclose abuse.

Risk factors:

> Victim: female; advanced age (especially older than 80); vulnerability due to a chronic disorder, functional impairment, or cognitive impairment

> Perpetrator: substance abuse, psychiatric disorder, history of violence, cohabitation with the elderly person, dependence on the elderly person for support

Strategy for patient encounter

The likely scenario is an elderly patient being abused by a relative. It will involve a high degree of suspicion in an elderly patient with unexplained injuries or failure to thrive. The specified tasks could engage history, physical exam, investigations, or management.

History

Note that if the possible abuser is with the patient, the patient may not be honest with answers. If this is the case, request to interview the patient alone. Ask the patient if they are afraid of anyone, if anyone hurts them, how they get their food, and who controls their money. Ask about their living arrangements and social contacts, and if anyone controls who they speak to.

Physical exam

Perform an examination of the head and neck, musculoskeletal system, and skin, looking for signs of abuse (e.g., bruises and cuts, broken bones, lost teeth, burns).

Investigations

Consider X-rays to look for healed fractures.

Management

In suspected abuse, ensure the immediate safety of the patient and refer the patient to adult protection services.

Duty to report

The duty to report risk of harm to an adult varies by jurisdiction (and is absent in some). If in doubt, it is best to discuss the case with a social worker or police.

165

Adult abuse, intimate partner abuse

MCC particular objectives

Assess the medium- and short-term risk to the victim.

Devise a safe and effective plan for the patient.

MCC differential diagnosis
with added evidence

INTIMATE PARTNER ABUSE

Signs and symptoms: disclosed abuse (physical, psychological or emotional, sexual, economic, social isolation); bruising, scars, healed fractures; recurrent symptoms or injuries; resistance by the partner to having the patient interviewed alone (usual)

> Note: victims do not always disclose abuse.

Risk factors: pregnancy; threat to leave; partner's history of violence or substance abuse

Strategy for patient encounter

The likely scenario is a patient experiencing intimate partner abuse. A high degree of suspicion is necessary, especially in patients with recurring symptoms or injuries. The specified tasks could engage history, physical exam, investigations, or management.

History

Note that if the possible abuser is with the patient, the patient may not be honest with answers. If this is the case, request to interview the patient alone. Ask the patient if they are afraid of anyone. Ask if they are, or have been, the victim of abuse. Ask specifically about physical, psychological, sexual, and economic abuse, and about social isolation. Ask about risk factors for escalating abuse: Has the pattern of abuse increased in frequency or intensity?

Some patients do not disclose abuse, even in the absence of the perpetrator. In suspected undisclosed abuse, ask about risk factors for abuse: Are you pregnant? Have you told the perpetrator you want to leave? Is the perpetrator violent or a substance abuser?

Establish whether the patient has a plan to protect themselves: What steps have you thought of? Do you know of resources available to help you?

Physical exam

Perform an examination of the head and neck, musculoskeletal system, and skin, looking for signs of abuse (e.g., bruises and cuts, broken bones, lost teeth, burns).

Investigations

Order X-rays for any apparent broken bones.

Management

Counsel the patient on making a plan for personal protection. If the patient is facing escalating abuse, alert them that they have a greater risk of permanent injury or death.

Elements of a plan for personal protection include: where to go for help (e.g., a shelter); how to get away; how to get money (e.g., friends, family); how to protect children; and packing a fast-exit suitcase to leave with a friend or family member.

Refer the patient to social services if appropriate. Social services can provide assistance with finances, relocation, and protecting and caring for children.

Duty to report

The duty to report risk of harm to an adult varies by jurisdiction (and is absent in some). If in doubt, it is best to discuss the case with a social worker or police.

166

Acute visual disturbance or loss

MCC particular objective
Recognize the need for urgent referral to an ophthalmologist.

MCC differential diagnosis
with added evidence

PAINLESS CONDITION

Vascular disorder (e.g., retinal artery occlusion, giant cell arteritis)
RETINAL ARTERY OCCLUSION (RAO)
This is an ophthalmologic emergency: delays will lead to permanent blindness. It primarily affects the elderly.

Signs and symptoms:

Central RAO: acute, persistent, painless, complete loss of vision or blurring in 1 eye

Branch RAO: vision loss in a section of 1 eye

Risks signalled by RAO (these also need attention): systemic disease and/or stroke from carotid artery disease, diabetes, hypertension, atrial fibrillation, hyperlipidemia, atherosclerosis, endocarditis

Investigations: funduscopic exam

Findings immediately after RAO: afferent pupillary defect

Findings hours to days after RAO: cherry red spot, "ground glass" retina, or pale optic disc

GIANT CELL ARTERITIS (TEMPORAL ARTERITIS)

This is the most common form of vasculitis.

Signs and symptoms: older than 50 (incidence increases with age); headaches; tenderness in both temples; jaw pain; acute vision loss (partial or complete); fever; fatigue; weight loss

> Polymyalgia rheumatica (associated condition): shoulder, neck, torso, hip girdle pain; morning stiffness

Risk factors: Scandinavian descent, female, history of polymyalgia rheumatica

Investigations before treatment: elevated ALP, ESR, CRP levels

Neurologic disorder (e.g., optic neuritis)

OPTIC NEURITIS

This condition is associated with multiple sclerosis, neuromyelitis optica, and prior viral illness.

Signs and symptoms: eye pain on extraocular movement; change in colour perception; decreased pupillary light reaction in the affected eye; contrast and brightness sensitivity; vision impairment exacerbated by heat or exercise; gradual resolution

> Acute attacks: vision deficits in 1 eye (from mildly decreased visual acuity to blindness)

Retinal disorder (e.g., retinal detachment)

RETINAL DETACHMENT

This is an ophthalmologic emergency: delays may cause permanent damage. The most common form is rhegmatogenous detachment following spontaneous posterior vitreous detachment.

Signs and symptoms: perceived flashes of light and floaters in 1 eye (floaters usually have sudden onset, and number in the hundreds to thousands); visual field defect; history of recent trauma, previous ophthalmologic surgery; previous eye conditions (uveitis, vitreous hemorrhage)

Other (e.g., conversion disorders)

CONVERSION DISORDER

This is a psychological disorder that affects all ages.

Signs and symptoms: onset of symptoms after trauma or a stressful event; weakness or paralysis; impaired ability to walk, swallow; tremors; loss of balance; speech dysfunction (slurred speech, inability to speak); numbness or loss of touch; vision problems (double vision, blindness); hearing impairment; seizures, convulsions, unresponsive episodes

Risk factors: family history of conversion disorder; family or personal history of mental health disorders (depression, mood disorder, anxiety disorder)

PAINFUL CONDITION

Glaucoma

ACUTE ANGLE-CLOSURE GLAUCOMA

Signs and symptoms: hazy or blurred vision; rainbowlike halos around bright lights; sudden vision loss; severe eye and head pain; nausea, vomiting

OPEN-ANGLE GLAUCOMA

This is a painless cause of vision loss.

Signs and symptoms: often asymptomatic; gradual decline in peripheral vision

Investigations: visual field test; tonometry (intraocular pressure); slit-lamp exam, including dilated fundus exam, to detect glaucomatous optic nerve changes

Inflammatory condition (e.g., uveitis, corneal ulcer)

UVEITIS

This is eye inflammation that affects the uvea.

Signs and symptoms: sudden-onset, worsening symptoms that affect 1 or both eyes; age 20 to 50 (most common, but it may also affect children); eye redness; pain; light sensitivity; blurred vision; floaters; decreased vision

> History of infection (e.g., cat-scratch disease, herpes zoster virus, syphilis, toxoplasmosis, tuberculosis, Lyme disease, West Nile virus), injury, autoimmune disease (e.g., sarcoidosis, ankylosing spondylitis), inflammatory disease (e.g., Crohn disease, ulcerative colitis), cancer that affects the eye (e.g., lymphoma)

Investigations: eye fluid analysis; angiography

CORNEAL ULCER

This is an open sore in the outer layer of the cornea, caused by infection, abrasions on the eye surface, or severely dry eyes.

Signs and symptoms: blurry vision; itching and discharge; photophobia

Investigations: fluorescein stain of the cornea; exam of scrapings from the ulcer; blood tests to detect inflammatory disorders

Other (e.g., trauma)

TRAUMA

Trauma may cause inflammation of the structures of the eye and optic nerve, or hemorrhage in the eye.

Signs and symptoms: history of trauma with sudden disturbance or loss of vision; eye pain

Investigations: imaging of the head to detect any vascular complication causing vision loss

Strategy for patient encounter

The likely scenario is a patient with acute vision loss in 1 eye. The specified tasks could engage history, physical exam, investigations, or management.

History

Start with open-ended questions about the visual loss or disturbance: When did it start? How did it start? What other symptoms do you have? Listen for associated trauma and eye pain.

Ask about a history of infection and autoimmune disease (uveitis).

Ask about risk factors for retinal artery occlusion (carotid artery disease, diabetes, hypertension, atrial fibrillation, hyperlipidemia, atherosclerosis, and endocarditis).

Physical exam

Examine the eyes for redness, ulceration, and signs of trauma. In suspected infection or ulceration, examine the eyes using fluorescein dye. Examine the visual fields. Record the visual acuity in both eyes. Perform a fundoscopic exam looking for changes to the optic disc.

Investigations

In suspected glaucoma, perform tonometry to measure intraocular pressure. In suspected giant cell arteritis (temporal arteritis), order an erythrocyte sedimentation rate (ESR), which is usually > 50 mm/hour in giant cell arteritis.

Management

All cases of acute vision loss (with the exception of corneal abrasion) require urgent referral to an ophthalmologist.

For corneal abrasion, apply topical antibiotic and patch the eye (**do not** patch the eye if a foreign body is still present, or if the abrasion is due to contact lens use). In suspected giant cell arteritis (temporal arteritis), start the patient on high-dose oral steroids and refer them urgently for temporal artery biopsy.

167

Chronic visual disturbance or loss

MCC particular objectives
Recognize populations at risk of chronic visual loss (e.g., elderly, diabetics).

Institute screening and prevention measures.

MCC differential diagnosis
with added evidence

GLAUCOMA
ACUTE ANGLE-CLOSURE GLAUCOMA
Signs and symptoms: hazy or blurred vision; rainbowlike halos around bright lights; sudden vision loss; severe eye and head pain; nausea, vomiting

OPEN-ANGLE GLAUCOMA
Signs and symptoms: patchy blind spots in peripheral or central vision; tunnel vision (advanced stages)

Investigations: visual field test; visual acuity; tonometry (intraocular pressure); dilated eye exam to detect optic nerve damage

CATARACT
Signs and symptoms: blurred or dimmed vision; poor vision at night; sensitivity to glare; halos around lights; double vision in a single eye; frequent need for new prescription glasses

Risk factors: increasing age; diabetes; excessive exposure to sunlight; smoking; obesity; hypertension; previous eye injury or inflammation; prolonged use of corticosteroids; alcohol abuse

Investigations: visual acuity, slit lamp exam, retinal exam

MACULAR DEGENERATION
AGE-RELATED MACULAR DEGENERATION
This condition has 2 types: dry and wet. Dry is more common. Wet threatens vision.

Signs and symptoms: symptoms in both eyes (usual); gradual changes in vision (usual) (wet condition may present as sudden-onset central visual distortion); decreased vision, blurred vision; problems recognizing faces (if degeneration is present in both eyes)

Risk factors: older than 50; family history of macular degeneration; Caucasian descent (more common); obesity; history of smoking; cardiovascular disease; dietary factors

Investigations: funduscopic examination to assess presence of drusen and hemorrhages; optical coherence tomography to detect intraretinal and subretinal fluid secondary to choroidal neovascular membrane

RETINOPATHY DUE TO CHRONIC ILLNESS

RETINOPATHY DUE TO CHRONIC ILLNESS IN GENERAL

Populations at risk include diabetics and the elderly.

DIABETIC RETINOPATHY (DR)

Signs and symptoms: asymptomatic until late stage of disease (macular edema or proliferative DR); impaired vision or vision loss; spots or dark floaters; blurred vision; fluctuating vision; impaired colour vision; dark or empty areas in vision

> Nonproliferative DR (earlier disease): "cotton wool" spots (nerve-fibre layer infarcts); intraretinal hemorrhages; hard exudates; intraretinal microvascular abnormalities and venous bleeding in severe cases
>
> Proliferative DR (late-stage disease): neovascularization (complications include tractional retinal detachment, vitreous hemorrhage, and vision loss if there is bleeding into the retina or if the retina is detached)

Risk factors: type 2 diabetes (more common than type 1); higher risk with more advanced diabetes

Strategy for patient encounter

The likely scenario is a diabetic patient with chronic vision loss (the key to this encounter is to recognize populations at risk of chronic visual loss, including elderly patients and diabetics). The likely tasks are history or management (with an emphasis on screening and prevention).

History

It is important to suspect chronic visual loss in elderly and/or diabetic patients. Ask about decreased ability to read, decreased night vision, light sensitivity, double vision, and spots or loss of visual field. If any of these symptoms is present, refer the patient to an optometrist or ophthalmologist for visual evaluation.

Management

Even in the absence of symptoms, it is important to screen diabetic patients regularly for the development of retinal disease: progression can be rapid, and therapy can reduce the rate of progression.

Refer diabetic patients to an optometrist or ophthalmologist for retinal photographs and ophthalmoscopy on dilated fundi.

Screen all type 2 diabetic patients annually if retinopathy is progressing, or every 2 to 3 years following a normal eye exam by an optometrist or ophthalmologist.

Screen pregnant women with diabetes (not gestational diabetes) in the first trimester. Monitor the patient closely throughout the pregnancy and for 1 year postpartum.

Perform a comprehensive eye exam on all type 1 diabetic patients within 5 years of their diagnosis.

Prevention

For diabetics, strict glycemic control early in the course of type 1 and 2 diabetes, and good blood pressure control, reduce the risk of retinopathy.

- goal for glycemic control: glycated hemoglobin (HbA_{1c}) $\leq 7\%$
- goal for blood pressure: $< 130/80$ mmHg

Smoking cessation also reduces the risk of macular degeneration and cataracts.

168

Vomiting and/or nausea

MCC particular objective

Recognize that important causes of vomiting can arise outside the gastrointestinal system.

MCC differential diagnosis
with added evidence

GASTROINTESTINAL SYSTEM

Esophagus, stomach, duodenum disorder (e.g., obstruction, gastroenteritis, reflux, gastroparesis, peptic ulcer disease)

GASTRIC OUTLET OBSTRUCTION

Most patients with this condition have cancer. Other causes include peptic ulcer disease, Crohn disease, pancreatitis, injuries, large gastric polyps, and tuberculosis.

Signs and symptoms: epigastric abdominal pain; postprandial vomiting, nausea; early satiety; abdominal distention and bloating; weight loss

Investigations: radiologic testing; endoscopy

GASTROENTERITIS

Signs and symptoms: abrupt-onset diarrhea; crampy abdominal pain; nausea, vomiting; fever; epigastric tenderness on abdominal examination

Risk factors: exposure to persons with similar symptoms or to large groups of people (common: most cases are viral); eating undercooked or contaminated foods, or raw fluids (these are risk factors for bacterial infection)

GASTROESOPHAGEAL REFLUX DISEASE

Signs and symptoms: burning chest pain radiating into the throat (often with a bitter taste in the mouth or regurgitation of food into the mouth; often worse with lying down; often better with standing up or taking antacids; worse with spicy food, coffee, alcohol, fatty foods, peppermint); acid damage to teeth

Risk factors: obesity, pregnancy

GASTROPARESIS

This is a gastric obstruction that is frequently associated with diabetes.

Signs and symptoms: history of diabetes (often); vomit containing food that was eaten several hours earlier; nausea, early satiety, bloating, weight loss and/or upper abdominal pain

PEPTIC ULCER DISEASE

Signs and symptoms: constant midepigastric pain, often relieved with eating or with antacids; weight loss

Investigations: test for *H. pylori*; endoscopy to detect ulcer or inflammation of the gastric lining

Small bowel, colon disorder (e.g., acute infectious enteritis, obstruction, inflammatory bowel disease)

ACUTE INFECTIOUS ENTERITIS

Examples include acute gastroenteritis caused by bacterial, viral or parasitic pathogens.

Signs and symptoms: duration < 1 week; diarrhea that occurs ≥ 3 times per day (or ≥ 200 g of stool per day); nausea, vomiting; fever; abdominal pain; weight loss; fatigue

SMALL BOWEL OBSTRUCTION (ACUTE)

This condition requires emergent surgery.

Signs and symptoms: abdominal distention; abdominal tenderness and pain (every 5 minutes); nausea, vomiting; dehydration (tachycardia, orthostatic hypotension, reduced urine output)

SMALL BOWEL OBSTRUCTION (RECURRENT)

Signs and symptoms: similar to acute obstruction, but with resolution, and followed by diarrhea; asymptomatic between recurrences with normal abdominal exam

INFLAMMATORY BOWEL DISEASE

Signs and symptoms: younger than 30 (usually); family history of inflammatory bowel disease; fluctuating symptoms with periods of exacerbation and remission; diarrhea (possibly with nocturnal waking); blood in the stool; abdominal pain; weight loss; fever; fatigue; right lower quadrant and periumbilical pain; extraintestinal manifestations (e.g., uveitis, arthritis)

> Crohn disease: right lower quadrant mass, inflammation of the eyes, arthritis

Investigations: elevated CRP (this suggests active inflammation); fecal calprotectin; colonoscopy with biopsy (this is a standard diagnostic procedure); CT scan or MRI (findings: diagnostic structural changes associated with inflammatory bowel disease)

Hepatobiliary disease or pancreatic disease (e.g., acute hepatitis, acute pancreatitis, acute cholecystitis)

ACUTE HEPATITIS

Signs and symptoms: viral-like illness; abdominal pain; jaundice; palpable, tender liver

> History of infection with hepatitis A, B, or C virus (HAV, HBV, HCV) or risk factors for these infections (autoimmune conditions, unprotected sex, intravenous drug abuse, blood transfusions, tattoos, body piercings, imprisonment, workplace exposure to body fluids); toxic ingestion (e.g., acetaminophen); adverse drug reaction (e.g., change of medication)
>
> HCV: often asymptomatic

Investigations: elevated AST, ALT, bilirubin; abnormal PT/INR; positive viral serologic tests (e.g., HAV, HBV, HCV)

ACUTE PANCREATITIS

Signs and symptoms: persistent, severe abdominal pain and tenderness in the right upper quadrant; pain that radiates to the back; nausea, vomiting; abdominal distention; hypoactive bowel sounds

> Severe symptoms: shortness of breath; epigastric tenderness on palpation; diffuse tenderness over the abdomen; fever; tachypnea; hypoxemia; hypotension

Investigations: elevated serum amylase, serum lipase

ACUTE CHOLECYSTITIS

Signs and symptoms: steady, severe right upper quadrant or epigastric pain (pain may radiate to the right shoulder or back); positive Murphy sign; nausea, vomiting; fever; anorexia; fatty food ingestion ≥ 1 hour prior to pain

Investigations: leukocytosis with increased band forms; abdominal ultrasound

Peritoneal irritation (e.g., appendicitis)

PERITONEAL IRRITATION IN GENERAL

Signs and symptoms: abdominal tenderness, bloating, pain with movement; fever; loss of appetite; nausea, vomiting; constipation and diarrhea; fatigue

Investigations: elevated WBCs due to infection or inflammation

APPENDICITIS

Signs and symptoms: child (often); periumbilical pain that migrates over several days to localize in the right lower quadrant; anorexia; fever; localized pain over the McBurney point on abdominal palpation

Investigations: elevated WBCs; ultrasound or CT scan for distended appendix

CENTRAL NERVOUS SYSTEM

Increased intracranial pressure (e.g., infection, trauma, tumour)

Examples of infections include meningitis, encephalitis, and abscesses. Examples of tumours include glioma, meningioma, and brain metastasis.

Signs and symptoms: intracranial pressure $\geq$ 20 mmHg; headache; depressed level of consciousness; vomiting (projectile vomiting when arising from sleep)

Vestibular nerve lesions

Examples of lesions include vestibular neuritis or labyrinthitis.

Signs and symptoms: rapid-onset severe vertigo; nausea, vomiting; gait instability; nystagmus that is unilateral, horizontal, or horizontal-torsional (this is suppressed with visual fixation); positive head thrust test

> Labyrinthitis: unilateral hearing loss

Brainstem lesions

BRAINSTEM LESIONS IN GENERAL

Signs and symptoms: impaired senses (vision, hearing, touch); speech impairments (difficulty speaking, voice change); motor impairments (gait instability); vertigo or dizziness causing nausea, vomiting; muscle weakness

MULTIPLE SCLEROSIS (EXAMPLE OF CONDITION CAUSING BRAINSTEM LESIONS)

Signs and symptoms: variable depending on lesion location

> Spinal cord: sensory or motor dysfunction; Lhermitte sign (paresthesias radiating down the extremities or trunk with neck flexion); bowel, bladder or erectile dysfunction

> Brainstem: double vision; swallowing, speech difficulties; vertigo; pseudobulbar palsy

> Cerebrum: cognitive impairment; depression; upper motor neuron signs; unilateral motor or sensory deficits

> Cerebellum: problems with balance and coordination; vertigo

> Other symptoms: tonic spasms; fatigue; pain; exercise intolerance; temperature sensitivity; painful unilateral loss of visual acuity

Risk factors: younger than 50, female

Investigations: brain and spinal cord MRI, including advanced MRI techniques, with established occurrence of multiple episodes; CSF fluid analysis

Psychiatric or psychological conditions

Signs and symptoms: personal or family history of psychiatric conditions (e.g., anxiety, major depressive disorder); excessive worry; loss of interest in friends and usual activities; changes in sleep habits; hallucinations or delusions; suicidal thoughts; history of adverse experience (emotional, physical, or sexual abuse; recent stress such as death of a friend or family member), or substance abuse

> Cyclic vomiting syndrome: emotional stress with recurrent nausea, vomiting, lethargy, pallor, abdominal pain, diarrhea, headache that lasts up to 10 days

OTHER CONDITION

Endocrine and/or metabolic condition (e.g., diabetes, hypercalcemia, pregnancy)

DIABETES

Diabetes can produce gastrointestinal symptoms, such as vomiting and nausea, in the context of gastroparesis or diabetic ketoacidosis.

Signs and symptoms (diabetes in general): personal or family history of diabetes; history of diabetic complications and/or inadequate monitoring; polydipsia, polyuria, and/or weight loss

Investigations: fasting glucose or HbA$_{1c}$ test

HYPERCALCEMIA

Signs and symptoms: constipation, polyuria, polydipsia, dehydration, anorexia, nausea, muscle weakness, altered sensory status

> History of sarcoidosis, malignancy, hyperparathyroidism, immobilization, use of diuretics (thiazide)

Investigations: blood test (hypercalcemia is total calcium ≥ 2.63 mmol/L or ionized calcium ≥ 1.4 mmol/L); albumin; PTH

PREGNANCY

Signs and symptoms: amenorrhea, especially during childbearing years (some experience spotting); sexual activity, especially without contraception or with inconsistent use of contraception; nausea, vomiting (common early sign); breast enlargement and tenderness; increased frequency of urination without pain or difficulty; fatigue

Investigations: blood or urine β-hCG

Cancer

Cancers that commonly cause nausea and vomiting include malignant bowel obstruction and cancer that affects the brain.

Sepsis (e.g., pyelonephritis, pneumonia)

SEPSIS IN GENERAL

Definition: infection with systemic inflammatory response, dysfunction of ≥ 1 organ system

Signs and symptoms: fever or hypothermia; tachycardia; tachypnea; infection (most common: pneumonia, abdominal infection, kidney infection, bacteremia)

> Severe: oliguria; mental status changes; shortness of breath; extreme hypotension, unresponsive to fluid replacement (this indicates septic shock)

Risk factors: very young, very old; compromised immune system; wounds, burns; catheterization, intubation

Investigations: CBC with differential; cultures (blood, CSF, urine) to detect causative organism; ABG to detect acidosis; elevated creatinine; chest X-ray to detect pulmonary edema

PYELONEPHRITIS

Signs and symptoms: frequent urination; painful urination; tenderness over the costovertebral angle

Investigations: urinalysis, urine culture

PNEUMONIA

Signs and symptoms: shortness of breath; cough; purulent sputum; chest pain on coughing or deep breaths; fatigue; tachypnea; tachycardia; decreased oxygen saturation; lung crackles on auscultation; lung dullness on percussion

> Children: fever
>
> Elderly: confusion, low body temperature

Risk factors: very old, very young; smoking; immune compromise (e.g., due to chronic illness); hospitalization

Investigations: chest X-ray to detect consolidation

Drugs and toxins (e.g., chemotherapy, food poisoning)

CHEMOTHERAPY

Nausea and vomiting are common side effects of chemotherapy, especially for highly emetic agents (e.g., combination of cyclophosphamide and doxorubicin in breast cancer; combination of anthracycline and cyclophosphamide in breast cancer; combination of vincristine and prednisone in non-Hodgkin lymphoma; cisplatin).

FOOD POISONING

Signs and symptoms: history of eating undercooked meat or poorly refrigerated food; symptoms that develop within 6 hours of contaminated food consumption

Strategy for patient encounter

The likely scenario is an adult patient who has been vomiting for several days. The specified tasks could engage history, physical exam, investigations, or management.

This clinical presentation has a very wide differential diagnosis. A key goal is to narrow down possible causes, and specifically to differentiate gastrointestinal from nongastrointestinal causes.

History

Start with open-ended questions about the patient's vomiting: When did the vomiting start? What did you notice when it started? What makes it better or worse? Listen for information about sudden versus gradual onset, constant versus intermittent symptoms, and triggering or alleviating factors.

Perform a complete review of the patient's gastrointestinal symptoms: Have you had a change in appetite or weight? Do you feel full quickly when you eat? Have your bowel habits changed? Have you had a fever with your symptoms?

Ask about symptoms of neurological disease: headaches, personality changes, vision changes, focal neurologic symptoms, and altered gait.

Ask about symptoms of cardiac ischemia: chest pain, shortness of breath, and exercise intolerance.

Ask about symptoms of relevant metabolic conditions: diabetes (polyuria, polydipsia, weight loss), hypercalcemia (constipation, polyuria, polydipsia, dehydration, anorexia, nausea, muscle weakness), and pregnancy (amenorrhea; breast enlargement and tenderness).

Physical exam

Obtain the patient's vital signs looking for indications of dehydration (including hypotension and tachycardia) and fever (this suggests infection or malignancy). Examine the skin for tenting (from dehydration). Examine the abdomen for tenderness (this suggests infection or blockage). In a suspected neurologic cause, examine the fundi for papilledema (this indicates increased intracranial pressure).

Investigations

Order tests for serum electrolytes, creatinine, calcium, glucose, and cortisol. Order more specialized tests and/or imaging if the history and physical exam suggest a nongastrointestinal cause (see the information this resource lists in the MCC differential diagnosis).

Management

Target the underlying cause. Pay special attention to conditions requiring immediate management (dehydration, increased intracranial pressure). Note that, in some patients, no cause will be found. Where appropriate, recommend the use of common antinausea or antiemetic medications.

169

Weakness (not caused by cerebrovascular accident)

MCC particular objectives

Distinguish muscular, nerve, and upper neurological disorders.

Characterize the distribution of the weakness, or localize the region of the weakness.

Determine the underlying cause.

MCC differential diagnosis
with added evidence

MUSCULAR

Primary muscle disease

CONGENITAL (E.G., MUSCULAR DYSTROPHY)

MUSCULAR DYSTROPHY (MD)

Common types of muscular dystrophy include Duchenne MD, Becker MD, facioscapulohumeral MD, and myotonic dystrophy.

Signs and symptoms: progressive muscular wasting, scoliosis, limited range of movement, muscle spasms, poor balance, waddling gait, calf deformation, walking difficulty, shortness of breath, cardiomyopathy

Investigations: muscle biopsy, increased creatine phosphokinase, EMG, genetic testing

ACQUIRED (E.G., MYOSITIS, MYASTHENIA GRAVIS)

MYOSITIS

This describes a group of inflammatory diseases including dermatomyositis, inclusion body myositis, and polymyositis.

Signs and symptoms: gradual-onset muscle weakness (dermatomyositis and polymyositis: core-muscle weakness; inclusion body myositis: weakness in the thighs, wrist, and fingers); difficulty swallowing

> Dermatomyositis: rash

MYASTHENIA GRAVIS

Signs and symptoms: ocular weakness (usually just this) with drooping eyelid(s), blurred vision, or double vision; oropharyngeal weakness (difficulty speaking; hoarseness; chewing and swallowing difficulty); limb weakness with difficulty climbing stairs, working with elevated arms; fluctuating weakness that is asymmetrical and worse with sustained exercise

Investigations: single fibre electromyography, serum anti-AChR antibody

Central nervous system

MALIGNANCY

BRAIN TUMOUR

Types of brain tumour include meningioma, astrocytoma, oligodendroglioma, glioblastoma, and Schwannoma.

Signs and symptoms: acute-onset headaches; older than 50; change in chronic headache pattern; increasing intensity and frequency of headaches; headaches that disturb sleep; unilateral headache pain, always on the same side; position-evoked crescendo headache; impaired vision; light-headedness

> Other symptoms: focal seizures, confusion, memory loss, personality change, loss of coordination, muscle weakness

Investigations: imaging for intracranial masses (MRI with contrast enhancement is best for tumours and abscesses); biopsy

SPINAL CORD TUMOUR

Signs and symptoms: back pain; bilateral numbness and/or weakness in the arms or legs; loss of bladder and/or bowel control

Investigations: spinal MRI or CT scan; biopsy

INFECTION (E.G., ENCEPHALITIS)

ENCEPHALITIS

Viral infection is the most common cause: herpes simplex virus, type 1 and type 2 (HSV-1, HSV-2); Epstein-Barr virus (EBV); varicella-zoster virus; Enteroviruses (e.g., Coxsackievirus); and insect-borne viruses (e.g., West Nile disease, Lyme disease).

Signs and symptoms: seizures, altered mental status (e.g., decreased level of consciousness, lethargy, personality change, behaviour change), fever, headache, nausea, vomiting

> Infants and neonates: poor feeding, irritability, lethargy

> Children and adolescents: irritability, movement disorder,

ataxia, stupor, coma, hemiparesis, cranial nerve defect, status epilepticus (severe symptom)

Adults: motor or sensory deficits; speech or movement impairment; flaccid paralysis

Investigations: blood tests (CBC, differential, platelets, electrolytes, glucose, BUN, creatinine, aminotransferases, coagulation); MRI (to detect brain edema; inflammation of the cerebral cortex, gray-white matter junction, thalamus, basal ganglia); CSF tests (perform lumbar puncture after results of MRI; order CSF protein, glucose, cell count, differential, Gram stain, bacterial culture); EEG (usually abnormal) to differentiate from nonconvulsive seizure activity

DEGENERATIVE

DIABETIC NEUROPATHY

Signs and symptoms: polydipsia, polyuria, and/or weight loss; autonomic neuropathy effects (indigestion, nausea, diarrhea, constipation, dizziness upon standing, urinating difficulty, erectile dysfunction, vaginal dryness)

HUNTINGTON DISEASE

Signs and symptoms: family history of Huntington disease; abnormal eye movements; tics (uncontrolled movement in the fingers, feet, face, trunk); myoclonus; chorea (progressive chorea in late-onset Huntington disease; older than 50); psychiatric symptoms (depression; apathy; anxiety; obsessions, compulsions; irritability; psychosis; paranoid and acoustic hallucinations; hypersexuality); cognitive symptoms (impaired executive function; loss of mental flexibility, concentration, judgement, memory, awareness); motor symptoms (bradykinesia, dystonia, muscle weakness); profuse sweating from autonomic disturbance

Investigations: DNA analysis (PCR or Southern blot); neuroimaging (MRI, CT scan, SPECT, PET scan) for progression monitoring

AUTOIMMUNE OR INFLAMMATORY (E.G., MULTIPLE SCLEROSIS)

MULTIPLE SCLEROSIS

Signs and symptoms: variable depending on lesion location

Spinal cord: sensory or motor dysfunction; Lhermitte sign (paresthesias radiating down the extremities or trunk with neck flexion); bowel, bladder or erectile dysfunction

Brainstem: double vision; swallowing, speech difficulties; vertigo; pseudobulbar palsy

Cerebrum: cognitive impairment; depression; upper motor neuron signs; unilateral motor or sensory deficits

Cerebellum: problems with balance and coordination; vertigo

Other symptoms: tonic spasms; fatigue; pain; exercise intolerance; temperature sensitivity; painful unilateral loss of visual acuity

Risk factors: younger than 50, female

Investigations: brain and spinal cord MRI, including advanced MRI techniques, with established occurrence of multiple episodes; CSF fluid analysis

TRAUMA

Examples of trauma include head trauma and spinal trauma.

VASCULAR

Signs and symptoms: history of vascular conditions, such as stroke, cerebellar arterial dissection, vasculitis, hemorrhage (burst aneurysm, arteriovenous malformation), hypertension, repeat subarachnoid bleeding

OTHER (E.G., GENETIC)

GENETIC CONDITION

Signs and symptoms: family history of neuropathy such as Charcot-Marie-Tooth disease (common)

> Charcot-Marie-Tooth disease: symptom onset in adolescence or early adulthood, with gradual progression of symptoms; motor and sensory deficits; weakness in the foot and lower leg muscles (typical); foot deformities (high arch, hammer toes)

Strategy for patient encounter

The likely scenario is a patient with unexplained weakness. The specified tasks could engage history, physical exam, investigations, or management.

History

The key question is whether the patient has true weakness as opposed to fatigue. As a general rule, patients with true weakness describe specific symptoms of dysfunction.

Start with open-ended questions about the onset of weakness: How quickly did the weakness develop? How constant is it? How has it progressed? What makes the weakness better or worse? Listen for evidence consistent with particular entities (e.g., weakness that is worse with sustained exertion in myasthenia gravis; sudden-onset weakness in infection; progressive weakness in degenerative disorders).

Ask about a family history of similar symptoms, and a personal history of HIV, Lyme disease, granulomatous disorders, and malignancy. Ask about any underlying systemic illnesses (e.g., diabetes).

Take a medication history, listening for neoplastic agents, steroids, and statins. Ask about alcohol abuse. Ask the patient whether their immunizations are up to date. Ask about possible occupational or toxic exposures.

Patients who are malingering or have a conversion disorder may describe inconsistent histories or weakness when performing some tasks but not others.

Physical exam

Physical examination is a key aspect of diagnosis. Perform a full neurological examination including sensation, strength, and reflexes, and assessment of the sphincter and cranial nerves.

Investigations

Order a complete blood count (CBC), and glucose or glycated hemoglobin (HbA$_{1c}$) tests (to check for diabetes). Order tests for electrolytes, creatine kinase (CK), creatinine, calcium, and liver function. Myasthenia gravis can be rapidly diagnosed in some patients through the bedside Tensilon test (however, this is rarely done clinically). In suspected Guillain-Barré syndrome or multiple sclerosis, perform a lumbar puncture to look for protein, cells, and oligoclonal bands. In suspected myelopathy or stroke, order an MRI or CT scan. In suspected myopathy, perform a muscle biopsy. Order electromyography (EMG) to assist in the diagnosis of Guillain-Barré syndrome, motor neuron disease, and myasthenia gravis. In suspected inherited disease, order genetic testing.

Management

Management depends on the specific entity identified. Immediately correct any electrolyte abnormalities. Optimally control any underlying disease. Discontinue any causative drugs. Refer the patient to neurology, physiotherapy, occupational therapy, or a stroke clinic as appropriate.

170

Weight gain, obesity

MCC particular objectives

Determine the degree and pattern of obesity.

Exclude primary treatable causes.

Assess the risk of associated morbidity and mortality.

MCC differential diagnosis
with added evidence

INCREASED ENERGY INTAKE

Dietary cause (e.g., high fat/sugar diet, overeating)

HIGH FAT/SUGAR DIET

Signs and symptoms: history of high intake of foods with refined carbohydrates and fats (e.g., fast food, processed foods), and beverages containing sugar (soda, juice, alcohol)

OVEREATING

Signs and symptoms: polyphagia or hyperphagia (increased appetite or excessive hunger; no satiety from consuming food) due to diabetes, depression, stress (common causes)

Social and behavioural cause (e.g., socioeconomic cause, psychosocial cause)

SOCIOECONOMIC CAUSE

There is a higher incidence of obesity in children and adults with lower socioeconomic status, perhaps due to lack of access to good nutrition because of expense or location.

PSYCHOSOCIAL CAUSE

Signs and symptoms: sleeping < 6 hours a night; chronic sleep disturbance; employed in shift work; depression or stress

Iatrogenic cause (e.g., drugs, hormones, hypothalamic surgery)

DRUGS

Drugs associated with weight gain include atypical antipsychotics (these are associated with marked weight gain), steroids, some selective serotonin reuptake inhibitors (SSRIs), amitriptyline, mood stabilizers (e.g., lithium, valproic acid, carbamazepine), and antiepileptics (e.g., valproate, gabapentin).

HORMONES

Signs and symptoms: history of hypothyroidism, polycystic ovary syndrome (common), or Cushing syndrome (rare)

DECREASED ENERGY EXPENDITURE (E.G., SEDENTARY LIFESTYLE, SMOKING CESSATION)

Signs and symptoms: history of recent change in exercise habits (e.g., new job that involves more sitting; loss of mobility from injury or illness), or recent smoking cessation

NEUROENDOCRINE CONDITION (E.G., HYPOTHYROIDISM, CUSHING SYNDROME, POLYCYSTIC OVARY SYNDROME)

HYPOTHYROIDISM

Signs and symptoms: history of hypothyroidism or symptoms of hypothyroidism (cold intolerance, decreased reflexes, dry skin, weight gain, impaired cognition)

Investigations: elevated thyrotropin (TSH)

CUSHING SYNDROME

Signs and symptoms: history of glucocorticoid therapy; cushingoid features (round, red face; pronounced abdominal weight; hump on the upper back; thin arms and legs; high blood pressure; stretch marks; acne)

Investigations: high cortisol levels on either a 24-hour urine cortisol test or dexamethasone suppression test

POLYCYSTIC OVARY SYNDROME

Signs and symptoms: symptom onset after puberty, with increased rate of hair growth and male-pattern hair growth; irregular menstruation; infertility; obesity; acne

Investigations: LH:FSH ratio (elevated: 2:1 or 3:1) (usual); elevated testosterone; ultrasound for ovarian cysts; normal prolactin levels; normal thyroid function

Genetic (e.g., Prader-Willi syndrome)

PRADER-WILLI SYNDROME

Survival past 50 years is low unless this condition is treated.

Signs and symptoms (adults and children in general): excess fat in the central body; small hands and feet; prominent nasal bridge; thin upper lip; downturned mouth; almond-shaped eyes; high narrow forehead; tapered fingers; soft, easily bruised skin; light skin and hair compared to family members; incomplete sexual development; frequent skin picking; delayed motor development

Prenatal and neonate: reduced fetal movement; abnormal

fetal position; excessive amniotic fluid; breech or cesarean birth; lethargy; hypotonia; poor sucking; hypogonadism

Children: delayed intellectual development; excessive sleeping; strabismus; scoliosis; cryptorchidism; speech delay; poor physical coordination; hyperphagia; excessive weight gain; sleep disorders; delayed puberty; short stature; obesity; extreme flexibility

Adults: infertility; hypogonadism; sparse pubic hair; obesity; hypotonia; learning and cognitive disabilities; diabetes (often)

Investigations: DNA-based methylation testing for Prader-Willi syndrome and Angelman syndrome

Epigenetic

Some causes are well understood, including Prader-Willi syndrome (this is usually paternally imprinted) and abnormalities of the *GNAS* locus.

There are likely other epigenetic causes that are poorly understood.

Investigations: genetic testing

Strategy for patient encounter

The likely scenario is an obese patient looking to lose weight. The specified tasks could engage history, physical exam, investigations, or management (counselling).

The key to this encounter is to identify the primary mechanism of weight gain: increased nutritional intake or decreased expenditure.

History

Start with open-ended questions about the extent and time frame of the weight gain: How much weight have you gained? How long have you been gaining weight? Ask if the weight gain is intentional or unintentional, and whether it began with a new medication or smoking cessation. Ask about the patient's diet and social environment.

Use open-ended questions to establish associated symptoms and past medical history: What conditions do you have? How has your health been generally? Listen for a history of, or symptoms consistent with, hypothyroidism (e.g., cold intolerance, dry skin, impaired cognition), Cushing syndrome (e.g., hump on the upper back, stretch marks, acne), and (in female patients) polycystic ovary syndrome (e.g., male-pattern hair growth, irregular menstruation, infertility).

Because obesity is a major risk factor for cardiovascular disease, ask about additional risk factors for cardiovascular disease including family history, diabetes, smoking, hypertension, dyslipidemia, and sleep apnea.

Physical exam

Obtain the patient's vital signs, looking for bradycardia (this suggests hypothyroidism) and hypertension (this suggests Cushing syndrome). Note the distribution of fat (truncal with a hump on the upper back in Cushing syndrome). Measure the waist circumference, or waist-to-hip ratio, and calculate the patient's body mass index (BMI). Assess the patient for acanthosis nigricans (hyperpigmentation often found in the armpits, groin, and folds of the neck), which suggests insulin resistance.

Investigations

Rule out hypothyroidism with a thyrotropin (TSH) level. If the physical exam suggests Cushing syndrome or polycystic ovary syndrome, order additional investigations (see the information this resource lists in the MCC differential diagnosis). Perform screening for comorbid conditions (glucose and lipid panel).

Counselling

Counsel the patient regarding exercise, diet, and behaviour modification. Discuss indications for—and risks and benefits of—antiobesity drugs and bariatric surgery. Demonstrate sensitivity to the social and psychosocial consequences of obesity.

Pearls

Remember that for a stable weight, calories in equal calories out.

TIP

Tailoring information to individual patients

The MCC identifies providing generic information as a common exam error.

To avoid this error, ask patients about aspects of their lives that might affect their condition. Provide information that targets their situation and engage the patient in figuring out next steps.

For example, diet and exercise changes might be relevant for this case:

- Ask what the patient ate yesterday for breakfast, lunch, and supper. Use this to personalize guidelines on dietary changes they need to make.

- Ask what the patient did for exercise last week. Discuss short-term goals with the patient: What could the patient do next week to exercise every day? (For example, when could the patient fit in a 30-minute walk?)

171

Weight loss, eating disorders, anorexia

MCC particular objective

Investigate for underlying medical conditions, where appropriate.

MCC differential diagnosis
with added evidence

DECREASED NUTRITIONAL INTAKE

Psychiatric disease (e.g., anorexia nervosa, bulimia)

ANOREXIA NERVOSA[1(pp338–339)]

Signs and symptoms: significantly low body weight; intense fear of gaining weight or persistent behaviour that interferes with gaining weight; excessive focus on body weight or shape in self-evaluation, or persistent lack of recognition of current low body weight

BULIMIA NERVOSA[1(p345)]

Signs and symptoms: recurrent binge eating, followed by behaviours to prevent weight gain (e.g., vomiting, abuse of laxatives, excessive exercise, fasting); binging and weight-loss behaviours that both occur ≥ 1 time per week for ≥ 3 months; excessive focus on body weight or shape in self-evaluation

Medical disease (e.g., chronic illness, esophageal cancer)

CHRONIC ILLNESS

Examples of chronic illness include kidney disease and adrenal insufficiency.

Signs and symptoms:

> Kidney disease: bilateral lower limb swelling; shortness of breath; paroxysmal nocturnal dyspnea; orthopnea

> Chronic primary adrenal insufficiency: abdominal pain; fatigue; hyperpigmentation; orthostatic light-headedness

ESOPHAGEAL CANCER

Signs and symptoms: none in early esophageal cancer (typical); difficulty swallowing; worsening indigestion or heartburn; chest pain; coughing; weight loss

Investigations: barium swallow imaging for esophageal assessment; endoscopy to examine the esophagus; biopsy; CT and PET scan to determine the stage of the cancer

Substance abuse or medications (e.g., alcohol, opiates, cocaine, amphetamines, anticancer drugs)

INCREASED ENERGY EXPENDITURE

Hormonal condition (e.g., hyperthyroidism)

HYPERTHYROIDISM

Signs and symptoms: history of hyperthyroidism or symptoms of hyperthyroidism (changes in menstrual patterns, enlarged thyroid, tachycardia, palpitations, diarrhea, muscle weakness, tremor, hyperactive reflexes, weight loss, sweating, thinning hair)

Investigations: decreased thyrotropin (TSH)

Chronic illness (e.g., chronic obstructive pulmonary disease, congestive heart failure)

CHRONIC OBSTRUCTIVE PULMONARY DISEASE

Signs and symptoms: wheezing; chest tightness; chronic productive cough; clubbing of fingers; cyanosis around the lips and in the extremities; decreased oxygen saturation; decreased capacity on pulmonary function testing

Risk factors: smoking; occupational exposure; intrinsic lung disease

Investigations: chest X-ray

CONGESTIVE HEART FAILURE

Signs and symptoms: history of heart disease (or risk factors for heart disease: diabetes, hypertension, hyperlipidemia, smoking) or hepatic vein thrombosis (Budd-Chiari syndrome); severe shortness of breath; elevated jugular venous pressure; edema in the abdomen and legs; pink phlegm; heart murmurs and extra cardiac sounds

Investigations: chest X-ray to detect pulmonary edema; NT-proBNP level; echocardiogram to distinguish forms of heart failure; cardiac stress testing, either with exercise or pharmacological agent

Malignancy

Signs and symptoms: weight loss, night sweats, fatigue, fever, organ-specific symptoms (e.g., bone pain)

Infection

Signs and symptoms: weight loss that develops over weeks or months (weight loss is clinically important if an adult loses > 5% of body weight or > 5 kg over 6 months)

If due to fungal infections: fever, night sweats, fatigue, cough, shortness of breath

If due to parasitic infections: fever, abdominal pain, bloating, diarrhea, eosinophilia, history of travel in developing countries

If due to viral infection (HIV): fever, shortness of breath, cough, lymphadenopathy, diarrhea, oral candidiasis (white oral plaques)

If due to tuberculosis: fever; night sweats; cough; hemoptysis; exposure to infected persons; poor, crowded living conditions

Investigations: stool test for ova and parasites; blood test to detect HIV; sputum culture to detect TB

Increased physical activity (e.g., runners)

CALORIC LOSS

Malabsorption (e.g., diarrhea)

CHOLESTASIS

This is slowed or blocked bile flow from the liver caused by acute hepatitis, alcoholic liver disease, primary biliary cirrhosis, pancreatitis, gallstones, and certain drugs.

Signs and symptoms: pale fatty stools; dark urine; itching; nausea; right upper quadrant abdominal pain; jaundice

CELIAC DISEASE

Signs and symptoms: family history of celiac disease, or signs and symptoms of celiac disease (chronic abdominal pain, rashes)

Investigations: positive serum anti-tTG (with IgA level); duodenal biopsy to detect villous blunting

INFLAMMATORY BOWEL DISEASE

Signs and symptoms: younger than 30 (usually); family history of inflammatory bowel disease; fluctuating symptoms with periods of exacerbation and remission; diarrhea (possibly with nocturnal waking); blood in the stool; abdominal pain; weight loss; fever; fatigue; right lower quadrant and periumbilical pain; extraintestinal manifestations (e.g., uveitis, arthritis)

> Crohn disease: right lower quadrant mass, inflammation of the eyes, arthritis

Investigations: elevated CRP (this suggests active inflammation); fecal calprotectin; colonoscopy with biopsy (this is a standard diagnostic procedure); CT scan or MRI (findings: diagnostic structural changes associated with inflammatory bowel disease)

Diabetes

Signs and symptoms: personal or family history of diabetes; history of diabetic complications and/or inadequate monitoring; polydipsia, polyuria, and/or weight loss

Investigations: fasting glucose or HbA_{1c} test

Strategy for patient encounter

The likely scenario is an adolescent girl with anorexia nervosa (the minimum age to play standardized patients is 16). The specified tasks could engage history, physical exam, investigations, or management.

The key to this encounter is to identify the primary mechanism of weight loss: decreased nutritional intake or increased expenditure.

History

Start with open-ended questions about the extent and time frame of the weight loss: How much weight have you lost? How long have you been losing weight? Ask if the weight loss is intentional or unintentional, and about the symptoms of anorexia nervosa and bulimia (e.g., fear of gaining weight and lack of perspective on current weight in anorexia nervosa; binge eating followed by vomiting in bulimia).

Ask open-ended questions to establish associated symptoms and medical history: What conditions do you have? How has your health been generally? Listen for a history of, or symptoms consistent with, chronic obstructive pulmonary disease (shortness of breath, wheezing, history of smoking), malignancy (weight loss, night sweats, fatigue, fever), malabsorption (abdominal pain, diarrhea), and diabetes (polydipsia, polyuria).

Physical exam

Obtain the patient's vital signs. Measure the patient's height and weight, and calculate their body mass index (BMI).

Listen to the lungs (wheezing in chronic obstructive pulmonary disease, rales in congestive heart failure). Listen to the heart (murmurs or extra sounds in congestive heart failure). Examine the legs for peripheral edema (this is a finding in congestive heart failure). Eating disorders often do not have specific physical findings. Patients with bulimia may show damage to tooth enamel from stomach acid.

Investigations

For all patients, rule out diabetes with a blood glucose test and hyperthyroidism with a thyrotropin (TSH) level. Additional investigations will depend on the specifics of the history (see the information this resource lists in the MCC differential diagnosis). Nutritional status can be further investigated by measuring serum albumin.

Management

If you identify decreased nutritional intake, refer the patient to a dietitian or specialized treatment program. In cases of anorexia nervosa, refer the patient for counselling and to an eating disorders clinic.

If you identify increased energy expenditure, management will depend on the specific diagnosis.

Pearls

Remember that for a stable weight, calories in equal calories out.

REFERENCE

1 American Psychiatric Association. Diagnostic and statistical manual of mental disorders. 5th ed. Arlington, VA: American Psychiatric Association; 2013. 991 p.

172

Intrauterine growth restriction (IUGR)

MCC particular objectives

Pay attention to:

- modifiable risk factors for IUGR early in pregnancy
- routine monitoring of fetal growth throughout pregnancy
- careful evaluation of a neonate who is small for their gestational age to detect a possible case of IUGR and assess potential causal conditions

MCC differential diagnosis
with added evidence
IUGR IN GENERAL

This is defined as in-utero growth below the tenth percentile for a baby's gestational age.

MATERNAL CAUSE (E.G., NUTRITIONAL STATUS)

Maternal causes and risk factors include previous IUGR; previous stillbirth; medical conditions (hypertension, diabetes mellitus, renal disease, autoimmune diseases); medications (anticonvulsants, anticoagulants, heparin, antineoplastics, cyclophosphamide); malnutrition; smoking; use of alcohol or illicit drugs; low prepregnancy weight; low socioeconomic status; younger than 16 or older than 35; use of assisted reproductive technology; and current pregnancy complications (e.g., preeclampsia, threatened miscarriage with heavy bleeding).

FETAL CAUSE (E.G., GENETIC SYNDROME, INTRAUTERINE INFECTION)

GENETIC SYNDROME

Signs and symptoms: family history of a genetic condition or syndrome; karyotype (aneuploidy) abnormalities such as trisomy 21 syndrome, trisomy 13 syndrome, trisomy 18 syndrome, Turner syndrome

INTRAUTERINE INFECTION

TOXOPLASMOSIS

Signs and symptoms: mild, flu-like symptoms lasting weeks to months; history of having cats or changing litter boxes while pregnant, or ingesting undercooked meat or contaminated water

Investigations: low avidity test in acute or recent infection; high avidity test in past infection

CYTOMEGALOVIRUS

Signs and symptoms: history of contact with infected blood and body fluids, including blood transfusions or sexual contact

Investigations: PCR; antigen test

RUBELLA

Signs and symptoms: low-grade fever; rash that begins on the face then spreads to other areas of the body; red or swollen sclera; history of contact with infected persons

Investigations: positive IgM 5 days after rash onset; low IgG rubella antibody on avidity testing for the first few months postinfection

VARICELLA-ZOSTER VIRUS

Signs and symptoms: rash of pruritic blisters ("dew drops on a rose petal") that eventually crust or scab, and that appear first on the face, chest, and back, and then spread over several days; history of fever, fatigue, anorexia, and/or headache 1 to 2 days before the rash (possible); contact with infected persons

> Shingles: unilateral blister rash with crusting and scabbing along a dermatome; history of pain, pruritus, and/or tingling 1 to 5 days before the rash (possible); history of chickenpox or direct contact with shingles blisters

MALARIA

Signs and symptoms: chills followed by fever, headache, and vomiting, then sweating, normal temperature, and fatigue (bouts occur every second or third day depending on the species of *Plasmodium*); weakness; enlarged liver and spleen; mild jaundice; tachypnea; history of living or travelling to an area with endemic malaria and not using insect repellent, antimalarial medications, or bed nets

Investigations: peripheral blood smear to detect parasites in RBCs; PCR to detect organism

SYPHILIS

Signs and symptoms: history of unprotected sex or high-risk sexual behaviours; painless, firm, round ulcers or chancres on the genitals or anus, or in the mouth; nonpruritic red-brown rash on the whole body or on parts of the body (e.g., soles, palms); alopecia; myalgia

> Late stage symptoms: paralysis, numbness, blindness, dementia, loss of coordination, gummatous lesions

Investigations: darkfield microscopy of lesion to detect *Treponema pallidum* spirochete; VDRL test and treponemal test

HERPES SIMPLEX VIRUS

Signs and symptoms: sexual contact with infected persons who may or may not have visible sores; painful blister(s) on the genitals and rectum, and in the mouth; repeated outbreaks taking several weeks to heal (common)

Investigations: PCR HSV DNA assay (most sensitive); cell culture; Tzanck preparation for cytologic diagnosis

HIV
Signs and symptoms: history of HIV; sexual contact with infected persons

PLACENTAL CAUSE (E.G., MATERNAL SMOKING)

PLACENTAL INSUFFICIENCY
Signs and symptoms: asymmetry sparing the brain, but affecting weight and length (usual); late pregnancy stage (usual); oligohydramnios

PLACENTAL MALFORMATIONS
Signs and symptoms: positive ultrasound for, or gross identification of, a single umbilical artery; velamentous or marginal cord insertion; circumvallate or bilobed placenta; hemangioma of the placenta

ABRUPTIO PLACENTAE
Signs and symptoms: vaginal bleeding; abdominal or back pain with tender uterus; hypotension; tachycardia; fetal distress, including absent heart rate or decelerations with normal fetal presentation
Risk factors: late maternal age; polyhydramnios; history of hypertension or other vascular disease (including coagulopathy); smoking; cocaine use; physical trauma (including abuse); previous abruption; multigestational pregnancy; uterine fibroids
Investigations: low fibrinogen; anemia

PLACENTAL ISCHEMIA OR INFARCTION
Signs and symptoms: preeclampsia; abruptio placentae; history of previous infarction

Strategy for patient encounter
The likely scenario is a pregnant patient with possible (border-line) IUGR based on prenatal ultrasound. The specified tasks could engage history, physical exam, investigations, or management (referral and counselling).

History
Determine risk factors for IUGR. Ask about a family history of genetically inherited disorders; lack of personal immunization for rubella and varicella-zoster virus; and infectious exposures, including toxoplasmosis (exposure to cats, especially cleaning cat litter boxes), Cytomegalovirus (contact with infected blood and body fluids, sexual contact), malaria (travel to endemic areas),

syphilis (sexual contact), herpes simplex (sexual contact), and HIV (sexual contact, intravenous drug use).

Use open-ended questions to determine the history of the current pregnancy and previous pregnancies: How has this pregnancy been going? What difficulties did you have with previous pregnancies? Listen specifically for indications of bleeding (in all pregnancies), IUGR (previous pregnancies), and trauma (current pregnancy).

Physical exam

The physical exam should include vital signs, measurement of fundal height, and assessment of fetal heart rate with a Doppler monitor.

(State you will perform these examinations. Since a standardized patient experiencing IUGR is unlikely, the examiner will likely interrupt, ask what you are looking for, and provide findings. State that you are looking for unstable vital signs, small fundal height for age of gestation, and low or irregular fetal heart rate.)

Investigations

Order blood tests for infectious causes (see the information this resource lists in the MCC differential diagnosis), and for biophysical profile.

Referral and counselling

Refer the patient to a high-risk obstetrics clinic. Counsel on smoking cessation.

173

Abnormalities of white blood cells

MCC particular objective

Differentiate life-threatening conditions that require immediate treatment (overwhelming sepsis, acute leukemia, febrile neutropenia) from nonurgent conditions.

MCC differential diagnosis
with added evidence

LEUKOCYTOSIS

LEUKOCYTOSIS IN GENERAL

Leukocytosis usually indicates infection or a nonmalignant etiology.

Reactive (e.g., bacterial infection, infectious mononucleosis)

BACTERIAL INFECTION

Signs and symptoms: white blood cell (WBC) count > 10 000/mm^3; fever

MONONUCLEOSIS

Signs and symptoms (classic triad): fever, pharyngitis, lymphadenopathy (usually posterior cervical)

> Additional signs and symptoms: fatigue and malaise; headache; abdominal pain; nausea, vomiting; rash; splenomegaly; palatal exanthems or petechiae

Investigations: CBC, lymphocytosis (> 50%); peripheral blood smear to detect atypical lymphocytes; heterophile antibody test (e.g., Monospot); EBV-specific serology testing (definitive)

Neoplastic (e.g., leukemia)

LEUKEMIA

Signs and symptoms: fever; chills; persistent fatigue and weakness; frequent or severe infections; weight loss; pallor; swollen lymph nodes; enlarged liver or spleen; easy bleeding and bruising; recurrent nosebleeds; petechiae; excessive sweating; bone pain or tenderness

Investigations: CBC; peripheral blood smear; flow cytometry; bone marrow aspiration and biopsy

LEUKOPENIA

Increased destruction (e.g., bacterial infection, HIV)

BACTERIAL INFECTION

Examples of bacterial infections include typhoid fever, rickettsia, brucellosis, and dengue fever.

Signs and symptoms: acute neutropenia; fever (this indicates serious infection), shaking chills, hypothermia; increased respiratory and heart rate

> Rickettsia: history of insect bites or contact (ticks, fleas); characteristic rash or petechiae; sudden-onset fever, severe headache, malaise

HIV

HIV develops into AIDS when the CD4 cell count is < 200 cells/mm^3 (reference range of CD4: 500–2000 cells/mm^3).

Signs and symptoms: flu-like symptoms in the first, acute phase; leukopenia in the second, latent, asymptomatic stage (200–499 CD4 cells/mm^3); lymphadenopathy

> AIDS: recurrent, severe opportunistic infections or malignancies

Risk factors: unprotected sex; intravenous (IV) drug use

Investigations: positive HIV-1 p24 antigen in the blood followed by HIV antibody testing (positive ELISA result); PCR to determine HIV RNA level or viral load

Decreased production (e.g., marrow suppression)

This is commonly due to chemotherapy and can cause anemia, neutropenia, and thrombocytopenia.

Signs and symptoms:

> Anemia: fatigue, pallor, dizziness, shortness of breath, tachycardia
>
> Neutropenia: infections, fever, chills, diarrhea, cough, rash, mouth sores
>
> Thrombocytopenia: bleeding, petechiae, easy bruising, hematuria, black stools

LEUKOCYTE DYSFUNCTION (E.G., HIV, CHRONIC GRANULOMATOUS DISEASE)

HIV—SEE ABOVE

CHRONIC GRANULOMATOUS DISEASE

This immunodeficiency produces recurrent or persistent bacterial and fungal infections, and granulomas.

Signs and symptoms: onset before age 2 (usual), but also during 20s; male (usual); failure to thrive (in infants), short stature (older patients); recurrent pyoderma (common) such as perianal, axillary, scalp abscesses; recurrent or persistent pneumonia, dermatitis, cutaneous disease, or infections; gastrointestinal complications (diarrhea); abscesses (spleen, liver, gingival); septicemia

Investigations: nitroblue tetrazolium (NBT) dye test (this confirms that neutrophils, monocytes, macrophages, and eosinophils are not producing superoxide anions); peripheral blood leukocytosis (> 8500 neutrophils/μL); anemia

Strategy for patient encounter

The likely scenario is a patient with elevated white blood cells (WBCs) on a routine complete blood count (CBC). The specified tasks could engage history, physical exam, investigations, or management.

This encounter will likely involve correlating a CBC with history and clinical presentation.

History

Start with open-ended inquiry, such as: How has your health been lately? Listen for symptoms of infection (fever, localized pain, redness) and malignancy (fever, weight loss, malaise). Ask about a recent history of infectious contacts and foreign travel. Ask about a known history of immunodeficiency (cancer, autoimmune disease, HIV, immunosuppressive therapy).

Physical exam

The physical exam will be guided by the clinical findings. In all cases of suspected infection, obtain the patient's vital signs (looking for fever and hypotension), and examine the head and neck for sites of infection and swollen lymph nodes. Listen to the lungs for evidence of pneumonia. Examine the abdomen for enlarged liver and spleen (these suggest mononucleosis or cancer).

Investigations

In suspected infection, perform a culture of the relevant sites. In suspected sepsis (the key finding is hypotension), admit the patient to intensive care, perform blood cultures, and start empirical antibiotic treatment.

Remember that febrile neutropenia requires urgent cultures (blood, urine, and, in some cases, cerebrospinal fluid), hospitalization, and empirical antibiotic treatment. These patients are usually neutropenic due to malignancy or chemotherapy.

Elevated neutrophils usually indicate infection. Elevated lymphocytes may be in response to viral infection or may be neoplastic. If blasts are present, or if lymphocytosis (more than 5000 monoclonal lymphocytes per mm^3) persists for several months, consider leukemia: order cell surface markers and consider a bone marrow biopsy (see additional tests that this resource lists in the MCC differential diagnosis).

Management
The scenarios that require emergency management include sepsis and febrile neutropenia. Other scenarios may require further testing or referral to specialists (e.g., a hematologist).

Pearls
Remember to consider mononucleosis in younger individuals with elevated WBCs and atypical lymphocytes.

174

Negligence

MCC particular objectives
When a patient claims negligent care, or the candidate is aware of negligent care:

- Consider the standard of care.
- Consider the possibility of injury from the care.
- Describe what action to take.

MCC differential diagnosis
None stated.

Strategy for patient encounter
The likely scenario is a patient discussing negligent care from another health care provider. The likely tasks are history and counselling.

History

The encounter will likely be an interview with a patient who has a complaint against another physician.

The interview needs to cover the elements required to prove negligence: a duty of care; a breach of care; harm; and a connection between the harm and the breach of care.

Ask open-ended questions, such as: What events have led to your concerns? Where did they take place? What health issues are you having now?

Listen for information relevant to the existence of a doctor-patient relationship. In some situations, this relationship would not exist—for example, in an emergency situation outside of a health care facility. In these situations, a physician who acted with reasonable care is generally protected from prosecution in Canada.

If there was a duty of care, listen for details about the care provided. The question is whether it deviated from reasonable steps a physician with a similar level of training would have taken. This can be subjective, and, in a real situation of possible breach of care, would likely involve assessment by a number of peers: take notes.

Listen for evidence that the patient has suffered harm, and for details that connect the harm to the care provided. Ask specific questions that help clarify the nature and timing of any harm.

Counselling

Most complaints can be resolved quickly and directly by a meeting between the physician and the patient, possibly

---

CHECKLIST

How to respond to a formal complaint

- Acknowledge in writing that you have received the complaint (same day).
- Gather facts: review medical notes, reports, records.
- Speak to the Canadian Medical Protective Association (CMPA) regarding further actions to be taken.
- Follow confidentiality rules.
- Taking into account the advice of the CMPA, write a response to the patient. Use the facts to address all specific aspects of the complaint. If appropriate, describe measures now in place to prevent similar events. Thank the patient for bringing their concerns to your attention.
- Recognize that complaints have value and use them to improve.

with a facilitator present (e.g., the physician's medical director). Counsel the patient to consider this as a first option.

If the patient wishes to pursue a formal complaint, explain next steps: you will inform the physician, and the physician will respond to the patient in writing (see the checklist on how to respond to a formal complaint).

Pearls
Most complaints stem from inadequate communication.

175

Obsessive-compulsive (OCD) and related disorders

MCC particular objective
Pay particular attention to possible etiology and coexisting conditions.

MCC differential diagnosis
with added evidence

OCD AND RELATED DISORDERS IN GENERAL
The *Diagnostic and Statistical Manual of Mental Disorders* (*DSM-5*) identifies OCD and related disorders as a group of disorders characterized by obsessions and repetitive behaviours. This group includes OCD, body-dysmorphic disorder, hoarding disorder, trichotillomania (hair pulling), and excoriation disorder (skin picking). OCD often occurs with other psychiatric disorders.

ADVERSE CHILDHOOD EXPERIENCES
These include abuse (physical, sexual, emotional); neglect (physical, emotional); exposure to domestic violence; and family dysfunction due to divorce (or separation), substance abuse, mental illness, or imprisonment.

GENETIC NEUROLOGICAL DYSFUNCTION

A family history of OCD is a risk factor for developing OCD.

OTHER PSYCHIATRIC DISORDERS (E.G., TIC DISORDER, ANXIETY DISORDERS, DEPRESSION, SUBSTANCE USE DISORDER)

TIC DISORDER

Signs and symptoms: symptom onset in childhood or adolescence; motor and/or vocal tics (examples of motor tics: eye blinking, facial grimacing, head jerking; examples of vocal tics: grunting, repeating what other say, repeating particular words or phrases)

> Tourette syndrome: presence of both motor and vocal tics (not necessarily concurrently); presence of tics for ≥ 1 year; presence of tics before age 12 (common)

> Chronic tic disorder: presence of either motor or vocal tics; presence of tics for ≥ 1 year

> Provisional tic disorder: presence of motor and/or vocal tics; presence of tics for < 1 year

Risk factors: male (3 to 4 times more common); family history of tic disorder

ANXIETY DISORDERS[1(pp189-234)]

Examples of anxiety disorders listed in the *Diagnostic and Statistical Manual of Mental Disorders* (*DSM-5*) include generalized anxiety disorder, panic disorder, separation anxiety disorder, social anxiety disorder, and specific phobia.

Signs and symptoms: anxiety about anticipated events; panic attacks (possible); symptoms with significant impact on day-to-day life

> Generalized anxiety disorder: excessive worry about a number of contexts (e.g., work, school); presence of other symptoms, such as fatigue, irritability, loss of concentration, muscle tension, sleep disturbance; family history of anxiety disorders; presence of symptoms for most of the time for ≥ 6 months

> Separation anxiety disorder: excessive anxiety (e.g., distress, worry, nightmares) about separation from a particular person; physical symptoms provoked by anxiety (e.g., headaches, stomach aches); presence of symptoms for ≥ 6 months (in adults)

> Social anxiety disorder: excessive anxiety about scrutiny by others and being negatively judged; avoidance of social situations; presence of symptoms for ≥ 6 months (typical, in adults)

> Specific phobia: excessive anxiety about an object or situation (e.g., insects, receiving an injection); presence of symptoms for ≥ 6 months

Panic disorder: recurrent unexpected panic attacks (surges of intense fear or discomfort that peak within minutes); worry and/or avoidance behaviours regarding future panic attacks for ≥ 1 month

MAJOR DEPRESSIVE DISORDER[1(pp160-161)]

Signs and symptoms: symptoms that are present most of the time for ≥ 2 weeks; symptoms with significant impact on day-to-day life

Key symptoms: depressed mood and/or loss of interest in usual activities

Other symptoms: significant weight change; sleep disturbance; slowed or agitated mental processes; loss of concentration; recurrent thoughts of death or suicide

Risk factors: family history of mental health disorders (depression, anxiety, suicide); personal history of other mental health disorders; substance abuse; chronic illness (e.g., cancer, stroke, chronic pain)

SUBSTANCE USE DISORDER[1(p483)]

Signs and symptoms: using a substance for longer or in larger quantities than intended; unsuccessful attempts to quit using it; substantial time spent in acquiring the substance and/or recovering from its use; increasing need for the substance; maintaining the substance use despite negative consequences (e.g., financial trouble; jeopardized relationships) and known dangers to physical and/or mental health; withdrawal symptoms on attempts to quit

OTHER MEDICAL CONDITIONS (E.G., INFECTIONS)

PEDIATRIC AUTOIMMUNE NEUROPSYCHIATRIC DISORDERS ASSOCIATED WITH STREPTOCOCCAL INFECTIONS (PANDAS)

This is an autoimmune disorder that damages the basal ganglia (which help control movement and behaviour) following a group A streptococcal infection.

It is a controversial diagnosis, in part because a causal link between group A streptococcal infection and OCD remains uncertain.

Signs and symptoms: OCD symptoms following a streptococcal infection (e.g., streptococcal pharyngitis), which may or may not have been diagnosed

Streptococcal pharyngitis: sudden-onset fever and sore throat; enlarged lymph nodes in the neck; swollen tonsils, possibly with white spots or pus; palatal petechiae

Strategy for patient encounter

The likely scenario is an adult patient presenting with OCD-related behaviours. The specified tasks could engage history, physical exam, investigations, or management.

History

Use open-ended inquiry about the patient's symptoms and their effect on the patient's functioning: Please tell me what you have been experiencing. How do your symptoms affect your daily life? Listen for evidence consistent with OCD and related disorders (e.g., obsessive thoughts, repetitive behaviours, tics, phobias, panic attacks, sleep disturbance, loss of concentration, anxiety); and for significant impact of the symptoms on the patient's relationships, employment, and/or education.

Obtain a psychosocial history, including childhood experiences, and current and past stressors.

Physical exam

Perform a general physical examination, focusing on the neurological and dermatological exams.

Investigations

Order a urine drug screen. Consider specific testing for infectious agents (e.g., streptococcal infection). Consider neurological imaging (e.g., head CT or MRI).

Management

Consider referring the patient to a psychiatrist or psychologist. Consider the psychosocial impact of the patient's symptoms and assess the need for family counselling. Initiate treatment with a selective serotonin reuptake inhibitor (SSRI).

REFERENCE

1 American Psychiatric Association. Diagnostic and statistical manual of mental disorders. 5th ed. Arlington, VA: American Psychiatric Association; 2013. 991 p.

Abbreviations

5-HIAA 5-hydroxyindoleacetic acid
ABG arterial blood gas
ACE inhibitor angiotensin-converting enzyme inhibitor
AChR antibody acetylcholine receptor antibody
ACL anterior cruciate ligament
ACTH adrenocorticotropic hormone
ADAMTS13 a disintegrin and metalloproteinase enzyme with a thrombospondin type 1 motif, member 13
ADH antidiuretic hormone
ADHD attention deficit hyperactivity disorder
AFB acid fast bacilli
AFP α_1-fetoprotein
AHase antihyaluronidase
AIDS acquired immune deficiency syndrome
ALP alkaline phosphatase
ALT alanine aminotransferase
ANA antinuclear antibody
ANCA antineutrophil cytoplasmic antibody
anti-DNase antideoxyribonuclease B
anti-NAD antinicotinamide adenine dinucleotidase
anti-TPO antithyroid peroxidase
AP X-ray anterior-posterior X-ray
aPTT activated partial thromboplastin time
ASA acetylsalicylic acid
ASD autism spectrum disorder
ASKas antistreptokinase
ASO antistreptolysin
AST aspartate aminotransferase
AV conduction atrioventricular conduction
BMI body mass index
BNP B-type natriuretic peptide
BUN blood urea nitrogen
C3 complement component 3
CA 125 cancer antigen 125
CBC complete blood count
CEA carcinoembryonic antigen

CHARGE syndrome syndrome with a collection of congenital abnormalities (mnemonic **CHARGE**): coloboma, heart defects, atresia choanae, growth retardation, genital abnormalities, and ear abnormalities)
CK creatine kinase
CKMB creatine kinase MB
CNS central nervous system
COX-2 inhibitors cyclooxygenase-2 inhibitors
CPR cardiopulmonary resuscitation
CRP C-reactive protein
CSF cerebrospinal fluid
CT scan computed tomography scan
DAT direct antiglobulin test
DHEA-S dehydroepiandrosterone-sulfate
DNA deoxyribonucleic acid
dsDNA double-stranded DNA
DSM-5 *Diagnostic and Statistical Manual of Mental Disorders,* fifth edition
EBV Epstein-Barr virus
ECG electrocardiogram
EDTA ethylenediaminetetraacetic acid
EEG electroencephalogram
EIA enzyme immunoassay
ELISA enzyme-linked immunosorbent assay
EMG electromyogram
EPO erythropoietin
ERCP endoscopic retrograde cholangiopancreatography
ESR erythrocyte sedimentation rate
FEV forced respiratory volume (FEV1: forced respiratory volume in 1 second)
FSH follicle stimulating hormone
GBM glomerular basement membrane
GFR glomerular filtration rate
GGT γ-glutamyltransferase
GI gastrointestinal
HAV hepatitis A virus
HbA$_{1c}$ glycated hemoglobin
HBV hepatitis B virus
hCG human chorionic gonadotropin
HCV hepatitis C virus
HDL high density lipoprotein cholesterol

HELLP syndrome syndrome with the following characteristics (mnemonic HELLP): **h**emolysis, **e**levated **l**iver enzymes, **l**ow **p**latelet count

HEV hepatitis E virus

Hib vaccine *Haemophilus influenzae* type B vaccine

HIV human immunodeficiency virus

HLA human leukocyte antigen

HPLC high performance liquid chromatography

HPV human papillomavirus

HSV herpes simplex virus

IAT indirect antiglobulin test

ICU intensive care unit

IgA immunoglobulin A

IGF-1 insulin-like growth factor-1

IgG immunoglobulin G

IgM immunoglobulin M

INR international normalized ratio

IUD intrauterine device

IUGR intrauterine growth restriction

IV intravenous

KUB X-ray kidneys-ureter-bladder X-ray

LDH lactate dehydrogenase

LDL low density lipoprotein cholesterol

LH luteinizing hormone

LSD lysergic acid diethylamide

MAOI monoamine oxidase inhibitor

MDMA 3,4-methylenedioxymethamphetamine (ecstasy)

MEK inhibitor mitogen-activated protein kinase kinase inhibitor

MRCP magnetic resonance cholangiopancreatography

MRI magnetic resonance imaging

NAAT nucleic acid amplification tests

NCV test nerve conduction velocity test

NSAID nonsteroidal antiinflammatory drug

NT-proBNP N-terminal prohormone of brain natriuretic peptide

OCD obsessive-compulsive disorder

Pap test Papanicolaou smear test

PCR polymerase chain reaction

PET scan positron emission tomography

Pr/Cr ratio protein to creatinine ratio

PSA prostate-specific antigen

PTH parathyroid hormone

PT/INR prothrombin time/international normalized ratio

PTSD posttraumatic stress disorder

PTT partial thromboplastin time

RBC red blood cell

RNA ribonucleic acid

RT-PCR reverse-transcription polymerase chain reaction

SIADH syndrome of inappropriate secretion of antidiuretic hormone

SNRI select norepinephrine reuptake inhibitor

SPECT single-photon emission computed tomography

SSRI select serotonin reuptake inhibitor

STEMI/NSTEMI ST-segment elevation myocardial infarction/non-ST-segment elevation myocardial infarction

STI sexually transmitted infection

T$_3$ triiodothyronine

T$_4$ thyroxine

TB tuberculosis

TORCH screen a group of blood tests to detect several infections (mnemonic TORCH): **to**xoplasmosis, **r**ubella, **c**ytomegalovirus, HIV, **h**erpes simplex virus

tPA tissue plasminogen activator

TPO thyroid peroxidase

TSH thyroid-stimulating hormone (thyrotropin)

tTG tissue transglutaminase

UTI urinary tract infection

UV ultraviolet light

VACTERL association a collection of associated congenital abnormalities (mnemonic VACTERL): **v**ertebrae, **a**nus, **c**ardiac, **t**rachea, **e**sophageal, **r**enal, **l**imb)

VDRL Venereal Disease Research Laboratory

V/Q scan ventilation-perfusion scan

WBC white blood cell

Index of clinical presentations by disorder classification and medical discipline

This index lists the MCC's clinical presentations by type of disorder and medical specialty.

With this index, you can answer questions such as: Which clinical presentations include psychiatric disorders? Which involve pediatrics?

Ethics and legal aspects of medicine

Family and preventive medicine

Gastrointestinal disorders

Hereditary, genetic, and congenital disorders

Immune system disorders

Infectious diseases

Ophthalmological disorders

Palliative care

Pediatrics

Pharmacology and toxicology

Poisoning

Psychiatric disorders

Respiratory disorders

Sleep-wake disorders

Subject index

This index lists entities included in the differential diagnoses of the MCC's clinical presentations. It lists these by the clinical presentations in which they appear, with the page number that begins each clinical presentation. With this index, you can answer a question such as: Which clinical presentations might involve a diagnosis of gastro-esophageal reflux disease?

It also lists the MCC's clinical presentations by topic, and other key subjects.

About the author

Dr. Christopher Naugler is a general
pathologist and family physician
with wide-ranging research, teach-
ing, and clinical experience. He
is a professor and the head of the
Department of Pathology and Laboratory Medicine at the University of
Calgary, and a clinician-scientist at
the Cumming School of Medicine.

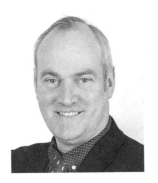